NATIONAL ACADEMIES

Sciences
Engineering
Medicine

NATIONAL
ACADEMIES
PRESS
Washington, DC

Federal Policy to Advance Racial, Etl and Tribal Health Equity

T0073682

Sheila P. Burke, Daniel E. Polsky, and Amy B. Geller, *Editors*

Committee on the Review of Federal Policies that Contribute to Racial and Ethnic Health Inequities

Board on Population Health and Public Health Practice

Health and Medicine Division

Consensus Study Report

NATIONAL ACADEMIES PRESS 500 Fifth Street, NW, Washington, DC 20001

This activity was supported by contract/task order HHSP233201499929B/75P0 0121F37110 between the National Academy of Sciences and the Office of Minority Health, an operating agency of the U.S. Department of Health and Human Services. Any opinions, findings, conclusions, or recommendations expressed in this publication do not necessarily reflect the views of any organization or agency that provided support for the project.

International Standard Book Number-13: 978-0-309-69774-3
International Standard Book Number-10: 0-309-69774-3
Digital Object Identifier: https://doi.org/10.17226/26834
Library of Congress Control Number: 2023945751

This publication is available from the National Academies Press, 500 Fifth Street, NW, Keck 360, Washington, DC 20001; (800) 624-6242 or (202) 334-3313; http://www.nap.edu.

Suggested citation: National Academies of Sciences, Engineering, and Medicine. 2023. *Federal policy to advance racial, ethnic, and tribal health equity.* Washington, DC: The National Academies Press. https://doi.org/10.17226/26834.

The **National Academy of Sciences** was established in 1863 by an Act of Congress, signed by President Lincoln, as a private, nongovernmental institution to advise the nation on issues related to science and technology. Members are elected by their peers for outstanding contributions to research. Dr. Marcia McNutt is president.

The **National Academy of Engineering** was established in 1964 under the charter of the National Academy of Sciences to bring the practices of engineering to advising the nation. Members are elected by their peers for extraordinary contributions to engineering. Dr. John L. Anderson is president.

The **National Academy of Medicine** (formerly the Institute of Medicine) was established in 1970 under the charter of the National Academy of Sciences to advise the nation on medical and health issues. Members are elected by their peers for distinguished contributions to medicine and health. Dr. Victor J. Dzau is president.

The three Academies work together as the **National Academies of Sciences, Engineering, and Medicine** to provide independent, objective analysis and advice to the nation and conduct other activities to solve complex problems and inform public policy decisions. The National Academies also encourage education and research, recognize outstanding contributions to knowledge, and increase public understanding in matters of science, engineering, and medicine.

Learn more about the National Academies of Sciences, Engineering, and Medicine at **www.nationalacademies.org**.

COMMITTEE ON THE REVIEW OF FEDERAL POLICIES THAT CONTRIBUTE TO RACIAL AND ETHNIC HEALTH INEQUITIES

SHEILA P. BURKE (*Cochair*), Adjunct Lecturer, John F. Kennedy School of Government, Harvard University; Senior Policy Advisor and Chair, Government Relations and Public Policy, Baker Donelson

DANIEL E. POLSKY (*Cochair*), Bloomberg Distinguished Professor of Health Policy and Economics, Department of Health Policy and Management, Johns Hopkins Bloomberg School of Public Health and Carey Business School, Johns Hopkins University

MADINA AGÉNOR, Associate Professor, Department of Behavioral and Social Sciences, Center for Health Promotion and Health Equity, Brown University School of Public Health

CAMILLE M. BUSETTE, Senior Fellow and Director, Race, Prosperity, and Inclusion Initiative, The Brookings Institution

MARIO CARDONA, Professor of Practice and Director of Policy, Children's Equity Project, Arizona State University[1]

JULIET K. CHOI, Chief Executive Officer, Asian & Pacific Islander American Health Forum

JUAN DE LARA, Associate Professor of American Studies and Ethnicity, University of Southern California

THOMAS E. DOBBS, III, Dean and Associate Professor, School of Population Health, University of Mississippi Medical Center

MEGAN D. DOUGLAS, Associate Professor, Department of Community Health and Preventive Medicine; Director, Research and Policy, National Center for Primary Care, Morehouse School of Medicine

ABIGAIL ECHO-HAWK, Director, Urban Indian Health Institute; Executive Vice President, Seattle Indian Health Board

HEDWIG LEE, Codirector, Center for the Study of Race, Ethnicity, and Equity; Professor of Sociology, Courtesy Joint Appointment with the Brown School, Washington University in St. Louis; Scholar in Residence of Sociology, Duke University

MARGARET P. MOSS, Professor, Director of First Nations House of Learning, University of British Columbia

SELA V. PANAPASA, Associate Research Scientist, Research Center for Group Dynamics, Institute for Social Research, University of Michigan

S. KARTHICK RAMAKRISHNAN, Professor of Public Policy, University of California, Riverside

---

[1] Resigned from the committee on October 5, 2022.

DIANE WHITMORE SCHANZENBACH, Margaret Walker Alexander Professor of Human Development and Social Policy; Director, Institute for Policy Research, Northwestern University

LISA SERVON, Kevin and Erica Penn Presidential Professor and Chair, Department of City and Regional Planning, University of Pennsylvania

VIVEK SHANDAS, Professor; Founder and Director, Sustaining Urban Places Research Lab, Portland State University

MELISSA A. SIMON, Vice Chair of Research and George H. Gardner Professor of Clinical Gynecology, Department of Obstetrics and Gynecology; Founder and Director, Center for Health Equity Transformation; Associate Director, Community Outreach and Engagement, Robert H. Lurie Comprehensive Cancer Center, Feinberg School of Medicine, Northwestern University

National Academy of Medicine Greenwall Fellow in Bioethics

KAVITA SHAH ARORA, Division Director, Division of General Obstetrics, Gynecology, and Midwifery; Associate Professor, University of North Carolina at Chapel Hill

Study Staff

AMY GELLER, Study Director
AIMEE MEAD, Associate Program Officer
L. BRIELLE DOJER, Research Associate
MAGGIE ANDERSON, Research Assistant
G. EKENE AGU, Senior Program Assistant
GRACE READING, Senior Program Assistant (*through November 2022*)
Y. CRYSTI PARK, Program Coordinator
ALINA BACIU, Senior Program Officer
MISRAK DABI, Senior Finance Business Partner
ROSE MARIE MARTINEZ, Senior Board Director
TASHA BIGELOW, Editor, Definitive Editing

Consultants

IGNATIUS BAU, Independent Consultant
AARON KLEIN, The Brookings Institution
BOBBY MILSTEIN, ReThink Health
REBECCA PAYNE, Rippel Foundation

Reviewers

This Consensus Study Report was reviewed in draft form by individuals chosen for their diverse perspectives and technical expertise. The purpose of this independent review is to provide candid and critical comments that will assist the National Academies of Sciences, Engineering, and Medicine in making each published report as sound as possible and to ensure that it meets the institutional standards for quality, objectivity, evidence, and responsiveness to the study charge. The review comments and draft manuscript remain confidential to protect the integrity of the deliberative process. We thank the following individuals for their review of this report:

JOSEPH ANTOS, American Enterprise Institute
DAVE A. CHOKSHI, New York University Grossman School of Medicine
JACK C. EBELER, Health and Medicine Division Committee
GLENN FLORES, University of Miami Miller School of Medicine
    and Holtz Children's Hospital, Jackson Health System
KRISTEN HARPER, Child Trends
EVE J. HIGGINBOTHAM, University of Pennsylvania
JAMES S. HOUSE, University of Michigan (emeritus)
JOSEPH KEAWE'AIMOKU KAHOLOKULA, University of Hawai'i
    at Mānoa
PAULA M. LANTZ, University of Michigan
APARNA MATHUR, Harvard University Kennedy School
JUSTIN GARRETT MOORE, Columbia University
JULIE MORITA, Robert Wood Johnson Foundation
JOHN A. RICH, Rush University
YVETTE ROUBIDEAUX, Colorado School of Public Health
ELIZABETH TOBIN-TYLER, Brown University

Although the reviewers listed above provided many constructive comments and suggestions, they were not asked to endorse the conclusions or recommendations of this report nor did they see the final draft before its release. The review of this report was overseen by **JOSE ESCARCE**, University of California, Los Angeles and **TRACY LIEU**, Kaiser Permanente, Northern California. They were responsible for making certain that an independent examination of this report was carried out in accordance with the standards of the National Academies and that all review comments were carefully considered. Responsibility for the final content rests entirely with the authoring committee and the National Academies.

Contents

Preface

The United States is a country rich in different cultures, perspectives, languages, and beliefs; that is one of its great strengths. It also is home to a society that values fairness and freedom. But a lack of fairness creates barriers that can keep people from having the opportunities to achieve their highest potential for health, whether they are a small business owner, student, or parent.

The report's purpose is to conduct a wide-ranging, though not comprehensive, assessment of the relationship between federal policies across multiple domains and health equity along ethnic and racial lines. National Academies studies have closely reviewed the effects of poverty, racism, and discrimination on health outcomes and examined the evidence demonstrating that low-income status and membership in racially or ethnically minoritized communities—both as separate factors and in interaction—result in these populations being more likely to live shorter lives and suffer other health inequities, at a great cost to families, communities, and our nation.[2]

This work, conducted at the request of the Office of Minority Health in the Department of Health and Human Services (charged with working toward a healthier nation), was intended to look at the effect of past and present federal policies that contribute to racial and ethnic inequities.

---

[2] See, for example, National Academies of Sciences, Engineering, and Medicine (NASEM). 2017. *Communities in action: Pathways to health equity.* Washington, DC: The National Academies Press; NASEM. 2019. *A roadmap to reducing child poverty.* Washington, DC: The National Academies Press; and, Institute of Medicine and National Research Council. 2013. *U.S. health in international perspective: Shorter lives, poorer health.* Washington, DC: The National Academies Press.

Why look at the past? Because it sets in motion processes that continue for decades and generations, operate across multiple domains, and interact in mutually reinforcing ways.

The breadth of the statement of task spanning all federal policies past and present gave this committee the opportunity to identify common cross-cutting themes actionable at the federal level for achieving health equity. We arrived at these themes and subsequent recommendations from our analysis of the evidence of the relationship between health equity and historical and current examples of federal policies.

We do call attention to how health inequities result from federal policies, but with a purpose to inform the federal policy change that can effectively address them. Our recommendations provide action steps for federal policy makers to advance the nation's path toward health equity.

Sheila P. Burke and Daniel E. Polsky, *Cochairs*
Committee on the Review of Federal Policies that
Contribute to Racial and Ethnic Health Inequities

Acknowledgments

The committee wishes to thank and acknowledge the many individuals and organizations that contributed to the study process and development of this report. To begin, the committee would like to thank the Department of Health and Human Services Office of Minority Health, the study sponsor, for its support of this work.

The committee found the perspectives of many individuals and groups immensely helpful in informing its deliberations through presentations and discussions at the public meetings. The following speakers provided their research, expertise, and perspectives: Maggie Blackhawk, Richard Cho, Loretta Christensen, Gail Christopher, RDML Felicia Collins, Janet Currie, J. Nadine Gracia, Cindy Mann, Kamilah Martin-Proctor, Stephanie Martinez-Ruckman, Barbara Masters, Tom Morris, Allison Orris, Liz Osborn, Sue Polis, John A. Rich, Ananya Roy, and Megan Ryerson. The committee also greatly benefited from hearing lived experiences and other input from many individuals and organizations on navigating federal programs and policies that contribute to racial and ethnic health inequities at its public comment sessions and through written comment.

The committee's work was enhanced by the expertise and writing contributions provided by Ignatius Bau, Aaron Klein, Bobby Milstein, and Rebecca Payne, who served as consultants.

The committee thanks the National Academies of Sciences, Engineering, and Medicine staff who contributed to producing this report, especially the extraordinary, creative, and tireless study staff Amy Geller, Alina Baciu, Aimee Mead, L. Brielle Dojer, Maggie Anderson, G. Ekene Agu, Grace Reading, Y. Crysti Park, and Rose Marie Martinez. The committee thanks the National Academies and Health and Medicine Division communications staff, including Mimi Koumanelis, Amber McLaughlin, Benjamin Hubbert, and Marguerite Romatelli. This project received valuable assistance from Megan Lowry (Office of News and Public Information); Misrak Dabi (Office of the Chief Financial Officer); and Monica Feit, Samantha Chao, Leslie Sim, Taryn Young, Lori Brenig, Rachael Nance, and Elizabeth Webber (Health and Medicine Division Executive Office). The committee received important research assistance from Anne Marie Houppert and Rebecca Morgan (National Academies Research Center). The committee also thanks Neha Dixit, Donna Doebler, and Kelly McHugh for their additional support.

Finally, the National Academies staff offers thanks to committee members' executive assistants and support staff, without whom scheduling the multiple meetings and conference calls would have been nearly impossible: Lianne Araki, Duane Haneckow, Lauren Kearns, Caitlin Keller, Jamey Longden, Mischa Makortoff, Kathleen Prutting, Hayley Smart, Liana Watson, and Sarah Wright.

Acronyms and Abbreviations

ACA	Affordable Care Act
ACO	accountable care organization
ACS	American Community Survey
ADA	Americans with Disabilities Act
AHRQ	Agency for Healthcare Research and Quality
AIAN	American Indian or Alaska Native
APA	Administrative Procedure Act
BIA	Bureau of Indian Affairs
BIE	Bureau of Indian Education
CARE	collective benefit, authority to control, responsibility, and ethics
CBO	Congressional Budget Office
CDC	Centers for Disease Control and Prevention
CEP	Community Eligibility Provision
CHIP	Children's Health Insurance Program
CHW	community health worker
CI	confidence interval
CLAS	culturally and linguistically appropriate services
CMS	Centers for Medicare and Medicaid Services
CNMI	Commonwealth of the Northern Mariana Islands
COFA	Compact of Free Association
COVID	coronavirus disease

CRA	Community Reinvestment Act of 1977
CTC	Child Tax Credit
CVD	cardiovascular disease
CWA	Clean Water Act
DACA	Deferred Action for Childhood Arrivals
DOE	Department of Education
DOD	Department of Defense
DOJ	Department of Justice
DOT	Department of Transportation
DPC	Domestic Policy Council
ECE	early childhood education
EHR	electronic health record
EITC	Earned Income Tax Credit
ELTRR	Equitable Long-Term Recovery and Resilience
EO	executive order
EPA	Environmental Protection Agency
ESEA	Elementary and Secondary Education Act
ESSA	Every Student Succeeds Act
FAFSA	Free Application for Federal Student Aid
FAIR	findability, accessibility, interoperability, and reusability
FAS	Freely Associated States
Fed	Federal Reserve
FHA	Federal Housing Administration
FDA	Food and Drug Administration
FDIC	Federal Deposit Insurance Corporation
FMAP	federal medical assistance percentage
FSM	Federated States of Micronesia
GAO	Government Accountability Office
GDP	gross domestic product
GI	green infrastructure
GPA	grade point average
HEA	Higher Education Act
HHS	Department of Health and Human Services
HiAP	Health in All Policies
HOLC	Home Owners' Loan Corporation
HRSA	Health Resources Services Administration

HSI	Hispanic serving institution
HUD	Department of Housing and Urban Development
IAP2	International Association for Public Participation's Spectrum of Public Participation
IDEA	Individuals with Disabilities Education Act
IHS	Indian Health Service
IRS	Internal Revenue Service
JIPA	George Floyd Justice in Policing Act
LGBTQ+	lesbian, gay, bisexual, transgender, queer (or questioning), and other sexual identities
MENA	Middle Eastern or North African
MSI	minority serving institution
NCLB	No Child Left Behind
NCD	noncommunicable diseases
NHIS	National Health Interview Survey
NHPI	Native Hawaiian or Pacific Islander
NIH	National Institutes of Health
NSLP	National School Lunch Program
OMB	Office of Management and Budget
OMH	Office of Minority Health
OSHA	Occupational Safety and Health Administration
OSTP	Office of Science and Technology Policy
PN	patient navigator
RETC	Racial, Ethnic, and Tribal Equity Council
RMI	Republic of the Marshall Islands
SBHC	school-based health center
SBP	School Breakfast Program
SDOH	social determinants of health
SEED OK	SEED for Oklahoma Kids
SFSP	Summer Food Service Program
SMM	severe maternal morbidity
SNAP	Supplemental Nutrition Assistance Program

SSA	Social Security Administration
SSI	Supplemental Security Income
STI	sexually transmitted infection
TCU	tribal college and university
USDA	United States Department of Agriculture
USPS	U.S. Postal Service
USPSTF	United States Preventive Services Task Force
VA	Department of Veterans Affairs
WIC	Special Supplemental Nutrition Program for Women, Infants and Children
WPS	Worker Protection Standard

Key Terms

The committee strived to use language that is respectful, accurate, and maximally inclusive. This relies on attempting to reflect preferences for how individuals and groups wish to be addressed, but there is not always consensus on preferred terms, and these preferences may evolve. The below terms are defined for the purpose of this report and adapted or informed by other several National Academies reports and government agency reports.[3]

Racial and Ethnic Population Terms

Specific Populations[4]

- **American Indian or Alaska Native:** For the purpose of this report, "American Indian" and/or "Alaska Native" is used when discussing

---

[3] NASEM. 2023. *Advancing antiracism, diversity, equity, and inclusion in STEMM organizations: Beyond broadening participation.* Washington, DC: The National Academies Press; NASEM. 2017. *Communities in action: Pathways to health equity.* Washington, DC: The National Academies Press; NASEM. 2021. *Sexually transmitted infections: Adopting a sexual health paradigm.* Washington, DC: The National Academies Press; HHS. n.d. *Healthy people 2030 social determinants of health.* https://health.gov/healthypeople/priority-areas/social-determinants-health (accessed March 7, 2023); Department of the Interior. 2017. *Who is an American Indian or Alaska Native?* https://www.bia.gov/faqs/who-american-indian-or-alaska-native (accessed March 15, 2023); CDC. 2022. *What is health equity?* https://www.cdc.gov/healthequity/whatis/index.html (accessed March 15, 2023); Wingrove-Haugland, E., and J. McLeod. 2021. Not "minority" but "minoritized." *Teaching Ethics* 21(1):1-11.

[4] It is important to note that race and ethnicity are not biological categories or otherwise verifiable. In addition, ethnicity is currently treated separately from race in most data collection efforts, but some consider this a flawed approach; for the purpose of this report, the committee treats them as separate categories.

individuals or the population served by policies or programs that relate to the U.S. federal government's trust responsibility and its government-to-government relationship with federally recognized Tribal Nations in the United States. Although American Indians and Alaska Natives are also often described along with other racial and ethnic groups, the term "American Indian and/or Alaska Native" is distinct because it is used in the context of legally enforceable obligations and responsibilities of the federal government to provide certain services and benefits to members or citizens (and, in some cases, descendants) of federally recognized Tribal Nations. "Indigenous" and "Native American" are also commonly used but are not specific enough to describe the special political status of American Indian and Alaska Native Tribal Nations.

- **Asian:** a person having origins in any of the original peoples of the Far East, Southeast Asia, or the Indian subcontinent; for example, Cambodia, China, India, Japan, Korea, Malaysia, Pakistan, the Philippine Islands, Thailand, and Vietnam. These individuals remain citizens of their home countries.
- **Asian American:** a resident of the United States who self-identifies as Asian or as one of the ethnic or detailed origin groups classified by the U.S. government as Asian; does not need to be a U.S. citizen or permanent resident.
- **African American:** U.S.-born people who have African ancestry (typically used for descendants of people from African who were enslaved) and may also refer to those who were not born in the United States but are now U.S. citizens or permanent residents. The committee elected to use "Black" unless the data specifically denote African American.
- **Black:** a person who was born in or outside of the United States and has origins in any of the Black ethnic groups of Africa. An umbrella term including African American, African, Afro-Caribbean, and other people of African descent.
- **Hispanic or Latino/a/x/e:** refers to a person of Mexican, Puerto Rican, Salvadoran, Cuban, or other Latin American and Caribbean cultural origin, regardless of race. The committee acknowledges that "Hispanic" is widely used in policy and research discussions when referring to this group. Nonetheless, the committee recognizes that Latin America and the Caribbean are home to many colonial and Indigenous languages and cultures. Therefore, the committee elected to use "Latino/a" unless the data specifically denote Hispanic.
- **Native Hawaiian or Pacific Islander:** a person having origins in any of the original peoples of Hawaii, Guam, American Samoa, Commonwealth of the Northern Mariana Islands, or other Pacific

Islands (that is, all sovereign/independent Pacific Island countries, including the Compact of Free Association States).
- **White:** a person having origins in any of the original peoples of Europe or the Middle East or North Africa (MENA). However, a movement exists to identify MENA people separately in the U.S. Census and elsewhere.

Additional Population Terms

- **Ethnicity:** In contrast to race, ethnicity has a stronger relationship with place. It is a socially constructed term used to describe people from a similar national or regional background who share common national, cultural, historical, and social experiences. An ethnic group likely contains people who share distinct beliefs, values, and behaviors. Race (even though it is not a valid biological construct) refers to phenotypic features that have been racialized, whereas ethnicity addresses social, cultural, and historical commonalities (see also Race).
- **Multiracial:** people who identify with more than one race.
- **Race:** a socially constructed, shorthand concept, dating back to the 15th century, which categorized populations into an arbitrary, hierarchical classification framework, largely based on phenotypic characteristics, such as skin color. Race, although not a valid biological concept, is a real social construction that is linked to racism and gives or denies benefits and privileges to racialized individual people and groups.
- **Tribal:** describes Tribal Nations in the United States but is also used as an adjective to describe circumstances related to them, such as tribal communities or tribal policies. It is not appropriate to use in the context of Native Hawaiians or Pacific Islanders.

Other Key Report Terms

Community: Any configuration of individuals, families, and groups whose values, characteristics, interests, geography, and/or social relations unite them in some way.

Equality: The treatment of all individuals in the same manner. It is important to emphasize that equity is not interchangeable with equality. Equality assumes a level playing field for everyone without accounting for historical and current inequities. See Health Equity for more details about why "equity" is used in this report.

Health: A state of complete physical, mental, and social well-being; not merely the absence of disease.

Health Equity: The state in which everyone has a fair opportunity to attain full health potential and well-being, and no one is disadvantaged from doing so because of social position or any other socially defined circumstance. Achieving health equity requires valuing everyone equally with focused and ongoing societal efforts to address avoidable inequalities and historical and contemporary injustices and eliminate health and health care disparities due to past and present causes. It is important to note that equity is not interchangeable with equality (see definition above).

Institutional Racism: policies and practices within institutions that, intentionally or not, produce outcomes that chronically favor White individuals and put individuals from minoritized racial and ethnic groups at a disadvantage.

Policy: For the purpose of this report, a policy is a law, regulation, procedure, administrative action, incentive, or voluntary practice of governments and other institutions that affects a whole population. Further, it is a course of action or inaction that government selects from among alternatives. Both formal and informal policies exist; formal policy has consequences for not following it when enforced (e.g., fines, withdrawal of funding or eligibility, criminal charges), whereas informal policy (e.g., guidelines, recommendations, funding opportunities for research and community-based initiatives, tax subsidies) does not have such consequences.

Racialized: the extension of racial meaning to resources, cultural objects, emotions, bodies, and organizations that have previously been seen as nonracial.

Racially and Ethnically Minoritized Individuals/Populations: Rather than referring to "racial and ethnic minorities," "members of minority groups," or "underrepresented minorities," this report uses "minoritized," which refers to people from groups that have been historically and systematically socially and economically marginalized or underserved based on their race or ethnicity as a result of racism (such as American Indian and Alaska Native, Asian, Black, Latino/a/x/e, and Native Hawaiian and Pacific Islander communities). The committee uses this term to make the distinction that being minoritized is not about the number of people in the population but rather about power and equity.

Racism: the combination of policies, practices, attitudes, cultures, and systems that affect individuals, institutions, and structures unequally and confer power and privilege to certain groups over others, defined according to social constructs of race and ethnicity.

Structural Racism: the totality of ways in which a society fosters racial and ethnic inequity and subjugation through mutually reinforcing systems, including housing, education, employment, earnings, benefits, credit, media, health care, and the criminal legal system. These structural factors organize the distribution of power and resources (i.e., the social determinants of health) differentially among racial, ethnic, and socioeconomic groups, perpetuating racial and ethnic health inequities. The key difference between institutional and structural racism is that structural racism happens *across* institutions, while institutional racism happens *within* institutions. "Systemic racism" is another term used to describe this.

Social Determinants of Health (SDOH): The conditions in the environments in which people live, learn, work, play, worship, and age that affect a wide range of health, functioning, and quality-of-life outcomes and risks. SDOH can both promote and harm health. For the purposes of this report, SDOH are organized by the Healthy People 2030 domains: economic stability, education access and quality, health care access and quality, neighborhood and built environment, and social and community context.

Structural Determinants of Health: Macrolevel factors, such as laws, policies, institutional practices, governance processes, and social norms that shape the distribution (or maldistribution) of the social determinants of health (e.g., housing, income, employment, exposure to environmental toxins, interpersonal discrimination) across and within social groups. Structural determinants of health, also referred to as the "determinants of the determinants of health," include structural racism and other structural inequities and thus influence not only population health but also health equity.

Abstract

Research demonstrates that many preventable disparities in health outcomes result from the structural disadvantage and diminished opportunity faced by racially and ethnically minoritized[1] populations and tribal communities. Extensive research on these health inequities demonstrates that these populations experience higher rates of illness and death for many different conditions, including heart disease, hypertension, and diabetes, and lower life expectancies compared to non-Hispanic White people.

Health equity is the state in which everyone has a fair opportunity to attain full health potential and well-being, and no one is disadvantaged from doing so because of social position or any other socially defined circumstance. Achieving health equity requires valuing everyone equally with focused and ongoing societal efforts to address avoidable inequalities and historical and contemporary injustices and eliminate health and health care disparities due to past and present causes. It is about fairness and ensuring that no one suffers inequitable outcomes in health and well-being, everyone's voice is heard, and everyone at the table has the power to inform action. When individuals thrive, families, communities, and the entire nation thrive.

There are many levels at which to intervene; however, the committee was asked by the Office of Minority Health to (1) examine *federal* policies that contribute to preventable and unfair differences in health status and outcomes experienced by all racially and ethnically minoritized populations in the United States and (2) provide conclusions and recommendations that

---

[1] See the Key Terms section for a definition of this term.

1

identify the most effective or promising approaches to policy change, with the goal of furthering racial and ethnic health equity. The committee also took into consideration relevant federal activities already underway.

The committee set out to identify how past and current federal policies (or features/components of federal policies) operate in ways that create, maintain, and amplify racial, ethnic, and tribal health inequities. Moreover, the committee identified key features of past and current policies that have served to reduce inequities to inform its recommendations to not only further reduce and eliminate inequities but also achieve equity, with a focus on policies and programs controlled or influenced by the executive and legislative branches of the federal government. Federal policy makers have worked on health equity issues in the past with significant progress; the goal of this report is to further that progress.

To guide its work, the committee adopted the following key principles:

1. Health is more than physical and mental well-being—it also includes well-being in social, economic, and other factors, all of which are necessary for human flourishing;
2. All federal policies have the potential to affect population health;
3. Evidence is informed by quantitative, qualitative, and community sources;
4. Federal policies should center health equity;[2] and
5. To advance health equity, structural and systems change are needed.

On the path to eliminating health inequities, both short-term strategies (e.g., mitigation by getting people what they need now to thrive) and long-term structural and systems change strategies that address the root causes (e.g., employment and economic development) will be needed. Based on its review of federal policies, the committee identified four action areas through which the federal government can better support states, localities, tribes, territories, and communities to advance health equity.

1. Implement Sustained Coordination Among Federal Agencies
2. Prioritize, Value, and Incorporate Community Voice in the Work of Government
3. Ensure Collection and Reporting of Data Are Representative and Accurate
4. Improve Federal Accountability, Enforcement, Tools, and Support Toward a Government That Advances Optimal Health for Everyone

---

[2]Centering equity means prioritizing the needs of racially and ethnically minoritized populations and considering the consequences of current and future policies for advancing or impeding health equity.

    This report provides 36 conclusions and 13 recommendations for action (see the Summary or full report for a full exposition of each conclusion and recommendation). Several of these recommendations build on actions already underway in the federal government and could be implemented in the short term. Some of the structural-level needs articulated in the recommendations will require broad societal-level change and long-term effort, as these are tied to accumulated inequities over generations that need to be unwound to achieve health equity. Both levels of action are required to make progress on eliminating—versus only mitigating—racial and ethnic health inequities.

Summary[1]

INTRODUCTION

Health equity is the state in which everyone has a fair opportunity to attain full health potential and well-being, and no one is disadvantaged from doing so because of social position or any other socially defined circumstance. Achieving health equity requires valuing everyone equally with focused and ongoing societal efforts to address avoidable inequalities and historical and contemporary injustices and eliminate health and health care disparities due to past and present causes. When individuals thrive, communities and the entire nation thrive.

Racial,[2,3] ethnic, and tribal health inequities and their root causes have been substantially documented, and the evidence is clear—advancing health equity needs to be approached using a holistic view of health, one that considers all that impacts it: economic stability, access to quality education and health care, and vibrant and livable communities (such as access to housing,

---

[1] This Summary does not include references. Citations for the discussion presented in the Summary appear in the subsequent report chapters, as does a detailed discussion of the policies and evidence reviewed to support the committee's conclusions and recommendations.

[2] The racial and ethnic categories discussed in this report should not be interpreted as being primarily biological or genetic. Race and ethnicity should be thought of in terms of social and cultural characteristics and ancestry and could be considered proxies for racism and social characteristics. Race and ethnicity are not biological categories or otherwise verifiable.

[3] Over time, terminology related to racial, ethnic, and tribal health equity has significantly evolved. The committee strived to use language that is respectful, accurate, and maximally inclusive; however, there is not always consensus on preferred terms, and these preferences may evolve. See the "Key Terms" and Chapter 1 discussion on terminology.

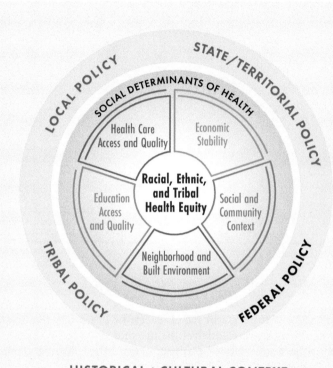

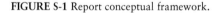

FIGURE S-1 Report conceptual framework.

transportation, and healthy environments; see Figure S-1 and Box S-1). There are many levels at which to intervene; however, the committee was asked to (1) focus on *federal* policies that contribute to preventable and unfair differences in health status and outcomes experienced by all racially and ethnically minoritized[4] populations in the United States and (2) provide

---

[4]Rather than referring to "racial and ethnic minorities," "members of minority groups," or "underrepresented minorities," this report uses the term "minoritized," which refers to people from groups that have been historically and systematically socially and economically marginalized or underserved based on their race or ethnicity as a result of racism (such as American Indian and Alaska Native, Asian, Black, Latino/a, and Native Hawaiian and Pacific Islander communities). The committee uses this term to make the distinction that being minoritized is not about the number of people in the population but rather about power and equity. (See the Key Terms section for additional terminology used in this report.)

BOX S-1
Factors That Shape Health Outcomes

Although family circumstances and personal choice play a role in health outcomes, the evidence suggests that improving the social and environmental conditions where people, families, and communities live, play, work, age, and pray—so that all people have the opportunity to make the healthy choice—is essential.

The Whitehall I study, which began in 1967, showed an inverse relationship between social class (based on the employment grade of British civil servants) and mortality from a variety of illnesses. In the decades since, the Whitehall II study and other research have further illustrated that social factors, such as race, ethnicity, zip code, education level, employment, and income, impact health outcomes and thereby create inequities.

Today, the social ecological or social determinants of health (SDOH) framework is a vital part of public health and health equity work. Healthy People 2030 defines SDOH as "the conditions in the environments where people are born, live, work, play, worship, and age that affect a wide range of health, functioning, and quality-of-life outcomes and risks." Healthy People 2030 acknowledges that targeting individual health behaviors cannot eliminate health inequity and so has an "increased and overarching focus on SDOH."

HHS has organized the SDOH in five areas:

- Economic stability
- Education access and quality
- Health care access and quality
- Neighborhood and built environment
- Social and community context

The committee used this categorization for its report.

---

conclusions and recommendations that identify the most effective or promising approaches to policy change with the goal of furthering racial and ethnic health equity (the committee was asked to review both promising and evidence-based solutions). The committee also took into consideration federal activities already underway. Although there are many examples of policies that have advanced health equity, the committee was not asked to review such policies. In the context of the significant progress advancing health equity by federal policy makers, this report provides a framework for federal action that builds on that progress to address continued barriers.

Although membership in a particular racial, ethnic, or tribal group does not predict a given outcome, and each of the broad categories of race and ethnicity has considerable heterogeneity, the available data on health outcomes and other measures of well-being tell a consistent story of wide disparities in health. Research demonstrates that the inequitable patterns of these social risk factors across race and ethnicity are in large part a consequence of structural disadvantages for minoritized communities that were, in no small measure, initiated by historical federal policy decisions. These decisions have guided the organization and governance of society and the distribution of resources. For example, the U.S. history of extermination, removal, and assimilation of American Indian people, enslavement of African and African American people, colonialism, and immigration policy have played a critical role in how the country is stratified, affecting contemporary outcomes across health, education, socioeconomic status, and other measures of well-being. There are higher rates of childhood asthma among low-income households, higher morbidity and mortality from chronic diseases among individuals with lower educational attainment, and higher exposure to air pollution among residents of disinvested communities—disproportionately individuals who are racially and ethnically minoritized. Moreover, the effects of the structural determinants of health on many health outcomes persist when accounting for income and education.

A policy could influence health inequities in many ways. For example, the report considered policies that are neutral in terms of racial, ethnic, or tribal inequity but have indirect equity implications (i.e., policies that aim to improve health or the factors that shape it without considering health equity may unintentionally improve equity or improve population health overall but fail to decrease, or even widen, gaps); policies that are intended to address inequities but fall short of this goal (i.e., they may be working but have aspects that can be improved or may have unintentionally worsened inequities); policies that intentionally worsened racial, ethnic, or tribal inequities (i.e., causing harm to some but not others); and the lack of policy in a given area. The report also describes federal policy levers, including implementation and enforcement.

Federal, state, local, tribal, and territorial policies have a complicated relationship. The federal government often sets priorities at all levels of government via funding and regulations. However, if federal policy makers want health equity to be prioritized at all levels of government, they need to set the standard of equity and lead with policies aligned with funding priorities that drive health for all. Practices consistent with this include providing supportive tools, coordination, and resources and incentivizing states, localities, tribal nations, and territories.

Report Key Principles

To guide its work, the committee adopted a set of principles informed by a large and growing body of research on the social determinants of health (SDOH) and input from experts, policy leaders, and other key stakeholders.

1. Health is more than physical and mental well-being—it also includes well-being in social, economic, and other factors, all of which are necessary for human flourishing;
2. All federal policies have the potential to affect population health;
3. Evidence is informed by quantitative, qualitative, and community sources;
4. Federal policies should center health equity;[5] and
5. To advance health equity, structural and systems change are needed.

With these principles in mind, it is important to emphasize that equity is not interchangeable with equality—equality is the treatment of all individuals in the same manner and assumes a level playing field for everyone without accounting for historical and current inequities.

Data Limitations

Although the statistics on racial and ethnic inequities in health outcomes are striking, they are complicated by problems such as inaccurate and missing data within and between minimum Office of Management and Budget (OMB) race and ethnicity categories. For example, for Native Hawaiian and Pacific Islander populations, aggregation of data under broad categories, such as "Asian," "Asian and Pacific Islander," or "Asian, Native Hawaiian, and Pacific Islander," masks the complexity of the challenges faced by these different populations. Given these limited and inaccurate data, the committee relied on a range of information to form a fuller understanding of the mechanisms that result in health inequities for these populations.

Role of Communities

Community voice and expertise have been critical for creating and implementing strategies to advance health equity, allowing many communities to flourish despite barriers. Including community leaders and organizations in the development and execution of federal policies that contribute to health equity is a key theme in this report. Although community participation is

---

[5] Centering equity means prioritizing the needs of racially and ethnically minoritized populations and considering the consequences of current and future policies for advancing or impeding health equity.

frequently touted as a value in policy making and program design processes, specificity is often lacking as to what constitutes community engagement or inclusion. These processes also typically lack accountability mechanisms to ensure meaningful community input.

Committee Approach

The committee's task was extremely broad, as many factors contribute to health inequities (see Figure S-1 and Box S-1). The committee could not review every relevant federal policy and program in the year it had to develop its report. To focus its review, the committee prioritized policies that (1) impact a large percentage of racially or ethnically minoritized populations; (2) have a body of literature or available data to assess them based on race and ethnicity; (3) continue to cause harm, based on the literature, even if those policies are historical; (4) illustrate how data gaps could fail to document health inequities (given that data gaps for these populations are well documented); and (5) were informed by available expertise from both the committee and invited speakers, verbal public comment at information-gathering meetings, and written public comment. Based on a combination of these considerations, the committee used its expert judgment to choose the policies to review and examined how they affected (both positively and negatively) racial, ethnic, or tribal health equity, with a focus on policies and programs controlled or influenced by the executive and legislative branches of the federal government.

The committee had to make difficult decisions regarding which policies to highlight in this report; omitting one does not mean it is any less important. Furthermore, the committee builds on the abundance of high-quality, evidence-based, and peer-reviewed reports from the National Academies and other organizations that have laid out the evidence for the root causes and mechanisms of health inequities or provided recommendations for specific federal actions to advance health equity. The topics, policies, and programs reviewed include the following:

- **Economic Stability:** The effect of incarceration and pretrial detention on income and wealth; the federal minimum wage; federal social benefit programs (e.g., Supplemental Nutrition Assistance Program [SNAP]); nonprofit sector partnerships; policies to support savings and wealth accumulation, such as baby bonds; and access to safe and affordable banking services, such as bank accounts and low-cost credit.
- **Education Access and Quality:** The Every Student Succeeds Act, the Individuals with Disabilities Education Act, the Higher Education Act, Section 504 of the Americans with Disabilities Act; early

childhood education programs, such as Head Start; K–12 school spending/funding; school-based programs (e.g., health centers and meals programs); and higher education programs (e.g., Pell Grants and minority serving institutions).

- **Health Care Access and Quality:** Medicaid and the Children's Health Insurance Program; policies and practices related to health literacy and language access; value-based payment; inclusion in clinical trials and the workforce; the Indian Health Service [IHS]; and maternal, territorial, and immigrant health.
- **Neighborhood and Built Environment:** Housing insecurity and segregation (e.g., redlining, housing on American Indian and Alaska Native [AIAN] reservations and for Native Hawaiian people, and federal rental assistance); disinvestment in infrastructure and the built environment (e.g., policies related to water, transportation, and aging and green infrastructure); environmental exposures that threaten health outcomes and well-being, particularly in the workplace (e.g., the Worker Protection Standard and exposure to pesticides); and food access and production (e.g., the Farm Bill and Food Distribution Program on Indian Reservations).
- **Social and Community Context:** Violence, public safety, and the criminal legal system, such as waiting periods for gun purchases, policies that increase accountability in policing and data collection, mass incarceration policies (e.g., long and mandatory minimum sentences); policies that acknowledge and provide redress for historical actions, practices, laws, and policies that caused enduring harm; and policies that build civic engagement and a sense of community and belonging.

Advancing health equity (or equity in areas that impact health, such as the environment, housing, and economic well-being) has garnered much attention recently from philanthropies, nonprofit organizations, and federal, state, and local governments. These efforts are described in this report, including Executive Order (EO) 13985, *Advancing Racial Equity and Support for Underserved Communities Through the Federal Government*, and the Equitable Long-Term Recovery and Resilience (ELTRR) plan released in November 2022. The committee built on these and other efforts and analyses in its report.

ACTION STEPS TO ADVANCE HEALTH EQUITY

Based on its review, the committee provides 36 conclusions in the five SDOH categories on their connection to health and conclusions for many of the reviewed policy areas (see Summary Annex for a listing of all report conclusions). The committee identified four action[6] areas through which the federal government can better support states, localities, tribes, territories, and communities to advance health equity.

1. Implement sustained coordination among federal agencies;
2. Prioritize, value, and incorporate community voice in the work of government;
3. Ensure collection and reporting of data are representative and accurate; and
4. Improve federal accountability, enforcement, tools, and support toward a government that advances optimal health for everyone.

On the path to eliminating health inequities, both short-term strategies (e.g., mitigation by getting people what they need now to thrive) and long-term structural and system change strategies that address the root causes (e.g., employment and economic development) will be needed. This report provides 13 recommendations for action with the goal of not only increasing access to important programs but also improving the effectiveness and coordination of government programs and policies. Several recommendations build upon actions underway in the federal government, as described in this report, and could be implemented in the short term. Additional details and considerations for each recommendation are available in Chapter 8.

Action 1: Implement Sustained Coordination Among Federal Agencies

The federal policy landscape is complex, with over 100 agencies in the executive branch, and the legislative and judiciary branches. Many federal policies affect health even if that is not their main focus. Coordination among federal agencies is critical to advance health equity. Some collaborative efforts are currently underway, such as the interagency ELTRR plan.

The importance of a whole-of-government approach to advance equity is central to EO 13985. Similar to a Health in All Policies approach, the committee recommends a parallel "whole person" and "whole community" approach. Just as health equity is not just about health care

---

[6] Barriers and opportunities related to these action areas are discussed in this report. Chapter 1 provides important background and context, and Chapter 2 discusses the connection between health equity and history, federal policy, and data. Chapters 3–7 review federal policies in specific SDOH areas—each providing an overview of its connection to health outcomes and inequities and a review of specific past or current policies that have implications for health equity.

access and quality, it is the responsibility of not only the Department of Health and Human Services (HHS) but also multiple agencies that affect individual health and well-being. Therefore, achieving racial, ethnic, and tribal health equity requires centering equity in federal policy creation, decision making, implementation, and regulation, such as through accountability standards, across the board.

The ELTRR plan includes 10 crosscutting recommendations to address agency coordination and infrastructure in service of eliminating inequities. However, changing systems and organizations is challenging—the problems often persist because of complex interdependencies, where solving one aspect reveals or creates new challenges. In addition, federal programs can have different legal responsibilities, many of which cannot be easily coordinated around or may need to be rethought through new legislation. Furthermore, advancing equity typically involves complex, long-term change management that requires sustained attention.

> **Recommendation 1: To improve health equity, the president of the United States should create a permanent and sustainable entity within the federal government that is charged with improving racial, ethnic, and tribal equity across the federal government. This should be a standing entity, sustained across administrations, with advisory, coordinating, and regulatory powers. The entity would work closely with other federal agencies to ensure equity in agency processes and outcomes.**

Multiple options to configure this entity exist, with pros and cons as described in this report.

Leadership for the Equitable Long-Term Recovery and Resilience Plan

A major component of the ELTRR plan is establishing an executive steering committee to guide and compel coordination across federal agencies at multiple levels. The group is expected to be composed of senior executive leaders from a significant number of representative departments and agencies; the Assistant Secretary for Health and one non-HHS agency lead (to be determined) will serve as cochairs. The committee affirms the crucial role of the executive steering committee:

> **Recommendation 2: The president of the United States should appoint a senior leader within the Office of Management and Budget (OMB) who can mobilize assets within OMB to serve as the cochair of the Equitable Long-Term Recovery and Resilience Steering Committee.**

This configuration is ideal because unlike HHS, OMB has the capacity and authority to oversee the implementation of the ELTRR plan across the executive branch, including overseeing agency performance.

Equity Audit and Scorecard

When policies and budgets to address racial, ethnic, and tribal health equity are designed and policy alternatives reviewed, data are needed for Congress to better prioritize and debate their potential to address or exacerbate inequitable outcomes. Scoring legislation for its effect on racial, ethnic, or tribal equity is not currently required. Without sufficient data or analysis to understand the disparate effects of policies across racial and ethnic groups, policies are often adopted that inadvertently reinforce inequities.

> Recommendation 3: The federal government should assess if federal policies address or exacerbate health inequities by implementing an equity audit and developing an equity scorecard. Specifically,
> a. Federal agencies should engage in a retrospective review of federal policies that had a historical impact on racial and ethnic health inequities that exist today to address contemporary impacts.
> b. The Office of Management and Budget should develop, and federal agencies should conduct, an equity audit of existing federal laws. The federal laws reviewed should be identified via public input obtained by a variety of means. The equity audit should include a review of how the laws are implemented and enforced by federal agencies and state and local governments. The audit should also include criteria related to equity in process, measurement, and outcomes.
> c. Congress should develop and implement an equity scorecard that is applied to all proposed federal legislation, similar to the requirement of a Congressional Budget Office score.
> d. The process and results from the equity audit and scorecard should be transparent and made publicly available.

If a health equity coordination entity is created per Recommendation 1, it could oversee and coordinate this process; however, such an entity is not required to implement this recommendation. The equity audit of existing federal policies in Recommendation 3b would build on the work by federal agencies under EOs 13985 and 14091, which direct each one to develop a health equity team to implement its equity initiatives. An important consideration for those implementing this recommendation is how accountability will be ensured after audits are conducted. For example, if a policy does not meet the equity criteria, a plan should be developed and put in place to ensure needed changes are enacted; action would also need to be taken if lack of enforcement was identified as contributing to inequity (e.g., enforcing civil rights protections). Regarding Recommendation 3c, various mechanisms can be used for the scorecard and could vary based on available data, evidence, and process. However, legislation is the "bare bones" of a policy or program, and implementation through regulations and adjustments in the field to address unanticipated complications determine its impact. Therefore, even when an equity score is applied to proposed legislation, an equity audit would still be required after implementation. Although existing policies could be audited in the short term, the equity scorecard for proposed legislation will likely require more advance planning to implement. The report discusses additional details, including potential categories of metrics and other important considerations.

The implementation of Recommendations 1, 2, and 3 will help ensure the equitable and effective distribution of resources and signal that racial, ethnic, and tribal equity is a national priority and advance equity in domestic policy development, implementation, and evaluation across domains including health, economic security, the criminal legal system, and education.

Action 2: Prioritize, Value, and Incorporate Community Voice in the Work of Government

It is essential to base federal policy for all SDOH on the best available evidence—this includes communities' experiences, knowledge/expertise, and needs. The reasons to value, prioritize, and incorporate community voice in the work of government are ethical and practical and include accountability and the achievement of intended outcomes. Affected communities need to be an integral part of the legislative process from beginning to end, as well as part of the process to decide how laws, regulations, programs, and policies are administered. Racial, ethnic, and tribal communities have been consistently left out of the federal policy-making process, and the effects have sometimes been egregiously inequitable. Community voices are needed to redress past harms; earn trust; secure partnership, buy-in, and collaboration; and ensure policies are fully responsive to their needs and advance health equity. A promising strategy to improve policies that do not currently promote health equity is to elevate and empower community voice and expertise to influence outcomes through the following design principles:

1. Prioritize meaningful community input by moving past simply keeping communities informed about policy and toward a more substantive level of input that involves consultation, involvement, collaboration, and empowerment whenever possible;
2. Ensure effectiveness, efficiency, and equity in the way that community input is collected;
3. Maximize coordination and sharing of information and insights on implementation across federal agencies while maintaining data privacy and client confidentiality; and
4. Within each federal agency, maximize coordinating and sharing information and insights on implementation among federal, state, local, and tribal government counterparts.

Although there are many technical and scientific advisory bodies at federal departments and agencies, few recognize the unique perspectives of communities—including the recipients and beneficiaries of federal programs and services—as "expertise" and (lived) experience as essential for designing, implementing, and evaluating those programs and services.

> Recommendation 4: The federal government should prioritize community input and expertise when changing or developing federal policies to advance health equity. Specifically,
> 1. The president of the United States should require federal agencies relevant to the social determinants of health to generate and sustain community representation and advisory practices that are integrated with accountability measures and enforcement mechanisms.
> 2. Congress should request a Government Accountability Office report to document across federal agencies whose work impacts the social determinants of health, as well as federal statistical agencies, that
>   a. Assesses how community advisory boards are positioned within their agencies, whom they are composed of, how often they meet, how they report back, and how that work influences the agencies' policies and programs; and
>   b. Identifies promising and evidence-based practices, gaps, and opportunities for community advisory boards that could be applied by other agencies.

As described in this report, several mechanisms for community input at the federal level are available to learn from, improve, and/or implement more broadly, such as community engagement associated with the decennial census, the White House Initiative on Asian Americans and Pacific Islanders Regional Interagency Working Group, and the Tribal Consultation and Urban Confer.

Action 3: Ensure Collection and Reporting of Data Are Representative and Accurate

To advance health equity, data need to better capture the experiences and needs of tribal and smaller racial and ethnic groups. A lack of representation in data collection, and sharing inaccurate or imprecise data about these communities, has meant that government agencies have been unprepared to understand, let alone reduce or eliminate, health inequities. High-quality data are required to understand the full extent of inequities and appropriately distribute resources. Federal government data collections have occurred without accountability or consideration of their effects and demands on communities (e.g., time and other resources), matters of tribal sovereignty, and community interest in the use of the data.

Data Equity for Small Minimum Reporting OMB Categories

Sample sizes in national surveys are often too small to obtain high-quality, reliable, nationally representative estimates required to monitor issues of health equity for all the minimum reporting OMB categories of race and ethnicity. The issues are more pronounced the smaller the category or survey. Omitting data for these minimum reporting OMB categories perpetuates inequities and promotes inaction—particularly when people are invisible in federal datasets. The data collected on these smaller minimum OMB categories are often biased due to incomplete representation, poorly designed sampling frames, inadequate collection approaches, language barriers (including failure to administer instruments in a person's primary language), and culturally inappropriate question design.

Recommendation 5: The Office of Management and Budget (OMB) should require the Census Bureau to facilitate and support the design of sampling frames, methods, measurement, collection, and dissemination of equitable data resources on minimum OMB categories—including for American Indian or Alaska Native, Asian, Black or African American, Hispanic or Latino/a, and Native Hawaiian or Pacific Islander populations—across federal statistical agencies. The highest

priority should be given to the smallest OMB categories—American Indian or Alaska Native and Native Hawaiian or Pacific Islander.

Although there are barriers to expanding sample sizes and collecting data on small or geographically remote populations (e.g., cost, data reliability, privacy), expanding sampling frames to generate statistically reliable estimates of the population at varying levels of geography is important for policy and program development. Decisions to do so will need to consider several factors, such as population size, the magnitude of the disparity based on scientific research, and cost and feasibility.

Detailed-Origin Categories and Data Disaggregation

Each OMB minimum reporting category has important differences based on origin and/or tribe. The need to collect and disseminate data at this level of disaggregation for racial and ethnic groups has been discussed for decades. Recently, the Census Bureau has made positive strides, and many others have provided recommendations for accomplishing this goal. This need is recognized across multiple racial, ethnic, and tribal populations. In addition to disaggregation for minimum category OMB groups by origin and/or tribe, these communities have many important intersecting identities, including communities of lesbian, gay, bisexual, transgender, queer (or questioning), and other sexual identities people, people of varying immigration statuses, people with disabilities, women, and children.

> **Recommendation 6: The Office of Management and Budget (OMB) should update and ensure equitable collection and reporting of detailed-origin and tribal affiliation data for all minimum OMB categories through data disaggregation by race, ethnicity, and tribal affiliation (to be done in coordination with meaningful tribal consultation), including populations who self-identify as American Indian or Alaska Native, Asian, Black or African American, Native Hawaiian or Pacific Islander, and Hispanic or Latino/a.**

In January 2023, OMB released a Federal Register notice with proposed changes to the collection of data on race and ethnicity. Several of the proposed changes are generally in line with the committee's recommendation (see report for more details). The report provides important considerations, including data privacy, checkboxes versus write-ins on surveys, expanding sampling frames to generate accurate statistical information on detailed-origin groups, and decisions regarding allocating resources to collect, analyze, and disseminate detailed origin with a view toward equity.

Measures of Social and Structural Inequities

Without proper social and environmental context, racial and ethnic health inequities may be incorrectly interpreted as the result of individual-level biological and behavioral factors, blaming individuals and groups for poor health outcomes. Including measures of racialized social and structural inequities at multiple levels of influence in national health surveys and other federal health data sources can facilitate contextualizing health inequities data and promote investigation of the effects of social and structural factors on these inequities.

> **Recommendation 7: The Centers for Disease Control and Prevention should coordinate the creation and facilitate the use of common measures on multilevel social determinants of racial and ethnic health inequities, including scientific measures of racism and other forms of discrimination, for use in analyses of national health surveys and by other federal agencies, academic researchers, and community groups in analyses examining health, social, and economic inequities among racial and ethnic groups.**

Such measures should pertain to racism and other forms of discrimination and include social, economic, educational, political, and legal indicators in a range of societal domains as well as measures of interpersonal racism, individual-level experiences of structural racism, and sociocontextual measures of structural racism (see the full report for examples). These measures should be usable at the state, county, and neighborhood levels and developed in partnership with academic researchers, community groups and members, and other key stakeholders. Some of this work is already underway, and the health equity coordinating entity recommended by the committee (Recommendation 1) could facilitate these efforts.

Budget Needs

Oversampling and targeted data collection are admittedly costly. However, identifying health, socioeconomic, and environmental inequalities, which negatively affect outcomes for these groups across the life span is essential for determining solutions to achieve health equity goals. Furthermore, context on social factors when interpreting racial and ethnic health inequities is crucial to understand the multiple levels of influence that impact health outcomes.

> **Recommendation 8: Congress should increase funding for federal agencies responsible for data collection on social determinants of health**

measures to provide information that leads to a better understanding of the correlation between the social environment and individual health outcomes.

These data will more accurately indicate the specific needs of underserved populations and improve overall equity in health and socioeconomic outcomes by identifying where policy change or interventions are needed to inform government investments to advance health equity.

Equitable Data Working Group

In April 2022, the Equitable Data Working Group (established under EO 13985) developed a report with recommendations for improvements in data equity and identified inadequacies in federal data collection programs, policies, and infrastructure across agencies. To ensure that this important work is enduring, the committee recommends:

> **Recommendation 9: The president of the United States should convert the Equitable Data Working Group, currently coordinated between the Office of Management and Budget (OMB) and the Office of Science and Technology Policy, into an Office of Data Equity under OMB with representation from the Domestic Policy Council, with an emphasis on small and underrepresented populations and with a scientific and community advisory commission, to achieve data equity in a manner that is coordinated across agencies and informed by scientific and community expertise.**

To benefit from the guidance of scientific and community experts, the federal government should make interagency coordination on data equity a permanent feature of its work across statistical agencies. By situating the Office of Data Equity under OMB, the federal government will be able to ensure cross-agency coordination and collaboration on data improvements that advance health equity in all federal agencies and policies.

Action 4: Improve Federal Accountability, Enforcement, Tools, and Support Toward a Government That Advances Optimal Health for Everyone

Although states and other levels of government need to tailor their health equity efforts to the needs of their populations, they need the federal-level tools and support to do so. Often, politics can stand in the way of or stall good policy, so processes and guardrails are needed to support state, local, tribal, and territorial needs. For example, guidance that has been vetted for health equity effects at the federal level needs to be in place for the implementation of policies and access requirements and to set expectations. Accountability mechanisms and processes can play a vital role in driving progress for health equity and require engaging with multiple diverse actors using dynamic accountability processes.

Program Implementation and Access

The committee's review illustrates numerous examples of barriers in implementation and access to federal programs that exacerbate inequities, such as administrative burden. In addition, state variation in program implementation (such as in Medicaid expansion and participation in social benefits programs, such as SNAP) can lead to differential access based on geography. Equitable implementation supports government efficiency and effectiveness and can decrease inequities and improve outcomes for all.

> **Recommendation 10: Congress and executive agencies should leverage the full extent of federal authority to ensure equitable implementation of federal policies and access to federal programs.**
> a. Relevant federal departments and agencies should design and implement policies to improve the administration of assistance programs to facilitate access to the benefits to which individuals and families are entitled. Such activities should include implementation and delivery processes, including administrative burden, eligibility, enrollment, enforcement, and client experience; and, where applicable, the creation of performance standards in federal programs administered by other (state, local, and tribal) governments.
> b. Congress should ensure that sufficient funding is made available to conduct these activities.

This recommendation builds on work already in progress by federal agencies to identify mechanisms to reduce administrative burden for underserved communities. To enable agencies to leverage the full extent of their authorities, additional funding may be needed—for example, for enforcement of civil rights protections.

Eligibility for Federal Program and Services

Access to federally funded programs for all people in the United States who meet requirements is essential to move toward health equity. For example, formerly incarcerated people and immigrants have restricted access to social service programs and incarcerated people cannot use Medicaid coverage; immigrants are not eligible for Medicaid until they have completed 5 years of legal U.S. residence. To increase access to federally funded programs for those who are categorically excluded, the committee recommends:

> Recommendation 11: The president of the United States should direct the Office of Management and Budget to review federal programs that exclude specific populations, such as immigrants and those with a criminal record and, in some cases, currently incarcerated people (e.g., Medicaid coverage), to assess the rationale and implications for equity of excluding these populations, including potential impacts on their families and communities. A report on the findings and suggested changes (when applicable) should be made publicly available.

The pros and cons, including cost and health equity implications, should be weighed for each excluded category in federally funded programs.

Advance American Indian and Alaska Native Health Equity

Although the committee was expansive in its attempt to incorporate all minoritized racial, ethnic, and tribal communities impacted by federal policies, it paid special attention to AIAN communities, who are often overlooked in large national reports. For most measures of health, AIAN people are worse off than other racial and ethnic groups; this includes life expectancy, suicide, homicide, and chronic diseases resulting in earlier and increased functional disability and death. As detailed in this report, the United States has a complex relationship with this population. A critically important aspect is that the 574 federally recognized tribes are sovereign nations and have a formal nation-to-nation relationship with the U.S. government with a trust responsibility that has not been fully upheld. The traumas that have unfolded over generations have resulted in untold cumulative harm, the effects of which are still being felt. Federal responsibility for AIAN health care was codified in 1976 to form the legislative authority for the IHS, which receives less funding per person than Medicaid, Medicare, Veterans Affairs, or federal prisons. Furthermore, AIAN voices in federal leadership and influence in the executive and legislative branches have been few, although several notable appointments were made recently.

> Recommendation 12: The federal government should undertake the following actions to advance health equity for American Indian

and Alaska Native communities in both urban and rural settings by raising the prominence of the agencies that have jurisdiction. Specifically,

   a. The president of the United States and Congress should raise the level of the Director of Indian Health Service (IHS) to an Assistant Secretary.
   b. Congress should authorize funding of IHS at need/parity with other health care programs. This funding should be made mandatory and include advance appropriations.
   c. The House of Representatives should re-establish an Indian Affairs Committee.

Although these actions will not address all barriers to health equity for the AIAN population, together, they will give more voice and prominence to AIAN people, which will help advance health equity for a population that is ignored and inadequately resourced.

Health Care Access

One major barrier to health equity is health care access, which includes health insurance coverage and the availability of and access to culturally appropriate, high-quality care, including preventive care, primary care, specialist care, chronic disease management, dental and vision care, mental health treatment, and emergency services. Lack of access to health insurance leads to adverse health outcomes and negative economic effects that exacerbate racial and ethnic inequities. However, health insurance is just one piece of the equation. Increasing access to high-quality, comprehensive, affordable, accessible, timely, respectful, and culturally responsive health care would advance racial and ethnic health equity.

Recommendation 13: The Departments of Health and Human Services, Defense, Veterans Affairs, Homeland Security, and Justice, as federal government purchasers and direct providers of health care, should undertake strategies to achieve equitable access to health care across the life span for the individuals and families they serve in every community. These strategies should prioritize access to effective, comprehensive, affordable, accessible, timely, respectful, and culturally appropriate care that addresses equity in the navigation of health care. While these strategies have a greater chance of success when everyone has adequate health insurance, there are ways the executive branch can improve and reinforce access to care for the adequately insured, the underinsured, and the uninsured.

There are a multitude of approaches that federal agencies can use to achieve this outcome, including ensuring access to health insurance coverage, primary care, enhancing inclusivity of language and communication/ health literacy, engendering trust in the health care system, and other innovations. Although it is not a panacea for health care access, health insurance coverage remains critical for all individuals residing in the United States. Examples of mechanisms to increase access include persuading nonexpansion Medicaid states to adopt federal financial support for their uninsured residents and federal directed strategies. The committee notes that AIAN people have a legal right to quality physician-led health care under treaty and trust responsibility. Further integration across the federal health system will also help achieve this recommendation—implementing Recommendation 1 would facilitate the needed integration.

CALL TO ACTION

This report points to both the positive and negative impacts federal policy has had on racial, ethnic, and tribal health equity. Although federal policy has played an important role in correcting past harms and advancing equity, substantial opportunities remain. The four action areas outlined in this report are connected and impact each other. For example, without representative and accurate data, it is difficult to identify where resources and tools are needed and policy efforts should be focused. Lack of community voice and expertise in policy development can lead to blind spots and cause unintended consequences. Staying vigilant for such unintended consequences of implemented policies is essential and needs to be built into feedback monitoring loops and measured in equity audits. Furthermore, as the federal government works to advance health equity, it should keep front and center the guiding principles in this report. Federal policy can play a key role in eliminating health inequities by collecting and employing accurate data, doing a better job of including and empowering communities who are most impacted, and coordinating and holding those who implement policy accountable. Implementing this report's recommendations will improve the circumstances in which people, families, and communities live, play, work, pray, and age so that all people living in the United States have the opportunity to meet their full health potential.

Summary Annex

Report Conclusions by Chapter

This Annex contains all of the report conclusions, organized by chapter. The discussions and evidence to support these conclusions are available in the corresponding chapter. There are conclusions on data gaps, the connection of the social determinants of health to health and health inequities, and the policy topics the committee reviewed.

CHAPTER 2: CONNECTION BETWEEN HEALTH EQUITY AND HISTORY, FEDERAL POLICY, AND DATA

- *Conclusion 2-1: The lack of oversampling of underrepresented racial, ethnic, and tribal populations in national health surveys and other relevant federal data collection efforts—for example, the Office of Management and Budget categories of American Indian or Alaska Native and Native Hawaiian or Pacific Islander—limits the availability of reliable data, and therefore meaningful action, by federal programs, researchers, and advocates to advance health equity for these communities.*
- *Conclusion 2-2: Disaggregated data on social, economic, health care, and health indicators that reflect the heterogeneity of racial and ethnic groups, including in relation to country of origin, are needed to inform targeted actions that promote health equity across and within groups.*

CHAPTER 3: ECONOMIC STABILITY

- *Conclusion 3-1: Evidence demonstrates that pretrial detention substantially reduces lifetime income, and strongly links incarceration with lower lifetime earnings and family income for incarcerated individuals. Given racial and ethnic inequities in incarceration and pretrial detention, there are opportunities in these areas to address racial and ethnic inequities in income and, thereby, health and well-being.*

- *Conclusion 3-2: Stagnation in the federal minimum wage, coupled with inflation, has left the real value of the minimum wage at a level not seen since the 1950s. Increases to the federal minimum wage raise incomes among low- and moderate-income families and lift families out of poverty. Since racially and ethnically minoritized populations and tribal communities are disproportionately represented in the groups that would be impacted by an increased federal minimum wage, such an increase is one method to address racial and ethnic inequities in economic stability and, therefore, health and well-being.*

- *Conclusion 3-3: Federal social benefit programs, such as the Supplemental Nutrition Assistance Program, Special Supplemental Nutrition Program for Women, Infants, and Children, and the Earned Income Tax Credit, significantly alleviate poverty and reduce the negative health consequences of poverty; however, there are barriers that prevent participation among many people who would otherwise qualify for these programs. Some racial, ethnic, and tribal populations have lower participation rates in these programs, contributing to racial and ethnic health inequity. Therefore, policies that address administrative barriers, hold programs accountable for participation rates, and improve administrative capacity can improve participation rates and reduce racial and ethnic health inequity.*

- *Conclusion 3-4: Federal social benefit programs, such as the Supplemental Nutrition Assistance Program, Special Supplemental Nutrition Program for Women, Infants, and Children, and the Earned Income Tax Credit, significantly alleviate poverty and reduce the negative health consequences of poverty. In some cases, eligibility for these and similar programs has been restricted for some groups, including childless adults, formerly incarcerated individuals, and immigrants. Because these groups disproportionately represent racially and ethnically minoritized populations, these restrictive policies contribute to racial and ethnic health inequity.*

- *Conclusion 3-5: Nonprofit sector partnerships play an important role in poverty alleviation and emergency food assistance that can influence racial and ethnic health inequities. Federal programs, such as the Emergency Food Assistance Program, help the non-profit sector more effectively serve those in need by providing food for distribution and grants for infrastructure and capacity building.*
- *Conclusion 3-6: Gaps in wealth for many racially and ethnically minoritized populations are linked to past and current federal policies, including redlining, disparate access to benefits of the 1944 GI Bill, and the financialization of the criminal legal system. Furthermore, policies that reward existing wealth, like the mortgage tax deduction, can exacerbate these gaps. Since wealth operates in tandem with income to enable access to healthier living conditions, quality health care, and amelioration of stress, these racial and ethnic inequities in wealth produce racial and ethnic inequities in health and well-being.*
- *Conclusion 3-7: Policies to support savings and wealth accumulation, for example, government subsidies of savings accounts for children, can increase wealth and narrow racial and ethnic differences in savings rates and wealth holding.*
- *Conclusion 3-8: Unequal access to safe and affordable financial services, including bank accounts and low-cost credit, is a driver of inequities. Enabling the provision of financial services that allow all Americans to spend, save, borrow, and plan will enable greater economic stability and increase health equity for low-income and racially and ethnically minoritized populations.*

CHAPTER 4: EDUCATION ACCESS AND QUALITY

- *Conclusion 4-1: There remain large differences in educational achievement and attainment between White and Asian students, on one hand, and Black, Latino/a, and American Indian and Alaska Native students, on the other. The empirical evidence that education is associated with health is strong. The causal evidence that more education can improve health is compelling given the many pathways through which education can affect health.*
- *Conclusion 4-2: There is strong evidence some federal policy changes and investments can improve educational outcomes and narrow differences in educational attainment and quality across racial and ethnic groups. However, the best mix of changes to policy and practice to improve student outcomes will vary across states, districts, schools, or groups of students. Thus, evidence-based policy, accountability, and community engagement play a critical role in improving federal policy for education as it relates to equity.*

- *Conclusion 4-3: Increases in per-pupil school spending have been shown to improve a range of student outcomes in the short and long run, including test scores, educational attainment, and earnings—all of which in turn are correlated with better health outcomes. Decreases in school spending lead to worse student outcomes, especially for children living in low-income neighborhoods and Black students. Federal policy could play a role to offset differences in cross-state spending and close spending gaps across racial and ethnic groups.*
- *Conclusion 4-4: In 1994, the federal government disqualified incarcerated people from Pell Grant eligibility, and in 2020, lawmakers reinstated Pell Grant access for incarcerated people enrolled in qualifying prison education programs. This is a promising example of how removing erected barriers to access for specific populations, such as incarcerated people, can address unequal access to federal programs that are linked to social determinants of health and health inequities.*
- *Conclusion 4-5: Minority serving institutions have demonstrated value on investment in economic outcomes for their students, and their effects on the racially and ethnically minoritized communities they serve merit research and measurement.*
- *Conclusion 4-6: Schools have unique opportunities to advance health, ranging from assisting in outreach and enrollment of eligible children in public health insurance programs and income support programs, to offering direct care through school-based health centers, to reducing food insecurity and improving dietary quality through school meals programs. Evidence shows that when schools adopt or improve these opportunities, both health and educational outcomes can be improved.*

CHAPTER 5: HEALTH CARE ACCESS AND QUALITY

- *Conclusion 5-1: Medicaid and the Children's Health Insurance Program are the most important federal policies that address the racial and ethnic inequities in access to affordable health care. The Medicaid expansions in eligibility incentivized in the 2010 Affordable Care Act have increased insurance coverage, improved health outcomes, and reduced racial and ethnic health inequities in access to preventive services, delayed care, and unmet health care needs.*
- *Conclusion 5-2: Among those eligible for Medicaid under the current federal eligibility criteria, racial and ethnic inequities in enrollment and participation remain. While acknowledging the important role of states, the federal government can play a role in addressing these issues, such as by reducing administrative burden*

and examining the racial and ethnic health equity implications of policies that exclude specific populations, such as immigrants and people involved with the criminal legal system.

- *Conclusion 5-3: State variation in implementation of the federal Medicaid law, most notably the state variation in the implementation of ACA Medicaid expansions, creates barriers to enrollment and differences in program eligibility and accessibility that have widened the gap in insurance coverage and access to care. The barriers disproportionately affect racially and ethnically minoritized populations, thus contributing to place-based racial and ethnic health inequities. While federal policies can address these barriers by limiting restrictive use of Medicaid flexibilities and effectively incentivize increasing access, these policy changes will require overcoming political and philosophical barriers related to Medicaid, federalism, and the role of government to ensure universal access to health care.*

- *Conclusion 5-4: Value-based payment and other programs intended to improve quality have, to date, not prioritized health equity. For example, such programs do not measure and incentivize reduction of racial and ethnic health inequities.*

- *Conclusion 5-5: A lack of inclusion and representation in clinical research may perpetuate health inequities because it limits the ability to identify issues of safety or effectiveness that might be specific to the populations that are not well represented. A lack of inclusion and representation in the health care workforce may perpetuate health inequities given the evidence that suggests better health outcomes when there is identity concordance between patients and providers.*

- *Conclusion 5-6: The Indian Health Service is the primary source of health care for many American Indian and Alaska Native people. The current structure and inadequate funding level of the Indian Health Service contributes to health inequities for American Indian and Alaska Native people.*

- *Conclusion 5-7: A lack of coordination, measurement, and prioritization of equity activities across the Department of Health and Human Services contributes to racial, ethnic, and tribal health inequities.*

- *Conclusion 5-8: Increasing access to high-quality, comprehensive, affordable, accessible, timely, respectful, and culturally appropriate health care would advance racial and ethnic health equity. Progress toward universal health care access can be achieved through many federal policy avenues, including but not limited to increasing access to public and private insurance coverage.*

CHAPTER 6: NEIGHBORHOOD AND BUILT ENVIRONMENT

- *Conclusion 6-1: Redlining and associated policies and structures resulted in residential segregation and neighborhood disinvestment, which have led to measurable health inequities present today. Safe, quality housing is necessary for maintaining an adequate standard of living, and there is a compelling link between housing and health equity. Increased federal investment in housing interventions for low-income people, such as the housing voucher program, could improve housing security and health outcomes for children and adults, especially among Black, Latino/a, American Indian and Alaska Native, and Native Hawaiian and Pacific Islander populations, and advance racial and ethnic health equity. Federal investment in housing would benefit from evidence-based guidelines to ensure that such investments do not contribute to future health inequities.*

- *Conclusion 6-2: The federal infrastructure policies governed by the Department of Housing and Urban Development, the Environmental Protection Agency, the Department of Transportation, and other agencies play critical roles to ensure health equity. Essential in these policies is the protection for those most vulnerable to the health effects of infrastructure investments, since, in many cases, federal funding propels infrastructure spending from state and local governments. While the role of federal funding may be limited in terms of the types of state and local infrastructure projects, there are missed opportunities for the federal government to monitor and address the health inequities tied to infrastructure. Coordination, monitoring, and guidance on infrastructure spending are lacking across federal agencies.*

- *Conclusion 6-3: There is a lack of coordination among relevant federal agencies to address workplace protection from pesticides, such as among the Occupational Safety and Health Administration, the Environmental Protection Agency, and the Centers for Disease Control and Prevention. Inadequate workplace protections from pesticides for agricultural workers disproportionately impact Latino/a workers, their children, and surrounding communities.*

- *Conclusion 6-4: Community voice through advocacy has played a positive role in shaping iterations of the Agriculture Improvement Act. However, given the bill's size and scope, an audit of the equity implications of the bill could identify additional areas of improvement, such as areas to expand further tribal self-determination and self-governance in relevant programs and other mechanisms to advance racial and ethnic health equity.*

CHAPTER 7: SOCIAL AND COMMUNITY CONTEXT

- *Conclusion 7-1: Community safety is critical for health and well-being. Racial and ethnic inequities in gun homicides and recent increases in firearm suicide among young Black adults suggest the need for more evidence-based policies that can prevent harm.*
- *Conclusion 7-2: There are clear racial and ethnic inequities in policing. Improved data collection is needed to increase accountability, better understand the extent of these inequities, and determine which policy changes may help reduce them.*
- *Conclusion 7-3: The criminal legal system is an important driver of health across the life course, as well as the health of communities and families. Racially and ethnically minoritized communities have experienced and continue to experience disproportionate contact with the criminal legal system. Evidence suggests that policies regarding mandatory minimum sentences, long sentences, and mass incarceration merit re-examination.*
- *Conclusion 7-4: Generations of Black, American Indian, Alaska Native, Native Hawaiian, Pacific Islander, Latino/a, and Asian communities have been negatively affected by past actions, practices, policies, and laws that inflicted lasting harm and undermined access to social, economic, and political resources and opportunities, contributing to current racial and ethnic health inequities. There is a need to continue to study and address the impacts of historical and contemporaneous laws and policies that sustain racial inequity.*
- *Conclusion 7-5: Research demonstrates that civic engagement and belonging have powerful effects on population health, well-being, and health equity. Civic infrastructure and civic engagement are important factors in building social cohesion and inclusionary decision making that lead to better design and implementation of policies that affect health equity.*
- *Conclusion 7-6: Important considerations when crafting federal action on health equity include leveraging existing policies and authority, considering the limitations of executive orders, and articulating elements that build belonging, community inclusion, and civic muscle into federal agency policy development processes.*

CHAPTER 8: ROADMAP TO HEALTH EQUITY

- *Conclusion 8-1: The widespread inequities in education, income, and other factors that impact health are the result of the disparate and harmful impact of trauma, laws, and policies at all levels of government, both past and present. Health inequities are prevalent, persistent, and preventable and federal policy is an important tool for correcting historical and contemporary harms.*

- *Conclusion 8-2: Federal policy can play a key role in eliminating health inequities by collecting and employing high-quality and accurate data, doing a better job of including and empowering communities that are most affected, and coordinating and holding those who implement policy accountable.*

1

Statement of Task and Approach

INTRODUCTION

In the United States, the opportunity to enjoy a healthy and prosperous life is often shaped by one's race and/or ethnicity.[1] As shown in this report, health outcomes and other measures of well-being are negatively affected by structural disadvantages, such as in education and income (see Box 1-1). Of course, no membership in a racial, ethnic, or tribal group predicts a given outcome, and each of the broad categories of race and ethnicity has considerable heterogeneity. However, the available data on health outcomes and other measures of well-being tell a story of structural disadvantage, preventable disparities in outcomes, and diminished opportunity. This report provides a framework for federal action that reviews contributing factors and identifies solutions—by building on past successes and addressing continued barriers—to structural racial, ethnic, and tribal health inequities.

THE URGENCY OF ADDRESSING HEALTH INEQUITIES

Although COVID-19 laid bare the reality of inequity in the United States, the disproportionate burden of poor health and inadequate access to health-protective social factors, such as economic stability, quality employment

---

[1] The racial and ethnic categories discussed in this report should not be interpreted as being primarily biological or genetic. Race and ethnicity should be thought of in terms of social and cultural characteristics and ancestry and could be considered proxies that invoke racism (how race impacts how others perceive/treat different populations) and social characteristics (adapted from 62 FR 58782; see also the committee's definition of key terms in the beginning of this report).

BOX 1-1
Factors That Shape Health Outcomes

The Whitehall I study, which began in 1967, showed an inverse relationship between social class (based on the employment grade of British civil servants) and mortality from a variety of illnesses. In the decades since, the Whitehall II study and other research have further illustrated that social factors, such as race, ethnicity, zip code, education level, employment, and income, impact health outcomes and thereby create significant inequities (Marmot et al., 1991; NASEM, 2017). Countless scholars have developed social ecological models of health and theories to explain the link between social and structural factors and health (IOM, 2003a; Link and Phelan, 1995; McGinnis and Foege, 1993; NASEM, 2017).

Today, the social ecological or social determinants of health (SDOH) framework is a vital part of public health and health equity work. Healthy People 2030 defines SDOH as "the conditions in the environments where people are born, live, work, play, worship, and age that affect a wide range of health, functioning, and quality-of-life outcomes and risks." Healthy People 2030 acknowledges that targeting individual health behaviors cannot eliminate health inequity and so has an "increased and overarching focus on SDOH" (HHS, n.d.).

HHS has organized the SDOH in five areas (HHS, n.d.):

- Economic stability
- Education access and quality
- Health care access and quality
- Neighborhood and built environment
- Social and community context

The committee used this categorization for its report. Chapters 3–7 each focuses on one of the SDOH and describes what each includes and how federal policies in those areas impact health outcomes.

---

and education, and quality and affordable health care, faced by racial and ethnic populations that are minoritized, long preceded the pandemic (for a description the term "minoritized" and why it is used, see the Terminology section of this chapter). "The existence of racial and ethnic disparities in morbidity, mortality, and many indicators of health for African Americans, Native Americans, Hispanics, and Asians/Pacific Islanders was first acknowledged by the federal government in the 1985 Report of the Secretary's Task Force on Black and Minority Health. Since then, research has sought to identify additional disparities and explain the mechanisms by which these disparities occur" (NASEM, 2017). Extensive research on these health inequities demonstrates that these populations experience higher rates of illness and death for many different conditions, including heart disease, hypertension, and diabetes, as well as lower life expectancies compared to non-Hispanic White people (CDC, 2021). Maternal health is another

---

BOX 1-2
U.S. Health Outcomes in Comparison to Other Nations

As one of the wealthiest nations in the world, and one that outspends in health care compared to other wealthy nations, the United States is among the least healthy countries compared to other wealthy and even middle-income countries (Gunja et al., 2023; IOM and NRC, 2013). It has the lowest life expectancy and highest suicide rates among the 11 Organisation for Economic Co-operation and Development nations (Gunja et al., 2023). Americans are living shorter and unhealthier lives despite immense wealth and health care spending. A key factor driving poor health compared to counterpart nations is the large racial, ethnic, and tribal health inequities and the federal policies and lack of policies driving these inequities. Eliminating inequities will improve the health of not only racial, ethnic, and tribal populations that are minoritized but also the entire population. Studies have documented that programs designed to benefit minoritized and underserved groups, such as people with disabilities or racialized groups, often benefit all of society (Blackwell, 2016). Eliminating racial and ethnic inequities will serve to not only revitalize the United States but also make it a thriving society that will allow for continued innovation in science and a strong economy (NASEM, 2017).

---

important area—mortality is 2–3 times higher among Black and American Indian and Alaska Native (AIAN) women (Petersen et al., 2019), and severe maternal morbidity (SMM) is higher among racial and ethnical people who are minoritized (Hill et al., 2022). An abundance of data points to social and structural determinants of health as the mechanism by which these disparities occur (NASEM, 2017, 2019e). Health inequity has consequences for the economy, national security, business viability, and public finances. For example, diminished health affects military readiness, and poor health impacts private businesses significantly (research from the Urban Institute shows that young adults who are less healthy and cannot find jobs in the mainstream economy are less productive and generate higher health care costs for businesses) (NASEM, 2017; Urban Institute, n.d.). Furthermore, health inequity has consequences for U.S. competitiveness in relation to other nations (see Box 1-2).

The Costs of Health Inequities

Public Health and Health Care

A plethora of evidence points to systemic and structural racism and discrimination as key elements of the mechanisms by which racial and ethnic health disparities occur (NASEM, 2017, 2019a, 2019c, 2019d, 2019e, 2022e). Therefore, a critical cost of racial inequity is poor health outcomes for significant portions of the nation. The following section lays out examples of the stark reality of the state of health for such populations due to the lack of opportunities afforded to them. These patterns of inequity transcend most health outcomes. The COVID-19 pandemic brought this crisis into the nation's consciousness as patterns of infection, hospitalization, and mortality took shape, mirroring the racial and ethnic health inequities seen everywhere else (CDC, 2022a; Hill and Artiga, 2022). In response to increasing understanding of the urgency of this crisis, many public health organizations, states, and other entities have declared racism a public health emergency, and the public health and health care sectors increasingly incorporate this understanding into how they approach their work (APHA, 2021).

These poorer health outcomes for groups that have been minoritized have important implications for health care spending. Research demonstrates that racial and ethnic inequities in health outcomes are responsible for significant avoidable expenditures (see below for estimates). Inequities in health care quality and access and other SDOH increase costs for health care consumers, providers, insurers, and taxpayers. Along with the increased burden of disease faced by racially and ethnically minoritized and tribal communities, inadequate or delayed care can lead to complications that require more extensive and expensive care, such as emergency department services or surgical interventions for heart disease (NASEM, 2017).

A 2009 analysis by the Joint Center for Political and Economic Studies found that 30.6 percent of direct medical care expenditures from 2003 to 2006 for African American, Asian, and Hispanic people were excess costs due to health inequalities and that eliminating inequalities in this same period for these populations would have saved $229.4 billion and more than $1 trillion in direct and indirect medical expenditures, respectively (LaVeist et al., 2009). That same year, the Urban Institute estimated that racial health inequity would cost health insurers $337 billion from 2009 to 2018 and that the annual costs would more than double by 2050 with increased representation of these populations among elderly people (Waidmann, 2009). Furthermore, a 2018 analysis by the W.K. Kellogg Foundation estimated that racial and ethnic health disparities amount to approximately $93 billion in excess medical care costs, $175 billion in economic impact of shortened life-spans (and 3.5 million lost life years associated with premature deaths), and $42 billion in lost productivity per year, as well as other costs, yielding $230 billion in projected economic gain per year if health disparities are eliminated by 2050 (Turner, 2018). A June 2022 analysis by Deloitte estimated that health inequities (in race, socioeconomic status, and sex/gender) account for $320 billion in annual health care spending and could eclipse $1 trillion by 2040 if left unaddressed (Dhar et al., 2022). The 2009 analysis by LaVeist et al. was updated in 2023; it found that in 2018, the estimated economic burdens of racial and ethnic health inequities and education-related health inequities were \$42–45 billion and \$940–978 billion, respectively. The analysis showed that most of the "economic burden was attributable to the poor health of the Black population; however, the burden attributable to American Indian or Alaska Native and Native Hawaiian or Other Pacific Islander populations was disproportionately greater than their share of the population" (LaVeist et al., 2023 p. 1).

Income Inequality

The economic and other costs individuals, families, and communities face due to racial and ethnic health inequities also perpetuate a cycle of accumulating disadvantage (see Chapter 3). High health care costs leave individuals and families struggling financially. Poor health and complications from chronic conditions impede the ability to work, jeopardizing access to employer-provided health coverage and the ability to provide for oneself and one's family. Using an SDOH framework (see Figure 1-2) for public health illustrates the importance of economic stability, the ability to *thrive* financially, and access to quality employment and benefits to health and well-being (see Chapter 3 for a detailed discussion). These costs impact not only racially and ethnically minoritized populations but also the United States overall due to the implications for health care spending.

Societal Division, Political Costs

The existence of racial and ethnic inequity is antithetical to ideas written into the Constitution that all "are created equal, that they are endowed by their Creator with certain unalienable Rights, that among these are Life, Liberty and the pursuit of Happiness" and to the prevailing conception of the United States as a country of equal opportunity for all.

Christopher described the nation's inability to abandon the false belief in a hierarchy of human value as a point of vulnerability. In her book *Rx Racial Healing: A Guide to Embracing our Humanity*, she argues that "current levels of societal division" make it crucial to engage in the work of truth, racial healing, and transformation, for which her book provides a framework (Christopher, 2022) and which can help foster collective action to address health equity. Such societal and political divisions have led to the politicization of health, health care, and other areas (Pew Research Center, 2020). The Truth and Reconciliation Commission following apartheid in South Africa (United States Institute of Peace, 1995) and Canada's more recent efforts to confront the traumatic history and legacy of its residential school system and its impact on Indigenous families and communities provide precedents for taking action (Crown-Indigenous Relations and Northern Affairs Canada, 2022). The racial justice protests that followed the murder of George Floyd in 2020, the January 6, 2021, attack on the U.S. Capitol, and studies illustrating the depth of the U.S. political divide (Dimock and Wike, 2021; Kort-Butler, 2022) support Christopher's argument. The UN's World Social Report 2020 draws similar conclusions about the negative consequences and vulnerability of inequity, including social unrest, discontent, destabilized political systems, threats to democracy, and violent conflict (United Nations, 2020).

ROOT CAUSES OF HEALTH INEQUITIES IN THE UNITED STATES

"The factors that make up the root causes of health inequity are diverse, complex, evolving, and interdependent in nature" (NASEM, 2017). The inequitable distribution of disease and well-being in the United States shows that social factors, such as economic stability, education access and quality, health care access and quality, neighborhood and built environment, and social and community context, as well as the upstream structural factors that impact them, including governance systems and processes and the nation's cultural and historical context, play a critical role in health outcomes (see Chapters 2–7 for detailed examples of these factors) (NASEM, 2017, 2023b; University of Wisconsin Population Health Institute, 2023). These social, environmental, economic, and cultural determinants of health are "the terrain on which structural inequities produce health inequities" and the conditions in which people live.

> For example, the effect of interpersonal, institutional, and systemic biases in policies and practices (structural inequities) is the "sorting" of people into resource-rich or resource-poor neighborhoods and K–12 schools (education itself being a key determinant of health) on the basis of race and socioeconomic status. Because the quality of neighborhoods and schools significantly shapes the life trajectory and the health of the adults and children, race- and class-differentiated access to clean, safe, resource-rich neighborhoods and schools is an important factor in producing health inequity. Such structural inequities give rise to large and preventable differences in health metrics. (NASEM, 2017, pp. 100–101)

Research demonstrates that the inequitable pattern of these social risk factors across race and ethnicity are in large part a consequence of structural disadvantages for minoritized communities that were, in no small measure, initiated by historical federal policies (NASEM, 2017). These decisions, some made centuries ago, have guided the organization and governance of society and the distribution of resources, affecting all generations since. The U.S. history of assimilation, removal, and extermination of

American Indian people, enslavement of African and African American people, colonialism, and immigration policy have been key to how the country is stratified, impacting outcomes across health, education, socioeconomic status, and other measures of well-being even today (see Chapter 2 for more information) (NASEM, 2017).

The outcomes are evident in the disproportionate burden of poor health faced by disadvantaged groups, such as low-income individuals and families, people living in historically segregated and disinvested areas, those without access to high-quality employment and educational opportunities, members of sovereign nations and tribes, and people who are American Indian, Alaska Native, Asian, Black, Latino/a, or Native Hawaiian, and Pacific Islander. Owing to the U.S. history and prevailing legacy of structural racism (see Key Terms for definition), patterns of inequity with regard to these social factors fall along racial and ethnic lines (see Chapter 2 for more details). There are higher rates of childhood asthma among low-income households, higher morbidity and mortality from chronic diseases among individuals with lower educational attainment, and higher exposure to air pollution among residents of disinvested communities—those in low-income, disinvested communities are disproportionately racially and ethnically minoritized. Moreover, the effects of the structural determinants of health on many health outcomes persists when accounting for income and education. For example, New York City data from 2008 to 2012 demonstrate that, among women who did not finish high school, SMM, a measure of life-threatening complications of pregnancy, labor, and delivery, was three times higher for Black than White women. SMM was 2.4 times higher among Black women with an undergraduate degree or higher compared to White women who did not finish high school (Angley et al., 2016). This report reviews the social and structural factors (e.g., policy) contributing to racial and ethnic health inequities and provides solutions for advancing racial, ethnic, and tribal health equity at the federal level.

The following four case examples illustrate some of the ways different populations are affected by health inequities via uneven access to the SDOH. These examples are not meant to be comprehensive; other racialized and ethnic groups and multiracial individuals experience similar inequities but unique outcomes, and these populations are highlighted in other parts of the report.

The Experience of Black Men

Health outcomes for Black men are an example of how structural racism—via the health care, criminal legal, education, and employment systems—is expressed as health vulnerabilities. Black men live an average of 74 years, 4.4 years less than the average for non-Hispanic White men, and face high rates of mortality from preventable chronic illness (HHS, 2023). Compared to other populations, young Black men are less likely to have a regular source of primary care, have insurance coverage, and rate communication with a provider as positive, and they often see the health care system as complicit with other aggressive and oppressive systems, such as the law enforcement system (Vasquez Reyes, 2020). Overall, Black Americans die at higher rates than White Americans of heart disease, stroke, cancer, asthma, influenza, pneumonia, HIV/AIDS, and homicide (HHS, 2023). Such negative health outcomes are exacerbated or caused by social inequities. "Young Black men have poor access to quality primary care which is especially devastating when we consider that many of these young men are often [affected] by racially inflected violence in their communities through their interactions with social institutions and systems."[2] Young Black men face unique burdens as a result of racist stereotypes about anger, violence, and criminality that society has imposed on their identities. These social stigmas lead to outcomes that expose them to poor health outcomes. For instance, about 1 in 1,000 Black men and boys in America can expect to die at the hands of police (Edwards et al., 2019). Furthermore, 1 in 3 Black boys born today will be sentenced to prison during his lifetime, compared to 1 in 17 White boys—which is due not to higher crime rates by Black boys but rather to social and structural factors at play (NAACP, 2021; NASEM, 2022d). These social and structural factors limit Black men's ability to live a healthy and prosperous life.

The Experience of American Indian and Alaska Native People

The lived experiences of AIAN people are also shaped by structural disadvantage and a history of extermination, removal, and assimilation in the interest of Euro-American expansion (Moss, 2019). For example, life expectancy in 2019 was 73.1—5.1 years lower than the White and 12.6 years lower than the Asian population (NIH, 2022). The AIAN population also saw a sharper decrease in life expectancy from 2019 to 2021 than any other racial or ethnic group (Goldman and Andrasfay, 2022). American Indians have rates of high infant mortality, maternal death, and diabetes, with the most resulting amputations and other complications (IHS, 2014). Despite these poor outcomes indicating an urgent need, access to and funding of treaty-mandated health care remain problematic. The Indian Health Service (IHS) receives less funding per person than Medicaid,

---

[2] Quote by John A. Rich, Rush University Medical Center, at Meeting 3 of the committee (see https://www.nationalacademies.org/event/08-01-2022/review-of-federal-policies-that-contribute-to-racial-and-ethnic-health-inequities-meeting-3-part-2 [accessed May 30, 2023]).

Medicare, VA, or federal prisons. Indian Country often has health care workforce shortages and inadequate health care and infrastructure funding (Heisler and McClanahan, 2020). For example, accessing medical care later in the calendar year can be problematic, as the IHS referred care program begins to run out of resources because it does not receive advance appropriations (Heisler and McClanahan, 2020). American Indian populations also have high rates of mental health and substance use challenges, resulting in some of the highest U.S. suicide and homicide rates. Violence is an especially pertinent issue for AIAN women, for whom murder is the third leading cause of death in some counties, according to the Centers for Disease Control and Prevention (CDC). Invisibility is another—of 5,712 cases of missing and murdered Indigenous women and girls reported in 2016, only 116 were logged in the U.S. Department of Justice federal missing persons database (Lucchei and Echo-Hawk, 2018). The erasure of American Indians in data collection cuts across the spectrum of measures for health and well-being; a common saying is "born Native but dying White." Thus, as serious as the picture that the data paint, the reality is likely much worse. In addition, tribes are domestic dependent nations, "Wards of the State," sovereigns, and at the "sufferance of Congress" for their status as federally recognized tribes due a federal trust responsibility stemming from the Marshall Trilogy from the early 1800s, which is the basis of Indian law today (NCAI, n.d.).

The Experience of Native Hawaiian and Pacific Islander People

The lived experience of Native Hawaiian and Pacific Islander (NHPI) people is also marked by long-standing historical trauma that has resulted in racial segregation, physical displacement, declining health, higher death rates, premature mortality, stereotyping, and inadequate data leading to a level of invisibility (Alexander, 1899; Bureau of East Asian and Pacific Affairs, 2005; Faucher, 2021; Galinsky et al., 2017; Kaholokula et al., 2020; Kana'iaupuni and Malone, 2006; Klest et al., 2013; Morey et al., 2022; Ogden et al., 2017; Panapasa et al., 2010; Tobin, 1967; Xiang et al., 2020). In 1997, the Office of Management and Budget (OMB) disaggregated the single Asian or Pacific Islander category into two independent categories and required federal programs to adopt the new standards by January 1, 2003. When data for NHPI are combined with Asian population data, this aggregation masks the true outcomes for NHPI people—who are composed of Indigenous, migrant, and immigrant groups—for all measures (Moon et al., 2022; Taparra and Pellegrin, 2022). This lack of data has damaging effects as inadequate basic national-level data limits knowledge on health outcomes, perpetuating invisibility and lack of representation, and depriving NHPI people of access to effective resources and interventions.

These factors underscore how structural inequities perpetuate disparities in population health outcomes. NHPI people continue to face a disproportionate burden of disability, morbidity, and mortality (Galinsky et al., 2017; Morey, 2014; Pillai et al., 2022). Compared to other populations, they are more likely to have elevated levels of asthma, heart disease, hypertension, and diabetes and least likely to have a healthy body weight (Galinsky et al., 2017). Overall, NHPI people have the highest end-stage kidney disease incidence rate among all races in the 50 states (921, 95 percent CI: 895–987, per million population per year)—2.7 times greater than White and 1.2 times greater than Black Americans. In the U.S. Pacific Island territories, the rate was 941 (95 percent CI: 895–987) (Xiang et al., 2020). Common factors that lead to health inequities in the Native Hawaiian population include poverty, low levels of high school completion, exposure to pollutants, poor physical environments, limited access to care, and discrimination (Liu and Alameda, 2011; Morey, 2014). Pacific Islander people in the Los Angeles County area report some of the highest levels of childhood and adult asthma, and their heavy concentration in the lawn care and construction industries also represents a high risk of ongoing exposure to pesticides and dangerous chemicals (LACDPH, 2022). In 2020, NHPI people in Los Angeles County were reported to have the highest mortality rate (1,324 per 100,000) and lowest life expectancy (73.5 years compared to 82.3 years for the county overall) (LACDPH, 2022).

Although these inequities are considerable, NHPI communities have the potential to thrive. As one of the most rapidly growing demographic groups in the country, they live in every state (Kehaulani Goo, 2015; OMH, 2023). NHPI people are increasingly attending college, often through athletic scholarships but also due to a growing recognition of education as a way forward for their children (Teranishi et al., n.d.; Tran et al., 2010). Community and faith-based organizations are assuming a greater role as stakeholders in community-based research activities and aggressively ensuring that relevant health, educational, housing, and economic information reaches the neighborhoods they serve (Burrage et al., 2023; Galinsky et al., 2019; McElfish et al., 2018; Panapasa et al., 2012).

The Experience of Latino/a Immigrants

The Latino/a population is the largest minoritized group in the United States, and 19.7 million people—34 percent of the total immigrant population—identify as Hispanic or Latino (Esterline and Batalova, 2022). Undocumented Latino/a people compared to documented have worse health outcomes for many measures (such as higher blood pressure, hypertension, depression, and anxiety), and undocumented Latina immigrants are more likely to have low-birthweight babies. Limited access to health care, health-protective resources (such as social and economic factors), and interactions with immigration enforcement actions are mechanisms that contribute to inequities within the population (Cabral and Cuevas, 2020). Furthermore, social mobility is limited, as is access to health care, placing undocumented Latino/a people at an increased risk for disease. Lack of legal status is a barrier to higher educational attainment—half of the Hispanic undocumented population aged 18+ has less than a high school education (Cabral and Cuevas, 2020). These issues transfer generationally as well. For parents who do not have experience navigating the health care and social systems, cultural and language barriers coupled with transportation and economic challenges hamper their ability to access public programs, such as health care, for their children (Aragones et al., 2021; Flores et al., 1998; Oropesa et al., 2016).

Additional Populations and Data Limitations

These four examples are only a small snapshot of the experiences of minoritized racial and ethnic populations. Much more is discussed elsewhere in this report. For example, the Asian American population has roots in more than 20 countries in East and Southeast Asia and the Indian subcontinent. There are groups within the Asian community who suffer greater health inequities than the group as a whole and have unique experiences, histories, cultures, languages, and needs. The Hmong people differ significantly from other Asian American populations in many social factors (such as income and education levels), which may put them at risk for poorer health (Lor, 2018). Black men were discussed, but Black women also face significant inequities—for example, maternal mortality is three times higher among Black than White mothers (CDC, 2022d; Hoyert, 2022), and their infant mortality rate is more than two times higher (CDC, 2022b). In addition, the Black population includes people with very different socioeconomic characteristics, such as individuals who immigrated from Sub-Saharan Africa versus those who represent multigenerational North American African Americans (see Chapter 2 for more information).

Although the statistics on racial and ethnic inequities in health outcomes—including those in the examples—are striking, they are complicated by problems such as data inaccuracy, sometimes intentionally missing data for certain populations, and failure to disaggregate data (see Chapter 2). In addition to these examples, failure to accurately record race for AIAN people in medical records erases them in the data (Espey et al., 2014; Jim et al., 2014). Some populations, such as people of Middle Eastern or North African descent, are entirely excluded from categories for race and ethnicity because they are counted as White under current federal standards even though they are routinely racialized as non-White. For NHPI populations, aggregation of data under broad categories, such as "Asian," "Asian and Pacific Islander," or "Asian, Native Hawaiian, and Pacific Islander," masks the complexity of the challenges faced by these different populations and reinforces racist and colonialist views of racial and ethnic minorities as monolithic. Another important consideration is that ethnicity is currently treated separately from race in most data collection efforts, but some consider this a flawed approach and advocate for using a mutually exclusive single race/ethnicity variable because not doing so can sometimes limit the ability to identify inequities and/or distort findings due to misclassification or missing data points. "For example, not providing a mutually exclusive race/ethnicity category for Latino individuals forces them to artificially choose a race" (Flores, 2020, p. 2). For the purpose of this report, the committee treats these as separate categories because that is how the majority of the data are collected.

The understanding that data on health outcomes for racially and ethnically minoritized populations are limited is a critical component of the committee's approach to its task (see the Committee's Approach section; see Chapter 2 for a detailed discussion on data limitations and opportunities). Given the limited and inaccurate data for specific populations, the committee relied on a variety of data to capture a fuller understanding of the mechanisms that result in health inequities for these different populations and made the intentional decision to center lived experiences and other forms of knowledge as data throughout this study.

Role of Communities

Although the illustrative examples provided here and elsewhere in the report are discouraging, racially and ethnically communities that are minoritized have flourished despite many barriers. For example, a 2017 National Academies report highlighted nine communities[3] that advanced health equity by addressing various SDOH—that is just a small sample of communities' work nationwide (NAM, n.d.; NASEM, 2017; RWJF, n.d.; TFAH, 2018). In addition, some communities have made significant gains on health outcomes. For example, although CDC reported in 2022 that over the last 2 years, the life expectancy of Black people declined to about 71 years old (6 years lower than their White counterparts), in certain communities, it is much higher—in Manassas Park, VA, and Weld County, CO, it is 96 years. Black people are living longer in some smaller jurisdictions as well (Brookings Metro and NAACP, n.d.).

---

[3] These include Blueprint for Action in Minneapolis, MN; IndyCAN in Indianapolis, IN; Magnolia Community Initiative in Los Angeles, CA; Mandela Marketplace in Oakland, CA; and WE ACT for Environmental Justice in Harlem, NY (NASEM, 2017).

In the majority of these examples, community voice and expertise played a strong role in creating and implementing strategies designed to advance health equity. Ensuring the inclusion of community leaders and organizations in federal policies that contribute to health equity is a key theme in this report (see Guiding Principles). Communities are defined as population groups residing in a specific zip code, census tract, or county or sharing another commonality, such as race or ethnicity, gender, or age (NASEM, 2017).

Although community participation is often touted as a value in policy making and program design processes, two problems persist: a lack of specificity as to what constitutes community engagement or inclusion and of accountability mechanisms to ensure that authentic community input has been integrated into the policy or program. Figure 1-1 illustrates the International Association for Public Participation's Spectrum of Public Participation (IAP2). This model is useful because it enables both specificity and accountability. To advance health equity, the role of communities—particularly those that suffer most from current health inequities—needs to move further to the right on this spectrum (CDC, 2011; NAM, 2022; NASEM, 2017; South et al., 2015; Wallerstein et al., 2020). Such an approach can help partners better understand and address the roots of health issues and protect against creating repressive partnerships (CDC, 2011; NAM, n.d.; Viswanathan et al., 2004).

INCREASING IMPACT ON THE DECISION →

	INFORM	CONSULT	INVOLVE	COLLABORATE	EMPOWER
PUBLIC PARTICIPATION GOAL	To provide the public with balanced and objective information to assist them in understanding the problem, alternatives, opportunities and/or solutions.	To obtain public feedback on analysis, alternatives and/or decisions.	To work directly with the public throughout the process to ensure that public concerns and aspirations are consistently understood and considered.	To partner with the public in each aspect of the decision including the development of alternatives and the identification of the preferred solution.	To place final decision making in the hands of the public.
PROMISE TO THE PUBLIC	We will keep you informed.	We will keep you informed, listen to and acknowledge concerns and aspirations, and provide feedback on how public input influenced the decision.	We will work with you to ensure that your concerns and aspirations are directly reflected in the alternatives developed and provide feedback on how public input influenced the decision.	We will look to you for advice and innovation in formulating solutions and incorporate your advice and recommendations into the decisions to the maximum extent possible.	We will implement what you decide.

© IAP2 International Federation 2018. All rights reserved. 20181112_v1

FIGURE 1-1 The International Association for Public Participation's Spectrum of Public Participation Model.
SOURCE: IAP2, 2018; Credit: © International Association for Public Participation www.iap2.org.

Although including community voice in decisions that will affect them is crucial, "communities exist in a milieu of national-, state-, and local-level policies, forces, and programs that enable and support or interfere with and impede the ability of community residents and their partners to address the conditions that lead to health inequity. Therefore, the power of community actors is a necessary and essential, but not sufficient, ingredient in promoting health equity" (NASEM, 2017)—supportive policies at all levels are also needed.

THE COMMITTEE'S APPROACH

The committee was asked to (1) review federal policies (e.g., social, economic, environmental) that contribute to preventable and unfair differences in health status and outcomes experienced by all U.S. racially and ethnically minoritized populations and (2) provide conclusions and recommendations that identify the most effective or promising approaches to policy change with the goal of furthering racial and ethnic health equity (see Box 1-3). The Department of Health and Human Services (HHS) Office of Minority Health (OMH) requested this study in response to a request in a Congressional Appropriations Report.[4] The committee was not asked to review the state of U.S. health inequities but does provide background on this throughout the report. Although there

---

BOX 1-3
Statement of Task: Committee on the Review of
Federal Policies That Contribute to Racial
and Ethnic Health Inequities

An ad hoc committee of the National Academies of Sciences, Engineering, and Medicine (National Academies) will provide an evidence-based, independent and objective analysis of federal policies that contribute to racial and ethnic health inequities, including those policies that impact the social determinants of health, as well as potential solutions. The review should focus on all racial and ethnic minority populations in the U.S. The analysis should identify the most effective or promising strategies to eliminate or modify policies to advance racial and ethnic health equity. The National Academies' committee will develop a report with conclusions and recommendations. Recommendations may include, but are not limited to, policy and budget considerations.

---

[4] House conference report (H. Rept. 116-450—Departments of Labor, Health and Human Services, and Education, and Related Agencies Appropriations Bill, 2021).

are many examples of federal policies that have advanced health equity, the committee was not asked to review such policies. However, because many successful policies can be changed to be even more effective or implemented more broadly, such policies are reviewed in this report (see Box 1-4).

BOX 1-4
Types of Policies

For the purpose of this report, a policy is a law, regulation, procedure, administrative action, incentive, or voluntary practice of governments and other institutions that affects a whole population (NASEM, 2017). Further, it is a course of action or inaction that government selects from among alternatives. A policy could influence health inequities in many ways. The committee grouped them into four categories:

1. Policies that are neutral in terms of racial, ethnic, or tribal inequity (that is, their purpose was not to address health equity) but have indirect equity implications. For example, the policy could address a social determinants of health challenge that disproportionately affects racial and ethnic groups that have been minoritized, such as antipoverty programs (see Chapter 3). While this type of policy does not address racial and ethnic health inequities directly, it does so indirectly. This report looks closely at these policies to examine inequities with uneven enforcement, unintended consequences, or a lack of recognition of specific community factors/needs.
2. Policies that were intended to reduce inequities and/or account for racism. The policies generally are working but have aspects that can be improved, such as expanding Medicaid coverage and funding early childhood education. On rare occasions, policies in this category may not be achieving the aim of reducing inequities. For example, the federal Medicaid sterilization policy was enacted in 1976 in response to coerced and nonconsensual sterilization practices that disproportionately affected low-income women of color. This policy was intended to be a protective mechanism by requiring patients to wait 30 days after signing a specific consent form before the procedure could occur. However, in contemporary medical practice, this policy now serves as a barrier to desired care (ACOG, 2021).
3. Policies that were intended to worsen racial, ethnic, or tribal inequities. For example, the U.S. history of extermination, removal, and assimilation of American Indians; the enslavement of African American people; colonialism; redlining; and immigration policy have played a critical role in how the country is stratified, affecting contemporary outcomes across health, education, socioeconomic status, and other measures of well-being.
4. A lack of policy in a given area, or status quo, is also a policy decision. Inaction in an area may be due to lack of political will, lack of funding, or lack of data, or lack of community input to raise the policy concern to the attention of policy makers.

BOX 1-4 Continued

Both formal and informal policies exist; formal policy has consequences for not following it when enforced (e.g., fines, withdrawal of funding or eligibility, criminal charges), whereas informal policy (e.g., guidelines, recommendations, funding opportunities for research and community-based initiatives, tax subsidies) does not have such consequences. This report reviews each of the above policy types and how policy makers can accelerate the use of evidence and data to advance health equity. (See Chapter 2 for a description of the types of federal policy levers, including implementation and enforcement.)

A range of views exist on the role and place of government in U.S. society. However, the committee focused on the evidence of how federal policies—or lack thereof—have contributed to health inequity and looked to federal policy levers for solutions, as this was its charge, with a focus on policies and programs in the executive and legislative branches of the federal government. Policies at other levels of government may be more or less important for contributions and/or solutions, but the committee does not comment on or address these issues, as they are not part of the Statement of Task. The following section reviews the terminology and key terms used in this report and the committee's approach to its Statement of Task.

Terminology

Over time, terminology related to racial, ethnic, and tribal health equity has significantly evolved (NASEM, 2021c). Lack of "person first" language, stigmatizing language, and omitting some populations from data collection have contributed to exclusion, lack of trust, and misinformation. Therefore, throughout this report, the committee strived to use language that is respectful, accurate, and maximally inclusive. It attempted to use language that reflects how individuals and groups wish to be addressed, but consensus does not always exist on preferred terms, and these preferences may evolve.

Rather than referring to "racial and ethnic minorities," "members of minority groups," or "underrepresented minorities," this report uses the term "minoritized," which makes the distinction that being minoritized is not about the number of people in the population but rather about power and equity and points to the intersectionality of being a minoritized member of a minoritized group (Wingrove-Haugland and McLeod, 2021). "Minoritized" demonstrates that dominant groups "minoritize members of subordinated groups rather than obscuring this agency" (Wingrove-Haugland

and McLeod, 2021). "Minoritization recognizes that systemic inequalities, oppression, and marginalization place individuals into 'minority' status rather than their own characteristics" (Sotto-Santiago, 2019). However, "minoritized" will not resonate with all. Some link this term to hierarchal thinking related to the dehumanization of specific populations. "While using minoritized risks creating a false equivalence that sees all instances of being minoritized as equal and discounting unique forms of oppression. . . . using this term carefully can ensure that its advantages outweigh these risks" (Wingrove-Haugland and McLeod, 2021).

This report uses "Black people" when referencing African American and other people who are part of the African diaspora, as the term is often understood to be broader and include persons whose cultural history is not grounded in the United States (NASEM, 2021c). Similarly, the committee has chosen "Latino/a" to refer to persons with cultural connections to Latin America, recognizing that some people may prefer "Hispanic," "Latinx," "Latine," or another term. The phrase "American Indian and Alaska Native" is preferred because this is the population recognized under treaty rights. See the frontmatter for definitions of key terms in this report.

In this report, as with many other published reports, the comparison group when looking at health inequities is typically non-Hispanic White people. Electing a culturally dominant group as the reference group can subtly imply the notion that dominant groups are the most "normal." However, this report does not do so because Whiteness should be the aspiration or it is centering Whiteness. Rather, this comparison is made because White people have not directly suffered the impacts of structural racism and other structural determinants of health due to race.

Societal understanding of gender identity is rapidly evolving. Gender-related terms are used, but when applicable, broader terms, such as "pregnant people" in place of "pregnant women," to acknowledge the diversity of gender identities and point to ways that our common language can be updated to accord greater respect to all people. "LGBTQ+" refers to individuals who are lesbian, gay, bisexual, transgender, and queer or questioning (NASEM, 2021c).

Sometimes the terms used in this report, however, are determined by the terms or definitions in data systems or a specific research study referred to or summarized. For example, if referencing data collected or analyzed for "Native Americans," that terminology is used.

Definitions

Definitions are available in the "Key Terms" section; definitions provided are how the terms are used in *this* report, and National Academies, government, and other reports may define them differently. One important distinction is that health disparities and health inequities are not the same. Health disparities are differences among specific population groups in the attainment of full health potential that can be measured by differences in incidence, prevalence, mortality, burden of disease, and other adverse health outcomes (NASEM, 2017). "Health *inequities*" implies that these differences are unfair and preventable (Meghani and Gallagher, 2008). Health equity is the state in which everyone has a fair opportunity to attain full health potential and well-being, and no one is disadvantaged from doing so because of social position or any other socially defined circumstance. Achieving health equity requires valuing everyone equally with focused and ongoing societal efforts to address avoidable inequalities and historical and contemporary injustices and eliminate health and health care disparities due to past and present causes (CDC, 2022c; NASEM, 2017). By these definitions, addressing inequities requires transformational changes, including in how resources are allocated, decisions are made, and goals and objectives are established; "business as usual" perpetuates inequities. It is important to emphasize that equity is not interchangeable with equality—equality is the treatment of all individuals in the same manner. Equality assumes a level playing field for everyone without accounting for historical and current inequities.

Report Conceptual Framework

Given the broad task provided to the committee (see Box 1-3), it developed a conceptual framework (Figure 1-2) to approach its analysis and this report. The framework uses Healthy People 2030's five categories for the SDOH (HHS, n.d.), recognizing the role that the inequitable distribution of SDOH, such as economic stability, health care access and quality, education access and quality, social and community context, and neighborhood and built environment, play in perpetuating racial and ethnic health inequities.

Moreover, the SDOH are shaped by structural determinants, including local, state, tribal, territorial, and federal policies and laws, and societal-level aspects of the historical and cultural context, such as structural racism. The latter refers to the totality of ways in which a society fosters racial and ethnic inequity and subjugation through mutually reinforcing systems, including housing, education, employment, earnings, benefits, credit, media, health care, and the criminal legal system (Bailey et al., 2017). These structural factors "organize the distribution of power and resources (i.e., the social determinants of health) differentially" among racial, ethnic, and socioeconomic groups, perpetuating health inequities (NASEM, 2019e). The key difference between institutional and structural racism is that structural racism happens *across* institutions; institutional racism happens *within* institutions ("systemic racism" is another term).

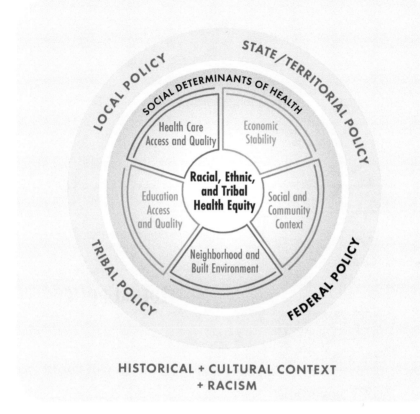

FIGURE 1-2 Report conceptual framework.

The intertwining relationships between the SDOH, laws and policies, government policy, and historical and cultural factors are more complex than can be clearly visualized in a single model. Historical and cultural factors at the larger societal level also impact laws and policies, which affect the SDOH and health inequities. Figure 1-3 illustrates the complexity of the relationships between the social and structural determinants introduced in Figure 1-2.

Although not represented in Figures 1-2 and 1-3, the committee also incorporated a life course lens in its analysis and throughout this report. Such approaches to examining health inequities incorporate both structural and developmental perspectives, considering how social and structural determinants of health, particularly exposures "during sensitive life stages" can "shift health trajectories" and "shape health within and across generations" (Jones et al., 2019).

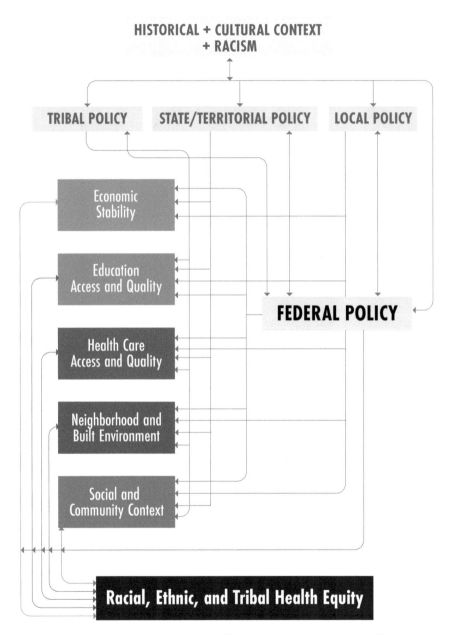

FIGURE 1-3 Report conceptual framework illustrating the complex relationships between social determinants, structural determinants, and racial, ethnic, and tribal health equity.

Key Principles

The committee adopted a set of principles to guide its work (see Box 1-5), alongside the conceptual framework (which provides a higher-level view of its approach). These principles are essential when embarking on health equity work and were informed by a large and growing body of research on the SDOH (IOM, 2003a; Link and Phelan, 1995; McGinnis and Foege, 1993; NASEM, 2017) and input from experts, policy leaders, and other key stakeholders gathered via public comment and information-gathering sessions.

1. **Health is physical and mental well-being, but it also includes well-being in social, economic, and other factors, all of which are necessary for human flourishing.**

The committee defined health as not only medical but also social supporting capacities for human flourishing (CDC, 2017). The implications of using this holistic approach are that federal policies can impact health both directly (e.g., access to medical care via Medicaid Expansion) or indirectly (e.g., reducing family economic insecurity via Earned Income Tax Credit [EITC]). In addition, all people should have the opportunity to attain health and well-being. "Rebuilding a healthy social contract for the U.S. requires focusing on health as a foundation for the 'safety and happiness' of the people. Those are the words used in the Declaration of Independence as a translation of the ancient Roman dictum *salus populi suprema lex esto* ('let the health of the people be the supreme law')" (Impact Initiative, n.d.). This pursuit needs to include all people, and this is rooted in the "concept of solidarity that is a deep but submerged strand in American history" (Impact Initiative, n.d.). This holistic view of health is needed for all people to flourish.

BOX 1-5
Report Key Principles

1. Health is more than physical and mental well-being—it also includes well-being in social, economic, and other factors, all of which are necessary for human flourishing.
2. All federal policies have the potential to affect population health.
3. Evidence is informed by quantitative, qualitative, and community sources (all of which should be equally valued).
4. Federal policies should center health equity.
5. To advance health equity, structural and systems change are needed.

2. Every federal policy has the potential to affect population health.

Given the role of federal policies in both impacting and securing health and well-being, a Health in All Policies (HiAP) approach is needed when assessing health equity. HiAP is informed by an SDOH framework and ". . . a collaborative approach that integrates and articulates health considerations into policy making across sectors to improve the health of all communities and people. HiAP recognizes that health is created by a multitude of factors beyond health care and, in many cases, beyond the scope of traditional public health activities" (CDC, 2016). Using this approach means that every federal policy has potential population health implications that need to be considered when evaluating it for health equity.

3. Evidence is informed by quantitative, qualitative, and community sources.

The committee used an inclusive (standards of) evidence approach. This meant drawing from both quantitative and qualitative historical and contemporary evidence from peer-reviewed sources and nonpartisan research organizations across disciplinary perspectives. The committee paid particular attention to community-informed research approaches that are often not included in the evidence base to inform, implement, or evaluate policy. Each of these sources of evidence should be valued and evaluated in building the knowledge base, which should be evaluated from a fundamental cause of disease approach,[5] focusing on structures and systems versus individual- or community-level actions as the causes of health inequities. This approach requires reviewing other factors that impact health equity, including the intersections of systems of stratification across, but not limited to, race, ethnicity, gender, sexual orientation, class, and ability. It also allows for evaluating the impact of policies (or absence of policies) on multiple domains of mental, physical, and behavioral health and well-being across diverse groups.

4. Center health equity in all federal policies.

The committee centered equity in every step of evaluating federal policies and developing recommendations for future policy assessment and

---

[5] Using a fundamental cause of disease approach means that individually based risk factors need to be contextualized by examining what puts people at risk of risks; social factors, such as socioeconomic status and social support, are considered "fundamental causes" of disease that "because they embody access to important resources, affect multiple disease outcomes through multiple mechanisms, and consequently maintain an association with disease even when intervening mechanisms change" (Link and Phelan, 1995, p. 80).

creation. Centering equity means prioritizing the needs of racially and ethnically minoritized populations and considering the consequences of current and future policies for advancing or impeding health equity. Multiple tools exist to assess current policies for equity and project the impacts of future policies (for example, see Ashley et al., 2022; Martin and Lewis, 2019; MITRE, n.d.; OMB, 2021; Urban Institute, n.d.).

Although a cost–benefit analysis of policies is beyond the scope of the report, centering equity also requires affirmatively advancing civil rights, racial justice, and equal opportunity as key structural, political,[6] and social determinants of health; elevating community experience, voice, and expertise; and using that voice to inform policy. Tensions and tradeoffs exist (e.g., prioritizing equity over efficiency, recognizing that communities are diverse and can have opposing views and needs, respecting data sovereignty, and making data available to the public) when working with diverse communities. However, multiple evidence-based processes have been established for collective decision-making processes across groups with diverse identities and views (e.g., public deliberation) (Blacksher et al., 2021; Bose et al., 2017; Christiano, 1997).

The committee centered equity when examining structures and systems in understanding impacts of policies on health inequities, with two subprinciples.

(4a): **Eliminate and prevent harm:** When evaluating current policies across multiple domains, the committee first identified characteristics of federal policies or their implementation that are maintaining, causing, or amplifying racial/ethnic health disparities either directly or indirectly, as measured by available evidence. The committee's focus on eliminating and preventing harm was strongly informed by the precautionary principle in environmental science, which contains four principles: (1) taking preventive action in the face of uncertainty, (2) shifting the burden of proof to the proponents of a policy, (3) exploring a wide range of alternatives to possibly harmful actions, and (4) increasing public participation in decision making (Kriebel et al., 2001). In some situations, elimination may not be possible but mitigation can reduce harm and prevent further harms.

(4b): **Maximize potential for equity:** Policies were evaluated with an eye toward achieving health equity. The committee acknowledges that removing harm, reducing disparities, and/or improving health capacities are necessary first steps; reducing disparities is not the end goal.

---

[6] "Political determinants of health involve the systematic process of structuring relationships, distributing resources, and administering power, operating simultaneously in ways that mutually reinforce or influence one another to shape opportunities that either advance health equity or exacerbate health inequities" (Dawes, 2020, p. 44).

5. Structural and systems change are needed to advance health equity.

Achieving health equity will require structural and systems changes. This means that not only must policies address structure and create systems change but also the structure and components of policies need to be interrogated and also potentially changed. Because of this, the committee used an approach where the sum of policy parts is greater than the whole. It is often said that, "The whole is greater than the sum of the parts," but this may not always be the case for policies. They have multiple components as they relate to setting and prioritizing objectives; coordinating policy and implementation; and monitoring, analysis, and evaluation. Even well-intentioned policies aimed at improving well-being can have a negative impact based on how they are created, implemented, or monitored. Policies targeted at low-income people, for example, may impose higher levels of administrative burden (e.g., complex, opaque, rigid, or repetitive requirements) than services more likely to be universal (OMB, 2021). Later chapters show, for example, how eligibility criteria or lack of enforcement can turn health-promoting into health-harming policies, particularly for racially and ethnically minoritized populations, creating health inequities.

Approach to the Report and Recommendations

The task provided to the committee was extremely but necessarily broad—review federal policies that contribute to racial, ethnic, and tribal inequities. The number of factors that contribute to health inequities are large and fall in many domains (see Figure 1-2 and Box 1-1). At its first meeting, Rear Admiral (RDML) Felicia Collins, director of OMH (the sponsor of this report), provided the charge to the committee. She was clear that the charge included reviewing all the SDOH but left it to the committee to determine how to approach its task and what to include in its review. RDML Collins also requested that the committee use the Healthy People 2030 SDOH framework. The committee could not review every federal policy and program that might contribute to racial, ethnic, and tribal health inequities within the five SDOH domains in the year it had to develop its report. For example, Congress has enacted hundreds of statutes during each of its 118 biennial terms and more than 30,000 statutes since 1789, and federal agencies each have numerous policies under their authority (GovInfo, n.d.; Govtrack, n.d.).

To focus its review to best achieve the Statement of Task, the committee took a multi-phased approach: gathering information, developing criteria for selecting policies to review, and reviewing prioritized policies.

For information gathering, the committee reviewed the published literature (including grey literature), held information-gathering meetings (see Appendix B), put out a call for public input (including lived experiences), and reviewed key policies in each of the five SDOH domains (see Chapters 3–7).

To identify the federal policies reviewed in this report, the committee developed the following set of considerations for prioritization. First, prioritize policies that impact a large percentage of minoritized racial or ethnic populations. Second, prioritize policies that have a body of literature or available data to assess them based on race and ethnicity. Third, prioritize historical policies that, based on the literature, continue to harm racially and ethnically minoritized and tribal populations. Fourth, given that data gaps for racially and ethnically minoritized and tribal populations are a well-documented problem (see Chapter 2), prioritize policies that illustrate how these data gaps could fail to document health inequities. Finally, the committee also prioritized expertise from itself and invited speakers, verbal public comments at information-gathering meetings, and written public comments (see Appendix B and Box 1-7). Based on a mix of these considerations, the committee used its expert judgment to choose the federal policies to review in the following chapters. The review examined how the policy affected (both positively and negatively) racial, ethnic, or tribal health equity.

Based on its review, the committee was able to identify aspects of federal policy that cut across domains and contribute to health inequities or could advance health equity. These crosscutting themes formed the foundation of the report recommendations, with the key principles as a guide (see Box 1-5), When the committee identified barriers to health equity for a specific federal policy, if the literature reviewed promising or evidence-based solutions, the committee provided a discussion of those solutions (the committee was asked in its Statement of Task to review both promising and evidence-based solutions—see Box 1-3). The committee is not unique in its approach to recommendations. The Federal Plan for Equitable Long-Term Recovery and Resilience (ELTRR) (November 2022) also lays out a crosscutting approach and recommendations for federal agencies to cooperatively strengthen the vital conditions necessary for improving individual and community resilience and well-being nationwide (see the next section for more information) (ELTRR Interagency Workgroup, 2022).

Although the committee had to make difficult decisions regarding which policies to highlight, omitting a particular policy does not mean it is any less important. The committee focused on those policies (or lack thereof in a given area) that would best illustrate how policies (or particular components) can hinder or advance racial, ethnic, and tribal health equity. The committee applied the key principles and concepts and took into account the important interplay between federal policy with states, tribes, territories, and localities and the policy tools available at the federal level (see Chapter 2 for more on this topic). Similarly, many painful historical actions, practices, policies, and laws have led to trauma for specific groups in relation to federal policy; this report could not cover them all.

An abundance of high-quality evidence-based and peer-reviewed reports, from the National Academies and other evidence-based organizations, has either laid out the evidence for the root causes and mechanisms of health inequities or provided actionable recommendations for specific policy actions that could be taken to change federal policies to advance health equity (for example, see, IOM, 2003a, 2003b; IOM and NRC, 2013; NASEM, 2017, 2018a, 2018b, 2019a, 2019b, 2019c, 2019d, 2019e, 2021a, 2021b, 2022a, 2022b, 2022c, 2022d, 2022e). The committee builds off of this work and looks to the future, rather than repeating existing analysis. The committee also provides recommendations from other reports that have not been acted on and endorses them because they still merit attention and action. In addition, other National Academies studies in progress or recently released overlap with the committee's charge, so the committee focused more on policies not covered by those reports (for example, the Committee on Unequal Treatment Revisited: The Current State of Racial and Ethnic Disparities in Healthcare,[7] the Committee on the Review of Policies and Programs to Reduce Intergenerational Poverty,[8] and the 2023 report *Closing the Opportunity Gap for Young Children* [NASEM, 2023a]).

As noted in the guiding principles, the committee focused on identifying institutional- and structural-level factors that impact population health. Therefore, it focused its efforts on providing recommendations on crosscutting approaches that would impact a wide range of policies (see Chapter 8). Per the guiding principles, the committee considered policies that leave populations that have been racially and ethnically minoritized behind, cause harm, undermine civil rights, racial justice, and equal opportunity, omit community voice and evidence, and/or do not consider health equity. It provides recommendations at both the institutional (for example, addressing administrative burden across programs) and structural (for example, addressing accountability) levels. The committee does provide select policy-specific recommendations (it focused on those policies most proximal to health outcomes, such as health care access and quality).

This report focuses mainly on the U.S. 50 states, but racial and ethnic groups that have been minoritized live in U.S. territories as well. The territories' governing systems vary—for example, individuals born in Commonwealth of the Northern Mariana Islands (CNMI), Guam, Puerto Rico, and U.S. Virgin Islands are U.S. citizens, and those born in American Samoa are U.S. nationals. Their eligibility for federally subsidized programs varies by territory and program. Residents of all five territories may participate in Medicaid, CHIP, Medicare, and Social Security, but

---

[7] See https://www.nationalacademies.org/our-work/unequal-treatment-revisited-the-current-state-of-racial-and-ethnic-disparities-in-healthcare (accessed March 7, 2023).

[8] See https://www.nationalacademies.org/our-work/policies-and-programs-to-reduce-intergenerational-poverty (accessed March 22, 2023).

BOX 1-6
Executive Order 13985—Summary of Actions for Embedding Equity in the Everyday Business of Government

- Reduce administrative burdens and simplify government services.
- Engage with stakeholders and communities who have been historically excluded from policy-making processes.
- Narrow wealth gaps through federal contracting and procurement.
- Deliver equity through grantmaking.
- Build accountability for equity through data collection and reporting.

---

none except those in CNMI is eligible for Supplemental Security Income (MACPAC, 2021). Addressing health equity in U.S. territories is important, and the report provides several examples of how federal policy varies in territories; however, the necessary deep analysis is beyond the scope of this report.

CURRENT LANDSCAPE

Advancing health equity (or equity in areas that impact health, such as the environment, housing, and economic well-being) has garnered much attention recently from philanthropies, nonprofit organizations, and federal, state, and local governments. The following section summarizes some of these efforts. The committee strived to build off these and other existing efforts and analyses in its report.

Executive Orders

The most relevant executive order Executive Order (EO) is 13985,[9] *Advancing Racial Equity and Support for Underserved Communities Through the Federal Government* (January 2021). It notes that "equal opportunity is the bedrock of American democracy, and our diversity is one of our country's greatest strengths" but that entrenched inequities in U.S. law and policy (and private and public institutions) have "denied that equal opportunity to individuals and communities." The EO called on the Domestic Policy Council to coordinate the efforts outlined in the EO and embed equity principles, policies, and approaches across the federal government in coordination with the National Security Council and National Economic Council (see Box 1-6). Although the EO does not explicitly

---

[9] Exec. Order No. 13985, 86 FR 7009 (January 2021).

state "health" equity as its goal, the proposed actions span all federal agencies. As discussed, health equity is impacted by a large range of factors, including economic stability and access to housing and a safe environment—and therefore the EO is strongly tied to health. OMB was tasked with partnering with agency heads to study methods for assessing whether agency policies and actions create or exacerbate barriers to full and equal participation by all eligible individuals (see OMB, 2021). Findings and recommendations from the OMB report highlight that federal programs and services should be viewed through an equity lens. Some of the report findings include the following:

- Bringing together expertise and experience from across sectors can be a powerful catalyst for learning and solutions.
- The federal government can learn from and improve upon existing equity assessments, demographic data collection processes, and tools, particularly models that have supported state and local governments.
- Intersectionality matters—federal policies, grants, and programs should always account for how people's multiple identities interact with intersecting systems of oppression (OMB, 2021).

To meet the goals of EO 13985, each federal agency was tasked with developing an equity plan within 1 year (agencies released their plans in April 2022, and these are available online)[10] (DPC, 2023; The White House, 2022a). The EO also highlights the need for "engagement with members of underserved communities" and that the agencies "should consult with members of communities that have been historically underrepresented in the federal government and underserved by or subject to discrimination in federal policies and programs." Another major aspect of the EO was establishing the Equitable Data Working Group (see Chapter 2 for more information) (Equitable Data Working Group, 2022). A follow-up EO (14091)[11] was issued on February 16, 2023, stating that federal agency and department Equity Action Plans will be updated annually and that each agency and department will designate and provide resources to Agency Equity Teams for implementation. The updated EO also adds increased requirements for engagement with and investments in impacted communities, addresses emerging risks from technology, and continues data equity and transparency efforts (The White House, 2023). The EO and resulting efforts are discussed throughout this report, with several key initiatives and OMB findings outlined in Chapter 8.

---

[10] See https://www.whitehouse.gov/equity/#equity-plan-snapshots (accessed March 15, 2023).
[11] Exec. Order No. 14091, 88 FR 10825 (February 2023).

Other relevant EOs have been created by the current and past administrations:

- 13175 (November 2000), *Consultation and Coordination with Indian Tribal Governments*[12]
- 13995 (January 2021), *Ensuring an Equitable Pandemic Response and Recovery*, which called for establishing a Presidential COVID-19 Health Equity Task Force[13,14]
- 14008 (January 2021), *Tackling the Climate Crisis at Home and Abroad*[15]
- 14031 (May 2021), *Advancing Equity, Justice, and Opportunity for Asian Americans, Native Hawaiians, and Pacific Islanders*[16]
- 14050 (October 2021), *White House Initiative on Advancing Educational Equity, Excellence, and Economic Opportunity for Black Americans*[17]
- 14053 (November 2021), *Improving Public Safety and Criminal Justice for Native Americans and Addressing the Crisis of Missing or Murdered Indigenous People*[18]
- 14070 (April 2022), *Continuing to Strengthen Americans' Access to Affordable, Quality Health Coverage*[19]
- 14075 (June 2022), *Advancing Equality for Lesbian, Gay, Bisexual, Transgender, Queer, and Intersex Individuals*[20]

Other Federal Government Reports, Initiatives, and Background

One example of a federal initiative to advance health equity is Opportunity Zones. EO 13853, signed by President Trump, established the White House Opportunity and Revitalization Council to carry out the administration's

---

[12] This order established regular and meaningful consultation and collaboration with tribal officials to develop federal policies that have tribal implications, strengthen the U.S. government-to-government relationships with Indian tribes, and reduce the imposition of unfunded mandates. Exec. Order No. 13175, 65 FR 67249 (November 2022)

[13] Exec. Order No. 13995, 86 FR 7193 (January 2021).

[14] Recommendations from the task force included (1) invest in community-led solutions to address health equity, (2) enforce a data ecosystem that promotes equity-driven decision making, and (3) increase accountability for health equity outcomes. Its accountability framework highlighted that (1) community expertise and effective communication needs to be elevated in health care and public health; (2) data should accurately represent all populations and their experiences to drive equitable decisions; and (3) health equity should be centered in all processes, practices, and policies (Presidential COVID-19 Health Equity Task Force, 2021).

[15] Exec. Order No. 14008, 86 FR 7619 (January 2021).

[16] Exec. Order No. 14031, 86 FR 29675 (May 2021).

[17] Exec. Order No. 14050, 86 FR 58551 (October 2021).

[18] Exec. Order No. 14053, 86 FR 64337 (November 2021).

[19] Exec. Order No. 14070, 87 FR 20689 (April 2022).

[20] Exec. Order No. 14075, 87 FR 37189 (June 2022).

plan to target, streamline, and coordinate federal resources to be used in Opportunity Zones and other economically distressed communities (Opportunity and Revitalization Council, 2019).

Another example is the Federal Plan for ELTRR released in November 2022 by the HHS Office of the Assistant Secretary for Health and the Office of Disease Prevention and Health Promotion (ODPHP), on behalf of an interagency workgroup composed of over 35 federal departments and agencies. The plan was developed "to address the deep disparities in health, well-being, and economic opportunity that were laid bare during the COVID-19 pandemic" (ODPHP, 2022). The workgroup identified opportunities for collaboration to maximize available resources across government agencies and improve community resilience[21] with the vision of "all people and places thriving, no exceptions." The plan uses the seven "Vital Conditions for Health and Well-Being" as the guiding framework. The vital conditions are the following:

- Belonging and Civic Muscle
- Thriving Natural World
- Basic Needs for Health and Safety
- Humane Housing
- Meaningful Work and Wealth
- Lifelong Learning
- Reliable Transportation

The vital conditions align with the Healthy People 2030 five SDOH categories that the committee used to guide its work (see Committee Approach section). This effort began during the Trump administration, ended during the Biden administration, and has been embraced by federal agencies (see Chapter 7). The plan includes 78 recommendations for interagency action and maps out how federal entities can connect through mutual interests and existing authorities. Most recommendations tie to a specific vital condition; 10 address crosscutting infrastructure and governance.

Another example of a government initiative related to health equity is Justice 40, a whole-of-government initiative with the goal "that 40 percent

---

[21] Key actions for the plan include (1) align federal government departments and agencies to strengthen the Vital Conditions for Health and Well-Being; (2) foster community-centered collaboration within and outside of government to ensure an equitable, thriving future; (3) adapt steady-state and other federal investments within agency authority to transform systems that enable resilience and well-being; and (4) achieve equity and aspire to eliminate disparities by focusing sustained resources on communities that have been underserved or disadvantaged. The next steps include (1) form an executive steering committee, (2) retain the ELTRR Interagency Workgroup, (3) establish a measurement framework and indicators, (3) systematically link plan efforts to related executive orders and priorities, (4) leverage regional expertise and networks, and (5) engage with and gather input from nongovernmental partners (ELTRR Interagency Workgroup, 2022).

of the overall benefits of certain federal investments flow to disadvantaged communities that are marginalized, underserved, and overburdened by pollution" stemming from EO 14008 (The White House, 2022b). The current administration has also taken a whole-of-government approach to addressing climate change.

The federal government's focus on health equity is also evident in a January 2021 report: *Something Must Change: Inequities in U.S. Policy and Society* (U.S. House Committee on Ways and Means, 2021b). It examines how racism, ableism, and other social, structural, and political determinants negatively impact health and economic equity. On March 4, 2021, the chair of the committee announced the creation of its Racial Equity Initiative to "address the role of racism and other forms of discrimination in perpetuating health and economic inequalities in the United States" to build on the framework A Bold Vision for a Legislative Pathway Toward Health and Economic Equity that the committee also issued in January 2021 (U.S. House Committee on Ways and Means, 2021a, n.d.).

Several ongoing court cases also could have significant impacts on health equity, including the unfolding effects of overturning *Roe v. Wade*,[22] and *Braidwood Management v. Becerra*[23] (on Affordable Care Act [ACA] coverage of services recommended by the U.S. Preventive Services Task Force[24]), which could have important implications for coverage with $0 cost sharing for preventive health care services. A relevant recent case is *Students for Fair Admissions Inc. v. President & Fellows of Harvard College*,[25] which ended race-based considerations in higher education, including in medical school and other health professions school admissions. Another recent case, *Haaland v. Brackeen* (the Indian Child Welfare Act),[26,27] could have had major consequences for both tribes' right to exist as political entities and family separation—however, the law was upheld with the June 15, 2023, Supreme Court decision.

---

[22] *Roe v. Wade*, 410 U.S. 113.

[23] *Braidwood Management Inc. v. Xavier Becerra*, 4:20-cv-00283, (N.D. Tex.).

[24] Under Section 2713 of ACA, self-funded health plans and insurers offering nongrandfathered group or individual market health plans must cover services given an "A" or "B" rating from the U.S. Preventive Services Task Force, Advisory Committee on Immunization Practices–recommended vaccines, Health Resources and Services Administration (HRSA)–recommended preventive care and screening recommendations for children, and HRSA Women's Preventive Services Initiative–recommended services, including contraceptives (Child Welfare Information Gateway, n.d.).

[25] *Students for Fair Admissions, Inc. v. President & Fellows of Harvard College* 600 U.S. ____ (2023).

[26] *Haaland v. Brackeen* (Docket No. 21-376).

[27] The Indian Child Welfare Act is a 43-year-old federal law that protects the well-being and best interests of Indian children and families by upholding family integrity and stability and keeping children connected to their community and culture and affirms the tribal sovereignty of First Nations.

STUDY PROCESS AND REPORT OVERVIEW

Information-Gathering Process

The committee gathered information in a variety of ways. It held three information-gathering sessions between June and September of 2022 (agendas are available in Appendix B; all meetings were virtual) on a range of topics, including racial and ethnic health inequities; socioeconomic differences in health; housing, transportation, and health policy; federal Indian law and constitutional law; community infrastructure challenges and solutions; policy levers; and interagency collaboration. In addition, the committee held two public comment sessions to solicit feedback on key questions that broadly asked about the impacts, both positive and negative, of health policies and their effects on health equity and the lived experiences of racially and ethnically minoritized groups. The committee held deliberative meetings and received public submissions of materials throughout the study.[28] The committee made a call for public comments via the project website (see Box 1-7 for a summary of topics raised), listserv, and outreach to relevant organizations. Its online activity page also provided information to the public about its work and facilitated communication with the public.[29]

Report Overview

Throughout this report, the committee provides conclusions, and the report ends with recommendations for action, guided by the conceptual framework and guiding principles introduced in this chapter. The committee organized its recommendations under four core action areas to advance racial, ethnic, and tribal health equity:

1. Implement Sustained Coordination Among Federal Agencies
2. Prioritize, Value and Incorporate Community Voice in the Work of Government
3. Ensure Collection and Reporting of Data Are Representative and Accurate
4. Improve Federal Accountability, Enforcement, Tools, and Support Toward a Government That Advances Optimal Health for Everyone

These themes are explored in detail in the following chapters. Chapter 2 provides an overview of the state of health inequities and of some of the underlying structural determinants and contextual factors that have led to these outcomes. It also describes the role of data collection, shortcomings of the data system, opportunities for improvement to advance federal policy, and

---

[28] Public access materials can be requested from PARO@nas.edu.
[29] See http://nationalacademies.org/health-equity-policies (accessed September 22, 2022).

BOX 1-7
Public Comment Summary

The committee put out a request for public comments in both written and verbal (at information-gathering meetings) form. The request sought input on federal policies that contribute to racial and ethnic health inequities and potential solutions. The committee also requested comments regarding lived experiences navigating federal programs and systems, including barriers and solutions, from community members and organizations. The committee posed the following questions for the public to consider:

- What are examples of federal policies that create racial and ethnic health inequities?
- What are examples of federal policies that promote racial and ethnic health equity?
- What are the most important considerations when prioritizing action regarding federal policies to advance racial and ethnic health equity?

Over 100 unique written responses were received, in addition to over 40 verbal comments. Respondents included nonprofit organizations, institutions, community members providing lived experiences, and academics. The comments covered a large number of topics and included background information on the state of health inequities, examples of inequitable policies, and potential solutions. Respondents expressed strong support for a number of topics that affect racially and ethnically minoritized and tribal populations to be addressed and comments covered a large range of issues, such as the following:

- Access:
  - Improved cultural and linguistic access to services
  - Administrative burden and eligibility requirements of federal programs
- Data and representation:
  - Representation of diverse populations in clinical trials
  - Federal grant eligibility requirements and the need to diversify recipients
  - The need for sexual orientation and gender identity data (e.g., state Medicaid program)
- Planning and implementation:
  - Improved planning and implementation of federal policies (e.g. environmental justice issues, school finance, exclusionary zoning and location affordability)
  - Access to digital information
  - Siloed public health funding
- Lack of federal policies:
  - School finance
  - Exclusionary zoning and location affordability
  - Structural racism
  - Reparations for descendants of enslaved people
- Health care:
  - Health insurance coverage for racially and ethnically minoritized populations, such as
    - Related services not defined as medical care (such as housing and food insecurity)
    - Gender-affirming care
    - Undocumented persons

BOX 1-7 Continued

- o Reproductive health and equity
- o The need for mental health facilities and services, especially for communities that experience social and economic marginalization
- o Universal health care
- o Bias in medical innovation
- o Public fund for copays and fees for health care
- o Incorporation of homeopathic remedies
- o Mobile health care clinics
- o Development of a health and allied health workforce that reflects the racial and ethnic diversity of the patients they serve
- o Access to free clinical trials of promising therapies
- o Lack of trust in the health care profession
- o Women's health protections
- o Overexposure to fluoride
- o Funding for Black-led HIV service providers
- o Role of nurse practitioners for advancing health equity
- o Need for social workers to work in health care and community settings
- o Medication access
- o Systemic barriers to the use of naturopathic medicine
- o Access to care and workforce shortages in rural areas
- o Prevention and mitigation of tobacco use
- Specific health conditions:
  - o Long COVID-19
  - o Diabetes, prediabetes, and diet-related illnesses
  - o Obesity
  - o Rare neurological conditions
  - o Mental health and substance use disorder crises
- Economic stability:
  - o Life insurance policy discrimination
  - o Social security disability programs
  - o Tax reform
  - o Medicaid estate recovery and asset testing rules
- Community and built environment:
  - o Housing access and affordability
  - o Transportation access and availability
  - o Trichloroethane groundwater pollution
  - o Environmental justice
  - o Nutrition access
- Specific populations:
  - o Inequities for persons with disabilities due to ableism and inaccessibility of facilities and digital information
  - o Sexual discrimination and intersection with race and ethnicity
  - o Barriers for immigrants for access and participation in public programs
  - o Aging and the intersection of race and ethnicity
  - o Native American and Alaska Native/tribal:
    - Underfunding of Indian health services
    - Compliance issues with tribal treaties
    - Returning federal land and reforming the federal tribe recognition process

---

BOX 1-7 Continued

- Early child care and education:
  - ○ Child care access
  - ○ Diversifying and accessibility to scholarships and internships
- Civic infrastructure:
  - ○ Access to voting
  - ○ Community involvement in policy making
- Inequities in the criminal legal system:
  - ○ Remove for-profit prisons
  - ○ Federal drug laws
  - ○ Deaths in police custody

The comments submitted provided the committee with useful insights on these various topics that contribute to racial and ethnic health inequities and highlighted how broad the task was. The committee is thankful for the time and effort that was put into these submissions.

---

an overview of the role of government in policy making. Chapters 3–7 cover federal policies in a specific SDOH area—each providing an overview of its connection to health outcomes and inequities and then reviewing specific past or current policies that have implications for health equity. Chapter 3 reviews economic stability and focuses on income, poverty, wealth, and financial services. Chapter 4 reviews levers for federal engagement in early childhood, K–12, and higher education. Chapter 5 reviews health care access and quality by exploring the role of federal programs and policies, such as Medicaid, IHS, value-based payment, and issues around the health care workforce, health literacy, and maternal health. Chapter 6 reviews the neighborhood and built environment and federal policies related to housing insecurity and segregation, disinvestment in infrastructure and the built environment, environmental exposures that threaten health outcomes, particularly in the workplace, and food access and production. Chapter 7 examines social and community context and covers a number of historical and current federal policies that have led to trauma and healing, the criminal legal system, and belonging and civic infrastructure. Finally, Chapter 8 provides recommendations for action organized by the four action areas, with the goal of not only increasing access to important programs but also improving the effectiveness and coordination of government programs and policies.

CONCLUDING OBSERVATIONS

Recent attention given to racial, ethnic, and tribal health inequities across sectors and all levels of government suggests this report is being released during a time of policy interest in the committee's findings, conclusions, and recommendations. However, the committee's exploration of the complexities of the challenge makes it clear that although successful advances have been made over time, eliminating these health inequities will take concerted effort, commitment, and action sustained over decades. Implementing the committee's recommendations will be a powerful first step to meeting this critical challenge.

REFERENCES

ACOG (American College of Obstetricians and Gynecologists). 2021. ACOG committee opinion no. 827: Access to postpartum sterilization. *Obstetrics & Gynecology* 137(6):169–176.

Alexander, W. D. 1899. *A brief history of the Hawaiian people*. New York, NY: American Book Company.

Angley, M., C. Clark, R. Howland, H. Searing, W. Wilcox, and S. H. Won. 2016. *Severe maternal morbidity*. New York, NY: New York City Department of Health and Mental Hygiene Bureau of Maternal, Infant, and Reproductive Health.

APHA (American Public Health Association). 2021. *Analysis: Declarations of Racism as a Public Health Crisis*. https://www.apha.org/-/media/Files/PDF/topics/racism/Racism_Declarations_Analysis.ashx (accessed June 13, 2023).

Aragones, A., C. Zamore, E. Moya, J. Cordero, F. Gany, and D. Bruno. 2021. The impact of restrictive policies on Mexican immigrant parents and their children's access to health care. *Health Equity* 5(1):612–618.

Ashley, S., G. Acs, S. Brown, M. Deich, G. MacDonald, D. Marron, R. Balu, M. Rogers, M. McAfee, J. Kirschenbaum, T. Ross, A. Gardere, and S. Treuhaft. 2022. *Scoring federal legislation for equity: Definition, framework, and potential application*. Washington, DC: Urban Institute and PolicyLink.

Bailey, Z. D., N. Krieger, M. Agénor, J. Graves, N. Linos, and M. T. Bassett. 2017. Structural racism and health inequities in the USA: Evidence and interventions. *The Lancet* 389(10077):1453–1463.

Blacksher, E., V. Y. Hiratsuka, J. W. Blanchard, J. R. Lund, J. Reedy, J. A. Beans, B. Saunkeah, M. Peercy, C. Byars, J. Yracheta, K. S. Tsosie, M. O'Leary, G. Ducheneaux, and P. G. Spicer. 2021. Deliberations with American Indian and Alaska Native people about the ethics of genomics: An adapted model of deliberation used with three tribal communities in the United States. *AJOB Empirical Bioethics* 12(3):164–178.

Blackwell, A. G. 2016. The curb-cut effect. *Stanford Social Innovation Review* 15(1):28–33.

Bose, T., A. Reina, and J. A. R. Marshall. 2017. Collective decision-making. *Current Opinion in Behavioral Sciences* 16:30–34.

Brookings Metro, and NAACP. n.d. *The Black Progress Index*. https://www.brookings.edu/interactives/black-progress-index/ (accessed March 6, 2023).

Bureau of East Asian and Pacific Affairs. 2005. *Report Evaluating the Request of the Government of the Republic of the Marshall Islands Presented to the Congress of the United States of America*. https://2001-2009.state.gov/p/eap/rls/rpt/40422.htm (accessed June 13, 2023).

Burrage, R. L., K. J. Mills, H. C. Coyaso, C. K. Gronowski, and M. T. Godinet. 2023. Community resilience and cultural responses in crisis: Lessons learned from Pacific Islander responses to the COVID-19 pandemic in the USA. *Journal of Racial and Ethnic Health Disparities* (online ahead of print):1–14.

Cabral, J., and A. G. Cuevas. 2020. Health inequities among Latinos/Hispanics: Documentation status as a determinant of health. *Journal of Racial and Ethnic Health Disparities* 7(5):874–879.

CDC (Centers for Disease Control and Prevention). 2011. *Principles of community engagement,* 2nd edition. Washington, DC: U.S. Department of Health and Human Services.

CDC. 2016. *Health in All Policies.* https://www.cdc.gov/policy/hiap/index.html#:~:text=Health%20 in%20All%20Policies%20(HiAP,of%20all%20communities%20and%20people (accessed March 6, 2023).

CDC. 2017. *Well-Being Concepts.* https://www.cdc.gov/hrqol/wellbeing.htm (accessed May, 2023).

CDC. 2021. *Racism and Health.* https://www.cdc.gov/minorityhealth/racism-disparities/index. html (accessed March 6, 2023).

CDC. 2022a. *Hospitalization and Death by Race/Ethnicity.* https://www.cdc.gov/coronavirus/2019-ncov/covid-data/investigations-discovery/hospitalization-death-by-race-ethnicity.html (accessed March 6, 2023).

CDC. 2022b. *Infant Mortality.* https://www.cdc.gov/reproductivehealth/maternalinfanthealth/ infantmortality.htm (accessed March 6, 2023).

CDC. 2022c. *What Is Health Equity?* https://www.cdc.gov/healthequity/whatis/index.html (accessed March 15, 2023).

CDC. 2022d. *Working Together to Reduce Black Maternal Mortality.* https://www.cdc.gov/ healthequity/features/maternal-mortality/index.html (accessed June 13, 2023).

Child Welfare Information Gateway. n.d. *Indian Child Welfare Act (ICWA).* https://www. childwelfare.gov/topics/systemwide/diverse-populations/americanindian/icwa/ (accessed May 19, 2023).

Christiano, T. 1997. The significance of public deliberation. In *Deliberative democracy: Essays on reason and politics,* edited by J. Bohman and W. Rehg. Cambridge, MA: The MIT Press. Pp. 243–278.

Christopher, G. C. 2022. *Rx racial healing: A guide to embracing our humanity.* Washington, DC: Association of American Colleges and Universities.

Crown-Indigenous Relations, and Northern Affairs Canada. 2022. *Government of Canada Supports Indigenous Communities Across the Country to Address the Ongoing Legacy of Residential Schools.* https://www.canada.ca/en/crown-indigenous-relations-northern-affairs/ news/2022/05/government-of-canada-supports-indigenous-communities-across-the-country-to-address-the-ongoing-legacy-of-residential-schools.html (accessed March 6, 2023).

Dawes, D. E. 2020. *The political determinants of health,* 1st ed. Baltimore, MD: Johns Hopkins University Press.

Dhar, A., J. Bhatt, N. Batra, B. Rush, W. Gerhardt, and A. Davis. 2022. *US health care can't afford health inequities.* https://www2.deloitte.com/us/en/insights/industry/health-care/ economic-cost-of-health-disparities.html (accessed June 13, 2023).

Dimock, M., and R. Wike. 2021. *America is exceptional in its political divide.* Washington, DC: Pew Research Center.

DPC (Domestic Policy Council). 2023. *Delivering on Equity, Access, and Opportunity, for the American People.* https://www.whitehouse.gov/wp-content/uploads/2023/02/Equity-EO-Agency-Highlights.pdf (accessed March 15, 2023).

Edwards, F., H. Lee, and M. Esposito. 2019. Risk of being killed by police use of force in the United States by age, race–ethnicity, and sex. *Proceedings of the National Academy of Sciences* 116(34):16793–16798.

ELTRR (Equitable Long-Term Recovery and Resilience) Interagency Workgroup. 2022. *Federal plan for equitable long-term recovery and resilience for social, behavioral, and community health.* Washington, DC: Department of Health and Human Services.

Equitable Data Working Group. 2022. *A vision for equitable data: Recommendations from the Equitable Data Working Group.* Washington, DC: The White House.

Espey, D. K., M. A. Jim, T. B. Richards, C. Begay, D. Haverkamp, and D. Roberts. 2014. Methods for improving the quality and completeness of mortality data for American Indians and Alaska Natives. *American Journal of Public Health* 104(Suppl 3): S286–294.

Esterline, C., and J. Batalova. 2022. *Frequently Requested Statistics on Immigrants and Immigration in the United States.* https://www.migrationpolicy.org/article/frequently-requested-statistics-immigrants-and-immigration-united-states (accessed March 6, 2023).

Faucher, J. 2021. Nuclear displacement: Effects of America's nuclear tests on Pacific Islanders. *PANDION: The Osprey Journal of Research and Ideas* 2(1, Article 8).

Flores, G. 2020. Language barriers and hospitalized children: Are we overlooking the most important risk factor for adverse events? *JAMA Pediatrics* 174(12):e203238.

Flores, G., M. Abreu, M. A. Olivar, and B. Kastner. 1998. Access barriers to health care for Latino children. *The Archives of Pediatrics & Adolescent Medicine* 152(11):1119–1125.

Galinsky, A. M., C. E. Zelaya, C. Simile, and P. M. Barnes. 2017. Health conditions and behaviors of Native Hawaiian and Pacific Islander persons in the United States, 2014. *Vital and Health Statistics Series. Series 3, Analytical and Epidemiological Studies* (40):1–99.

Galinsky, A. M., C. Simile, C. E. Zelaya, T. Norris, and S. V. Panapasa. 2019. Surveying strategies for hard-to-survey populations: Lessons from the Native Hawaiian and Pacific Islander national health interview survey. *American Journal of Public Health* 109(10):1384–1391.

Goldman, N., and T. Andrasfay. 2022. Life expectancy loss among Native Americans during the COVID-19 pandemic. *medRxiv.* https://doi.org/10.1101/2022.03.15.22272448.

GovInfo. n.d. *United States Statutes at Large.* https://www.govinfo.gov/app/collection/statute/2016 (accessed March 7, 2023).

Govtrack. n.d. *Statistics and Historical Comparison.* https://www.govtrack.us/congress/bills/statistics (accessed March 7, 2023).

Gunja, M., E. Gumas, and R. Williams, II. 2023. *U.S. health care from a global perspective, 2022: Accelerating spending, worsening outcomes.* New York, NY: Commonwealth Fund.

Heisler, E. J., and K. P. McClanahan. 2020. *Advance appropriations for the Indian Health Service: Issues and options for Congress.* Washington, DC: Congressional Research Service.

HHS (U.S. Department of Health and Human Services). 2023. *Profile: Black/African Americans.* https://minorityhealth.hhs.gov/omh/browse.aspx?lvl=3&lvlid=61 (accessed June, 2023).

HHS. n.d. *Healthy People 2030 Social Determinants of Health.* https://health.gov/healthypeople/priority-areas/social-determinants-health (accessed March 7, 2023).

Hill, L., and S. Artiga. 2022. *COVID-19 cases and deaths by race/ethnicity: Current data and changes over time.* Menlo Park, CA: Kaiser Family Foundation.

Hill, L., S. Artiga, and U. Ranji. 2022. *Racial disparities in maternal and infant health: Current status and efforts to address them.* Washington, DC: Kaiser Family Foundation.

Hoyert, D. L. 2022. *Maternal mortality rates in the United States, 2020.* Atlanta, GA: National Center for Health Statistics, Centers for Disease Control and Prevention.

IAP2 (International Association for Public Participation). 2018. *IAP2 Spectrum of Public Participation.* https://cdn.ymaws.com/www.iap2.org/resource/resmgr/pillars/Spectrum_8.5x11_Print.pdf (accessed March 9, 2023).

IHS (Indian Health Service). 2014. *Trends in Indian health: 2014 edition.* Washington, DC: Indian Health Service.

Impact Initiative. n.d. *Health.* https://jhdimpact.org/health/ (accessed March 6, 2023).

IOM (Institute of Medicine). 2003a. *The future of the public's health in the 21st century.* Washington, DC: The National Academies Press.

IOM. 2003b. *Unequal treatment: Confronting racial and ethnic disparities in health care.* Washington, DC: The National Academies Press.

IOM and NRC (National Research Council). 2013. *U.S. health in international perspective: Shorter lives, poorer health.* Washington, DC: The National Academies Press.

Jim, M. A., E. Arias, D. S. Seneca, M. J. Hoopes, C. C. Jim, N. J. Johnson, and C. L. Wiggins. 2014. Racial misclassification of American Indians and Alaska Natives by Indian Health Service contract health service delivery area. *American Journal of Public Health* 10(Suppl 3):S295–302.

Jones, N. L., S. E. Gilman, T. L. Cheng, S. S. Drury, C. V. Hill, and A. T. Geronimus. 2019. Life course approaches to the causes of health disparities. *American Journal of Public Health* 109(S1):S48–S55.

Kaholokula, J., R. E. S. Miyamoto, A. H. Hermosura, and M. K. Inada. 2020. Prejudice, stigma, and oppression on the behavioral health of Native Hawaiians and Pacific Islanders. In *Prejudice, stigma, privilege, and oppression: A behavioral health handbook.* 1st ed., edited by L. T. Benuto, M. P. Duckworth, A. Masuda, and W. O'Donohue. Cham, Switzerland: Springer Nature. Pp. 107–134.

Kanaʻiaupuni, S.M., and N. Malone. 2006. This land is my land: The role of place in Native Hawaiian identity. *Hūlili: Multidisciplinary Research on Hawaiian Well-being* 3(1):281–307.

Kehaulani Goo, S. 2015. *After 200 years, Native Hawaiians make a comeback.* Washington, DC: Pew Research Center.

Klest, B., J. J. Freyd, and M. M. Foynes. 2013. Trauma exposure and posttraumatic symptoms in Hawaii: Gender, ethnicity, and social context. *Psychological Trauma: Theory, Research, Practice, and Policy* 5(5):409–416.

Kort-Butler, L. A. 2022. Pandemic, politics, and public opinion about crime. *Criminal Justice Review* Oct: 07340168221131379. https://doi.org/10.1177/07340168221131379.

Kriebel, D., J. Tickner, P. Epstein, J. Lemons, R. Levins, E. L. Loechler, M. Quinn, R. Rudel, T. Schettler, and M. Stoto. 2001. The precautionary principle in environmental science. *Environmental Health Perspectives* 109(9):871–876.

LACDPH (Los Angeles County Department of Public Health). 2022. *Patterns in mortality and life expectancy in Los Angeles County, 2010–2019.* Los Angeles, CA: Office of Health Assessment & Epidemiology.

LaVeist, T. A., D. J. Gaskin, and P. Richard. 2009. *The economic burden of health inequalities in the United States.* Washington, DC: Joint Center for Political and Economic Studies.

LaVeist, T. A., E. J. Pérez-Stable, P. Richard, A. Anderson, L. A. Isaac, R. Santiago, C. Okoh, N. Breen, T. Farhat, A. Assenov, and D. J. Gaskin. 2023. The economic burden of racial, ethnic, and educational health inequities in the US. *Journal of the American Medical Association* 329(19):1682.

Link, B. G., and J. Phelan. 1995. Social conditions as fundamental causes of disease. *Journal of Health and Social Behavior* (Spec No.):80–94.

Liu, D. M., and C. K. Alameda. 2011. Social determinants of health for Native Hawaiian children and adolescents. *Hawaiʻi Medical Journal* 70(11 Suppl 2):9–14.

Lor, M. 2018. Systematic review: Health promotion and disease prevention among Hmong adults in the USA. *Journal of Racial and Ethnic Health Disparities* 5(3):638–661.

Lucchei, A., and A. Echo-Hawk. 2018. *Missing and murdered Indigenous women and girls.* Seattle, WA: Urban Indian Health Institute.

MACPAC (Medicaid and CHIP Payment and Access Commission). 2021. *Fact sheet: Medicaid and CHIP in the territories.* Washington, DC: Medicaid and CHIP Payment and Access Commission.

Marmot, M. G., G. D. Smith, S. Stansfeld, C. Patel, F. North, J. Head, I. White, E. Brunner, and A. Feeney. 1991. Change in health inequalities among British civil servants: The Whitehall II study. *Lancet* 337(8754):1387–1393.

Martin, C., and J. Lewis. 2019. *The state of equity measurement: A review for energy-efficiency programs.* Washington, DC: Urban Institute.

McElfish, P. A., C. R. Long, J. K. Kaholokula, N. Aitaoto, Z. Bursac, L. Capelle, M. Laelan, W. I. Bing, S. Riklon, B. Rowland, B. L. Ayers, R. O. Wilmoth, K. N. Langston, M. Schootman, J. P. Selig, and K. H. K. Yeary. 2018. Design of a comparative effectiveness randomized controlled trial testing a faith-based diabetes prevention program (WORD DPP) vs. a Pacific culturally adapted diabetes prevention program (PILI DPP) for Marshallese in the United States. *Medicine (Baltimore)* 97(19):e0677.

McGinnis, J. M., and W. H. Foege. 1993. Actual causes of death in the United States. *Journal of the American Medical Association* 270(18):2207–2212.

Meghani, S. H., and R. M. Gallagher. 2008. Disparity vs. inequity: Toward reconceptualization of pain treatment disparities. *Pain Medicine* 9(5):613–623.

MITRE. n.d. *A Framework for Assessing Equity in Federal Programs and Policy.* https://www.mitre.org/news-insights/publication/framework-assessing-equity-federal-programs-and-policy (accessed March 7, 2023).

Moon, P. K., T. Chakoma, Y. Ma, and U. C. Megwalu. 2022. Thyroid cancer incidence, clinical presentation, and survival among Native Hawaiian and other Pacific Islanders. *Otolaryngology—Head and Neck Surgery* online ahead of print (1945998221118538).

Morey, B. N. 2014. Environmental justice for Native Hawaiians and Pacific Islanders in Los Angeles County. *Environmental Justice* 7(1):9–17.

Morey, B. N., R. C. Chang, K. B. Thomas, Tulua, C. Penaia, V. D. Tran, N. Pierson, J. C. Greer, M. Bydalek, and N. Ponce. 2022. No equity without data equity: Data reporting gaps for Native Hawaiians and Pacific Islanders as structural racism. *Journal of Health Politics, Policy and Law* 47(2):159–200.

Moss, M. 2019. *Trauma Lives on in Native Americans by Making Us Sick—While the US Looks Away.* https://www.theguardian.com/commentisfree/2019/may/09/trauma-lives-on-in-native-americans-while-the-us-looks-away (accessed March 6, 2023).

NAACP (National Association for the Advancement of Colored People). 2021. *Criminal Justice Fact Sheet.* https://naacp.org/resources/criminal-justice-fact-sheet (accessed June 13, 2023).

NAM (National Academy of Medicine). 2022. *Assessing meaningful community engagement: A conceptual model to advance health equity through transformed systems for health.* Washington, DC: National Academy of Medicine.

NAM. n.d. *Community-driven health equity action plans.* https://nam.edu/programs/culture-of-health/community-driven-health-equity-action-plans/ (accessed March 6, 2023).

NASEM (National Academies of Sciences, Engineering, and Medicine). 2017. *Communities in action: Pathways to health equity.* Washington, DC: The National Academies Press.

NASEM. 2018a. *Exploring tax policy to advance population health, health equity, and economic prosperity: Proceedings of a workshop—in brief.* Washington, DC: The National Academies Press.

NASEM. 2018b. *Proactive policing: Effects on crime and communities.* Washington, DC: The National Academies Press.

NASEM. 2019a. *Integrating social care into the delivery of health care: Moving upstream to improve the nation's health.* Washington, DC: The National Academies Press.

NASEM. 2019b. *Minority serving institutions: America's underutilized resource for strengthening the stem workforce.* Washington, DC: The National Academies Press.

NASEM. 2019c. *The promise of adolescence: Realizing opportunity for all youth.* Washington, DC: The National Academies Press.

NASEM. 2019d. *A roadmap to reducing child poverty.* Washington, DC: The National Academies Press.

NASEM. 2019e. *Vibrant and healthy kids: Aligning science, practice, and policy to advance health equity.* Washington, DC: The National Academies Press.

NASEM. 2021a. *Population health in rural america in 2020: Proceedings of a workshop.* Washington, DC: The National Academies Press.

NASEM. 2021b. *Racial equity addendum to critical issues in transportation.* Washington, DC: The National Academies Press.

NASEM. 2021c. *Sexually transmitted infections: Adopting a sexual health paradigm.* Washington, DC: The National Academies Press.

NASEM. 2022a. *Addressing structural racism, bias, and health communication as foundational drivers of obesity: Proceedings of a workshop series.* Washington, DC: The National Academies Press.

NASEM. 2022b. *The impact of juvenile justice system involvement on the health and well-being of communities of color: Proceedings of a workshop.* Washington, DC: The National Academies Press.

NASEM. 2022c. *Racial equity, Black America, and public transportation, volume 1: A review of economic, health, and social impacts.* Washington, DC: The National Academies Press.

NASEM. 2022d. *Reducing racial inequality in crime and justice: Science, practice, and policy.* Washington, DC: The National Academies Press.

NASEM. 2022e. *Structural racism and rigorous models of social inequity: Proceedings of a workshop.* Washington, DC: The National Academies Press.

NASEM. 2023a. *Closing the opportunity gap for young children.* Washington, DC: The National Academies Press.

NASEM. 2023b. *Using population descriptors in genetics and genomics research: A new framework for an evolving field.* Washington, DC: The National Academies Press.

NCAI (National Congress of American Indians). n.d. *Tribal governance.* https://www.ncai.org/policy-issues/tribal-governance#:~:text=Tribal%20governments%20are%20an%20important,the%20authority%20to%20self%2Dgovern. (accessed March 11, 2023).

NIH (National Institutes of Health). 2022. *Life Expectancy in the U.S. Increased Between 2000–2019, But Widespread Gaps Among Racial and Ethnic Groups Exist.* https://www.nih.gov/news-events/news-releases/life-expectancy-us-increased-between-2000-2019-widespread-gaps-among-racial-ethnic-groups-exist#:~:text=In%20 2019%2C%20overall%20life%20expectancy,73.1%20for%20the%20AIAN%20 population. (accessed March 11, 2023).

ODPHP (Office of Disease Prevention and Health Promotion). 2022. *Announcing the Federal Plan for Equitable Long-Term Recovery and Resilience!* https://health.gov/news/202211/announcing-federal-plan-equitable-long-term-recovery-and-resilience (accessed May, 2023).

Ogden, C. L., T. H. Fakhouri, M. D. Carroll, C. M. Hales, C. D. Fryar, X. Li, and D. S. Freedman. 2017. Prevalence of obesity among adults, by household income and education—United States, 2011–2014. *Morbidity and Mortality Weekly Report* 66(50):1369–1373.

OMB (Office of Management and Budget). 2021. *Study to identify methods to assess equity: Report to the president.* Washington, DC: Office of Management and Budget.

OMH (Office of Minority Health). 2023. *Profile: Native Hawaiians/Pacific Islanders.* https://minorityhealth.hhs.gov/omh/browse.aspx?lvl=3&lvlid=65#:~:text=According%20 to%20the%202019%20U.S.,percent%20of%20the%20U.S.%20population (accessed March 7, 2023).

Opportunity and Revitalization Council. 2019. *Report to the President from the White House Opportunity and Revitalization Council.* https://opportunityzones.hud.gov/sites/opportunityzones.hud.gov/files/documents/OZ_One_Year_Report.pdf (accessed March 8, 2023).

Oropesa, R. S., N. S. Landale, and M. M. Hillemeier. 2016. Legal status and health care: Mexican-origin children in California, 2001–2014. *Population Research and Policy Review* 35(5):651–684.

Panapasa, S. V., M. K. Mau, D. R. Williams, and J. W. McNally. 2010. Mortality patterns of Native Hawaiians across their lifespan: 1990–2000. *American Journal of Public Health* 100(11):2304–2310.

Panapasa, S., J. Jackson, C. Caldwell, S. Heeringa, J. McNally, D. Williams, D. Coral, L. Taumoepeau, L. Young, S. Young, and S. Fa'asisila. 2012. Community-based participatory research approach to evidence-based research: Lessons from the Pacific Islander American health study. *Progress in Community Health Partnership* 6(1):53–58.

Petersen, E. E., N. L. Davis, D. Goodman, S. Cox, C. Syverson, K. Seed, C. Shapiro-Mendoza, W. M. Callaghan, and W. Barfield. 2019. Racial/ethnic disparities in pregnancy-related deaths—United States, 2007–2016. *Morbidity and Mortality Weekly Report* 68(35):762.

Pew Research Center. 2020. *America Is Exceptional in the Nature of Its Political Divide.* https://www.pewresearch.org/fact-tank/2020/11/13/america-is-exceptional-in-the-nature-of-its-political-divide/ (accessed March 17, 2023).

Pillai, D., N. Ndugga, and S. Artiga. 2022. *Health Care Disparities Among Asian, Native Hawaiian, and Other Pacific Islander (NHOPI) People.* https://www.kff.org/racial-equity-and-health-policy/issue-brief/health-care-disparities-among-asian-native-hawaiian-and-other-pacific-islander-nhopi-people/ (accessed March 16, 2023).

Presidential COVID-19 Health Equity Task Force. 2021. *Final Report and Recommendations.* https://www.minorityhealth.hhs.gov/assets/pdf/HETF_Report_508_102821_9am_508Team%20WIP11-compressed.pdf (accessed March 8, 2023).

RWJF (Robert Wood Johnson Foundation). n.d. *RWJF Culture of Health Prize: Communities Leading the Way.* https://www.rwjf.org/en/grants/grantee-stories/culture-of-health-prize.html (accessed March 3, 2023).

Sotto-Santiago, S. 2019. Time to reconsider the word minority in academic medicine. *Journal of Best Practices in Health Professions Diversity* 12(1):72–78.

South, J., J. Stansfield, and K. Fenton. 2015. Putting communities at the heart of public health. *Perspectives in Public Health* 135(6):291–293.

Taparra, K., and K. Pellegrin. 2022. Data aggregation hides Pacific Islander health disparities. *The Lancet* 400(10345):2–3.

Teranishi, R. T., A. Le, R. A. E. Gutierrez, R. Venturanza, I. Hafoka, D. Toso-Lafaele Gogue, and L. Uluave. n.d. *Native Hawaiians and Pacific Islanders in higher education: A call to action.* Washington, DC: APIA Scholars.

TFAH (Trust for America's Health). 2018. *Advancing health equity: What we have learned from community-based health equity initiatives.* Washington, DC: Trust for America's Health.

Tobin, J. A. 1967. The resettlement of the Enewetak people: A study of a displaced community in the Marshall Islands, PhD diss., Tobin, J. A.: University of California, Berkeley, U.S.

Tran, J. H., M. Wong, E. K. Wright, J. Fa'avae, A. Cheri, E. Wat, K. L. Camacho, and M. A. Foo. 2010. Understanding a Pacific Islander young adult perspective on access to higher education. *Californian Journal of Health Promotion* 8:23–38.

Turner, A. 2018. *The business case for racial equity: A strategy for growth.* Battle Creek, MI: W.K. Kellogg Foundation.

U.S. House Committee on Ways and Means. 2021a. *A bold vision for a legislative pathway toward health and economic equity.* Washington, DC: U.S. House of Representatives.

U.S. House Committee on Ways and Means. 2021b. *Something must change: Inequities in U.S. Policy and society.* Washington, DC: U.S. House of Representatives.

U.S. House Committee on Ways and Means. n.d. *Equity Work.* https://democrats-waysandmeans.house.gov/committee-activity/equity-work (accessed March 7, 2023).

United Nations. 2020. *World social report 2020: Inequality in a rapidly changing world.* Washington, DC: United Nations.

United States Institute of Peace. 1995. *Truth Commission: South Africa.* Washington, DC: United States Institute of Peace.

University of Wisconsin Population Health Institute. 2023. *County Health Rankings Model.* https://www.countyhealthrankings.org/explore-health-rankings/county-health-rankings-model (accessed June, 2023).

Urban Institute. n.d. *Quantitative Data Analysis.* https://www.urban.org/research/data-methods/data-analysis/quantitative-data-analysis/microsimulation (accessed March 7, 2023).

Vasquez Reyes, M. 2020. The disproportional impact of COVID-19 on African Americans. *Health and Human Rights* 22(2):299–307.

Viswanathan, M., A. Ammerman, E. Eng, G. Garlehner, K. N. Lohr, D. Griffith, S. Rhodes, C. Samuel-Hodge, L. L. S. Maty, L. Webb, S. F. Sutton, T. Swinson, A. Jackman, and L. Whitener. 2004. *Community-based participatory research: Assessing the evidence: Summary, AHRQ evidence report summaries.* Rockville, MD: Agency for Healthcare Research and Quality.

Waidmann, T. A. 2009. *Estimating the cost of racial and ethnic health disparities.* Washington, DC.

Wallerstein, N., J. G. Oetzel, S. Sanchez-Youngman, B. Boursaw, E. Dickson, S. Kastelic, P. Koegel, J. E. Lucero, M. Magarati, K. Ortiz, M. Parker, J. Peña, A. Richmond, and B. Duran. 2020. Engage for equity: A long-term study of community-based participatory research and community-engaged research practices and outcomes. *Health Education & Behavior* 47:380–390.

The White House. 2022a. *Fact sheet: Biden-Harris Administration Announces New Actions to Support Indian Country and Native Communities Ahead of the Administration's Second Tribal Nations Summit.* https://www.whitehouse.gov/briefing-room/statements-releases/2022/11/30/fact-sheet-biden-harris-administration-announces-new-actions-to-support-indian-country-and-native-communities-ahead-of-the-administrations-second-tribal-nations-summit/ (accessed June, 2023).

The White House. 2022b. *Justice40.* https://www.whitehouse.gov/environmentaljustice/justice40/ (accessed March 7, 2023).

The White House. 2023. *Executive Order on Further Advancing Racial Equity and Support for Underserved Communities Through the Federal Government.* https://www.whitehouse.gov/briefing-room/presidential-actions/2023/02/16/executive-order-on-further-advancing-racial-equity-and-support-for-underserved-communities-through-the-federal-government/ (accessed March 15, 2023).

Wingrove-Haugland, E., and J. McLeod. 2021. Not "minority" but "minoritized." *Teaching Ethics* 21(1):1–11.

Xiang, J., H. Morgenstern, Y. Li, D. Steffick, J. Bragg-Gresham, S. Panapasa, K. L. Raphael, B. M. Robinson, W. H. Herman, and R. Saran. 2020. Incidence of ESKD among native Hawaiians and Pacific Islanders living in the 50 U.S. states and Pacific Island territories. *American Journal of Kidney Diseases* 76(3):340–349.

2

Connection Between Health Equity and History, Federal Policy, and Data

INTRODUCTION

This chapter begins by outlining U.S. governmental structures and power and how policies play out today, followed by a description of the historical and contemporary factors that have contributed to health inequities and the state of these health inequities. The chapter also discusses important factors that intersect with race and ethnicity, including sex, gender, sexuality, age, disability status, geographical considerations, and citizenship, that have implications for health equity. Finally, the committee reviews the state of data sources for racial, ethnic, and tribal populations and outlines critical gaps and data needs.

GOVERNMENTAL STRUCTURES AND POWER

This section provides a brief overview of federalism and available policy levers and the unique governing aspects for American Indian and Alaska Native (AIAN) people. Policy has four main levers. (1) Laws/statutes are passed by Congress and signed by the president. (2) Rules/regulations—when Congress enacts legislation, it frequently delegates rulemaking authority to federal agencies, which establish specific requirements (this generally requires a public notice and comment period). (3) Guidance is supplemental materials that provide clarity on laws or rules. Guidance with broad applicability may be published in the Federal Register, but some may only appear on agency websites, and it generally does not require notice and public comment. The Administrative Procedure Act (APA) guides agency rulemaking; agencies have to establish an administrative record that lays out the legal, scientific, technical, economic, and policy basis for the rule. Rules go through an extensive "clearance" process within each agency and at the White House before they are released. According to APA and Supreme Court precedent, agencies must provide a reasoned explanation when they want to change established policy. (4) Finally, on the implementation side, enforcement is through a combination of public and private efforts, such as the enforcement of civil rights statutes.

One additional lever is the Executive Order (EO), which is issued by the president, acting in their capacity as head of the executive branch, directing a federal official or administrative agency to engage in or refrain from a course of action. It is an often-used approach for swift policy implementation. It is appealing in that it lays out priorities for a given administration, takes immediate effect, and does not require input or review from Congress or other constituents. It is an effective tool to demonstrate action on promises made to constituents, create momentum, and bring focus to an effort across one or many agencies. Staff are compelled to take action, so attention and resources are quickly redirected to carrying out these orders. They are also precarious because they become viewed as the darling of a given administration and can fall prey to shifts in political leadership. As a tool, they are a less enduring form of policy implementation and risk a subsequent administration easily drafting a new EO ending or undoing the authority of the original. The limitations need to be carefully considered when trying to address long-held systemic barriers to equity. A review of active EOs may reveal progress toward equity goals that would benefit from actions to stabilize and make permanent the changes beyond a given administration. EOs can advance and contribute to health equity. For example, EO 13985[1] *Advancing Racial Equity and Support for Underserved Communities Through the Federal Government* is focused on advancing equity. However, EO 13950[2] *Combatting Race and Sex Stereotyping* is an important example of how federal policy could negatively impact efforts aimed at improving health equity (it was revoked in January 2021), as it prohibited federal contractors and subcontractors from providing certain workplace diversity training and programs.

Federalism

The committee has been charged with reviewing the effects of federal policies on health equity, but federal policies cannot be viewed in a vacuum because they interact with or act on other levels of government—state, tribal, territorial, and local. In addition, power is shared between states and the federal government, with states generally taking the lead on most issues.

---

[1] Exec. Order No. 13985, 86 FR 7009 (January 2021).
[2] Exec. Order No. 13950, 85 FR 60683 (September 2020).

Federalism "refers to the division and sharing of power between the national and state governments" and is a fundamental principle upon which the U.S. government was established (Congress, n.d.). The Constitution divides governmental power between the federal and state governments, limiting federal authority to issues of national interest. Through the 10th Amendment to the Constitution, "[t]he federal government is delegated certain enumerated powers while all other powers not otherwise prohibited by the Constitution are reserved to the states" (Cornell Law School, n.d.-b; NGA, 2018). The enumerated powers include the power to tax and spend, regulate interstate commerce, standardize immigration/naturalization, establish and maintain a military, and declare war. All other powers, broadly defined as "police powers," which include the authority to protect public health and safety, are left to the states. It is through the principle of federalism that the concept of states as laboratories of democracy was established. In *New State Ice Co v. Liebmann* (1932),[3] Supreme Court Justice Louis Brandeis described how a single "courageous State may, if its citizens choose, serve as a laboratory; and try novel social and economic experiments without risk to the rest of the country."

Theoretically, federalism establishes a unified national government while preserving localized governing and decision making. However, the interplay between the federal and state, and state and local, authority is often contentious and used as a tactic to voice opposition. States cite federalism when pushing against federal actions aimed at constraining state autonomy. Federalism provides both protections and challenges on the path to furthering health equity; it created and, in many ways, continues to perpetuate racial inequities. For example, it informed Supreme Court attitudes toward slavery as a state right. In *Dred Scott v. Sanford* (1857),[4] which involved moving an enslaved person from a state that allowed slavery to one that outlawed it, the court's views of federalism led it to find against the enslaved person (Maltz, 1992).

In the 21st century, federalism played a key role in the passage and evolution of the Patient Protection and Affordable Care Act (ACA). It expanded health care coverage, with the federal government providing financing and establishing a floor for regulating the insurance markets; states enacted regulations that shaped access and other aspects of implementation (Collins and Lambrew, 2019). A 2019 Commonwealth Fund analysis found that ACA's combination of federal standards and subsidies and state regulatory authority significantly improved coverage and access nationally and narrowed regional differences. "However, the law's federalist structure, established in statute and altered through regulations and court decisions,

---

[3] 285 U.S. 262 (1932).
[4] 60 U.S. 393 (1857).

resulted in disparities in coverage and access across states" (Collins and Lambrew, 2019). One important change that led to this outcome is the 2012 Supreme Court's decision in *NFIB v. Sebelius*,[5] which made optional the requirement that states extend Medicaid to all adults with incomes below 138 percent of the federal poverty level. The court found that this individual mandate[6] was not valid under the Commerce Clause because Congress cannot use that power to require someone to purchase health insurance. However, the court upheld the mandate as a valid use of congressional taxing power (treating the penalty for not purchasing insurance as a tax) and upheld Medicaid expansion by judicially prohibiting the Secretary from withdrawing existing Medicaid funds from states that refuse compliance. "More broadly, policy decisions about the allocation of state versus federal governing responsibility in health care have implications for the relative performance of states as well as the overall health of the U.S. population" (Collins and Lambrew, 2019).

States have what is generally called "police powers" to protect the public's health and sometimes delegate it to local governments. Federal authority to govern health resides primarily in the ability to tax and spend and regulate interstate and foreign commerce, through congressional power via the Commerce Clause of the Constitution; it and the Public Health Service Act give federal health agencies broad authority.

Government responsibilities for public health reside largely at the state level, with the federal government providing resources, generally paired with program requirements, and technical assistance to states and to local public health entities. In other domains, such as education and transportation, the relationship between the federal department and agency and the state-level equivalents reflects a similar division of authority.

Federal-level policies aimed at furthering equity, such as the Civil Rights Act, and especially Title VI, place specific requirements on state governments as a condition of receiving federal support. Examples include Department of Education funding to the states (DOE, 2020) and Federal Highway Administration funding to the state departments of transportation (FHWA, n.d.). These requirements may help further the goal of health equity because they are intended to prevent discrimination, such as by prioritizing environmental justice in transportation planning (AASHTO, n.d.). Federal civil rights law provides a set of minimum standards on which states can build by enacting further protections (Pepin and Weber, 2019). One example is

---

[5] *National Federation of Independent Business v. Sebelius*, 567 U.S. 519 (2012).

[6] The individual mandate of ACA imposed a "penalty" or "tax" on certain individuals who failed to obtain health insurance through their employer, the government, or a private company and expanded Medicaid to specified individuals below the poverty line. Federal funding to states' Medicaid programs was conditioned on acceptance of these terms.

state application of standards to protect individuals with a criminal record from discrimination that may make it difficult, if not impossible, to find employment or housing. Beyond civil rights law, federal agencies may use a range of strategies to encourage state innovation and experimentation to identify the most effective solutions. This includes the Centers for Medicare & Medicaid Services (CMS) State Innovation Models and Medicaid waiver programs (Kissam et al., 2019; Vleet and Paradise, 2014) (see Chapter 5). On a negative note, in the context of the COVID-19 pandemic, federal government action under the Commerce Clause has been complicated by a range of factors, including judicial challenges. Federal action in the domains of housing, transportation, and public health has been heavily contested by both the federal judiciary and states. For example, some states banned sharing infectious disease data with the federal government (Rai, 2021) or criticized the CDC-imposed moratorium on evictions (Stennett, 2021). Federalism may also have hampered an effective COVID-19 response because of minimal coordination among states to agree on standard public health approaches to address the threat they all faced (Kettl, 2021). A federal judge vacated the federal mask requirement on public transportation in April 2022 based on a narrow interpretation of U.S. Code "Regulations to Control Communicable Diseases"[7] (Jost, 2022).

Role of the Judiciary in Determining the Responsibility of the Federal Government

Given the separation of powers among the executive, legislative, and judicial branches, these dynamics also unfold in a complex judiciary context. For example, the Supreme Court decision to jettison decades-old precedent on abortion in *Dobbs v. Jackson Women's Health Organization* (2022)[8] was made based on arguments that the decision should be returned to the domain of the states. A similar decision can be found in voting rights, with the Supreme Court's ending of preclearance requirements for specific states under the Voting Rights Act in *Shelby County v. Holder* (2013).[9] For ACA, the judicial interpretation of federalism found the Commerce Clause was insufficient to support federal ability to compel individuals to carry insurance, but federal tax and spend power prevailed, as the tax penalty in the individual mandate was upheld (Aaron, 2012). ACA's Medicaid expansion was also challenged in court, and the Supreme Court found that although the federal government could withhold new funds for that expansion, it could not take away existing Medicaid funds (Cornell Law School, n.d.-a).

---

[7] 42 U.S.C. 264.
[8] *Dobbs v. Jackson Women's Health Organization*, 597 U.S. ___ (2022).
[9] *Shelby County v. Holder*, 570 U.S. 529 (2013).

The role of the federal government could be viewed in a top-down frame, as a central government imposing its will, or in a collaborative frame, which could have created a pandemic response that brought states and their federal partners together to confront a shared threat.

American Indian and Alaska Native People: Federal Trust Responsibility

The relationship between American Indians and the federal government is termed the federal trust responsibility: the government is responsible for supporting those and their descendants who ceded land to the United States by force, coercion, or mutual treaty-making. Treaties between tribes and the United States confirm each nation's rights and privileges. This includes protection for AIAN from attacks upon their lands; health care; education; sovereignty and religious freedom; confirmation and protection of certain rights, including self-government and jurisdiction over their own lands. Tribes ceded title to vast amounts of land in exchange for these protections and services but reserved certain lands and rights. However, the slate of federal policy periods that followed this doctrine undermined it, leading to the inequities AIAN people face today.

Tribes are neither states nor foreign countries. When AIAN people are enrolled members of the 574 federally recognized tribes, which are sovereign nations, they have a formal nation-to-nation relationship with the U.S. government (Schwartz, 2023). "Sovereignty" is a legal term meaning the authority to self-govern. "Hundreds of treaties, along with the Supreme Court, president, and Congress, have repeatedly affirmed that Tribal Nations retain their inherent powers of self-government and created a fundamental contract between tribes and the United States" (NCAI, n.d.).

Tribes are the only group to be dual citizens originating from within what is now the United States, which sets them apart from other groups who are minoritized. They share similar adversities with the additional, unique challenges of having been described historically as "Wards of the Nation," been tied currently or ancestrally to reservation bases, and suffered under federal policy periods aimed at solving the "Indian problem" (Moss, 2019). For example, they are the only population listed in U.S. Code, as Title 25-INDIANS (25 U.S.C).[10] However, obstacles to self-governance are based on three areas that have been identified in recent years: (1) outmoded bureaucratic processes, (2) lack of federal agency coordination, and (3) regulations and laws that prevent tribal governments from equitable access to federal programs on par with state and local governments (NCAI, n.d.).

---

[10] The Code of Federal Regulations Title 25 contains the codified federal laws and regulations that are in effect as of the date of the publication pertaining to American Indians (Native Americans), including gaming/casinos, arts and crafts, education, and health (U.S. Code, 2011 Edition).

U.S. federal Indian policies/eras that were implemented from the late 1700s through 1978 to solve the "Indian problem" and allow for Euro-American expansion included exterminating, removing, assimilating, and relocating AIAN people (Moss, 2019). These policy periods and their off-shoot policies can be mapped directly onto the definition of genocide from the United Nations in Article 2 of the Convention on the Prevention and Punishment of the Crime of Genocide (". . . a crime committed with the intent to destroy a national, ethnic, racial or religious group, in whole or in part") (UN, 1948). There are five parts:

1. Killing members of the group;
2. Causing serious bodily or mental harm to members of the group;
3. Deliberately inflicting on the group conditions of life calculated to bring about its physical destruction in whole or in part;
4. Imposing measures intended to prevent births within the group; and
5. Forcibly transferring children of the group to another group (UN, 1948).

By this definition, the United States perpetrated genocide within its borders specifically on *this* population. This is important to understand as policy makers contemplate the contribution of federal policies to health inequities.

"Invasion is a structure not an event" (Wolfe, 1999, p. 2). This quote, well known in Indian Country, indicates that the structures left behind by this history make it extremely hard to move toward health equity, as AIAN people are often blamed for their circumstances, including changing their health and wellness circumstances and abilities. The three most problematic policy periods creating and continuing colonial structures were specifically meant to either "get rid of the Indian problem" or "kill the Indian, save the man/or child." They were (1) Removal and Reservations (1830–1886), (2) Assimilation (1887–1932), and (3) Termination (1946–1960).

Termination is when the federal government recognized tribes' sovereignty, trusteeship over reservations, and the exclusion of state law's applicability. This era saw a reversal in policies from the self-government era, when the federal government resolved to end the special trustee relationship (House Resolution No. 108, 83rd Congress. August 1, 1953). In addition to eliminating the right to be sovereign nations, the policy terminated federal support of most health care and education programs. On its face, the resolution seemed well intended—to liberate tribes from federal control. However, it became another means of controlling and erasing AIAN rights. The government-to-government relationship was unilaterally severed by Congress—over 100 tribes were cut from the list of those with federal recognition. Those now "unrecognized" tribes were no longer considered Indian in the eyes of Congress and the federal government.

Numerous examples illustrate how federal policies have impacted the health and well-being of the AIAN population. For example, President Washington ordered the outright killing of AIAN people, and President Lincoln ordered the largest mass execution by the U.S. government on U.S. soil on Dakhóta Nations in Minnesota 6 days before the Emancipation Proclamation in 1862 (University of Minnesota, n.d.). The United States withheld citizenship for AIAN people until 1924 (the last racial group to gain citizenship) and, until the 1950s, forced exile to reservations and outlawed AIAN religious and cultural practices. The Indian Health Service (IHS) undertook coerced or nonconsensual sterilization of AIAN women into the 1970s (Torpy, 2000). For decades, many Indian children were removed to boarding schools or adoption and/or foster to White families. Historical trauma (trauma persisting from previous generations) coupled with some of the highest contemporaneous traumas for AIAN people have resulted in substantial health inequities (see Chapter 7). The traumas that have unfolded over generations, and done so "invisibly," resulted in untold cumulative harm, the effects of which are still felt today.

However, "the sovereignty that the Indian tribes retain is of a unique and limited character. It exists only *at the sufferance of Congress* and is subject to complete defeasance."[11] Tribal Nations would argue that they retain inherent sovereignty for being on this land for 1,000s of years before contact. Another way this has been described legally is that a tribe is only a tribe if Congress confirms it. By extension, an Indian is only an Indian if Congress confirms it. Congress designates tribes, and tribes designate membership. These tribes are then called "federally recognized."

Hawaii, Pacific Islands, and Territories

People from Hawaii, the Pacific Islands, and U.S. territories have varied histories, cultures, and membership in or ties to the United States. These relationships are briefly described here (see Chapter 7 for additional historical information).

Until January 17, 1893, Native Hawaiians, Kānaka Maoli, were a self-governing people; between 1893 and 1898, a provisional government comprised mainly of Americans was in place. Aboriginal people have lived on Hawaii for more than 1,000 years, but the U.S. overthrow of the Kingdom of Hawaii in 1893 and its annexation in 1898 without the consent of the people means no federally recognized native governing body exists (Kanaʻiaupuni and Malone, 2006). Native Hawaiians do not have a government-to-government relationship (which is based on treaties) comparable to AIAN people (Davis, 2021), and residents of Hawaii are subject to Hawaiian state and U.S. federal laws. Hawaii has sent congressional delegations to the Senate and House of Representatives since it became a state in 1959. Although Native Hawaiians

---

[11] *United States v. Wheeler*, 435 U.S. 313, 98 S. Ct. 1079 (1978).

never relinquished their sovereignty (see Chapter 7 for additional details) and the United States provided a formal Apology Resolution (U.S. Public Law 103–150), Native Hawaiians are not seen as sovereign under U.S. federal law and do not have self-governance rights. Some have engaged in a movement to have their status as Native people revived (though not all Native Hawaiians agree this is the best path—some argue for complete independence from the United States, federal recognition and Indigenous status, or more control over Native Hawaiian assets, such as crown and ceded lands) (Greene, 2021; Nation of Hawai'i, n.d.; Pacheco, 2005). "However, the Department of the Interior has a special political and trust relationship with the Native Hawaiian Community that exists even without a formal government-to-government relationship (43 CFR 50)" (DOI, 2022). Other federal statutes, regulations, and reports[12] outline certain responsibilities of the federal government to Native Hawaiians, such as the Hawaiian Homes Commission Act (see Chapter 6) and its land trust obligation and the Native Hawaiian Health Care Improvement Act[13] (see Chapter 5).

Puerto Rico and the U.S. Virgin Islands are unincorporated territories (meaning that only select parts of the Constitution apply to their residents); Puerto Rico is also commonwealth (it has a political union with the United States). Individuals born in both places are considered U.S. citizens, but residents cannot vote in federal elections; the federal government also does not collect income tax from residents (except for federal employees). Puerto Rico residents are subject to most federal laws.

Guam is also an unincorporated territory. Individuals born in Guam are considered U.S. citizens. Residents elect a delegate to the House of Representatives, who serves for a term of 2 years and has limited voting abilities, but cannot vote in federal elections. Residents of Guam also caucus for presidential primary candidates.

American Samoa is an unincorporated, unorganized territory. Congress has not established a system of government for it. Individuals born in American Samoa are U.S. nationals rather than citizens (they may apply for citizenship). Residents cannot vote in federal elections.

The Northern Mariana Islands are a commonwealth. The U.S. president is head of state of the Northern Mariana Islands, which receives funds from the U.S. government. Individuals born in the Northern Mariana Islands are considered U.S. citizens, but residents cannot vote in federal elections.

The Compacts of Free Association govern the relationships between the United States and the Republic of the Marshall Islands (RMI), Federated States of Micronesia (FSM), and Republic of Palau. The compacts grant the United States the choice to operate military bases in Freely Associated States (FAS—the RMI, FSM, and Republic of Palau) and make decisions

---

[12] For examples, see https://www.doi.gov/hawaiian/lawreport (accessed May 31, 2023).
[13] 42 U.S.C. 11701-11714.

related to their security. Citizens of the FAS have the right to reside and work in the United States and its territories as lawful nonimmigrants or "habitual residents," meaning they can freely travel, live, and work in the United States without a visa and with no time restraints. They do not have their own militaries and are eligible to join the U.S. military (CRS, 2022).

HISTORICAL AND CURRENT STRUCTURAL RACISM: FUNDAMENTAL CONTRIBUTORS TO HEALTH INEQUITY

As discussed in Chapter 1, federal policies can prevent, address, and contribute to health equity. Not all policies are designed to address health inequities—a policy or program could be simply neutral. In addition, most policies do not intend to increase inequities; it is an unanticipated outcome. However, historical policies have shaped the current state of health inequities.

The United States has a deep history that has contributed significantly to the health inequities seen today. Settler colonialism, when European settlers infected Native Americans (and made infection rates worse due to lack of quarantine) with new epidemic diseases (Patterson and Runge, 2002), was followed by violence from warfare, forced displacement, and enslavement to control Native populations (Fisher, 2017). Hundreds of thousands of people were captured from Africa, forced into slavery in U.S. and other colonies, and exploited to work in the production of crops, textiles, and a host of other industries (Library of Congress, n.d.). During Reconstruction after the Civil War, the Freedmen's Bureau, which provided services to newly freed people, was dissolved (United States Senate, n.d.); the bureau was not able to carry out its initiatives and could not provide long-term protection for African American people (Maltz, 1992). Rather than address this, the government framed African American people as innately diseased due to presumed biological inferiority (Hogarth, 2019). Racism was built into the structure of society, not only influencing how future policy and practices are designed but also shaping culture, ideology, norms, and values in ways that serve to maintain racial order and hierarchies in which Black, AIAN, and other minoritized people are deemed inherently inferior (Downs, 2012).

Although the 13th Amendment abolished slavery and hundreds of treaties were signed to protect Native Americans, racial violence took on different forms through new policies and practices, affecting the health and well-being of all racially and ethnically minoritized populations (e.g., Jim Crow and Japanese internment camps) (Downs, 2012; U.S. Commission on Civil Rights, 2018). Even today, with federal recognition of past racial harm and efforts to create policies and laws to ameliorate and prevent harm, policies are still created that negatively affect the health and well-being of communities that have historically been disenfranchised and underserved, as discussed in Chapters 3–7. See Chapter 7 for more on how historical and current policies have led to both trauma and healing for racialized populations.

Structural Racism, Laws and Policies, and
Racial and Ethnic Health Inequities

Racism is a key determinant of racial and ethnic health inequities and operates at all levels of society (Williams et al., 1997, 2019). Racism systematically excludes, Black, AIAN, Latino/a, and other targeted people from power, status, and other social, economic, and political resources and opportunities, which contributes to health inequities (Baah et al., 2019; Williams et al., 2019). Racism has long been studied in the social science, law, and the humanities, but in recent years, population health researchers have increasingly examined the role of not only interpersonal but also structural racism in shaping population health outcomes across and within racial and ethnic groups (Bailey et al., 2017; Gee and Ford, 2011; Williams et al., 2019). "Specifically, investigators have found that structural racism—defined as the historically contingent and persistent ways in which social systems and institutions generate and reinforce inequities in access to power, privilege, and other resources" (Agénor et al., 2021, p. 428) among racial and ethnic groups deemed to be superior and inferior (Bailey et al., 2017; Gee and Ford, 2011; Williams et al., 2019)—negatively affects health outcomes, including breast cancer, premature mortality, birth outcomes, and cardiovascular disease (CVD), among Black people (Bailey et al., 2017; Krieger et al., 2013, 2014; Krieger et al., 2017b; Lukachko et al., 2014; Williams et al., 2019). Additionally, scholars have shown that structural racism, including genocide and immigration policies, undermines the physical and mental health of AIAN and Latino/a people, respectively (Bailey et al., 2017; Gee and Ford, 2011; Viruell-Fuentes et al., 2012).

Agénor and colleagues (2021, p. 429) explain that

> . . . .structural racism—which evolves and stems from historical processes such as genocide, slavery, and immigrant exclusion—operates through and is embedded in contemporary federal- and state-level laws and policies pertaining to various social systems and institutions, such as housing, education, health care, employment, criminal justice, voting rights, and immigration (Bell, 2017; Bonilla-Silva, 1997; Delgado and Stefancic, 2017; Higginbotham Jr., 1974; Pager and Shepherd, 2008). Past and present laws and policies overtly and covertly, directly and indirectly, and actively and passively (through both inaction and colorblindness) determine the inequitable allocation of social, economic, political, and environmental resources and harms across racial/ethnic groups today (Bell, 2017; Bonilla-Silva, 1997; Delgado and Stefancic, 2017; Higginbotham Jr., 1974; Pager and Shepherd, 2008).

Policies that explicitly or implicitly favor or disadvantage certain racial and ethnic groups (e.g., historical and contemporary housing and banking laws, and practices such as redlining, mortgage lending, zoning) result in minoritized racial and ethnic groups being more likely than White people to live in systematically underserved neighborhoods (Agénor et al., 2021).

As a result, they live in neighborhoods that lack access to high-quality infrastructure, social and health services, and educational and employment opportunities (Agénor et al., 2021; Badger, 2013; Bailey et al., 2017; Gee and Ford, 2011; Pager and Shepherd, 2008; Rugh and Massey, 2010; Williams et al., 2019).

Criminal legal system laws, policies, and practices also disproportionately affect minoritized racial and ethnic groups (see Chapter 7). This leaves Black, AIAN, and Latino/a people (who tend to be the target of overpolicing, arrest, and incarceration negative racial stereotypes) disproportionately represented in prisons and jails (Alexander et al., 2012; Bailey et al., 2017; NAACP, 2014; Pager and Shepherd, 2008). Consequently, voting rights laws that disenfranchise people with convictions disproportionately affect Black and other minoritized groups, which has implications for the composition of the electorate that make laws and set policy agendas (Alexander et al., 2012). "Furthermore, given pervasive racist stereotypes that erroneously depict Black people as dangerous criminals, stand-your-ground laws systematically threaten their rights and lives by selectively allowing. . . . [someone] to harm or kill a Black person by claiming self-defense, even in the absence of an actual threat (Morris, 2016)" (Agénor et al., 2021, p. 429).

Minimum-wage, income-related housing, and predatory lending laws disproportionately affect minoritized groups (Agénor et al., 2021). This leads to Black, AIAN, and Latino/a people having lower levels of wealth and income than their White counterparts (Bailey et al., 2017; Bell, 2017; Delgado and Stefancic, 2017; Pager and Shepherd, 2008; Williams, 1999). This is the result of laws and policies that prevent the intergenerational transfer of wealth among Black and other underserved communities, as well as structural and interpersonal racism in the education system and employment sector. Because of biases—conscious or unconscious—that inaccurately depict Black people as threatening or violent, discipline that uses force is more likely to be directed at Black students than their White counterparts in both elementary and high schools (Agénor et al., 2021; Gregory, 1995; Morris, 2016; Riddle and Sinclair, 2019). Immigration laws also disproportionately target Black and Latino/a people and lead to the social exclusion of minoritized groups by "prohibiting entry, facilitating deportation, and limiting access to social, economic, and political opportunities and resources as well as legal rights" (Agénor et al., 2021, p. 429) for groups considered to be undesirable (Gee and Ford, 2011; Viruell-Fuentes et al., 2012).

Theory and empirical research suggest that these historical and contemporary federal and state laws disadvantage people from minoritized groups shape racial and ethnic health inequities through various social, economic, physical, and psychological mechanisms into low-quality neighborhoods, schools, and jobs and other circumstances, including chronic and acute psychosocial stressors (Bailey et al., 2017;

Gee and Ford, 2011; Komro et al., 2012; Williams, 1999; Williams and Collins, 2001; Williams et al., 1997, 2016, 2019). "For example, research shows that racial residential segregation, which is linked to housing and banking laws, policies, and practices that disproportionately disadvantage Black people and people from other marginalized racial and ethnic groups, is negatively associated with low-birthweight and preterm birth among Black women and higher rates of breast and lung cancer mortality among Black people compared with White people (Gee and Ford, 2011; Williams and Collins, 2001; Williams et al., 2019)" (Agénor et al., 2021). Living in a neighborhood with high levels of stop and frisk—which occurs more often in Black and Latino/a neighborhoods and affects AIAN people disproportionately (ACLU, 2020; NAACP, 2014; NYCLU, 2019), is correlated with several negative mental and physical health outcomes, including psychological distress, diabetes, and high blood pressure (Sewell and Jefferson, 2016).

These examples illustrate not only how structural determinants of health are embedded within institutions across society but also how different manifestations and dimensions of racism interact, reinforce, and even replace each other to maintain inequalities and make them seem natural and even quotidian rather than a consequence of historical and contemporary processes (Gee and Hicken, 2021).

STATE OF HEALTH INEQUITIES IN THE UNITED STATES

Despite data gaps that prevent accurate and full documentation of health and well-being for many racially and ethnically minoritized populations, data that are available suggest persistent and sometimes growing health inequities. The inequities discussed in this report reflect historical and contemporary structural disadvantage that have led to different social and economic opportunities (see Figure 2-1)—for a comprehensive, in-depth assessment of the root causes of health inequities, see *Communities in Action: Pathways to Health Equity* (NASEM, 2017). The report identified root causes that can be organized into two clusters (p. 7):

(1) Intrapersonal, interpersonal, institutional, and systemic mechanisms (also referred to as structural inequities) that organize the distribution of power and resources differentially across lines of race, gender, class, sexual orientation, gender expression, and other dimensions of individual and group identity.

(2) The unequal allocation of power and resources—including goods, services, and societal attention—which manifests itself in unequal social, economic, and environmental conditions, also called the determinants of health.

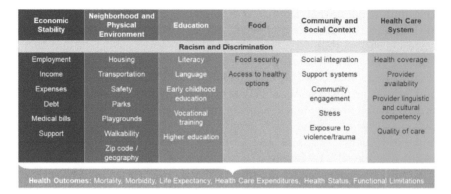

Economic Stability	Neighborhood and Physical Environment	Education	Food	Community and Social Context	Health Care System
Racism and Discrimination					
Employment	Housing	Literacy	Food security	Social integration	Health coverage
Income	Transportation	Language	Access to healthy options	Support systems	Provider availability
Expenses	Safety	Early childhood education		Community engagement	Provider linguistic and cultural competency
Debt	Parks	Vocational training		Stress	
Medical bills	Playgrounds	Higher education		Exposure to violence/trauma	Quality of care
Support	Walkability				
	Zip code / geography				
Health Outcomes: Mortality, Morbidity, Life Expectancy, Health Care Expenditures, Health Status, Functional Limitations					

FIGURE 2-1 Social and economic factors drive health outcomes.
SOURCE: Artiga, 2020; licensed under CC BY-NC-ND 4.0 (https://creativecommons.org/licenses/by-nc-nd/4.0/).

Furthermore, the report concluded that "health inequities are the result of more than individual choice or random occurrence. They are the result of the historical and ongoing interplay of inequitable structures, policies, and norms that shape lives" (NASEM, 2017, p. 8) and that interventions targeting the above factors hold the greatest promise for promoting health equity. Although family circumstances and personal choice play a role in health outcomes, the evidence suggests that improving the social and environmental circumstances where people, families, and communities live, work, play, age, and pray—so that all people have the opportunity to make the healthy choice—is essential. This includes supporting parents, families, and communities via federal policy.

Racial, ethnic, and tribal health inequities take on many forms, such as higher rates of chronic disease and premature death. Despite progress to narrow the gaps in some racial, ethnic, and tribal health outcomes, there are still ongoing and persistent inequities tied to the social and structural determinants of health. For example, in the AIAN population, non-Hispanic AIAN people are 1.8 times more likely to be killed by the police compared to non-Hispanic White people and diabetes prevalence remains high; in addition, the COVID pandemic put this population further behind compared to other racial and ethnic groups, with an estimated loss in life expectancy at birth of 4.5 years in 2020 and 6.4 years in 2021 relative to 2019 (ASPE, 2019; GBD 2019 Police Violence U.S. Subnational Collaborators, 2021; Goldman and Andrasfay, 2022). The following section provides an overview of a sample of these health inequities.

Racial and ethnic groups are also not homogenous. Take, for example, the experience of the Hispanic and Latino/a population, specifically when examining data in disaggregated form (Fernandez et al., 2023). In general, data show that people from Puerto Rico have worse health outcomes than every other Hispanic and Latino/a group in the United States (Aguirre-Molina et al., 2001; Díaz et al., 2020). An analysis of childhood adversity and mental health measures from the National Heart, Lung, and Blood Institute Hispanic Community Health Study/Study of Latino/a people demonstrates this trend as well (Cooper et al., 2021). People from Puerto Rico have the highest age-adjusted mortality rate, at 605.7/100,000, followed by people from Mexico (523.7), Cuba (489.1), Central American (393.2), and South American (315.5) (Fernandez et al., 2023). Health outcomes for Hispanic people vary based on birthplace, place of ancestry, immigrant status, length of time in the United States, where they live, age, gender, and socioeconomic compositions (Fernandez et al., 2023). "Broad statements about Hispanics as a group often do not translate into better comparable health outcomes among all Hispanics" (Fernandez et al., 2023, p. 163).

Another example is Asian American people, who are the fastest-growing U.S. immigrant group and projected to become the largest by 2065 (Kim et al., 2021). However, research on this population is lacking and has not kept pace with the changing demographics (Đoàn et al., 2019; Kim et al., 2021). Kim and colleagues (2021) explain that this may result in part from the myth of the model minority stereotype for this population. However, the Asian population is one of the most diverse groups in the United States, with widely varying backgrounds across more than 37 ethnocultural groups. The Asian population also has the largest within-group wealth gap; the lowest income levels show the least growth 1970–2016 compared to other racial and ethnic groups (Kim et al., 2021).

This heterogeneity applies to other population groups as well (e.g., the AIAN, Black, and Native Hawaiian and Pacific Islander [NHPI] populations) and impacts all measures of health. This report uses available data, which typically do not sufficiently break out the heterogenous places of origin within race and ethnicity. These masked differences have large health care implications, and disaggregating data would allow for more individualized or tailored approaches to addressing health equity (see Data Gaps and Opportunities later in this chapter).

Life Expectancy

From 2000 to 2019, overall U.S. life expectancy increased by 2.3 years, but this gain was not consistent across racial and ethnic groups or by geography. In 2019, the life expectancy was 85.7 years for the Asian, 82.2 for the Latino, 78.9 for the White, 75.3 for the Black, and 73.1 for the AIAN populations (NIH, 2022). AIAN people experienced the sharpest decline of any racial and ethnic group for 2019–2021 (Goldman and Andrasfay, 2022). Researchers have noted that estimates that do not disaggregate the Asian population from the NHPI populations likely mask important differences in life expectancy. "Regional studies generally show worse outcomes for NHPI populations, further underscoring the need to study these groups individually" (NIH, 2022). A study measuring population- and race-specific age-standardized mortality rates found, on average, 74,402 excess deaths (all-cause mortality) for Black people compared to White people each year for 2016–2018 (Benjamins et al., 2021). Annual excess deaths varied considerably by location—at the city level, this ranged from 6 in El Paso to 3,804 in Chicago. These higher rates of death translate into years of life lost. A study by Amiri and colleagues (2022) examined years of potential life lost by race and ethnicity in Washington State and found that relative to non-Hispanic White people, non-Hispanic Black, AIAN, Asian or other Pacific Islander, multiracial, and Hispanic decedents had significantly higher rates. Disparities were reduced, but not eliminated, when controlling for sociodemographic factors, and controlling for place-based risk factors did not further lessen differences. A 2023 study by Caraballo and colleagues calculated excess age-adjusted all-cause mortality, cause-specific mortality, age-specific mortality, and years of potential life lost rates (per 100,000 individuals) for Black people in comparison to White people in a cross-sectional study using 1999–2020 Centers for Disease Control and Prevention (CDC) data; the Black population experienced more than 1.63 million excess deaths and more than 80 million excess years of life lost. After a period of improvement for the gap in the age-adjusted mortality rate, it plateaued and then worsened in 2020. The analysis showed similar trends in rates of excess years of potential life lost (Caraballo et al., 2023).

Maternal Health and Infant Mortality

Maternal Health

Gunja et al. (2023) found that the United States had the highest rate of maternal mortality of 13 high-income countries in its analysis, even though over 80 percent of these deaths are preventable (Trost et al., 2022). Severe maternal morbidity rates have also been increasing in recent years, with higher rates than other high-income countries (Ahn et al., 2020; Hoyert, 2022), with stark racial and ethnic inequities in maternal health (see Figure 2-2). Black, AIAN, and NHPI people have higher rates of inadequate prenatal care compared to White people (Hill et al., 2022; March of Dimes, 2022). Black and AIAN pregnancy-related mortality rates are over three and two times higher respectively compared to White rates, with racial disparities increasing by age (Hoyert, 2022; Petersen et al., 2019). Several factors may contribute to these inequities, including access to care, quality of care, prevalence of chronic diseases, structural racism, and implicit biases (CDC, 2023a) manifested in a complex and multifactorial manner (see Figure 2-1).

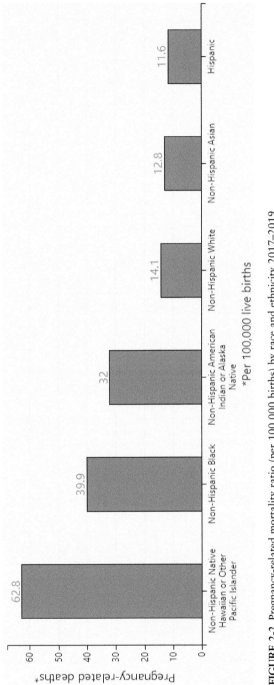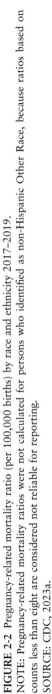

FIGURE 2-2 Pregnancy-related mortality ratio (per 100,000 births) by race and ethnicity 2017–2019.
NOTE: Pregnancy-related mortality ratios were not calculated for persons who identified as non-Hispanic Other Race, because ratios based on counts less than eight are considered not reliable for reporting.
SOURCE: CDC, 2023a.

For example, lack of federally mandated paid family leave,[14] lack of insurance coverage, geographic inequities in access to care, lack of a culturally congruent workforce, and a lack of trust in the patient–provider relationship and health care system are shown to contribute to these inequities (IOM, 2003; NASEM, 2019). The National Academies convened a 2021 workshop, "Advancing Maternal Health Equity and Reducing Maternal Morbidity and Mortality," to address this urgent issue (NASEM, 2021a). Although recent federal attention to these inequities is promising (see Chapter 5), they both reflect and result from the complex, intersectional, and cross-sectoral issues discussed in this report.

Infant Mortality

Infant mortality is the death of an infant before their first birthday. Stark racial inequities have persisted for decades, even with continued advancements in medical care (Hill et al., 2022). Racially and ethnically minoritized people are more likely to experience certain birth risks and adverse birth outcomes compared to White people. Black, Hispanic, AIAN, and NHPI people had higher shares of preterm or low-birthweight infants and received late or no prenatal care compared to White people in 2020 (Hill et al., 2022). Asian people were also more likely to have low-birthweight babies than White people. Similarly, Black, NHPI, and AIAN infants were two times as likely to die as White infants (Ely and Driscoll, 2022) (see Figure 2-3). Asian infants had the lowest mortality rate. "Notably, disparities in maternal and infant health persist even when controlling for certain underlying social and economic factors, such as education and income, pointing to the roles racism and discrimination play in driving disparities" (Hill et al., 2022).

Chronic Disease

Chronic diseases[15] and illnesses can cause financial stress, disability, and even death. According to CDC, chronic conditions—such as heart disease, stroke, cancer, type 2 diabetes, obesity, and arthritis—"are among the most common, costly, and preventable of all health problems and leading drivers

---

[14] The United States is one of only six countries, and the only Organisation for Economic Co-operation and Development member, that does not mandate paid family leave at the federal level (BPC, 2022). The Family and Medical Leave Act provides only unpaid leave and job protection, only covers employers with 50 or more employees, and does not cover part-time employees (DOL, n.d.). This disproportionately harms underserved racial and ethnic low-income families, as they are less likely to be able to afford to take leave.

[15] Chronic diseases are defined broadly as conditions that last 1 year or more and require ongoing medical attention, limit activities of daily living, or both.

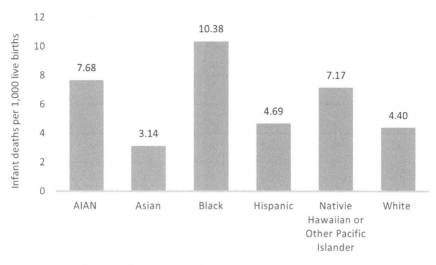

FIGURE 2-3 Infant mortality (per 1,000 live births) by maternal race and Hispanic Origin, United States, 2020.
NOTES: AIAN = American Indian or Alaska Native. Persons of Hispanic origin may be of any race but are categorized as Hispanic for this analysis; other groups are non-Hispanic.
SOURCE: Data from Ely and Driscoll, 2022.

of the nation's $4.1 trillion in annual health care costs" (CDC, 2022). A recent study, using National Health Interview Survey data (1999–2018), found persistent racial and ethnic inequities in multimorbidity (defined as the presence of two or more concurrent chronic health conditions) in the United States over a 20-year period (Caraballo et al., 2022). Annual prevalence of important chronic conditions was persistently higher among Black Americans compared with Asian, Latino/Hispanic, and White people. The following paragraphs discuss two common U.S. chronic diseases—obesity and cardiovascular disease (CVD).

Obesity

Obesity can be thought of as a collection of diseases with multiple causes, contributors, and clinical expressions (in contrast to the common belief that it is typically caused by eating too much and moving too little) (NASEM, 2022a). Examples include dysregulation of hormones involved in thyroid function, hunger, and appetite satiety. This alternate view points out that contributors are extrinsic—outside of a person—and can lead to obesity in the presence of causes that are preventable, modifiable, and treatable. Examples include poor sleep quality, food insecurity, and exposure to energy-dense foods (NASEM, 2022a). A 2021 study found that socioeconomic status, health behaviors, neighborhood environments, and early childhood health factors explained substantial racial and ethnic differences in obesity (Min et al., 2021). This framing is important because it affects relevant interventions. A CDC analysis of 2017–2018 U.S. data found that the age-adjusted prevalence was highest for non-Hispanic Black adults (49.6 percent) overall, followed by Hispanic (44.8 percent), non-Hispanic White (42.2 percent), and non-Hispanic Asian (17.4 percent) adults (Hales et al., 2020). Racial and ethnic disparities in obesity exist by the age of two (Pan et al., 2016). A study found that African American children had the highest prevalence of risk factors, whereas Asian children had the lowest (the sample size for Pacific Islander children was too small, so their data were not included in this study) (Isong et al., 2018). The rate of infant weight gain during the first 9 months was a major contributor to the gap, which accounted for 14.9–70.5 percent of explained disparities between White children and racially and ethnically minoritized peers. Another important contributor to these inequities—especially between White and Hispanic children—was socioeconomic status. A higher proportion of African American (56.7 percent), Hispanic (51.3 percent), and American Indian (50.1 percent) children belonged to households earning less than $25,000 per year compared with White (19.8 percent) and Asian (17.7 percent) children. The study found that early childhood risk factors, such as lack of fruit and vegetable consumption and amount of television viewing, were less important in explaining racial and ethnic differences (Isong et al., 2018).

Cardiovascular Disease

CVD is the leading cause of morbidity and mortality globally. Racial and ethnic inequities have been extensively documented, and although management of CVD has led to improved mortality, striking inequities in outcomes have persisted and widened among racial and ethnic groups (Glynn et al., 2019; Mazimba and Peterson, 2021; Singh et al., 2015). Black Americans experience the highest mortality rates attributable to CVD and stroke, with almost 30 and 45 percent higher mortality, respectively, than non-Hispanic White Americans (Churchwell et al., 2020). Recent data for NHPI people are limited; however, in 2014, they were 10 percent more likely to be diagnosed with coronary heart disease than non-Hispanic White people (OMH, 2021b). CVD is the leading cause of death among AIAN people, with over one-third of CVD deaths occurring before the age of 65 (Breathett et al., 2020). American Indian people are 1.5 times as likely to be diagnosed with coronary heart disease compared with the White population (Javed et al., 2022). Furthermore, hypertension prevalence rates reported among AIAN women (age 18–44) are significantly higher compared to non-Hispanic White women

(12 percent versus 8.2 percent) (Hutchinson and Shin, 2014). Several studies and papers find that these inequities are not fully explained by socioeconomic status, and several studies point to structural racism as a contributor (Churchwell et al., 2020; Javed et al., 2022; Mazimba and Peterson, 2021).

Intersections and Considerations

Although the committee was asked to focus on racial, ethnic, and tribal health inequity specifically, these populations have intersectional identities along multiple other axes that are also an important part of the picture when addressing policy needs (Cooper, 2015), including sex, gender, sexuality, age, disability status, geographical considerations, and citizenship. Inequalities exist in these dimensions for all racial and ethnic groups, and each could be reviewed separately; however, the committee considers only at the intersection of these factors with race and ethnicity (for example, the intersection of being Black and being a woman) in alignment with its statement of task. Experiences and health outcomes cannot be considered in a vacuum with regard to race and ethnicity but are impacted by these other aspects (Ritzer and Stepnisky, 2022). These identities combine in complex and interwoven ways to create novel interaction effects (Crenshaw, 1991). The committee provides several examples to illustrate the complex intersectional factors that need to be considered when developing or changing policy to advance racial, ethnic, and tribal health equity. One cross cutting consideration is the adverse consequences of limited English proficiency on health equity—see Chapter 5 for more information.

Disability

The intersection of race and disability represents a complex and interconnected history of oppression, stigma, and discrimination, resulting in disproportionate rates of disability among racially and ethnically minoritized people and inequities in health care access, health outcomes, and quality of life (Morgan et al., 2022; Varadaraj et al., 2021). Furthermore, racial inequities exist among people with disabilities, even those with the same medical condition or disability. For example, Black, AIAN, and other minoritized populations with autism are diagnosed later and more likely to be misdiagnosed (Morgan et al., 2022). Native American and Black people have the highest rates of disability among working-age adults, followed by White, NHPI and Hispanic, and Asian people (CDC, 2020; Courtney-Long et al., 2017; Siordia et al., 2017). Due to long-standing structural determinants of health, both racially and ethnically minoritized people and people with disabilities carry disproportionate burdens of ill health, face more significant barriers to accessing quality health care, are more likely to be unemployed and have lower incomes, and experience discrimination from health care professionals (Gulley et al., 2014; Lagu et al., 2022; National Disability Institute, 2020; Peterson-Besse et al., 2014).

Law and federal policy have played a substantial role in advancing and institutionalizing racism and ableism. For example, forced and coerced abortion and sterilization are recurring themes for the disability community. In 1927, the Supreme Court case *Buck v. Bell*[16] set a legal precedent that states may sterilize residents of public institutions. The court argued that imbecility, epilepsy, and feeblemindedness are hereditary and that residents should be prevented from passing these to the next generation. *Buck v. Bell* has not been overturned, but its reasoning has been discredited. In another example, a landmark 1999 Supreme Court case, *Olmstead v. L.C.*[17] found that the unjustified segregation of people with disabilities is a form of un-lawful discrimination under the Americans with Disabilities Act and led to developing new opportunities for individuals to live and work in their communities instead of institutionalizing them.

One current federal policy example is Supplemental Security Income (SSI). It provides essential economic assistance to people with disabilities, including 1.1 million children and their families (SSA, 2022). In addition to important financial support for low-income families, in many states, qualify-ing for SSI makes recipients eligible for Medicaid and other social supports (Musumeci and Orgera, 2021). Black, Hispanic, and AIAN people make up disproportionate shares of SSI enrollees compared to White people (Musumeci and Orgera, 2021). The delivery of these vital programs can be hampered by racial and ethnic inequities in Social Security Administration (SSA) policies and processes, creating inequities in individuals' and families' ability to access and maintain SSI benefits. Administrative, literacy, citizenship, and financial barriers to applying for and maintaining SSI benefits disproportionately af-fect racially and ethnically underserved individuals and families. Eligibility is limited to U.S. citizens except in very limited circumstances (SSA, 2023).[18] SSA's complex rules for financial eligibility and stringent definition of dis-ability, which requires substantial documentation to prove, pose barriers to participation. Of the 29 percent of nonelderly adults with Medicaid who have a disability, only 41 percent have SSI (Musumeci and Orgera, 2021). Furthermore, only 35 percent of medical determinations were approved upon initial application; those that were appealed via an administrative law judge

---

[16] *Buck v. Bell*, 274 U.S. 200 (1927).

[17] 527 U.S. 581; 119 S.Ct. 2176 (1999).

[18] SSA determines income based on an expansive definition that includes earned and unearned cash and noncash, including "in kind" support, such as food and shelter provided or paid by another person. The amount of SSI that a person is eligible to receive cannot ex-ceed the maximum federal benefit rate ($794/month in 2021) minus their calculated income (SSA, n.d.).

hearing or a higher appeals level, processes that are challenging to navigate without legal representation, were successful 40 percent of the time. During the reapplication and appeals process for SSI, individuals may be at risk for income insecurity. Federal SSA policy includes provisions that suspend or terminate benefits to children who become involved in the criminal legal or child welfare systems; these are disproportionately members of racially and ethnically minoritized populations. Restrictive SSA criteria for asthma and sickle cell disease, illnesses that disproportionately affect Black children, create inequity (NASEM, 2020a). Because eligibility determination relies on other systems—schools, health care providers, child welfare, criminal legal system, and others—the structural racism and inequities that may affect those systems are likely to shape the administration of benefits (Community Legal Services of Philadelphia, 2020).

Sex and Gender

Sex and gender affect health and health outcomes in complex ways. Sex can impact disease risk and progression and treatment outcomes through genetic, epigenetic, and physiological pathways, including differences in reproductive autonomy, hormonal milieu, and metabolism (Crimmins et al., 2019; WHO, 2021). Much as race is a social construct,[19] gender norms, access to resources due to the socialization of gender, perception of illness and health behaviors, access to health care, and biases in the health care system all affect health and health outcomes. For example, in a study assessing the influence of social support on nutritional risk, White women who lacked social support were less likely to be affected by poor nutrition than Black women who did (Locher et al., 2005). Black women are more likely than White women to develop CVD, and nearly 60 percent more likely to have high blood pressure (a risk factor for CVD) (CDC, 2023b; Nayak et al., 2020); however, research shows differences in referrals for cardiac care that are most evident for African American women, then African American men, compared with White men and women (IOM, 2003; Schwartz et al., 1999).

Furthermore, much of the discussion surrounding racial and ethnic health inequities mirrors that on the effect of sex/gender on health outcomes, including the importance of research that distinguishes between females and women from males and men, the historical role and power dynamics between men and women, and the role of policy across the same multiple domains that impact health outcomes. A salient example is AIAN women who are disproportionally affected by violence; 84 percent experience physical and sexual violence in their lifetime, with a majority of it perpetrated by

---

[19] Genetic ancestry affects human health (for example, sickle cell); however, this is distinct from the impact of race, which is a social construct that has its foundations in systemic racism.

non-American Indian offenders (Rosay, 2016). Federal policies regarding public safety on reservation and village lands has resulted in an environment where tribal authorities are often unable to prosecute non-Indian offenders. Assumptions have been made that the violence only exists on tribal lands; however, a study of AIAN women in Seattle found that 94 percent of them had been sexually assaulted and or coerced into sex in their lifetime, with only 8 percent of those who reported to local law enforcement seeing their perpetrator convicted (Urban Indian Health Institute, 2018).

Societal prejudices and stereotypes of AIAN women and girls contribute to rape culture that creates further barriers to prevention, intervention, and justice. These factors mesh into a crisis of epic proportions, with women and girls going missing and being murdered at disproportional rates. A first-of-its-kind study in 2018 found that this was occurring at high rates in 71 cities across the country. However, it noted that the data were severely limited due to law enforcements' noncollection and nonreporting of race and ethnicity, effectively making the crisis invisible. The study additionally found lack of media coverage; what did occur was rife with stereotypes of sex workers and runaways (Lucchei and Echo-Hawk, 2018). Through tribal advocacy and congressional support, recent legislation (Violence Against Women Act)[20] was passed to address this crisis. Yet, a 2021 Government Accountability Office report found the implementation was lacking and many of the tasks had yet to be completed by the Department of Justice, illustrating the need for accountability mechanisms in congressional and White House–mandated equity efforts (GAO, 2021).

Racially and Ethnically Minoritized LGBTQ+ People

As noted, structural racism can be experienced differently by different groups and compound other forms of structural discrimination, including structural sexism, heterosexism, and cisgenderism. Given the co-occurrence and mutual reinforcement of these three factors, racially and ethnically minoritized LGBTQ+ people often experience greater health inequities than their heterosexual and White counterparts (Hatzenbuehler et al., 2013; IOM, 2011; NASEM, 2020b), which plays out in sexual and reproductive health. For example, HIV and other sexually transmitted infections (STIs) are higher in many LGBTQ+ populations compared to their heterosexual and cisgender peers. Gay, bisexual, and other men who have sex with men have the highest incidence of HIV; they account for 66 percent of new infections each year even though they are only 2 percent of the population. However, the highest burden is among Black and Latino gay, bisexual, and other men who have sex with men (HIV.gov, 2023). Studies show that

---

[20] Title IV of the Violent Crime Control and Law Enforcement Act, H.R. 3355.

decades of not only sexual orientation–related but also racial and ethnic oppression, discrimination, and disenfranchisement compound STI risk and transmission (NASEM, 2021c). Moreover, STI rates among transgender women, particularly Black and Latina women, are some of the highest in the United States (Becasen et al., 2019; Poteat et al., 2014). Racially and ethnically minoritized transgender women possess multiple marginalized statuses and thus experience multiple forms of discrimination, including racism, sexism, and cisgenderism, all of which compound one another and simultaneously increase STI risk and undermine access to prevention, diagnosis, and treatment (NASEM, 2021c). Data on STIs among sexual minority women are not routinely collected, but existing data show that racially and ethnically minoritized women—who face sexual orientation–related stigma and racism—may experience a higher burden compared to their White counterparts (NASEM, 2021c).

In recent years, researchers have begun explicitly assessing the simultaneous impact of structural racism and other forms of structural discrimination, including structural heterosexism, on the health of racially and ethnically minoritized LGBTQ+ people. For example, English and colleagues (2022) examined associations between structural racism, structural heterosexism (modeled using anti-LGBTQ policies), and mental and behavioral health among Black and White young sexual minority men. The researchers found that for Black sexual minority men, state-level structural racism and state anti-LGBTQ+ policies were both independently positively associated with anxiety, heavy drinking, and other factors; the positive associations between structural racism and several psychological and behavioral health outcomes were stronger in states with more anti-LGBTQ+ policies, underscoring the compounding impact of both structural racism and heterosexism. In contrast, no association appeared between structural racism or heterosexism among White sexual minority men (English et al., 2022). However, policies such as sexual orientation–related nondiscrimination laws can be protective for Black LGBTQ+ populations, including Black lesbian and bisexual women; Everett and Agénor (2023) found that higher numbers of state-level sexual orientation–related nondiscrimination laws were associated with lower risk of maternal hypertension. These laws were also associated with a lower risk of maternal hypertension among White women, regardless of sexual orientation (Everett and Agénor, 2023). Passing, implementing, and enforcing laws and policies that prevent discrimination and advance equity are necessary, but LGBTQ+ racially and ethnically minoritized communities have many strengths that can be leveraged to advance health equity. For example, a 2020 survey of 38 LGBTQ+-identified people of color in New York City (guided by the health equity promotion model) found common strengths identified by participants were safety, acceptance, and support; interconnectedness and resource sharing;

and advocacy, collective action, and community potential (Hudson and Romanelli, 2020). Moreover, Agénor et al. found, in two different studies, that social support from other LGBTQ+ people of color, health information sharing within LGBTQ+ communities of color, peer advocacy during clinical encounters, and receiving care from health care providers who shared their lived experiences facilitated access to and receipt of needed sexual and reproductive health care among transmasculine young adults of color (Agénor et al., 2022a,b).

Rurality

In the context of "place" as a social determinant of health (SDOH), residence in a rural area is strongly linked with poor health outcomes. Over at least the past 50 years, this has evolved into one the strongest determinants of excess mortality (Cosby et al., 2019). The population-based mortality disparity is on par with race and level of education as a predictor of early death (NASEM, 2018a). Poverty and rurality have a strong interaction as well (USDA, 2022). This rural health penalty is not equally distributed; measures of poor health and poverty are more concentrated among Black, Hispanic, and AIAN than White populations (Cosby et al., 2019; James et al., 2017). Death from heart disease, cancer, and stroke are considerably higher among rural Black people compared to those living in urban areas (Probst et al., 2020).

Resource constraints that drive health and economic inequities are often more severe in rural areas, demonstrated by the lack of transportation resources, inadequate economic opportunity, diminished access to health care, and a preponderance of food insecurity in rural areas (NASEM, 2021b; Romanello et al., 2022). Rural hospital closures are more likely in communities with higher percentages of Black and Hispanic residents, exacerbating pre-existing inequities (NASEM, 2018a). AIAN people in rural areas are affected by these same resource imbalances and further impacted by a woefully underfunded IHS (see Chapter 5 for more information on the IHS) (Heisler and McClanahan, 2020; NASEM, 2017).

Rurality is a strong predictor of poor health outcomes and health inequities (James et al., 2017). Areas with persistent poverty are not evenly distributed but are concentrated in the mid-South and AIAN reservations and villages. Although mirroring those in more populous areas, racial and ethnic inequities are more concentrated (NASEM, 2021b). Different strategies to address health inequities and to improve the overall level of care in rural areas are needed given the pre-existing deficit of wealth and public infrastructure. These approaches need to be community driven and funded in ways that acknowledge the unique implementation challenges of working with small populations.

Citizenship and Immigration Status

Citizenship and immigration status are powerful determinants of health status and life chances (NASEM, 2018b). U.S. citizenship is mostly understood as a legal membership at the national level, with such membership granted through birthright based on the Constitution's 14th Amendment, 1924 Citizenship Act,[21] and Immigration and Nationality Act of 1965.[22] Federal law limits certain benefits and opportunities to U.S. residents that have significant implications for health outcomes, including on employment in most federal government jobs, voting in national elections, priorities in bringing family members to the United States, and protections from threats to immigration status renewal based on public charge considerations and deportations based on criminal convictions even for legal permanent residents (NASEM, 2015, 2018b). U.S. citizenship also forms the basis of access to many benefits and protections at the state level, including for government employment and voting (Citizenship and Immigration Services, 2020).

In addition to U.S. citizenship status, immigration status also plays a powerful role in limiting access to federal programs that can address key SDOH and increasing risks to immigration enforcement actions that may more directly impact health status (NASEM, 2015, 2018b). The federal government has exclusive authority to allow persons to enter the United States, deport or remove people, and provide work authorization and the ability to remain in the country for specified periods (American Immigration Council, 2021). The highest levels protections are accorded to legal permanent residents (often referred to as "green card" holders); they are able to access most federal benefits and state benefits without risk of deportation or removal, with renewal of status virtually guaranteed (American Immigration Council, 2021). Other statuses are temporary, tied to such factors as employment (H visas), education (F and M visas), and visitors on business or tourism (B visas), and they vary with respect to the ability to obtain work authorization and access to federal benefits. Finally, the federal government also provides certain persons with temporary protected status based on emergency conditions in their countries of origin, Deferred Action for Childhood Arrivals based on age and year of entry, and asylee or pending asylee status (American Immigration Council, 2021); see Chapter 5 for more information. These temporary statuses also vary greatly in the kinds of federal benefits and, by extension, state and local benefits they provide. Finally, people with no or expired legal status are ineligible for most federal benefits and protections and subject to detention or deportation (Colbern and Ramakrishnan, 2021). These immigration enforcement actions affect

---

[21] Pub. L. 68–175.
[22] Pub. L. 89–236.

the health status of not only the particular individuals involved but also family members living in multigenerational and multistatus households (Castañeda and Melo, 2014).

DATA GAPS AND OPPORTUNITIES

High-quality and accurate data are needed for several reasons in relation to racial, ethnic, and tribal health equity and policy making. One key reason is accountability—if data are poor, inequities can be hidden (intentionally and unintentionally) or ignored, and progress cannot be monitored (NCQA, 2021a; Rubin et al., 2018). The ability to conduct equity assessments to identify the impact of federal policies on health equity and then identify and remove barriers to accessing government programs is also contingent on having data available (Equitable Data Working Group, 2022). Accurate and high-quality data are also needed to guide the development and implementation of interventions. In addition, data can point to both health improvement and declines to guide resource allocation. If data are unavailable or inaccurate for a certain population, they may not receive the resources they need (Erickson et al., 2021; NCQA, 2021a; Rubin et al., 2018). Self-reported data on race and ethnicity are also important aspects, as they better reflect how people identify themselves.

Since 1977, the Office of Management and Budget (OMB) has issued minimum standards for maintaining, collecting, and presenting federal data on race and ethnicity. These were last revised in 1997, when the federal government separated "Asian or Pacific Islander" into "Native Hawaiian or Other Pacific Islander," changed "Hispanic" to "Hispanic or Latino," allowed respondents to self-identify with more than one race, and required federal agencies to report data on multiple racial categories rather than combining them into a general category of "multiracial" (OMB, 1997). These minimum standards inform all federal race and ethnicity data collection efforts and are critical to understanding patterns, conditions, and outcomes, including those related to health and health care and the SDOH. Not all federal agencies collect and report high-quality and accurate data on these minimum racial, ethnic, and tribal population categories, which is a significant barrier to achieving data equity. This lack of data also contributes to health inequities, as policy decisions are not fully informed by the data.

The OMB revised 1997 standards included minimum categories for race for AIAN, Asian, Black or African American, Native Hawaiian or Other Pacific Islander, and White, with individuals able to select one or more categories (OMB, 1997; OMH, 2021a). However, although these standards were to be effective/fully enforced by 2003, OMB has not done so (e.g., NHPI are often not separately reported and are combined with

Asian) (AAPI Data and National Council of Asian Pacific Americans, 2022; OMB, 1997). In addition, the OMB minimum categories for ethnicity are Hispanic or Latino/a and Not Hispanic or Latino/a.

In January 2023 of the Federal Register, OMB proposed important changes to the data collection on race and ethnicity, with a published notice on "Initial Proposals for Updating OMB's Race and Ethnicity Statistical Standards."[23] that follows over a decade of constituent engagement and questionnaire testing by the Census Bureau. Until a revision, however, the 1997 standards remain in place. Some of the important proposed changes include the following (see also Chapter 8):

1. Collect race and ethnicity information using one combined question, rather than have a question on Hispanic ethnicity separate from the question on race.
2. Add "Middle Eastern or North African" (MENA) as a new minimum category.
3. Require the collection of detailed race and ethnicity categories by default, "unless an agency determines that the potential benefit of the detailed data would not justify the additional burden to the agency and the public or the additional risk to privacy or confidentiality."
4. Update terminology deemed to be inaccurate or archaic, including removing "Negro" from the Black of African American definition; removing "Far East" from the Asian definition—replacing with "East Asian"; removing the phrase "who maintain tribal affiliation or community attachment" in the AIAN definition; and removing "Other" in the Native Hawaiian and Other Pacific Islander definition.

The committee provides input on these proposed changes in Chapter 8.

The Department of Health and Human Services (HHS) has used the OMB minimum standards in most of its data collection efforts since 1997. Data are collected through surveillance systems, national surveys, administrative programs, and clinical trials. In 2011, HHS developed new standards for data collection of race and ethnicity to understand better the heterogeneous racial and detailed-origin subgroups that comprise the broader OMB categories (ASPE, 2011). The new HHS race standard disaggregates the Asian (Asian Indian, Chinese, Filipino, Japanese, Korean, Vietnamese, and other Asian) and Native Hawaiian or Other Pacific Islander (Native Hawaiian, Guamanian or Chamorro, Samoan, and other Pacific Islander) categories into more fine-grained detailed groups that correspond to ethnicity and country or place of origin. In addition, the new

---

[23] See https://www.federalregister.gov/documents/2023/01/27/2023-01635/initial-proposals-for-updating-ombs-race-and-ethnicity-statistical-standards (accessed March 8, 2023).

HHS ethnicity standard disaggregates the Hispanic or Latino/a category as follows: Mexican, Mexican American, or Chicano/a; Puerto Rican; Cuban; and other Hispanic, Latino/a, or Spanish origin (OMH, 2021a).

In contrast, the new HHS race standards do not disaggregate the Black or African American category by ethnicity, country, or place of origin (e.g., African, Caribbean, Haitian, Nigerian). Since 2000, the proportion of Black immigrants in the United States has increased steadily, from about 600,000 in 2000 to 2.0 million in 2019, with African immigrants representing the largest share of arrivals in 2019 and the Caribbean representing the most common region of birth. Because of pronounced social, economic, and health differences between U.S.-, African-, and Caribbean-born Black U.S. individuals, it is important for data collection efforts to capture the heterogeneity of the population. Not doing so undermines efforts to address the specific and unique needs of diverse communities and promote health equity for all Black populations (Tamir, 2022). Similarly, the AIAN category does not recognize distinct Tribal Nations (OMH, 2021a).

Given the relative recency of the revised HHS race and ethnicity standards, the vast majority of data on health and health care outcomes across and within racial and ethnic groups continue to use the OMB minimum standards. Unfortunately, the most reported groups remain non-Hispanic Black, non-Hispanic White, and Hispanic or Latino/a, for reasons discussed below (including the lack of capacity to report more granular data due to sample sizes too small to produce reliable estimates).

In addition to HHS data collection, the 2020 census collected detailed data on ethnicity or enrolled tribal affiliation for each of the OMB racial and ethnic categories. This represents a huge opportunity for (1) examining within-group disparities among OMB racial and tribal groups and (2) redesigning primary sampling units and more targeted data collection of hard-to-survey groups because of the more detailed 2020 census data on race and ethnicity population distribution (Census Bureau, 2019).

Gaps in Race and Ethnicity Federal Data Collection Efforts

Continued gaps in federal data collection on race and ethnicity pose a problem and contribute to data inaccuracy. These gaps, which have ramifications for data equity efforts, include (1) lack of disaggregation of diverse groups, (2) lack of oversampling, (3) inability to capture intersections with other social identity factors, (4) lack of granular data on small racial and ethnic groups, and (5) gaps in contextual data. Accurate data are necessary to inform knowledge and action on racial and ethnic health inequities and their social determinants.

The first major barrier is that data on OMB-defined historically under-represented groups are not disaggregated (Panapasa et al., 2011). They reflect a conglomeration of various ethnicities, countries or places of origin, or Tribal Nations. Failing to capture the diversity within OMB-defined racial and detailed-origin groups obscures significant within-group health inequities and hampers efforts to mitigate or eliminate health inequities between and within racial groups. These differences result from social and economic inequities based on ethnicity, country or place of origin, immigrant or refugee status, geography, language, skin color, historical context, or federal recognition.

This lack of disaggregation reflects both historical and contemporary norms, values, and practices rooted in racism, xenophobia, colonialism, and imperialism that view and treat racially and ethnically minoritized populations as monoliths and erase the complexity, nuances, and specificities of their social positions and lived experiences (see earlier sections of this chapter for more information). Multiracial people are a very heterogeneous population. They represent diverse social and economic positions, racial and ethnic backgrounds, histories, countries or place of origin, skin colors, cultures, tribal affiliations, and health and health care needs. All these concerns are masked by the lack of data disaggregated by race or ethnicity for this multifaceted group (Holland and Palaniappan, 2012; NCAI, 2021; Rodríguez, 2021; Rubin et al., 2018; Urban Indian Health Institute, 2020; Williams and Jackson, 2000; Zambrana et al., 2021). Data disaggregation can be costly with added confidentiality issues; however, prioritizing these populations is essential.

The second gap is the lack of oversampling, especially of AIAN and NHPI populations, in national health surveys and other relevant federal data collection efforts to produce reliable statistics on these minimum OMB categories (Faircloth et al., 2015; Galinsky et al., 2019; Panapasa et al., 2011; Wu and Bakos, 2017). In addition, adequate granular/detailed data are not collected on the minimum OMB categories (such as Asian, Native Hawaiian, and Pacific Islander) or by geography. This leads to inadequate data on the health of these diverse communities and precludes meaningful action to achieve health equity (Islam et al., 2010; Johnson et al., 2010; Nguyen et al., 2022). To offset the failure of federal agencies to oversample, researchers supported by federal data collection efforts and other funders conduct smaller specific group studies to address data gaps. However, the data on these smaller groups are extrapolated to other Asian, Native Hawaiian, and Pacific Islander groups or interpreted as representative of the total population; these smaller studies are not robust, are based on convenience samples, and suffer from bias, limiting generalizability to the population group (Holland and Palaniappan, 2012; Shah and Kandula, 2020; Yom and Lor, 2022). Despite barriers to expanding sample sizes and collecting data on small or geographically remote populations (e.g., cost, data reliability, privacy), expanding sampling frames to generate statistically reliable estimates of the population at varying levels of geography is important for policy and program development. Decisions to do so will need to consider a number of factors, such as population size, the magnitude of the disparity based on scientific research, and cost and feasibility (see Chapter 8 for a recommendation and more details on oversampling).

The third gap is the lack of data on the intersection of race and ethnicity and racism with other axes of social identity and inequality, including gender, ableism, sexism, cisgenderism, sexual orientation, heterosexism, socioeconomic position and classism, nativity and xenophobia, and age and ageism. Together, these issues impact the health and health care outcomes of multiply marginalized individuals and populations (e.g., LGBTQ+ people, older adults, youth, low-income people) in compounding and unique ways (Bowleg, 2012, 2017; Collins and Bilge, 2020). However, the vast majority of federally collected health data are only reported in relation to a single axis of social identity or inequality at a time, thus rendering invisible the specific health experiences and needs of multiply marginalized groups and undermining the development and implementation of tailored actions that promote their health. Moreover, health surveys and other federal data collection efforts tend to include only some of the measures needed for an intersectional analysis of racial and ethnic health inequities. For example, although the National Health Interview Survey, the nation's leading source of population health data from CDC, does collect information on sexual orientation identity, it does not include other measures of sexual orientation (e.g., sexual behavior) or gender identity. This inhibits the ability of researchers, policy makers, and program planners to identify racially or ethnically minoritized LGBTQ+ people in the data and formulate policies, programs, and practices that promote their health (Zambrana et al., 2021).

Moreover, substantial within- and across-group disparities are masked, and inappropriate interpretations and conclusions can be drawn when race and ethnicity data are not cross-tabulated with other social indicators. For example, poor average health outcomes among Black populations are often erroneously attributed to socioeconomic inequities alone. However, analyses that stratify data for racial and ethnic groups by socioeconomic status often show a more complex picture, implicating other factors related to interpersonal, institutional, and structural racism as essential drivers of health inequities (Williams and Jackson, 2000).

Relatedly, efforts are inadequate to collect data on persons speaking a language other than English at home and limited English proficiency. The census has reliable questions, but these are not typically administered as part of federal data-collection efforts (Flores, 2020).

The fourth gap pertains to the absence, or masking, of subgroups in data collection and reporting efforts. In particular, OMB standards do not include Arabs and Arab Americans or people of MENA descent as a distinct racial or ethnic category (Wiltz, 2014). These individuals have to select a category that may not reflect their personal or social identity, culture, history, or lived experience. Due to the lack of relevant options, some may select the "White" or "other" options, which erases their identity and experience, erases their existence in the data, prevents generating data on their health outcomes and needs, and obscures data for other populations (Rubin et al., 2018). Similarity, ethnicity is treated separately from race in most data collection efforts, forcing Latino/a individuals to artificially choose a race in some cases (Flores, 2020).

Additionally, smaller populations, such as AIAN and NHPI populations, are often entirely excluded from data collection and reports due to their small numbers, limiting access to resources (mandated under treaty and trust responsibility for the AIAN population) (Panapasa et al., 2011). Survey data collection on the Pacific Islander jurisdictions is limited as well (Erickson et al., 2021; Friedman et al., 2023). National datasets routinely relegate these groups to the "other" racial category, which grossly misrepresents and denies their existence. This conceals their social, economic, and health experiences and needs and undermines attempts to create relevant, tailored action to improve the health of the various and diverse groups included in this nebulous "catchall" category (Holland and Palaniappan, 2012; NCAI, 2021).

Relatedly, the federal definition of AIAN,[24] which is limited to those registered in federally recognized Tribal Nations, not only underestimates but also misclassifies AIAN people who do not fit this definition. This further undermines the generation of high-quality and accurate data (NCAI, 2021; Rubin et al., 2018; Urban Indian Health Institute, 2020). One added complication, either unknown by data collectors or ignored in the categorization, is that in the eyes of the federal government, the tribes are first and foremost political bodies or domestic dependent nations (see earlier in this chapter for more details). An additional complication in reporting correctly and comprehensively on the AIAN population is that researchers conducting studies or collecting data might be unaware of this unique political status and lump them in with all other groups, usually as "other." Use of data categories needs to respect the sovereign status of Tribal Nations to determine their own citizenship; federal, state, and county collection of tribal enrollment status is inappropriate without the express permission of a specific tribe. Collecting tribal affiliation is more appropriate, as it does not denote tribal citizenship and is cognizant of the historical context of disenrollment, descendants, and federal initiatives that separated AIAN people from their communities; however, it must be respectful of AIAN data sovereignty (Urban Indian Health Institute, 2020).

Due to extermination, reservation, termination, and assimilation policies, the AIAN population was splintered and now includes enrolled members, those purposively lost through assimilation, those "unenrolled,"

---

[24] Native Hawaiians are defined as descendants of the aboriginal people of State of Hawaii. Congress has not formally recognized them as a Tribal Nation.

and those who died/were killed. With these losses, any accountability and the capacity to generate accurate population counts were lost. Although the Self-Determination Era (characterized by an explosion in civil rights activism) began in 1975, AIAN people have seen few gains in health or SDOH. The same spirit of purposeful, targeted, strategic measures that caused these inequalities needs to now be applied to reversing the harmful policies' effects.

Data related to inequities and resiliencies are severely lacking for the AIAN population, which directly impacts the allocation of resources legally owed through the treaty and trust responsibility. The COVID-19 pandemic, which disproportionately affected AIAN people (Arrazola, 2020; Hatcher et al., 2020), provides a poignant example of how inadequate data can drive health inequity. AIAN-specific data on infection rates and mortality were mostly missing, with great variation between states (Erickson et al., 2021; GAO, 2022). As a result, resource allocation to address disproportionate health needs was inadequate, as federal agencies, including CDC, relied heavily on these faulty data. Disaggregation of data is a priority of AIAN communities, but it is increasingly difficult to disaggregate small samples; in addition, the population is small because of past genocide and the current lack of proper data collection.

A fifth gap is that data that reflect groups' social, economic, and historical contexts are not collected. In particular, national health surveys and other federal research efforts (e.g., clinical trials—see Chapter 5) fail to include measures of historical and contemporary structural, institutional, community, and interpersonal racism and xenophobia, which shape racial and ethnic health inequities (Brown and Homan, 2023).[25] As a result, available information on these inequities cannot be accurately contextualized, interpreted, and acted upon using health data alone. Additionally, although the census and other federal (e.g., administrative) data sources provide essential information on the SDOH of racial and ethnic health inequities (e.g., poverty, mortality, income, housing, education, and environmental risks), these data are typically not readily linked to or integrated with national survey, administrative, or clinical trial health data. This limits their usability and uptake in public health and health equity research (Knight et al., 2021; Rodríguez, 2021). The measures used would depend on the topic or SDOH area under study[26] (for examples of such measures, on a variety of SDOH, see Adkins-Jackson et al., 2022;

---

[25] For example, measures on explicit rules and laws, nonexplicit rules and laws, and area-based or institutional nonrule measures and expanding the use of structural measures that extend beyond the current psychosocial individual-level measures (Krieger, 2020).

[26] For example, to study the impact of structural racism on myocardial infarction, Lukachko and colleagues (2014) used the following indicators "(1) political participation; (2) employment and job status; (3) educational attainment; and (4) judicial treatment. State-level racial disparities across these domains were proposed to represent the systematic exclusion of Blacks from resources and mobility in society" (p. 42).

Agénor et al., 2021; Alson et al., 2021; Dougherty et al., 2020; Follis et al., 2023; Greenfield et al., 2021; Hardeman et al., 2022; Krieger, 2020; Krieger et al., 2016, 2017a; Mesic et al., 2018; Siegel et al., 2022; Wallace et al., 2015; Williams, 2016).

The census and other federal sources of data on SDOH do not include measures of historical or contemporary structural racism (see earlier). This would include measures of laws, policies, and institutional practices that minoritize Black, AIAN, Latina/o, and other communities across multiple social systems. Policies, such as Jim Crow laws, redlining practices, environmental zoning laws, and school funding policies, underlie and continue to drive racial and ethnic social and economic and ensuing health inequities (Chapters 3–7 provide examples). This undermines the ability of policy makers, researchers, and program officials to identify how historical and contemporary structural and social inequities shape racial and ethnic health inequities and, in turn, thwart action on these root causes at the federal, state, territorial, tribal, and local levels (Rodríguez, 2021). Moreover, failing to contextualize racial and ethnic health inequities by the historical and contemporary structural and social inequities that shape them fosters their interpretation as innate, inherent, and immutable. It supports an inaccurate view that they reflect individual-level biological and behavioral factors rather than the societal effects of racism and other forms of discrimination (Knight et al., 2021; NASEM, 2023).

Challenges in Race and Ethnicity Federal Data Collection Efforts

Contemporary race and ethnicity data collection practices stem from accounting, statistics, and epidemiology, which originated with the counting and monitoring of enslaved people and "imperial subjects" and were deployed in the context of eugenics in order to advance and justify slavery, colonialism, and imperialism (Gampa et al., 2020). In addition, due to structural inequities that undermine Black, AIAN, and other minoritized people's access to education and employment, they have been systematically excluded from and underrepresented in the fields charged with collecting data on race and ethnicity, including data science, statistics, demography, and epidemiology (Downs, 2021). Data collection efforts and their interpretation, presentation, and use reflect the priorities, preferences, and objectives of White and Western perspectives, which diverge in important ways from the lived experiences of racialized people and communities (Knight et al., 2021). Conversely, race and ethnicity and data collection have been and can be used to undermine the health and well-being of minoritized individuals and groups. Historical and contemporary race and ethnicity data collection efforts have been used to actively surveil, exclude, and criminalize underserved communities (e.g., Black, Native, Asian, Latino/a,

Pacific Islander, and Arab communities) directly in conflict with reducing or eliminating health inequities and promoting health equity (Knight et al., 2021; Rodríguez, 2021).

As described by the Equitable Data Working Group, "federal collaborations with state, local, territorial and tribal governments can yield high-quality demographic data when all partners see value in its collection and use" (Equitable Data Working Group, 2022, p. 10). However, current race and ethnicity measures and data collection, interpretation, translation, and dissemination efforts do not reflect the relevant communities' priorities, preferences, perspectives, and needs, which undermines their utility for informing community-centered actions that advance racial and ethnic health equity (Rubin et al., 2018; Urban Indian Health Institute, 2020). In addition, research studies that seek to investigate and address these issues in collaboration with impacted communities are usually sidelined from funding or publication in top-tier medical and public health journals, which further undermines the data and evidence available to inform equity-focused, community-centered solutions (Mervis, 2019).

To benefit Black, AIAN, NHPI, and other minoritized communities and advance health equity, race and ethnicity data collection efforts have to explicitly inform the equitable allocation of health-promoting resources to underresourced communities through laws, policies, programs, and community efforts. Additionally, care is required as data are disaggregated to avoid identifying and undermining the privacy of individual survey or study participants, particularly from small racial and ethnic groups while also achieving statistical reliability (Rubin et al., 2018; Urban Indian Health Institute, 2020). Disseminating point estimates by population group could include margins of error at the 95 percent confidence interval, with no predetermined cutoff on sample size as long as data privacy concerns are addressed.

A unique challenge for AIAN population data is the astounding levels of misidentification of race by health professionals, researchers, and medical examiners, for example, who collect data (Haozous et al., 2014). *Trends in Indian Health*, the official report of the IHS, includes multiple indications in the report acknowledging that the numbers are problematic, especially as received from states' data misreporting of race (IHS, 2014). Furthermore, no report has been published since 2014. As bad as the known numbers for all aspects of AIAN health are for life expectancy, COVID-19 exposures, and death, for example, the actual burden of disease is underreported (Haozous et al., 2014).

Health Care Data

Opportunities exist to improve the plethora of health care data collected to improve data equity. These data reflect the individual, provider to

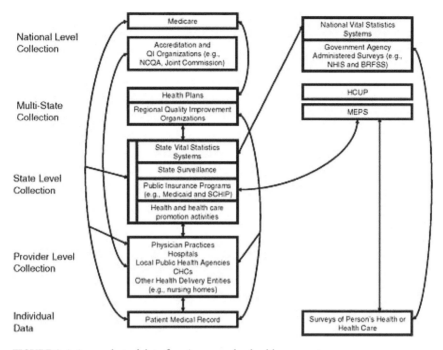

FIGURE 2-4 A snapshot of data flow in a complex health care system.
NOTE: BRFSS = Behavioral Risk Factor Surveillance System; CHC = community health center; HCUP = health care cost and utilization project; MEPS = Medical Expenditure Panel Survey; NCQA = National Committee for Quality Assurance; NHIS = National Health Interview Survey; QI = quality improvement; SCHIP = State Children's Health Insurance Plan.
SOURCE: IOM, 2009.

state/multistate, and national levels (see Figure 2-4) and are from various sources, including from surveys, billing records, and medical records. Entities collecting these data include payers and providers (hospitals, providers, clinics). A 2009 Institute of Medicine report provided recommendations on standardizing race, ethnicity, and language data to improve health care quality. In addition, the data can be used for multiple purposes: provider payment (see Chapter 5 discussion on value-based payment), a primary source for clinical trials and health services research, quality improvement initiatives, and incentives to improve individual behaviors.

Although health care data are rich, several gaps or issues are noted in the IOM (2009) report that continue to be relevant today:

- The entities listed above do not collect data on the entire population or have the capabilities to do so.
- Data are fragmented and not integrated.

- Health information technology can help streamline data collection and integration, but the maturity of technology varies across health care systems.
- Redundancy exists in the collection of race, ethnicity, and language data.
- Comparison groups cannot be equivalently stratified, given the lack of data standardization.

In addition, a 2022 systematic review of SDOH data in electronic health records yielded quality problems, such as misclassification bias of race, ethnicity, or country-of-origin data and incomplete data (Cook et al., 2022). Given these gaps and validity issues, data standardization in health care systems is important to achieving data equity. Several efforts are underway. In 2022, CMS' Office of Minority Health released its framework for health equity 2022–2032, and one of the priorities is to expand the collection, reporting, and analysis of standardized data (McIver, 2022, p. 2). Several collaborations are cited, including partnership with HHS to improve interoperability and demographic and SDOH data standards.[27] In addition, the National Committee for Quality Assurance updated guidance for health plans to stratify quality data by race and ethnicity beginning in measurement year 2020 (NCQA, 2021b), and the Joint Commission, which accredits over 22,000 health care organizations, released new requirements to reduce health care disparities (Joint Commission, 2023); these include not only having the medical record reflect care, treatment, and services but also including race and ethnicity. CMS and the Joint Commission, recognizing the important role of these data in advancing health, are making early but limited efforts to ensure that these are captured for a subset of patients.

The United States Preventive Services Task Force (USPSTF),[28] the national organization that promulgates recommendations on clinical preventive services, has launched an initiative to address structural racism that can serve as a model for other regulatory agencies. Given the intrinsic deficiencies in representation of racial and ethnic minorities in clinical trials (see Chapter 5), prevention guidelines shared by USPSTF will reflect those same deficiencies. Disease processes manifest differently among various racial and ethnic groups,

---

[27] For example, interoperability with 2011 HHS Data Standards, U.S. Core Data for Interoperability standards, HHS Disparities Action Plan, CMS Accountable Health Communities Model, Consumer Assessment of Health Care Providers & Systems, and Standardized Patient Assessment Data Elements.

[28] Title IX of the Public Health Service Act mandated the creation of USPSTF to "review the scientific evidence related to the effectiveness, appropriateness, and cost-effectiveness of clinical preventive services for the purpose of developing recommendations for the health care community, and updating previous clinical preventive recommendations, to be published in the Guide to Clinical Preventive Services" (USPSTF, 2019). Each year, the task force makes a report to Congress that identifies critical evidence gaps in research related to clinical preventive services and recommends priority areas that deserve further examination (USPSTF, 2019).

due to genetic variation and the effects of structural racism (Gee and Ford, 2011; NASEM, 2022b). Disproportionately adverse clinical outcomes in diseases, such as cancer and CVD, reflect the different environmental exposures, health care access, and life experiences among racial and ethnic minorities (NASEM, 2017). Recommendations based on primarily White cohorts of study participants are not generalizable[29] to all populations (NASEM, 2022b). In 2021, USPSTF identified systemic racism as a factor undermining the utility of its current recommendations and the integrity of the recommendation development process. It has six core actions to address racism in future recommendations (Doubeni et al., 2021, p. 628):

1. Consider race primarily as a social and not a biological construct, and use consistent terminology throughout recommendation statements to reflect this view.
2. Promote racial and ethnic diversity in addition to gender, geographic, and disciplinary diversity in USPSTF membership and leadership, and foster a culture of diversity and inclusivity as an enduring value of USPSTF. This will be assessed annually before soliciting nominations for new members and internally assigning leadership roles.
3. Commission a review of the evidence, including an environmental scan and interviews with clinicians, researchers, community leaders, policy experts, other guideline developers, and patients from groups that are disproportionately affected to summarize the evidence on how systemic racism undermines the benefits of evidence-based clinical preventive services and causes preventable deaths.
4. Iteratively, update USPSTF methods to integrate the best evidence and consistently address evidence gaps for Black, Indigenous, and Hispanic/Latino populations. This includes measures to identify and track strategies to demonstrate progress in addressing health inequities regarding clinical preventive services.
5. Use a consistent and transparent approach to communicate gaps in the evidence related to systemic racism in preventive care in recommendation statements and the USPSTF annual report to Congress. This includes an ongoing assessment of how the effects of systemic racism on the quality of the evidence and receipt of clinical preventive services perpetuate health inequities.
6. Collaborate with other guideline-making bodies, professional societies, policy makers, and patient advocacy organizations on efforts to reduce the influence of systemic racism on health.

---

[29] For example, Black men are at greater risk than White men for lung cancer at lower pack-years of smoking. Therefore, as USPSTF is now recommending lowering the pack-year level to start screening, this may reduce racial inequities in lung cancer health outcomes if implemented with fidelity (Doubeni et al., 2021).

Developments to Improve Data Equity in Federal Agencies

In the last two decades, the federal government has made progress in advancing data equity by issuing EOs and creating interagency working groups to achieve improvements in data design, collection, analysis, and dissemination. For example, each administration, starting in 1999, has issued an EO establishing a commission that encourages greater participation of Asian American and Pacific Islander populations or businesses in federal programs, with improvements in data collections on program use as a key priority.[30] Other EOs have also prioritized data collection improvements, including those pertaining to Hispanic American (EOs 13230,[31] 13555,[32] 13935,[33] and 14045[34]), Black (EOs 13621[35] and 14050[36]), and AIAN (EOs 13336,[37] 13592,[38] 14049,[39] and 14053[40]) people. Most recently, the Biden administration has issued several EOs that address improvements in data collection and dissemination of data to advance racial equity, including 13985 (updated by EO 14091[41] *Further Advancing Racial Equity and Support for Underserved Communities Through the Federal Government*), 14035[42] *Diversity, Equity, Inclusion, and Accessibility in the Federal Workforce*, and 14058[43] *Transforming Federal Customer Experience and Service Delivery to Rebuild Trust in Government*. In addition, the Equitable Data Working Group (established under EO 13985) studies and provides recommendations to the Assistant to the President for Domestic Policy to identify inadequacies "in existing Federal data collection programs, policies, and infrastructure across agencies, and strategies for addressing any deficiencies identified" and "support agencies in implementing actions, consistent with applicable law and privacy interests, that expand and refine the data available to the federal government to measure equity and capture the diversity of the American people" (The White House, 2021).

---

[30] See, for example, EOs 13125 (Clinton; 64 FR 31105 [June 1999]), 13216 and 13339 (George W. Bush; 66 FR 31373 [June 2001] and 69 FR 28035 [May 2004], respectively), 13515 (Obama; 74 FR 53635 [October 2009]), 13872 (Trump; 84 FR 22321 [May 2019]), and 14031 (Biden; 86 FR 29675 [June 2021]).

[31] Exec. Order No. 13230, 66 FR 52841 (October 2001).

[32] Exec. Order No. 13555, 75 FR 65415 (October 2010).

[33] Exec. Order No. 13935, 85 FR 42683 (July 2020).

[34] Exec. Order No. 14045, 86 FR 51581 (September 2021).

[35] Exec. Order No. 13621, 77 FR 45471 (August 2012).

[36] Exec. Order No. 14050, 86 FR 58551 (October 2021).

[37] Exec. Order No. 13336, 69 FR 25293 (May 2004).

[38] Exec. Order No. 13592, 76 FR 76603 (December 2011).

[39] Exec. Order No. 14049, 86 FR 57313 (October 2021).

[40] Exec. Order No. 14053, 86 FR 64337 (November 2021).

[41] Exec. Order No. 14091, 88 FR 10825 (February 2023).

[42] Exec. Order No. 14035, 86 FR 34593 (June 2021).

[43] Exec. Order No. 14058, 86 FR 71357 (December 2021).

The working group, cochaired by senior OMB leadership and the Office of Science and Technology Policy, issued a set of recommendations in April 2022 to advance data equity, including making "data disaggregation the norm while protecting privacy," catalyzing "existing federal infrastructure to leverage underused data," and building "capacity for robust equity assessment for policymaking and program implementation" (Equitable Data Working Group, 2022, p. 3; The White House, 2022). Some researchers and community organizations have characterized the Biden administration's actions as a *functional approach* to data equity (focused on the extent to which data collections advance racially equitable outcomes), in contrast to a *process approach* (focused on the methods that are used to produce more equitable data collections, including community consultation on data design and development, collection and compilation, processing and analysis, and dissemination and preservation) (AAPI Data and National Council of Asian Pacific Americans, 2022). Given a delay of more than 2 years in the release of detailed-origin population counts from the 2020 census, community organizations have pushed for timely dissemination as an important aspect of data equity (AAPI Data and National Council of Asian Pacific Americans, 2022).

In addition to the standards set by the federal government, community organizations and researchers focused on data equity are pushing for even higher standards that follow on data stewardship principles. In 2016, a wide-ranging group of stakeholders, "representing academia, industry, funding agencies, and scholarly publishers," published an article in the Nature journal *Scientific Data* outlining a set of principles on data stewardship known as FAIR (findability, accessibility, interoperability, and reusability) (Wilkinson et al., 2016). These recommendations placed "specific emphasis on enhancing the ability of machines to automatically find and use the data, in addition to supporting its reuse by individuals" and prompted the creation of several FAIR implementation networks to improve data collections (GoFair). In 2020, *Data Science Journal* published a supplementary set of data stewardship principles to address "concerns about secondary use of data and limited opportunities for benefit-sharing" among Indigenous communities (Carroll et al., 2020). The authors, representing a broad and diverse set of Indigenous data scholars and practitioners, encourage adoption of CARE principles (collective benefit, authority to control, responsibility, and ethics) as well to produce "data that reflect the realities of Indigenous Peoples, be useful for Indigenous purposes, and remain under Indigenous control, while promoting knowledge discovery and innovation" (Carroll et al., 2020, p. 8). These two principles seek to ensure advancements in data equity in not only functional (improving the production and availability of data collections that advance racial equity) but also process (ensuring racial and ethnic equity in the ways that data are collected, stored, analyzed, and disseminated) terms.

Data Gaps and Opportunities Conclusions

Conclusion 2-1: The lack of oversampling of underrepresented racial, ethnic, and tribal populations in national health surveys and other relevant federal data collection efforts—for example, the Office of Management and Budget categories of American Indian or Alaska Native and Native Hawaiian or Pacific Islander—limits the availability of reliable data, and therefore meaningful action, by federal programs, researchers, and advocates to advance health equity for these communities.

Conclusion 2-2: Disaggregated data on social, economic, health care, and health indicators that reflect the heterogeneity of racial and ethnic groups, including in relation to country of origin, are needed to inform targeted actions that promote health equity across and within groups.

CONCLUDING OBSERVATIONS

This chapter provides an overview of the role of government, and the complex relationship between states, examples of health inequities and some of their root causes, and data gaps and opportunities. A common theme is inadequate data in many areas, preventing a full understanding of the extent of health inequities to inform policy actions. However, the chapter also shows the rich information that has been collected that points to the mechanisms for how the social and structural determinants of health have contributed to health inequities and are therefore key areas to focus federal action to advance health equity. Chapters 3–7 take deeper dives into SDOH and how they can positively and negatively impact health equity via federal policies: economic stability, education access and quality, health care access and quality, neighborhood and built environment, and the social and community context.

REFERENCES

AAPI Data, and National Council of Asian Pacific Americans. 2022. *2022 Asian American, Native Hawaiian, and Pacific Islander (AA and NHPI) roadmap for data equity in federal agencies.* Washington, DC: National Council of Asian Pacific Americans.

Aaron, H. J. 2012. *The Supreme Court ruling on the Affordable Care Act—a bullet dodged.* https://www.brookings.edu/blog/up-front/2012/06/28/the-supreme-court-ruling-on-the-affordable-care-act-a-bullet-dodged/ (accessed March 11, 2023).

AASHTO (American Association of State Highway and Transportation Officials). n.d. *Environmental Justice & Transportation.* https://environment.transportation.org/education/environmental-topics/environmental-justice/environmental-justice-overview/ (accessed March 8, 2023).

ACLU (American Civil Liberties Union). 2020. *Racial disparities in stops by the Metropolitan Police Department: 2020 data update.* Washington, DC: American Civil Liberties Union.

Adkins-Jackson, P. B., T. Chantarat, Z. D. Bailey, and N. A. Ponce. 2022. Measuring structural racism: A guide for epidemiologists and other health researchers. *American Journal of Epidemiology* 191(4):539–547.

Agénor, M., C. Perkins, C. Stamoulis, R. D. Hall, M. Samnaliev, S. Berland, and S. Bryn Austin. 2021. Developing a database of structural racism–related state laws for health equity research and practice in the United States. *Public Health Reports* 136(4):428–440.

Agénor, M., S. R. Geffen, D. Zubizarreta, R. Jones, S. Giraldo, A. McGuirk, M. Caballero, and A. R. Gordon. 2022a. Experiences of and resistance to multiple discrimination in health care settings among transmasculine people of color. *BMC Health Services Research* 22(1):369.

Agénor, M., D. Zubizarreta, S. Geffen, N. Ramanayake, S. Giraldo, A. McGuirk, M. Caballero, and K. Bond. 2022b. "Making a way out of no way": Understanding the sexual and reproductive health care experiences of transmasculine young adults of color in the United States. *Qualitative Health Research* 32(1):121–134.

Aguirre-Molina, M., C. W. Molina, and R. E. Zambrana. 2001. *Health issues in the Latino community.* San Francisco, California: Jossey-Bass.

Ahn, R., G. P. Gonzalez, B. Anderson, C. J. Vladutiu, E. R. Fowler, and L. Manning. 2020. Initiatives to reduce maternal mortality and severe maternal morbidity in the United States: A narrative review. *Annals of Internal Medicine* 173(11_Supplement):S3–S10.

Alexander, M., P. Holmes, and A. Green. 2012. *The new Jim Crow: Mass incarceration in the age of colorblindness.* New York, NY: The New Press.

Alson, J. G., W. R. Robinson, L. Pittman, and K. M. Doll. 2021. Incorporating measures of structural racism into population studies of reproductive health in the United States: A narrative review. *Health Equity* 5(1):49–58.

American Immigration Council. 2021. *How the United States immigration system works.* Washington, DC: American Immigration Council.

Amiri, S., S. L. Stanley, J. T. Denney, and D. Buchwald. 2022. Disparities in years of potential life lost among racial and ethnic groups in Washington State. *Archives of Public Health* 80(1):211.

Arrazola, J., M. M. Masiello, S. Joshi, A. E. Dominguez, A. Poel, C. M. Wilkie, J. M. Bressler, J. McLaughlin, J. Kraszewski, K. K. Komatsu, X. Peterson Pompa, M. Jespersen, G. Richardson, N. Lehnertz, P. LeMaster, B. Rust, A. Keyser Metobo, B. Doman, D. Casey, J. Kumar, A. L. Rowell, T. K. Miller, M. Mannell, O. Naqvi, A. M. Wendelboe, R. Leman, J. L. Clayton, B. Barbeau, S. K. Rice, S. J. Rolland, V. Warren-Mears, A. Echo-Hawk, A. Apostolou, and M. Landen. 2020. COVID-19 mortality among American Indian and Alaska Native persons—14 states, January–June 2020. *Morbidity and Mortality Weekly Report* 69:1853–1856.

Artiga, S. 2020. *Health Disparities Are a Symptom of Broader Social and Economic Inequities.* https://www.kff.org/policy-watch/health-disparities-symptom-broader-social-economic-inequities/ (accessed June 9, 2023).

ASPE (Assistant Secretary for Planning and Evaluation). 2011. *HHS implementation guidance on data collection standards for race, ethnicity, sex, primary language, and disability status.* Washington, DC: Office of the Assistant Secretary for Planning and Evaluation.

ASPE. 2019. *The special diabetes program for Indians: Estimates of Medicare savings.* Washington, DC: Office of the Assistant Secretary for Planning and Evaluation.

Baah, F. O., A. M. Teitelman, and B. Riegel. 2019. Marginalization: Conceptualizing patient vulnerabilities in the framework of social determinants of health—an integrative review. *Nursing Inquiry* 26(1):e12268.

Badger, E. 2013. *The Dramatic Racial Bias of Subprime Lending During the Housing Boom.* https://www.bloomberg.com/news/articles/2013-08-16/the-dramatic-racial-bias-of-subprime-lending-during-the-housing-boom (accessed June 1, 2023).

Bailey, Z. D., N. Krieger, M. Agénor, J. Graves, N. Linos, and M. T. Bassett. 2017. Structural racism and health inequities in the USA: Evidence and interventions. *The Lancet* 389(10077):1453–1463.

Becasen, J. S., C. L. Denard, M. M. Mullins, D. H. Higa, and T. A. Sipe. 2019. Estimating the prevalence of HIV and sexual behaviors among the U.S. transgender population: A systematic review and meta-analysis, 2006–2017. *American Journal of Epidemiology* 109(1):e1–e8.

Bell, D. A. 2017. *Race, racism and American law*, 3rd ed. New York, NY: New York University Press.

Benjamins, M. R., A. Silva, N. S. Saiyed, and F. G. De Maio. 2021. Comparison of all-cause mortality rates and inequities between Black and White populations across the 30 most populous U.S. cities. *JAMA Network Open* 4(1):e2032086.

Bonilla-Silva, E. 1997. Rethinking racism: Toward a structural interpretation. *American Sociological Review* 62(3):465–480.

Bowleg, L. 2012. The problem with the phrase women and minorities: Intersectionality—an important theoretical framework for public health. *American Journal of Epidemiology* 102(7):1267–1273.

Bowleg, L. 2017. Intersectionality: An underutilized but essential theoretical framework for social psychology. In *The Palgrave handbook of critical social psychology*. New York, NY: Palgrave Macmillan/Springer Nature. Pp. 507–529.

BPC (Bipartisan Policy Center). 2022. *Paid Family Leave Across OECD Countries*. https://bipartisanpolicy.org/explainer/paid-family-leave-across-oecd-countries/ (accessed June 9, 2023).

Breathett, K., M. Sims, M. Gross, E. A. Jackson, E. J. Jones, A. Navas-Acien, H. Taylor, K. L. Thomas, and B. V. Howard. 2020. Cardiovascular health in American Indians and Alaska Natives: A scientific statement from the American Heart Association. *Circulation* 141(25):e948-e959.

Brown, T. H., and P. Homan. 2023. The future of social determinants of health: Looking upstream to structural drivers. *The Milbank Quarterly* 101(S1):36–60.

Caraballo, C., J. Herrin, S. Mahajan, D. Massey, Y. Lu, C. D. Ndumele, E. E. Drye, and H. M. Krumholz. 2022. Temporal trends in racial and ethnic disparities in multimorbidity prevalence in the United States, 1999–2018. *American Journal of Epidemiology* 135(9):1083–1092.e1014.

Caraballo, C., D. S. Massey, C. D. Ndumele, T. Haywood, S. Kaleem, T. King, Y. Liu, Y. Lu, M. Nunez-Smith, H. A. Taylor, K. E. Watson, J. Herrin, C. W. Yancy, J. S. Faust, and H. M. Krumholz. 2023. Excess mortality and years of potential life lost among the Black population in the U.S., 1999–2020. *JAMA* 329(19):1662–1670.

Carroll, S. R., I. Garba, O. L. Figueroa-Rodríguez, J. Holbrook, R. Lovett, S. Materechera, M. Parsons, K. Raseroka, D. Rodriguez-Lonebear, R. Rowe, R. Sara, J. D. Walker, J. Anderson, and M. Hudson. 2020. The CARE principles for Indigenous data governance. *Data Science Journal* 19.

Castañeda, H., and M. A. Melo. 2014. Health care access for Latino mixed-status families: Barriers, strategies, and implications for reform. *American Behavioral Scientist* 58(14):1891–1909.

CDC (Centers for Disease Contril and Prevention). 2019. *Pregnancy-Related Deaths: Saving Women's Lives Before, During and After Delivery*. https://www.cdc.gov/vitalsigns/maternal-deaths/index.html#:~:text=Overview,a%20year%20afterward%20(postpartum) (accessed March 18, 2023).

CDC. 2020. *Adults with Disabilities: Ethnicity and Race*. https://www.cdc.gov/ncbddd/disabilityandhealth/materials/infographic-disabilities-ethnicity-race.html (accessed March 11, 2023).

CDC. 2022. *Health and Economic Costs of Chronic Diseases*. https://www.cdc.gov/chronicdisease/about/costs/index.htm (accessed June 9, 2023).

CDC. 2023a. *Pregnancy Mortality Surveillance System.* https://www.cdc.gov/reproductivehealth/ maternal-mortality/pregnancy-mortality-surveillance-system.htm#:~:text=Since%20 the%20Pregnancy%20Mortality%20Surveillance,100%2C000%20live%20births%20 in%202018. (accessed May 31, 2023).
CDC. 2023b. *Women and Heart Disease.* https://www.cdc.gov/heartdisease/women.htm (accessed March 11, 2023).
Census Bureau. 2019. *Understanding and Using American Community Survey Data.* Washington, DC: US Department of Commerce.
Churchwell, K., M. S. V. Elkind, R. M. Benjamin, A. P. Carson, E. K. Chang, W. Lawrence, A. Mills, T. M. Odom, C. J. Rodriguez, F. Rodriguez, E. Sanchez, A. Z. Sharrief, M. Sims, and O. Williams. 2020. Call to action: Structural racism as a fundamental driver of health disparities: A presidential advisory from the American Heart Association. *Circulation* 142(24):e454–e468.
Citizenship and Immigration Services. 2020. *Should I Consider U.S. Citizenship?* https://www. uscis.gov/citizenship/learn-about-citizenship/should-i-consider-us-citizenship (accessed March 11, 2023).
Colbern, A., and S. K. Ramakrishnan. 2021. *Citizenship Reimagined: A New Framework for State Rights in the United States.* Cambridge, United Kingdom: Cambridge University Press.
Collins, P. H., and S. Bilge. 2020. *Intersectionality*, 2nd ed. Cambridge, UK: Polity Press.
Collins, S. R., and J. M. Lambrew. 2019. *Federalism, the Affordable Care Act, and health reform in the 2020 election.* New York, NY: The Commonwealth Fund.
Community Legal Services of Philadelphia. 2020. *Racial disparities in access to Supplemental Security Income benefits for children.* Philadelphia, PA: Community Legal Services of Philadelphia.
Congress. n.d. *Intro.7.3 Federalism and the Constitution.* https://constitution.congress.gov/ browse/essay/intro.6-2-3/ALDE_00000032/ (accessed March 8, 2023).
Cook, L. A., J. Sachs, and N. G. Weiskopf. 2022. The quality of social determinants data in the electronic health record: A systematic review. *Journal of the American Medical Informatics Association* 29(1):187–196.
Cooper, B. 2015. Intersectionality. In *The Oxford handbook of feminist theory*, edited by L. D. a. M. Hawkesworth. Online: Oxford Academic.
Cooper, D. K., M. Bámaca-Colbert, E. K. Layland, E. G. Simpson, and B. L. Bayly. 2021. Puerto Ricans and Mexican immigrants differ in their psychological responses to patterns of lifetime adversity. *PLOS ONE* 16(10):e0258324.
Cornell Law School. n.d.-a. *National Federation of Independent Business v. Sebelius (2012).* https:// www.law.cornell.edu/wex/national_federation_of_independent_business_v._sebelius_(2012) (accessed March 11, 2023).
Cornell Law School. n.d.-b. *Tenth Amendment.* https://www.law.cornell.edu/constitution/ tenth_amendment (accessed March 8, 2023).
Cosby, A. G., M. M. McDoom-Echebiri, W. James, H. Khandekar, W. Brown, and H. L. Hanna. 2019. Growth and persistence of place-based mortality in the United States: The rural mortality penalty. *American Journal of Public Health* 109(1):155–162.
Courtney-Long, E. A., S. D. Romano, D. D. Carroll, and M. H. Fox. 2017. Socioeconomic factors at the intersection of race and ethnicity influencing health risks for people with disabilities. *Journal of Racial and Ethnic Health Disparities* 4:213–222.
Crenshaw, K. 1991. Mapping the margins: Intersectionality, identity politics, and violence against women of color. *Stanford Law Review* 43(6):1241–1299.
Crimmins, E. M., H. Shim, Y. S. Zhang, and J. K. Kim. 2019. Differences between men and women in mortality and the health dimensions of the morbidity process. *Clinical Chemistry* 65(1):135–145.

CRS (Congressional Research Service). 2022. *The Compacts of Free Association*. https://crsreports.congress.gov/product/pdf/IF/IF12194/1#:~:text=The%20Marshall%20Islands%2C%20Micronesia%2C%20and%20Palau%20signed%20Compacts%20of%20Free,)%2C%20becoming%20effective%20in%201986 (accessed March 11, 2023).

Davis, J. 2021. *Native Hawaiian Law*. https://blogs.loc.gov/law/2021/05/native-hawaiian-law/ (accessed March 11, 2023).

Delgado, R., and J. Stefancic. 2017. Chapter II. Hallmark critical race theory themes. In *Critical race theory: An introduction*, 3rd ed. New York, NY: New York University Press. Pp. 19–43.

Díaz, D. H. S., G. Garcia, C. Clare, J. Su, E. Friedman, R. Williams, J. Vazquez, and J. P. Sánchez. 2020. Taking care of the Puerto Rican patient: Historical perspectives, health status, and health care access. *MedEdPORTAL* 16:10984.

Đoàn, L. N., Y. Takata, K. K. Sakuma, and V. L. Irvin. 2019. Trends in clinical research including Asian American, Native Hawaiian, and Pacific Islander participants funded by the U.S. National Institutes of Health, 1992 to 2018. *JAMA Network Open* 2(7):e197432.

DOE (Department of Education). 2020. *Education and Title VI*. https://www2.ed.gov/about/offices/list/ocr/docs/hq43e4.html (accessed March 8, 2023).

DOL (Department of Labor). n.d. *FMLA Frequently Asked Questions*. https://www.dol.gov/agencies/whd/fmla/faq#2https://www.dol.gov/agencies/whd/fmla (accessed May, 2023).

DOI (Department of the Interior). 2022. *Director's Order No. 227*. https://www.fws.gov/sites/default/files/documents/076566-USFWS-DO.pdf (accessed June 1, 2023).

Doubeni, C. A., M. Simon, and A. H. Krist. 2021. Addressing systemic racism through clinical preventive service recommendations from the U.S. Preventive Services Task Force. *JAMA* 325(7):627.

Dougherty, G. B., S. H. Golden, A. L. Gross, E. Colantuoni, and L. T. Dean. 2020. Measuring structural racism and its association with BMI. *American Journal of Epidemiology* 59(4):530–537.

Downs, J. 2012. *Sick from freedom: African-American illness and suffering during the CIVIL WAR and reconstruction*, 1st ed: Oxford University Press.

Downs, J. 2021. *Maladies of empire: How colonialism, slavery, and war transformed medicine*. Cambridge, MA: Harvard University Press.

Ely, D. M., and A. K. Driscoll. 2022. Infant mortality in the United States, 2020: Data from the period linked birth/infant death file. *National Vital Statistics Reports* 71(5):1-18.

English, D., C. A. Boone, J. A. Carter, A. J. Talan, D. R. Busby, R. L. Moody, D. J. Cunningham, L. Bowleg, and H. J. Rendina. 2022. Intersecting structural oppression and suicidality among Black sexual minority male adolescents and emerging adults. *Journal of Research on Adolescence* 32(1):226–243.

Equitable Data Working Group. 2022. *A vision for equitable data: Recommendations from the Equitable Data Working Group*. Washington, DC: The White House.

Erickson, S., K. Flannery, G. Leipertz, D. Wang, A. Small, N. Ly, A. Dominguez, and A. Echo-Hawk. 2021. *Data genocide of American Indians and Alaska Natives in COVID-19 data*. Seattle, WA.

Everett, B. G., and M. Agénor. 2023. Sexual orientation–related nondiscrimination laws and maternal hypertension among Black and White U.S. women. *Journal of Women's Health* 32(1):118–124.

Faircloth, S. C., C. M. Alcantar, and F. K. Stage. 2015. Use of large-scale data sets to study educational pathways of American Indian and Alaska Native students. *New Directions for Institutional Research* 2014(163):5–24.

Fernandez, J., M. García-Pérez, and S. Orozco-Aleman. 2023. Unraveling the Hispanic health paradox. *Journal of Economic Perspectives* 37(1):145–168.

FHWA (Federal Highway Administration). n.d. *What Is Title VI?* https://www.fhwa.dot.gov/civilrights/programs/docs/Title%20VI%20Basics.pdf (accessed March 8, 2023).

Fisher, L. D. 2017. "Why shall wee have peace to bee made slaves": Indian surrenderers during and after King Philip's War. *Ethnohistory* 64(1):91–114.

Flores, G. 2020. Language barriers and hospitalized children: Are we overlooking the most important risk factor for adverse events? *JAMA Pediatrics* 174(12):e203238.

Follis, S., K. Breathett, L. Garcia, M. Jimenez, C. W. Cené, E. Whitsel, H. Hedlin, E. D. Paskett, S. Zhang, C. A. Thomson, and M. L. Stefanick. 2023. Quantifying structural racism in cohort studies to advance prospective evidence. *SSM-Population Health* 22:101417.

Friedman, J., H. Hansen, and J. P. Gone. 2023. Deaths of despair and Indigenous data genocide. *The Lancet* 401:874–876.

Galinsky, A. M., C. Simile, C. E. Zelaya, T. Norris, and S. V. Panapasa. 2019. Surveying strategies for hard-to-survey populations: Lessons from the Native Hawaiian and Pacific Islander national health interview survey. *American Journal of Public Health* 109(10):13841391.

Gampa, V., K. Bernard, and M. J. Oldani. 2020. Racialization as a barrier to achieving health equity for Native Americans. *AMA Journal of Ethics* 22(10):E874–881.

GAO (Government Accountability Office). 2021. *Missing or murdered Indigenous women: New efforts are underway but opportunities exist to improve the federal response. GAO publication no. 22-104045.* Washington, DC: Government Accountability Office.

GAO. 2022. *THHS actions needed to enhance data access.* Washington, DC: United States Government Accountability Office.

GBD 2019 Police Violence U.S. Subnational Collaborators. 2021. Fatal police violence by race and state in the USA, 1980–2019: A network meta-regression. *The Lancet* 398(10307):1239–1255.

Gee, G. C., and C. L. Ford. 2011. Structural racism and health inequities. *Du Bois Review: Social Science Research on Race* 8(1):115–132.

Gee, G. C., and M. T. Hicken. 2021. Structural racism: The rules and relations of inequity. *Ethnicity & Disease* 31(Suppl):293–300.

Glynn, P., D. M. Lloyd-Jones, M. J. Feinstein, M. Carnethon, and S. S. Khan. 2019. Disparities in cardiovascular mortality related to heart failure in the United States. *Journal of the American College of Cardiology* 73(18):2354–2355.

GoFair. n.d. *Current Implementation Networks.* https://www.go-fair.org/implementation-networks/overview/ (accessed March 22, 2023).

Goldman, N., and T. Andrasfay. 2022. Life expectancy loss among Native Americans during the COVID-19 pandemic. *medRxiv.*

Greene, A. 2021. *What Is the Hawai'i Sovereignty Movement?* https://www.afar.com/magazine/understanding-the-hawaii-sovereignty-movement (accessed June 1, 2023).

Greenfield, B. L., J. H. L. Elm, and K. A. Hallgren. 2021. Understanding measures of racial discrimination and microaggressions among American Indian and Alaska Native college students in the southwest United States. *BMC Public Health* 21(1).

Gregory, J. F. 1995. The crime of punishment: Racial and gender disparities in the use of corporal punishment in U.S. public schools. *The Journal of Negro Education* 64(4):454.

Gulley, S. P., E. K. Rasch, and L. Chan. 2014. Difference, disparity, and disability: A comparison of health, insurance coverage, and health service use on the basis of race/ethnicity among U.S. adults with disabilities, 2006–2008. *Medical Care* 52(10 Suppl 3):S9–S16.

Gunja, M., E. Gumas, and R. Williams, II. 2023. *U.S. health care from a global perspective, 2022: Accelerating spending, worsening outcomes.* New York, NY: Commonwealth Fund.

Hales, C. M., Margaret D. Carroll, Cheryl D. Fryar, and C. L. Ogden. 2020. *Prevalence of obesity and severe obesity among adults: United States, 2017–2018.* Atlanta, GA: CDC.

Haozous, E. A., C. J. Strickland, J. F. Palacios, and T. G. Solomon. 2014. Blood politics, ethnic identity, and racial misclassification among American Indians and Alaska Natives. *Journal of Environmental and Public Health* 2014:321604.

Hardeman, R. R., P. A. Homan, T. Chantarat, B. A. Davis, and T. H. Brown. 2022. Improving the measurement of structural racism to achieve antiracist health policy. *Health Affairs* 41(2):179–186.

Hatcher, S. M., C. Agnew-Brune, M. Anderson, L. D. Zambrano, C. E. Rose, M. A. Jim, A. Baugher, G. S. Liu, S. V. Patel, M. E. Evans, T. Pindyck, C. L. Dubray, J. J. Rainey, J. Chen, C. Sadowski, K. Winglee, A. Penman-Aguilar, A. Dixit, E. Claw, C. Parshall, E. Provost, A. Ayala, G. Gonzalez, J. Ritchey, J. Davis, V. Warren-Mears, S. Joshi, T. Weiser, A. Echo-Hawk, A. Dominguez, A. Poel, C. Duke, I. Ransby, A. Apostolou, and J. McCollum. 2020. COVID-19 among American Indian and Alaska Native persons—23 states, January 31–July 3, 2020. *Morbidity and Mortality Weekly Report*(69):1166–1169.

Hatzenbuehler, M. L., J. C. Phelan, and B. G. Link. 2013. Stigma as a fundamental cause of population health inequalities. *American Journal of Epidemiology* 103(5):813–821.

Heisler, E. J., and K. P. McClanahan. 2020. *Advance appropriations for the Indian Health Service: Issues and options for Congress.* Washington, DC: Congressional Research Service.

Higginbotham, A. L., Jr. 1974. Review of race, racism and American law by Derrick A. Bell, Jr. *University of Pennsylvania Law Review* 122(4):1044–1069.

Hill, L., S. Artiga, and U. Ranji. 2022. *Racial disparities in maternal and infant health: Current status and efforts to address them.* Washington, DC: Kaiser Family Foundation.

HIV.gov. 2023. *What Is the Impact of HIV on Racial and Ethnic Minorities in the U.S.?* https://www.hiv.gov/hiv-basics/overview/data-and-trends/impact-on-racial-and-ethnic-minorities/ (accessed March 10, 2023).

Hogarth, R. A. 2019. The myth of innate racial differences between White and Black people's bodies: Lessons from the 1793 yellow fever epidemic in Philadelphia, Pennsylvania. *American Journal of Epidemiology* 109(10):1339–1341.

Holland, A. T., and L. P. Palaniappan. 2012. Problems with the collection and interpretation of Asian-American health data: Omission, aggregation, and extrapolation. *Annals of Epidemiology* 22(6):397–405.

Hoyert, D. L. 2022. *Maternal mortality rates in the United States, 2020.* Atlanta, GA: National Center for Health Statistics, Centers for Disease Control and Prevention.

Hudson, K. D., and M. Romanelli. 2020. "We are powerful people": Health-promoting strengths of LGBTQ communities of color. *Qualitative Health Research* 30(8):1156–1170.

Hutchinson, R. N., and S. Shin. 2014. Systematic review of health disparities for cardiovascular diseases and associated factors among American Indian and Alaska Native populations. *PLOS ONE* 9(1):e80973.

IHS (Indian Health Service). 2014. *Trends in Indian health: 2014 edition.* Washington, DC: Indian Health Service.

IOM (Institute of Medicine). 2003. *Unequal treatment: Confronting racial and ethnic disparities in health care.* Washington, DC: The National Academies Press.

IOM. 2009. *Race, ethnicity, and language data: Standardization for health care quality improvement.* Washington, DC: The National Academies Press.

IOM. 2011. *The health of lesbian, gay, bisexual, and transgender people: Building a foundation for better understanding.* Washington, DC: The National Academies Press.

Islam, N. S., S. Khan, S. Kwon, D. Jang, M. Ro, and C. Trinh-Shevrin. 2010. Methodological issues in the collection, analysis, and reporting of granular data in Asian American populations: Historical challenges and potential solutions. *Journal of Health Care for the Poor and Underserved* 21(4):1354–1381.

Isong, I. A., S. R. Rao, M.-A. Bind, M. Avendaño, I. Kawachi, and T. K. Richmond. 2018. Racial and ethnic disparities in early childhood obesity. *Pediatrics* 141(1).

James, C. V., R. Moonesinghe, S. M. Wilson-Frederick, J. E. Hall, A. Penman-Aguilar, and
K. Bouye. 2017. Racial/ethnic health disparities among rural adults—United States,
2012–2015. *Morbidity and Mortality Weekly Report Surveillance Summaries* 66(23):1.

Javed, Z., M. Haisum Maqsood, T. Yahya, Z. Amin, I. Acquah, J. Valero-Elizondo, J. Andrieni,
P. Dubey, R. K. Jackson, M. A. Daffin, M. Cainzos-Achirica, A. A. Hyder, and K. Nasir.
2022. Race, racism, and cardiovascular health: Applying a social determinants of health
framework to racial/ethnic disparities in cardiovascular disease. *Circulation: Cardiovascular Quality and Outcomes* 15(1):e007917.

Johnson, P. J., K. T. Call, and L. A. Blewett. 2010. The importance of geographic data aggregation in assessing disparities in American Indian prenatal care. *American Journal of Public Health* 100(1):122–128.

Joint Commission. 2023. *R3 Report Issue 36: New Requirements to Reduce Health Care Disparities.* https://www.jointcommission.org/standards/r3-report/r3-report-issue-36-new-requirements-to-reduce-health-care-disparities/#.ZAliTHbMKUk (accessed March 8, 2023).

Jost, T. S. 2022. *Federal Judge Eliminates the CDC'S Public Transportation Mask Mandate.* https://www.commonwealthfund.org/blog/2022/federal-judge-eliminates-cdcs-public-transportation-mask-mandate (accessed March 11, 2023).

Kanaʻiaupuni, S. M., and N. Malone. 2006. This land is my land: The role of place in Native Hawaiian identity. *Hūlili: Multidisciplinary Research on Hawaiian Well-Being* 3(1):281–307.

Kettl, D. F. 2021. *How American-Style Federalism Is Hazardous to Our Health.* https://www.governing.com/now/how-american-style-federalism-is-dangerous-to-our-health (accessed March 11, 2023).

Kim, J. H. J., Q. Lu, and A. L. Stanton. 2021. Overcoming constraints of the model minority stereotype to advance Asian American health. *American Psychologist* 76(4):611–626.

Kissam, S. M., H. Beil, C. Cousart, L. M. Greenwald, and J. T. Lloyd. 2019. States encouraging value-based payment: Lessons from CMS's state innovation models initiative. *The Milbank Quarterly* 97(2):506–542.

Knight, H. E., S. R. Deeny, K. Dreyer, J. Engmann, M. Mackintosh, S. Raza, M. Stafford, R. Tesfaye, and A. Steventon. 2021. Challenging racism in the use of health data. *The Lancet Digital Health* 3(3):e144–e146.

Komro, K., R. O'Mara, and A. C. Wagenaar. 2012. Mechanisms of legal effect: Perspectives from public health: A methods monograph. *Public Health Law Research Methods Monograph Series.*

Krieger, N. 2020. Measures of racism, sexism, heterosexism, and gender binarism for health equity research: From structural injustice to embodied harm—an ecosocial analysis. *Annual Review of Public Health* 41:37–62.

Krieger, N., J. T. Chen, B. Coull, P. D. Waterman, and J. Beckfield. 2013. The unique impact of abolition of Jim Crow laws on reducing inequities in infant death rates and implications for choice of comparison groups in analyzing societal determinants of health. *American Journal of Public Health* 103(12):2234–2244.

Krieger, N., J. T. Chen, B. A. Coull, J. Beckfield, M. V. Kiang, and P. D. Waterman. 2014. Jim Crow and premature mortality among the U.S. Black and White population, 1960–2009: An age-period-cohort analysis. *Epidemiology* 25(4):494–504.

Krieger, N., P. D. Waterman, J. Spasojevic, W. Li, G. Maduro, and G. Van Wye. 2016. Public health monitoring of privilege and deprivation with the index of concentration at the extremes. *American Journal of Public Health* 106(2):256–263.

Krieger, N., J. M. Feldman, P. D. Waterman, J. T. Chen, B. A. Coull, and D. Hemenway. 2017a. Local residential segregation matters: Stronger association of census tract compared to conventional city-level measures with fatal and non-fatal assaults (total and firearm related), using the index of concentration at the extremes (ICE) for racial, economic, and racialized economic segregation, Massachusetts (U.S.), 1995–2010. *Journal of Urban Health* 94(2):244–258.

Krieger, N., J. L. Jahn, and P. D. Waterman. 2017b. Jim Crow and estrogen-receptor-negative breast cancer: U.S.-born black and white non-Hispanic women, 1992–2012. *Cancer Causes & Control* 28(1):49–59.

Lagu, T., C. Haywood, K. Reimold, C. DeJong, R. Walker Sterling, and L. I. Iezzoni. 2022. "I am not the doctor for you": Physicians' attitudes about caring for people with disabilities: Study examines physician attitudes about caring for people with disabilities. *Health Affairs* 41(10):1387–1395.

Library of Congress. n.d. *Immigration and Relocation in U.S. History*. https://www.loc.gov/classroom-materials/immigration/african/ (accessed March 11, 2023).

Locher, J. L., C. S. Ritchie, D. L. Roth, P. S. Baker, E. V. Bodner, and R. M. Allman. 2005. Social isolation, support, and capital and nutritional risk in an older sample: Ethnic and gender differences. *Social Science & Medicine* 60(4):747–761.

Lucchei, A., and A. Echo-Hawk. 2018. *Missing and murdered Indigenous women and girls*. Seattle, WA: Urban Indian Health Institute.

Lukachko, A., M. L. Hatzenbuehler, and K. M. Keyes. 2014. Structural racism and myocardial infarction in the United States. *Social Science & Medicine* 103:42–50.

Maltz, E. M. 1992. Slavery, federalism, and the structure of the Constitution. *American Journal of Legal History* 36(4):466–498.

March of Dimes. 2022. Prenatal Care. https://www.marchofdimes.org/peristats/data?reg=99&top=5&stop=24&lev=1&slev=1&obj=1 (accessed July 5, 2023).

Mazimba, S., and P. N. Peterson. 2021. JAHA spotlight on racial and ethnic disparities in cardiovascular disease. *Journal of the American Heart Association* 10(17):e023650.

McIver, L. 2022. *CMS framework for health equity 2022–2032*. Baltimore, MD: Centers for Medicare & Medicaid Services.

Mervis, J. 2019. *Study Identifies a Key Reason Black Scientists Are Less Likely to Receive NIH Funding*. https://www.science.org/content/article/study-identifies-key-reason-black-scientists-are-less-likely-receive-nih-funding (accessed June 9, 2023).

Mesic, A., L. Franklin, A. Cansever, F. Potter, A. Sharma, A. Knopov, and M. Siegel. 2018. The relationship between structural racism and black–white disparities in fatal police shootings at the state level. *Journal of the National Medical Association* 110(2):106–116.

Min, J., H. Goodale, H. Xue, R. Brey, and Y. Wang. 2021. Racial-ethnic disparities in obesity and biological, behavioral, and sociocultural influences in the United States: A systematic review. *Advances in Nutrition* 12(4):1137–1148.

Morgan, E. H., R. Rodgers, and J. Tschida. 2022. Addressing the intersectionality of race and disability to improve autism care. *Pediatrics* 149(Supplement 4).

Morris, M. 2016. *Pushout: The criminalization of Black girls in schools*. New York, NY: The New Press.

Moss, M. 2019. *Trauma Lives on in Native Americans by Making Us Sick—While the U.S. Looks Away*. https://www.theguardian.com/commentisfree/2019/may/09/trauma-lives-on-in-native-americans-while-the-us-looks-away (accessed March 6, 2023).

Musumeci, M., and K. Orgera. 2021. *Supplemental Security Income for people with disabilities: Implications for Medicaid*. Washington, DC: Kaiser Family Foundation.

NAACP (National Association for the Advancement of Colored People). 2014. *Born suspect: Stop-and-frisk abuses and the continued fight to end racial profiling*. Washington, DC: National Association for the Advancement of Colored People.

NASEM (National Academies of Sciences, Engineering, and Medicine). 2015. *The integration of immigrants into American society*. Washington, DC: The National Academies Press.

NASEM. 2017. *Communities in action: Pathways to health equity*. Washington, DC: The National Academies Press.

NASEM. 2018a. *Achieving rural health equity and well-being: Proceedings of a workshop*. Washington, DC: The National Academies Press.

NASEM. 2018b. *Immigration as a social determinant of health: Proceedings of a workshop.* Washington, DC: The National Academies Press.

NASEM. 2019. *Vibrant and healthy kids: Aligning science, practice, and policy to advance health equity.* Washington, DC: The National Academies Press.

NASEM. 2020a. *Addressing sickle cell disease: A strategic plan and blueprint for action.* Washington, DC: The National Academies Press.

NASEM. 2020b. *Understanding the well-being of LGBTQI+ populations.* Washington, DC: The National Academies Press.

NASEM. 2021a. *Advancing maternal health equity and reducing maternal morbidity and mortality: Proceedings of a workshop.* Washington, DC: The National Academies Press.

NASEM. 2021b. *Population health in rural America in 2020: Proceedings of a workshop.* Washington, DC: The National Academies Press.

NASEM. 2021c. *Sexually transmitted infections: Adopting a sexual health paradigm.* Washington, DC: The National Academies Press.

NASEM. 2022a. *Engaging communities in addressing structural drivers of obesity: Proceedings of a workshop—in brief.* Washington, DC: The National Academies Press.

NASEM. 2022b. *Improving representation in clinical trials and research: Building research equity for women and underrepresented groups.* Washington, DC: The National Academies Press.

NASEM. 2023. *Using population descriptors in genetics and genomics research: A new framework for an evolving field.* Washington, DC: The National Academies Press.

Nation of Hawai'i. n.d. *Restoring the Ahupua'a: Waimānalo Stream, from Mountain to Ocean.* https://www.nationofhawaii.org/ (accessed June 9, 2023).

National Disability Institute. 2020. *Race, health, and disability.* Washington, DC: National Disability Institute.

Nayak, A., A. J. Hicks, and A. A. Morris. 2020. Understanding the complexity of heart failure risk and treatment in Black patients. *Circulation: Heart Failure* 13(8):e007264.

NCAI (National Congress of American Indians). 2021. *NCAI Policy Research Center: Improving Outcomes for Indian Country with Research.* https://www.ncai.org/policy-research-center/research-data/data (accessed June 9, 2023).

NCAI. n.d. *Tribal Governance.* https://www.ncai.org/policy-issues/tribal-governance#:~:text=Tribal%20governments%20are%20an%20important,the%20authority%20to%20self%2Dgovern. (accessed March 11, 2023).

NCQA (National Committee for Quality Assurance). 2021a. *Federal action is needed to improve race and ethnicity data in health programs.* Washington, DC: National Committee for Quality Assurance.

NCQA. 2021b. *HEDIS 2022: See What's New, What's Changed and What's Retired.* https://www.ncqa.org/blog/hedis-2022-see-whats-new-whats-changed-and-whats-retired/ (accessed March 11, 2023).

NGA (National Governors Association). 2018. *Principles for State–Federal Relations.* https://www.nga.org/advocacy-communications/policy-positions/principles-for-state-federal-relations/ (accessed March 8, 2023).

Nguyen, K. H., K. P. Lew, and A. N. Trivedi. 2022. Trends in collection of disaggregated Asian American, Native Hawaiian, and Pacific Islander data: Opportunities in federal health surveys. *American Journal of Public Health* 112(10):1429–1435.

NIH (National Institutes of Health). 2022. *Life Expectancy in the U.S. Increased Between 2000–2019, But Widespread Gaps Among Racial and Ethnic Groups Exist.* https://www.nih.gov/news-events/news-releases/life-expectancy-us-increased-between-2000-2019-widespread-gaps-among-racial-ethnic-groups-exist#:~:text=In%202019%2C%20overall%20life%20expectancy,73.1%20for%20the%20AIAN%20population (accessed March 11, 2023).

NYCLU (New York Civil Liberties Union). 2019. *Stop-and-frisk in the De Blasio era.* New York, NY: New York Civil Liberties Union.

OMB (Office of Management and Budget). 1997. Revisions to the standards for the classification of federal data on race and ethnicity. *Federal Register* 62(210):58782–58790.

OMH (Office of Minority Health). 2021a. *Explanation of Data Standards for Race, Ethnicity, Sex, Primary Language, and Disability.* https://minorityhealth.hhs.gov/omh/browse. aspx?lvl=3&lvlid=54 (accessed March 11, 2023).

OMH. 2021b. *Heart Disease and Native Hawaiians/Pacific Islanders.* https://minorityhealth. hhs.gov/omh/browse.aspx?lvl=4&lvlid=79 (accessed March 11, 2023).

Pacheco, A. 2005. *Past, Present, and Politics: A Look at the Native Hawaiian Sovereignty Movement.* Senior thesis, Pacheco, A. Seattle, WA: University of Washington. https:// digital.lib.washington.edu/researchworks/handle/1773/2262 (accessed June 9, 2023).

Pager, D., and H. Shepherd. 2008. The sociology of discrimination: Racial discrimination in employment, housing, credit, and consumer markets. *Annual Review of Sociology* 34:181–209.

Pan, L., D. S. Freedman, A. J. Sharma, K. Castellanos-Brown, S. Park, R. B. Smith, and H. M. Blanck. 2016. Trends in obesity among participants aged 2–4 years in the Special Supplemental Nutrition Program for Women, Infants, and Children—United States, 2000–2014. *Morbidity and Mortality Weekly Report* 65(45):1256–1260.

Panapasa, S. V., K. M. Crabbe, and J. K. Kaholokula. 2011. Efficacy of federal data: Revised Office of Management and Budget standard for Native Hawaiian and Other Pacific Islanders examined. *AAPI Nexus* 9(1–2):212–220.

Patterson, K. B., and T. Runge. 2002. Smallpox and the Native American. *American Journal of Public Health* 323(4):216–222.

Pepin, D., and S. B. Weber. 2019. Civil rights law and the determinants of health: How some states have utilized civil rights laws to increase protections against discrimination. *The Journal of Law, Medicine & Ethics* 47(2_suppl):76–79.

Petersen, E. E., N. L. Davis, D. Goodman, S. Cox, C. Syverson, K. Seed, C. Shapiro-Mendoza, W. M. Callaghan, and W. Barfield. 2019. Racial/ethnic disparities in pregnancy-related deaths—United States, 2007–2016. *Morbidity and Mortality Weekly Report* 68(35):762.

Peterson-Besse, J. J., E. S. Walsh, W. Horner-Johnson, T. D. Goode, and B. Wheeler. 2014. Barriers to health care among people with disabilities who are members of underserved racial/ethnic groups: A scoping review of the literature. *Medical Care:*S51–S63.

Poteat, T., S. L. Reisner, and A. Radix. 2014. HIV epidemics among transgender women. *Current Opinion in HIV and AIDS* 9(2):168–173.

Probst, J. C., W. E. Zahnd, P. Hung, J. M. Eberth, E. L. Crouch, and M. A. Merrell. 2020. Rural–urban mortality disparities: Variations across causes of death and race/ethnicity, 2013–2017. *American Journal of Public Health* 110(9):1325–1327.

Rai, S. 2021. *University of Florida Researchers Pressured to Destroy COVID-19 data, Told Not to Criticize DeSantis: Report.* https://thehill.com/homenews/state-watch/584909-university-of-florida-researchers-pressured-to-destroy-covid-19-data/ (accessed June 9, 2023).

Riddle, T., and S. Sinclair. 2019. Racial disparities in school-based disciplinary actions are associated with county-level rates of racial bias. *Proceedings of the National Academy of Sciences* 116(17):8255–8260.

Ritzer, G., and J. Stepnisky. 2022. *Contemporary sociological theory and its classical roots: The basics,* 6th ed. Los Angeles, CA: Sage Publications.

Rodríguez, S. T. 2021. *Three steps to improving data to help combat the public health emergency of structural racism.* Washington, DC: Urban Institute.

Romanello, M., C. Di Napoli, P. Drummond, C. Green, H. Kennard, P. Lampard, D. Scamman, N. Arnell, S. Ayeb-Karlsson, L. B. Ford, K. Belesova, K. Bowen, W. Cai, M. Callaghan, D. Campbell-Lendrum, J. Chambers, K. R. van Daalen, C. Dalin, N. Dasandi, S. Dasgupta, M. Davies, P. Dominguez-Salas, R. Dubrow, K. L. Ebi, M. Eckelman, P. Ekins, L. E. Escobar, L. Georgeson, H. Graham, S. H. Gunther, I. Hamilton, Y. Hang, R. Hänninen, S. Hartinger, K. He, J. J. Hess, S.-C. Hsu, S. Jankin, L. Jamart, O. Jay, I. Kelman, G. Kiesewetter, P. Kinney, T. Kjellstrom, D. Kniveton, J. K. W. Lee, B. Lemke, Y. Liu, Z. Liu, M. Lott, M. L. Batista, R. Lowe, F. MacGuire, M. O. Sewe, J. Martinez-Urtaza, M. Maslin, L. McAllister, A. McGushin, C. McMichael, Z. Mi, J. Milner, K. Minor, J. C. Minx, N. Mohajeri, M. Moradi-Lakeh, K. Morrissey, S. Munzert, K. A. Murray, T. Neville, M. Nilsson, N. Obradovich, M. B. O'Hare, T. Oreszczyn, M. Otto, F. Owfi, O. Pearman, M. Rabbaniha, E. J. Z. Robinson, J. Rocklöv, R. N. Salas, J. C. Semenza, J. D. Sherman, L. Shi, J. Shumake-Guillemot, G. Silbert, M. Sofiev, M. Springmann, J. Stowell, M. Tabatabaei, J. Taylor, J. Triñanes, F. Wagner, P. Wilkinson, M. Winning, M. Yglesias-González, S. Zhang, P. Gong, H. Montgomery, and A. Costello. 2022. The 2022 report of the Lancet countdown on health and climate change: Health at the mercy of fossil fuels. *The Lancet* 400(10363):1619–1654.

Rosay, A. B. 2016. Violence against American Indian and Alaska Native women and men. National Institute of Justice. *National Institute of Justice Journal* 277:38–45.

Rubin, V., D. Ngo, Á. Ross, D. Butler, and N. Balaram. 2018. *Counting a diverse nation: Disaggregating data on race and ethnicity to advance a culture of health.* Oakland, CA: Policy Link.

Rugh, J. S., and D. S. Massey. 2010. Racial segregation and the American foreclosure crisis. *American Sociological Review* 75(5):629–651.

Schwartz, M. A. 2023. *The 574 federally recognized Indian tribes in the United States.* Washington, DC: Congressional Research Service.

Schwartz, L. M., S. Woloshin, and H. G. Welch. 1999. Misunderstandings about the effects of race and sex on physicians' referrals for cardiac catheterization. *The New England Journal of Medicine* 341(4):279–283; discussion 286–277.

Sewell, A. A., and K. A. Jefferson. 2016. Collateral damage: The health effects of invasive police encounters in New York City. *Journal of Urban Health* 93(S1):42–67.

Shah, N. S., and N. R. Kandula. 2020. Addressing Asian American misrepresentation and underrepresentation in research. *Ethnicity & Disease* 30(3):513–516.

Siegel, M., M. Rieders, H. Rieders, J. Moumneh, J. Asfour, J. Oh, and S. Oh. 2022. Measuring structural racism and its association with racial disparities in firearm homicide. *Journal of Racial and Ethnic Health Disparities* [Epub ahead of print]:1–16.

Singh, G. K., M. Siahpush, R. E. Azuine, and S. D. Williams. 2015. Widening socioeconomic and racial disparities in cardiovascular disease mortality in the United States, 1969–2013. *International Journal of Maternal and Child Health and AIDS* 3(2):106–118.

Siordia, C., R. A. Bell, and S. L. Haileselassie. 2017. Prevalence and risk for negative disability outcomes between American Indians-Alaskan Natives and other race-ethnic groups in the southwestern United States. *Journal of Racial and Ethnic Health Disparities* 4(2):195–200.

SSA (Social Security Administration). 2022. *Annual Report of the Supplemental Security Income Program.* https://www.ssa.gov/OACT/ssir/SSI22/ssi2022.pdf (accessed July 5, 2023).

SSA. 2023. *Supplemental Security Income (SSI) for Noncitizens.* https://www.ssa.gov/pubs/EN-05-11051.pdf (accessed March 17, 2023).

SSA. n.d. *Supplemental Security Income (SSI).* https://www.ssa.gov/ssi/text-income-ussi.htm (accessed March 17, 2023).

Stennett, D. 2021. DeSantis refuses new state eviction moratorium, but CDC extends federal ban for 2 months. *Orlando Sentinel* (August 4).

Tamir, C. 2022. *Key findings about Black immigrants in the U.S.* Washington, DC: Pew Research Center.

Torpy, S. J. 2000. Native American women and coerced sterilization: On the Trail of Tears in the 1970s. *American Indian Culture and Research Journal* 24(2):1–22.

Trost, S., J. Beauregard, G. Chandra, F. Njie, J. Berry, A. Harvey, and D. A. Goodman. 2022. *Pregnancy-related deaths: Data from maternal mortality review committees in 36 U.S. states, 2017–2019.* Atlanta, GA: Centers for Disease Control and Prevention.

UN (United Nations). 1948. *The Convention on the Prevention and Punishment of the Crime of Genocide.* https://www.un.org/en/genocideprevention/documents/Genocide%20Convention-FactSheet-ENG.pdf (accessed March 11, 2023).

United States Code. 2011 Edition. *25 U.S.C., Title 25—Indians.* https://www.govinfo.gov/content/pkg/USCODE-2011-title25/html/USCODE-2011-title25.htm (accessed March 11, 2023).

United States Senate. n.d. *Freedmen's Bureau Acts of 1865 and 1866.* https://www.senate.gov/artandhistory/history/common/generic/FreedmensBureau.htm (accessed March 11, 2023).

University of Minnesota. n.d. *U.S.–Dakota War of 1862.* https://cla.umn.edu/chgs/holocaust-genocide-education/resource-guides/us-dakota-war-1862 (accessed March 11, 2023).

Urban Indian Health Institute. 2018. *Our bodies, our stories.* Seattle, WA: Urban Indian Health Institute.

Urban Indian Health Institute. 2020. *Best Practices for American Indian and Alaska Native Data Collection.* https://www.uihi.org/resources/best-practices-for-american-indian-and-alaska-native-data-collection/ (accessed June 9, 2023).

U.S. Commission on Civil Rights. 2018. *Broken promises: Continuing federal funding shortfall for Native Americans.* Washington, DC: U.S. Commission on Civil Rights.

USDA (United States Department of Agriculture). 2022. *Rural Poverty & Well-Being.* https://www.ers.usda.gov/topics/rural-economy-population/rural-poverty-well-being/ (accessed March 17, 2023).

USPSTF (United States Preventive Services Task Force). 2019. *Congressional mandate establishing the U.S. Preventive Services Task Force.* Rockville, MD: U.S. Preventive Services Task Force.

Varadaraj, V., J. A. Deal, J. Campanile, N. S. Reed, and B. K. Swenor. 2021. National prevalence of disability and disability types among adults in the U.S., 2019. *JAMA Network Open* 4(10):e2130358.

Viruell-Fuentes, E. A., P. Y. Miranda, and S. Abdulrahim. 2012. More than culture: Structural racism, intersectionality theory, and immigrant health. *Social Science & Medicine* 75(12):2099–2106.

Vleet, A. V., and J. Paradise. 2014. *The State Innovation Models (SIM) program: An overview.* Washington, DC: KFF.

Wallace, M. E., P. Mendola, D. Liu, and K. L. Grantz. 2015. Joint effects of structural racism and income inequality on small-for-gestational-age birth. *American Journal of Public Health* 105(8):1681–1688.

The White House. 2021. *Executive order on advancing racial equity and support for underserved communities through the federal government.* https://www.whitehouse.gov/briefing-room/presidential-actions/2021/01/20/executive-order-advancing-racial-equity-and-support-for-underserved-communities-through-the-federal-government/ (accessed March 17, 2023).

The White House. 2022. *The Release of the Equitable Data Working Group Report.* https://www.whitehouse.gov/ostp/news-updates/2022/04/22/the-release-of-the-equitable-data-working-group-report/ (accessed June 9, 2023).

WHO (World Health Organization). 2021. *Gender and Health.* https://www.who.int/news-room/questions-and-answers/item/gender-and-health (accessed March 22, 2023).

Wilkinson, M. D., M. Dumontier, I. J. Aalbersberg, G. Appleton, M. Axton, A. Baak, N. Blomberg, J.-W. Boiten, L. B. Da Silva Santos, P. E. Bourne, J. Bouwman, A. J. Brookes, T. Clark, M. Crosas, I. Dillo, O. Dumon, S. Edmunds, C. T. Evelo, R. Finkers, A. Gonzalez-Beltran, A. J. G. Gray, P. Groth, C. Goble, J. S. Grethe, J. Heringa, P. A. C. 'T Hoen, R. Hooft, T. Kuhn, R. Kok, J. Kok, S. J. Lusher, M. E. Martone, A. Mons, A. L. Packer, B. Persson, P. Rocca-Serra, M. Roos, R. Van Schaik, S.-A. Sansone, E. Schultes, T. Sengstag, T. Slater, G. Strawn, M. A. Swertz, M. Thompson, J. Van Der Lei, E. Van Mulligen, J. Velterop, A. Waagmeester, P. Wittenburg, K. Wolstencroft, J. Zhao, and B. Mons. 2016. The FAIR guiding principles for scientific data management and stewardship. *Scientific Data* 3(1):160018.

Williams, D. R. 1999. Race, socioeconomic status, and health. The added effects of racism and discrimination. *Annals of the New York Academy of Sciences* 896(1):173–188.

Williams, D. R. 2016. *Measuring Discrimination Resource.* https://scholar.harvard.edu/files/davidrwilliams/files/measuring_discrimination_resource_june_2016.pdf (accessed March 8, 2023).

Williams, D. R., and C. Collins. 2001. Racial residential segregation: A fundamental cause of racial disparities in health. *Public Health Reports* 116(5):404–416.

Williams, D. R., and J. S. Jackson. 2000. Race/ethnicity and the 2000 census: Recommendations for African American and other Black populations in the United States. *American Journal of Public Health* 90(11):1728.

Williams, D. R., Y. Yan, J. S. Jackson, and N. B. Anderson. 1997. Racial differences in physical and mental health. *Journal of Health Psychology* 2(3):335–351.

Williams, D. R., N. Priest, and N. Anderson. 2016. Understanding associations between race, socioeconomic status and health: Patterns and prospects. *Health Psychology* 35(4):407–411.

Williams, D. R., J. A. Lawrence, and B. A. Davis. 2019. Racism and health: Evidence and needed research. *Annual Review of Public Health* 40:105–125.

Wiltz, T. 2014. *Counting Americans of Middle Eastern, North African descent.* Washington, DC: Pew Research Center.

Wolfe, P. 1999. *Settler colonialism and the transformation of anthropology: The politics and poetics of an ethnographic event.* New York, NY: Cassell.

Wu, S., and A. Bakos. 2017. The Native Hawaiian and Pacific Islander national health interview survey: Data collection in small populations. *Public Health Reports* 132(6):606–608.

Yom, S., and M. Lor. 2022. Advancing health disparities research: The need to include Asian American subgroup populations. *Journal of Racial and Ethnic Health Disparities* 9(6):2248–2282.

Zambrana, E., G. Amaro, C. Butler, M. DuPont-Reyes, and D. Parra-Medina. 2021. Analysis of Latina/o sociodemographic and health data sets in the United States from 1960 to 2019: Findings suggest improvements to future data collection efforts. *Health Education & Behavior* 48(3):320–331.

3

Economic Stability

INTRODUCTION

Economic stability is inextricably connected to physical and mental health. As one of the five social determinants of health (SDOH) categories, economic stability is broad and includes employment and income,[1] noncash benefits, such as Special Supplemental Nutrition Program for Women, Infants, and Children (WIC) and Supplemental Nutrition Assistance Program (SNAP), wealth,[2] and financial services, such as banking and credit scoring. Economic stability enables access to other SDOH, such as food security, housing stability, safe and healthy neighborhoods (see Chapter 6), education (Chapter 4), and social capital (Chapter 7). Access to these health-protective resources and conditions is one mechanism tying economic stability to health outcomes. Additionally, economic stability enables access to quality health care, which directly impacts health outcomes (see Chapter 5) (NASEM, 2017). Healthy People 2030 recognizes

---

[1] Income is "the amount of money earned in a single year from employment, government assistance, retirement and pension payments, and interest or dividends from investments or other assets" (NASEM, 2017, p. 118).

[2] Wealth can be understood as "economic assets accumulated over time" and calculated by taking assets, such as houses, land, cars, savings accounts, pension plans, stocks and other financial investments, and businesses, and subtracting debts and liabilities. Wealth can provide a more holistic understanding of financial resources than income. The intergenerational aspect of wealth is a critical component of being able to access wealth and particularly important in this context (NASEM, 2017, p. 118).

the impact of economic stability on health outcomes and considers how it can be affected by factors such as illness and disability (HHS, 2020). Although this chapter is titled "Economic Stability," the committee recognizes that enabling all people to thrive economically, rather than just achieve stability, is needed to advance equity and create a sustainable path to well-being.

Progress has been made toward improving the economic stability of U.S. households in recent decades. Median household incomes have been growing, and poverty rates have been decreasing (Creamer et al., 2022; Semega and Kollar, 2022; Wimer et al., 2022). On the other hand, median household wealth, an important source of protection against economic and health shocks, has been stagnant in recent decades (Horowitz et al., 2020). Additionally, millions of people still live in poverty despite progress made, and poverty is disproportionately experienced by racially and ethnically minoritized populations and tribal communities (KFF, n.d.; Krogstad, 2014). Racial, ethnic, and tribal inequities also exist in income and employment, wealth, and financial services, such as banking and credit scoring. These inequities stem in part from the legacy of structural racism and policies, such as redlining, territorial dispossession, and the disparate access to benefits of the 1944 GI Bill, that have harmed racially and ethnically minoritized and tribal populations. This chapter reviews these areas as opportunities for federal policy to be leveraged to improve economic stability for these populations and in turn advance health equity. Specifically, the chapter explores the following: the effect of incarceration and pretrial detention on income and wealth; the federal minimum wage; how administrative barriers and eligibility restrictions impact participation in federal social benefit programs; how nonprofit sector partnerships can play a role in poverty alleviation and emergency food assistance; the role of past policies, such as redlining and disparate access to benefits from the 1944 GI Bill, on inequities; policies to support savings and wealth accumulation, such as baby bonds; and access to safe and affordable banking services, such as bank accounts and low-cost credit. These examples include both policies that have intentionally perpetuated inequities (i.e., redlining) and policies that promote equity and can be improved for greater success (i.e., federal social benefit programs whose reach can be expanded by eliminating or reconsidering administrative barriers and eligibility restrictions). See Chapter 1 for an overview of the committee's process for selecting the policies reviewed in this report.

This chapter is unable to report on the Native Hawaiian and Pacific Islander (NHPI) population specifically due to the absence of data, rendering them invisible in this discussion. Additionally, data aggregation masks differences between NHPI and Asian people. Similarly, there is a lack of data, and in some cases inaccurate data, for American Indian and Alaska Native (AIAN) populations, masking the extent of the challenges faced by these communities (see Chapter 2 for more details). The frontmatter of this report includes a list of the committee's chosen terminology for the racial and ethnic groups discussed therein. However, sometimes the terms used in the report are determined by the language in data systems or a specific research study referred to or summarized. Although the committee chose to use "Latino/a" to refer to persons with cultural connections to Latin America, "Hispanic" appears frequently in this chapter due to its use in many of the research studies to which the chapter refers.

INCOME AND EMPLOYMENT

Income is associated with health outcomes across the life span, with higher income consistently predictive of better health. Babies born to low-income families have higher infant mortality compared to middle and higher income families. They also have lower birthweights compared to middle income families (Kennedy-Moulton et al., 2022). Lower-income adults die on average at earlier ages, and the gap in life expectancy has been growing in recent decades (NASEM, 2015). In between, there are gaps across income levels in access to health care services and differences in behavior, stress, and other factors that contribute to health inequities (Garfield et al., 2020; NASEM, 2017). When individuals are asked to assess their health status, lower-income individuals report worse health than higher-income individuals report (Schanzenbach et al., 2016b). Substantial evidence indicates that increasing incomes can improve health outcomes (Finkelstein et al., 2022). Those with more resources can invest in opportunities for health improvement, including medical care, housing and neighborhood amenities that promote good health, and other important determinants of health.

Income and race are correlated, with White and Asian people consistently having higher incomes than Black, Hispanic, and AIAN people (Semega and Kollar, 2022). Figure 3-1 shows 2021 Census data for mean and median household incomes by the reported race or ethnicity of the householder. The median for White households was just over $74,000, compared to just over $48,000 for Black households, just over $51,000 for AIAN households, and nearly $58,000 for Hispanic households. The median among Asian households was just over $100,000 (Semega and Kollar, 2022). Although mean household incomes are higher than median household incomes, differences across racial and ethnic groups are similar in percentage terms for both measures.

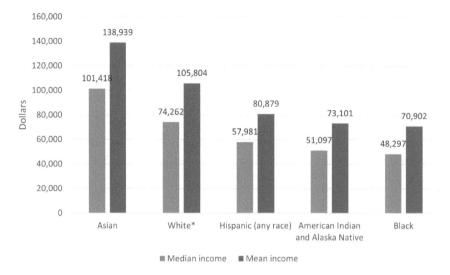

FIGURE 3-1 Median household income by race and ethnicity of householder, 2021.
NOTES: The data for Native Hawaiian and Pacific Islander populations are not reported separately, providing an inaccurate representation of this distinct racial Office of Management and Budget minimum category and masking inequities.
*In this table, "White" reflects income data reported under "White alone" in Semega and Kollar (2022). "White alone" indicates people who identified their race as White with no other race category. The separate category "White alone, not Hispanic" is not reported in this table.
SOURCE: Semega and Kollar, 2022.

One way to analyze changes over time is to compare how gaps in income relative to White households have evolved (see Figure 3-2). At the median, relative income among Black households has remained stagnant. It was 64 percent of White household income in 2002 and 65 percent in 2021. Hispanic household incomes went from 73 percent of White household incomes in 2002 to 78 percent in 2021. Income among AIAN households relative to White households went from 73 percent of White household incomes in 2002 to 69 percent in 2021. Asian households' relative incomes have increased from 17 percent higher than White households in 2002 to 37 percent higher in 2021 (Semega and Kollar, 2022).

Gaps in household incomes reflect differences across many characteristics, including household composition (Census Bureau, 2022), whether household members are employed and work full time or part time (Cajner et al., 2017; Federal Reserve Bank of St. Louis, n.d.), and salary and wage rates (Gould, 2020). For example, the unemployment rate—measured as the share of people in the labor force (not retired, students, or otherwise not seeking work) who are not employed—is consistently higher for Black

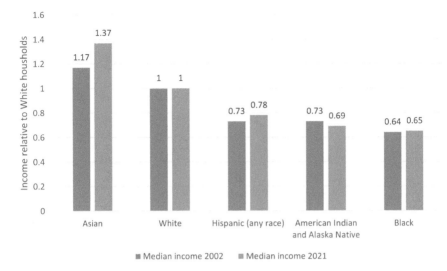

FIGURE 3-2 Relative median income, 2002 and 2021.
NOTES: The data for Native Hawaiian and Pacific Islander populations are not reported separately, providing an inaccurate representation of this distinct racial Office of Management and Budget minimum category and masking inequities.
*In this table, "White" reflects income data reported under "White alone" in Semega and Kollar (2022). "White alone" indicates people who identified their race as White with no other race category. The separate category "White alone, not Hispanic" is not reported in this table.
SOURCE: Semega and Kollar, 2022.

and Hispanic people than White and Asian people (see Figure 3-3). Between 1975 and 2021, it averaged more than twice as high for Black people than White people (Federal Reserve Bank of St. Louis, n.d.). Over this period, it ranged from about 30–90 percent higher among Hispanic people than White people (Federal Reserve Bank of St. Louis, n.d.). Research finds that factors such as age, education, marital status, and geography explain relatively little of the difference in unemployment rates between Black people and White people (in contrast to the larger explanatory power of these factors in differences in earnings, described below) but a higher share of the difference in unemployment rates between Hispanic people and White people (Cajner et al., 2017; Siripurapu, 2022).

Despite recent progress, large and troubling gaps remain among the employed in income and earnings across racial and ethnic groups. Many factors contribute to these gaps, including differences in education, age, family composition, occupation, time in the workforce, gender, geography, and incarceration rates (Bayer and Charles, 2016; Grodsky and Pager, 2001; Looney and Turner, 2018; Neal and Johnson, 1995). However, even accounting for these factors, sizable gaps in earnings across racial and ethnic groups persist

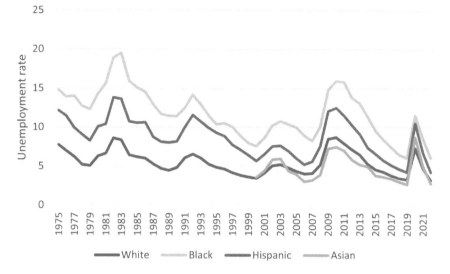

FIGURE 3-3 Unemployment rate, by race and ethnicity, 1975–2021.
NOTE: Data for American Indian and Alaska Native and Native Hawaiian and Pacific Is-
lander people were not available through the Federal Reserve Bank of St. Louis.
SOURCE: U.S. Bureau of Labor Statistics, Unemployment Rate—White [LNS14000003],
Unemployment Rate—Hispanic or Latino [LNS14000009], Unemployment Rate—Black or
African American [LNS14000006], Unemployment Rate—Asian [LNU04032183]; retrieved
from Federal Reserve Bank of St. Louis: https://fred.stlouisfed.org/series/LNS14000003,
March 3, 2023 (Federal Reserve Bank of St. Louis, n.d.).

(Bayer and Charles, 2016; Chetty et al., 2020). Between 2000 and 2019,
after statistically accounting for the effects of age, gender, education, and geography, the gap in wages between Black and White wage earners grew from
10.2 percent to 14.9 percent, but wage gaps between Hispanic and White
wage earners decreased from 12.3 percent to 10.8 percent (Gould, 2020).

Research demonstrates differential treatment by race in the job application process, pointing to labor market discrimination as one explanation
for these remaining gaps. In a 2004 study, fictitious resumes with randomly
assigned names that sounded "White" or "Black" were submitted to help-
wanted ads and received different responses based on the names' racial perception (Bertrand and Mullainathan, 2004). The study found that resumes
assigned names that sounded White were 50 percent more likely to be asked
to interview. The authors noted that the racial gap did not vary across occupation, industry, or employer size and found little evidence that names
were being used to infer social class instead of race. The authors conclude
that "differential treatment by race still appears to be prominent in the
U.S. labor market" (Bertrand and Mullainathan, 2004, p. 991). Additional
studies have similarly found that job applications with names that sound

Black have a lower response rate compared to names that sound White (Agan and Starr, 2018; Kline et al., 2022).

Differences in economic outcomes across racial and ethnic groups have followed different patterns among men and women (Altonji and Blank, 1999). Among men, across all racial and ethnic groups, wages and employment have declined over time and become more unequal. Men's labor force participation rates have declined for White, Hispanic, and Black men over the past 50 years, with White and Hispanic men participating in the labor force at higher rates and experiencing a smaller decline over time than Black men (Council of Economic Advisers, 2016). Inflation-adjusted hourly wages for men fell for each group between 1979 and 2016, but wage gaps have increased because Black and Hispanic men's wages dropped by 8.9 and 7.6 percent, respectively, compared to 1.4 percent for White men (Shambaugh et al., 2017). Although some of the differences in earnings between Black and White men (which is more often studied than the Hispanic–White gap) can be explained by easily measurable factors, such as age and education, the unexplained share has grown from about one-third in 1979 to about half in 2016 (Daly et al., 2017). Studies also show that significant portion of the wage gap between Hispanic and White male workers is attributable to education, a gap that has widened (Mora and Dávila, 2018).

The trends are somewhat different among women. Labor force participation rates increased for White, Hispanic, and Black women from 1971 through around 2000 but dropped since then. White and Black women's participation is nearly equal, with Hispanic women's participation about 10 points lower (Black et al., 2017). Women's occupations vary across racial and ethnic groups. For example, in 2021, 25.0 percent of employed Black women worked in service occupations, compared to 18.6 percent of White women and 29.7 percent of Hispanic or Latina women (BLS, 2023). Inflation-adjusted hourly wages increased for each group between 1979 and 2016, but gaps have increased because Black and Hispanic women's wages increased by 16.9 and 17.5 percent, respectively, compared to 33.7 percent for White women (Shambaugh et al., 2017). Similar to the pattern among men, both the gap and the share of the Black–White gap among women that is unexplained have grown over time (Daly et al., 2017).

Research has highlighted some similar and different explanations for the income gaps between White people and Black, Latino/a, and AIAN people. As discussed in Chapter 2, data on AIAN populations have been too often lacking. For example, only recently did the Census Bureau produce monthly data on AIAN unemployment, showing that rates are higher than for any other racial or ethnic group: 11.1 percent in January 2022, more than double that of White people (Maxim et al., 2022). Household composition is an important factor in the income gap, as 55 percent of AIAN mothers are the sole or primary earner in households with children under 18, compared

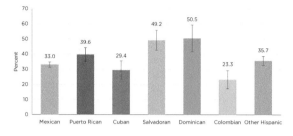

FIGURE 3-4 Share experiencing material hardship by detailed Hispanic origin: 2020 (in percent).
NOTE: Material hardship reflects whether individuals lived in households that experienced food, bill-paying, and/or housing hardship. The bars reflect the 90 percent confidence interval surrounding each estimate.
SOURCE: Scherer and Mayol-García, 2022.

to 37 percent of White mothers (Pathak, 2021). The income gap between White and AIAN people also reflects centuries of federal actions, practices, policies, and laws, such as forced assimilation, territorial dispossession, extermination, and failure to honor treaty obligations (discussed in Chapter 7).

"Hispanic," like all racial and ethnic classifications, encompasses individuals from many distinct and unique backgrounds. Mexico is the largest country of origin for Hispanic people in the United States, at 63 percent, but this means that more than one in three is from another country (Scherer and Mayol-García, 2022). Research has shown that Hispanic people from different countries have differing economic outcomes; this is sometimes lost when data are aggregated. For example, among Hispanic people from different countries of origin, there are differences in economic resilience[3] and security.[4] Figure 3-4 looks at material hardship during the recent COVID-19–induced recession: Salvadoran and Dominican people were more likely to experience hardship, while Colombian and Cuban people were less likely, indicating greater sources of economic resilience within those groups (Scherer and Mayol-García, 2022). Households were considered to have experienced material hardship if they experienced hardship in at least one of the following: food, bill-paying, or housing.

Although some federal policies have helped low-income and minoritized people, others have played a role in bringing about the income inequities this section describes. For example, incarceration (at the federal, state, or local level) has a lasting impact on income: Craigie et al. (2020) found

_____

[3] Economic resilience can be defined as the ability of an individual, household, or community to anticipate, withstand, adapt to, and recover from negative disruptions (Economic Development Administration, n.d.; National Association of Counties, 2013).
[4] Economic security can be defined as the ability to meet essential needs, such as food, shelter, clothing, health care, and education, sustainably (Global Social Development Innovations, n.d.).

that it is associated with a 52 percent reduction in annual earnings and with employment in low-paying jobs, impacting earnings growth for life (its impacts on income are just one aspect of incarceration's effect on equity; for a more comprehensive discussion, see Chapter 7). The Pew Charitable Trusts (2010) found that family income is 22 percent lower while a father is incarcerated and remains 15 percent lower the year after a father is released. They also found that incarceration is associated with reduced total or lifetime earnings of 2, 6, and 9 percent for White, Hispanic, and Black men, respectively (The Pew Charitable Trusts, 2010). These data have particularly important implications for racial and ethnic inequities, given that Black and Latino/a people make up nearly 65 percent of formerly imprisoned people in the United States (Craigie et al., 2020). AIAN people are also disproportionately incarcerated, at 38 percent over the national average, and overrepresented in the prison population of 19 states compared to other racial and ethnic populations (Fox et al., 2023; Wang, 2021).

Pretrial detention can also have a lasting impact on economic outcomes. Research has found that it substantially reduces individuals' subsequent earnings and that higher levels of pretrial detention may decrease intergenerational mobility in later years (Dobbie and Yang, 2021). This impacts racial and ethnic equity because Black and Hispanic people have significantly higher pretrial detention rates than White people (Dobbie and Yang, 2021). Federal policy changes relating to incarceration and pretrial detention therefore provide a potential opportunity to address racial and ethnic inequities in income and thereby health and well-being. Chapter 7 further discusses how federal policy can address racial and ethnic inequities in the criminal legal system. The wealth section of this chapter further discusses how inequities in the criminal legal system propagate racial and ethnic inequities in wealth through fines and fees.

Minimum wage laws are another example of how federal policy can address racial and ethnic inequities in income. Legal standards for minimum wages can be set at the local, state, and federal levels. The federal minimum wage is usually set in nominal terms, with periodic adjustments in law. This structure results in declines in real value during intervals between nominal adjustments (Lee, 1999); the rate of that decline is governed by inflation. The federal minimum wage last increased in July 2009, making this the longest period without an increase since it was established in 1938; in inflation-adjusted terms, it is at its lowest level since the 1950s (Cooper et al., 2022).

Thirty states and D.C. have minimum wages above the federal rate of $7.25/hour (NCSL, 2022). Several states have targeted minimum wages as high as $15 through law (including Illinois, New Jersey, and Rhode Island) or ballot initiative (Florida); others have lower targeted levels. Regional differences in factors such as cost of living and workforce composition create an environment where differences in minimum wage across states make sense (Dube, 2014). Although federal regulation lags behind states in many cases, numerous states have minimum wages at or below the federal level, and some have not set a minimum wage (in the latter two cases, the federal minimum wage applies and an increase could benefit individuals whose wages have not kept up with the cost of living) (DOL, 2023).

Increasing the minimum wage can help increase earnings for those at the lowest level and also reduce racial income disparities (Wursten and Reich, 2022); it would move some families out of poverty but likely also result in some job loss as workers become more expensive. The net effect would be a general reduction of the total number living in poverty, as the first effect is larger than the second. Incrementally increasing the federal minimum wage to $15 by 2027 could lift about 300,000 families above the poverty line, according to the mean estimate from the Congressional Budget Office, and increase real family incomes on net for families earning up to 300 percent of the poverty threshold (CBO, 2022). Real family income for higher-income families could see offsetting losses, primarily clustered among those earning above 600 percent of the poverty threshold (CBO, 2022). By raising incomes and lifting families out of poverty (which is disproportionately experienced by racially and ethnically minoritized populations) increases to the federal minimum wage could address racial and ethnic inequities in economic stability and therefore health and well-being.

Conclusion 3-1: Evidence demonstrates that pretrial detention substantially reduces lifetime income, and strongly links incarceration with lower lifetime earnings and family income for incarcerated individuals. Given racial and ethnic inequities in incarceration and pretrial detention, there are opportunities in these areas to address racial and ethnic inequities in income and, thereby, health and well-being.

Conclusion 3-2: Stagnation in the federal minimum wage, coupled with inflation, has left the real value of the minimum wage at a level not seen since the 1950s. Increases to the federal minimum wage raise incomes among low- and moderate-income families and lift families out of poverty. Since racially and ethnically minoritized populations and tribal communities are disproportionately represented in the groups that would be impacted by an increased federal minimum wage, such an increase is one method to address racial and ethnic inequities in economic stability and, therefore, health and well-being.

POVERTY

Poverty, defined by the Census Bureau as having income below a specific threshold that accounts for family size, unequally affects different racial and ethnic groups (Creamer et al., 2022). As shown in Figure 3-5,

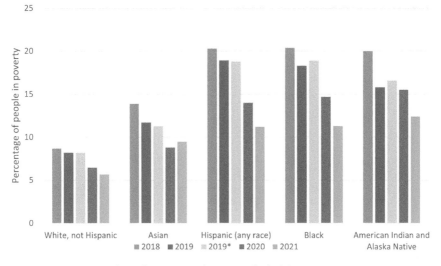

FIGURE 3-5 Percent of people in poverty by race and ethnicity.
NOTES: Data for Asian and Native Hawaiian and Pacific Islander (NHPI) populations are not shown separately, providing an inaccurate representation of the Asian and NHPI populations as distinct racial Office of Management and Budget minimum categories and masking differences between Asian and NHPI people. This table reflects poverty data for people who identified their race as White alone, not Hispanic, Asian alone, Hispanic (any race), Black alone, and American Indian and Alaska Native alone. Poverty measured by Supplemental Poverty Measure.
*Estimates reflect the implementation of revised Supplemental Poverty Measure methodology.
SOURCE: Creamer et al., 2022.

in 2021, more than 1 in 10 people who identify as Hispanic (of any race), Black, and AIAN had incomes below the poverty threshold. Just under 1 in 10 Asian people were in poverty, as were about 1 in 17 White (not Hispanic) people. Figure 3-6 shows the percent of children in poverty by race and ethnicity. The poverty rates in Figures 3-5 and 3-6 are based on the Census Bureau's Supplemental Poverty Measure, which accounts for income from a wide range of sources, including earnings and social benefits programs, such as Social Security, SNAP, the Earned Income Tax Credit (EITC), and, especially important in 2021, Economic Impact Payments distributed as part of COVID-19 relief packages. AIAN people have the highest poverty rate of all racial and ethnic groups[5] (Creamer et al., 2022), with consistently high childhood poverty rates among those living on a

---

[5] Creamer et al. (2022) note that "due to small sample size and sampling variability, caution should be used when examining rates and year-to-year changes for" the AIAN population (p. 5).

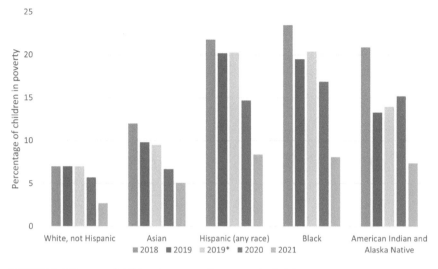

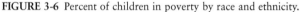

FIGURE 3-6 Percent of children in poverty by race and ethnicity.
NOTES: Data for Asian and Native Hawaiian and Pacific Islander (NHPI) populations are not shown separately, providing an inaccurate representation of the Asian and NHPI populations as distinct racial OMB minimum categories and masking differences between Asian and NHPI people. This table reflects poverty data for people who identified their race as White alone, not Hispanic, Asian alone, Hispanic (any race), Black alone, and American Indian and Alaska Native alone. Poverty measured by Supplemental Poverty Measure.
*Estimates reflect the implementation of revised Supplemental Poverty Measure methodology.
SOURCE: Creamer et al., 2022.

reservation (Akee, 2019). AIAN people have the highest poverty of all races for those 65 and older (NCOA, 2023).

Poverty is just one way to measure an individual's or household's limited access to economic resources. Many families that struggle with income volatility and lack access to necessary resources have incomes above the poverty threshold. For instance, two-thirds of food-insecure families have incomes above the poverty threshold (Schanzenbach et al., 2016a). Black, Hispanic, and American Indian populations have consistently higher rates of food insecurity (Coleman-Jensen et al., 2022; Schanzenbach and Pitts, 2020).

A range of social benefit programs significantly alleviate poverty. Programs differ in their designs in terms of the population targeted (e.g., retirees, people with disabilities, working parents), and the amount, type (cash or "in kind"—such as vouchers for food or housing), and duration of assistance. As a result, they have varying antipoverty effects on different groups (see Figure 3-7). For example, Social Security is most responsible for lifting incomes above the poverty line, but the impact is overwhelmingly on

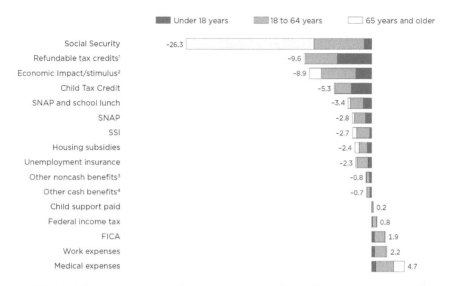

FIGURE 3-7 Change in number of people in poverty after including each element: 2021 (in millions).

NOTE: The figure illustrates the change in the number of people in poverty after the including each tax, benefit, or expenditure deduction; FICA = Federal Insurance Contributions Act, SNAP = Supplemental Nutrition Assistance Program, SSI = Supplemental Security Income.

[1] Refundable tax credits include the Earned Income Tax Credit, Child Tax Credit, and the Child and Dependent Care Credit.

[2] Includes the third stimulus payment. Details are available in Appendix B of source document.

[3] Other noncash benefits include utility assistance, Special Supplemental Nutrition Program for Women, Infants, and Children, and school lunch.

[4] Other cash benefits include workers' compensation, Temporary Assistance for Needy Families/general assistance, and child support received.

SOURCE: Creamer et al., 2022.

older adults who are the target (some younger adults and children may also be aided, such as by living in a family with an older recipient). The EITC and Child Tax Credit (CTC) lifted over 10 million out of poverty in 2018, with children and their parents the overwhelming beneficiaries (Bitler et al., 2020; CBPP, 2023a).

The 2021 expansion of the CTC through the American Rescue Plan Act[6] played an important role in this historic reduction of poverty (Hardy et al., 2023; IRS, 2023). The expansion increased the maximum credit amount; made the credit fully refundable, allowing families to claim it even if they did not have earned income or owe income taxes; and allowed families to receive part of the credit in 2021 through advance monthly payments

---

[6] Pub. L. 117–2, 135 Stat. 4 (Mar. 11, 2021).

(IRS, 2023). An analysis from the Center on Poverty and Social Policy at Columbia University revealed that monthly delivery of the credit more consistently reduced child poverty rates throughout the year than delivery of the credit in one lump sum after tax filing (Hamilton et al., 2022). These changes to the credit and their subsequent effect are especially critical for children; research demonstrates that poverty alleviation may be particularly important for children because it can improve their development and longer-term health and economic outcomes (Akee et al., 2018; Hardy et al., 2019; Hoynes et al., 2016).

A recent analysis from Child Trends found that child poverty declined by 59 percent from 1993 to 2019 (Thomson et al., 2022). As it declined at similar rates across racial and ethnic groups, inequities persisted. The analysis also found that the role of the social safety net[7] in decreasing poverty has increased for all racial and ethnic groups from 1993 to 2019, but the size of the effect varies across racial and ethnic groups; it has been consistently larger for Black and White children and smaller for Hispanic and Asian/Hawaiian/Pacific Islander children (Thomson et al., 2022). Other studies have found that the effects of specific programs also differ across racial and ethnic groups. For example, Social Security benefits are more likely to represent more than 90 percent of income among elderly Black, Asian, and Hispanic people than elderly White people (National Academy of Social Insurance, 2021). Looking at impacts on children, Bitler et al. (2023) find that EITC and CTC reduce poverty rates among Black and Hispanic children substantially more than White and Asian children, and SNAP reduces poverty rates most for Black children.

Some especially vulnerable groups may disproportionately experience poverty and have less access to antipoverty programs, including childless adults, formerly incarcerated individuals, and immigrants. Because these groups also disproportionately represent some racial and ethnic groups, their outcomes contribute to health inequities. Research demonstrates that poverty alleviation, through increased earnings and employment and programs such as EITC and SNAP, can improve health and narrow health disparities across racial, ethnic, and tribal groups. For example, EITC increases mothers' likelihood of employment and income levels and reduces their likelihood of being in poverty (Hoynes and Patel, 2015; Schanzenbach and Strain, 2020). It also improves their biological markers

---

[7] In this study the "social safety net" captured the impact of Supplemental Nutrition Assistance Program, Social Security, housing assistance, unemployment insurance, Supplemental Security Income, Temporary Assistance to Needy Families and Aid to Families with Dependent Children, the National School Lunch Program, WIC, and Low-Income Home Energy Assistance Program subsidies. It also captured the full tax system, including federal and state taxes owed, federal tax credits (including the refundable tax credits), payroll taxes, and stimulus payments in 2008 and 2009 (Thomson et al., 2022).

for stress and self-reported mental health (Evans and Garthwaite, 2014) and reduces smoking (Averett and Wang, 2013; Hoynes et al., 2015; Strully et al., 2010). EITC also improves infant health, increasing average birthweight (Baker, 2008; Strully et al., 2010) and decreasing low-birthweight births (Hoynes et al., 2015). This is important in part because improvements in birthweight subsequently lead to improved learning outcomes during childhood and improvements across a range of outcomes in adulthood, including wages, disability, health conditions, and human capital accumulation (Almond et al., 2018; Figlio et al., 2014). EITC also improves educational outcomes for children, measured by test scores, high school graduation, and college enrollment (Bastian and Michelmore, 2018; Chetty et al., 2011; Dahl and Lochner, 2012, 2017). Improvements in education have also been shown to improve health outcomes, as described in Chapter 4.

SNAP also has positive impacts on participants' health. SNAP improves health at birth; it has been shown to increase birthweights and reduce the incidence of low birthweight (Almond et al., 2008; East, 2020). SNAP access before age 5 improves health in adolescence (as reported by a parent), potentially through reduced school absences, doctor visits, and hospitalizations (East, 2020). Children with access to SNAP also have better health in adulthood, as measured by obesity, body mass index, and the absence of chronic conditions, such as diabetes and high blood pressure (Hoynes et al., 2016). Access to SNAP during childhood also affects education and economic outcomes, increasing high school graduation rates by 18 percentage points and improving a range of outcomes for women, including earnings, employment, family income, and educational attainment (Hoynes et al., 2016; Northwestern Institute for Policy Research, 2017), which may contribute to better health outcomes.

Participation in WIC has also been found to also improve birthweight and reduces the incidence of low birthweight (Currie and Rajani, 2015; Figlio et al., 2009; Hoynes et al., 2011; Rossin-Slater, 2013). In contrast, when local clinics close or stores end their participation in WIC, expectant mothers' participation declines, harming birth outcomes (Meckel, 2020; Rossin-Slater, 2013). Prenatal WIC participation reduces diagnoses for attention-deficit/hyperactivity disorder and other childhood mental health conditions and grade repetition (Chorniy et al., 2020).

Implications of the Research

The broad-ranging positive impacts of antipoverty programs underscore the importance of ensuring they are administered in a manner that allows eligible families to enroll and receive assistance. Although antipoverty programs are neutral in terms of racial and ethnic health equity, they do have indirect equity implications. Research and experimentation will be needed to facilitate full and equitable access to federal programs administered by states and localities. In addition, community organizations can play an important role in helping people sign up for and remain enrolled.

Monitoring Participation Rates can Facilitate Equitable Access to Federal Programs

Participation rates vary widely overall and across groups in social benefits programs. Although overall participation in SNAP has been high in recent years, it varies widely across groups. Recent estimates indicate that participation among Hispanic families lags far behind other groups (Bitler et al., 2023). Fewer than half of eligible older adults participate (Finkelstein and Notowidigdo, 2018). The Elderly Simplified Application Project is a federal demonstration project that allows streamlined administrative policies for elderly SNAP participants and has been shown to increase participation (Gothro et al., 2020; USDA, 2020a; Waxman, 2021); expanding it would increase participation in SNAP among older adults. Additionally, although data are limited, they indicate that outreach efforts, which could be incentivized by the federal government, may improve SNAP participation (Bleich et al., 2020; Gorman et al., 2013; Mabli, 2015).

WIC is very successful in its efforts to provide infants with access to needed food and breastmilk or formula, but it falls short along other dimensions. Participation rates decrease significantly as children age; 79.3 percent of eligible infants participate, dropping to 25 percent by age 4 (Gray et al., 2019; Schanzenbach and Thorn, 2020). Increasing WIC take-up could help improve outcomes for children and reduce racial and ethnic disparities in maternal and child health and food insecurity. Participation could be improved by establishing performance metrics for cross-enrollment of eligible SNAP and Medicaid participants into WIC, similar to the metrics for the National School Lunch Program (see Chapter 4). This could provide additional incentives for states to do the crucial outreach and institute the appropriate reforms in application and related processes needed to maintain high participation.

Estimates suggest that about 15 million households did not file a federal income tax return in 2019, for reasons such as not being required to do so based on their types and amounts of income (Gleckman and Maag, 2020). Increasing tax filing rates would likely increase participation in EITC and CTC (Goldin et al., 2022). The Internal Revenue Service (IRS) can take steps to increase filing rates, such as using data from administrative records to send out prepopulated tax returns and continuing the "simplified filing" process that allows families with very low incomes to provide a limited set of data to establish tax benefits without having to file full tax returns

(Tilly, 2022). States could also help to identify nonfilers by comparing SNAP and Medicaid rolls to the tax filing, so that nonfilers could be offered targeted assistance with tax filing.

Improving Administrative Capacity is Another Promising Approach to Facilitate Equitable Participation in Federal Programs

Administrative churn in programs such as SNAP occurs when otherwise eligible participants fail to recertify, are removed, and reapply as a new case within a short period, such as a few months or a year. Churn drives up administrative costs, because new cases are more expensive to process than recertifications. Churn also reduces the effectiveness of social programs when families lose benefits due to administrative burdens (Homonoff and Somerville, 2021). To address this problem, the federal government could monitor rates of churn and set performance standards. In addition, administrative burdens could be streamlined, and program integrity and effectiveness could be improved through federal investments in expansion of administrative capacity.

For SNAP, administrative burdens reduce recertification among eligible individuals (Homonoff and Somerville, 2021). Reforms that simplify recertification can increase retention (Gray, 2019). Federal policy could authorize, without the need for states to apply for waivers, administrative procedures that make it easier to enroll in and stay on SNAP, as was done during the COVID-19 federal health emergency. These included the extension of certification periods, reduced paperwork and interview burdens, telephonic signatures, and electronic filing of paperwork (CBPP, 2023b).

Maintaining Broad Eligibility Facilitates Equitable Participation in Federal Programs

In recent years, eligibility for antipoverty programs among some groups has been limited by some laws and regulations. Because of the many demonstrated benefits of these programs, any such limitations need to be carefully considered and their potential negative impacts, especially those that might disproportionately affect racial and ethnic minority groups, appropriately weighed. For example, a new "public charge" rule[8] took effect in 2020 (but was reversed in 2021) that significantly expanded the criteria for denying permanent residency, or green cards, to those who have or likely would participate in antipoverty programs. The rule caused eligible immigrant families to avoid enrolling for fear of consequences (Bernstein et al., 2020, 2021). When legal immigrants were barred from SNAP (then the Food Stamp

---

[8] Inadmissibility on Public Charge Grounds, 84 FR 41292 (August 2019).

Program) after the 1996 welfare reform law,[9] studies show that immigrant children's health worsened (East, 2020) and immigrant adults were less likely to have doctors' appointments (East and Friedson, 2020). Additionally, individuals convicted of drug-related felonies are permanently barred from SNAP, unless the state modifies or eliminates the ban. Denying food assistance to individuals who have completed their sentences makes it harder for them to reintegrate into society and increases recidivism rates (Tuttle, 2019). This ban disproportionately affects people who have been racially and ethnically minoritized (Bolen, 2021) and may also impact health inequities.

Support Nonprofit Sector Partnerships

Nonprofit sector partnerships play an important role in poverty alleviation and emergency food assistance that can influence racial and ethnic health inequities. Federal programs, such as the Emergency Food Assistance Program, help the nonprofit sector more effectively serve those in need by providing food for distribution and grants for infrastructure and capacity building (Cabili et al., 2013; Tiehen, 2002; USDA, 2020b). It is important to ensure that such programs provide an adequate supply of nutritious and culturally relevant foods. Additional targeted grants to invest in elements such as administration and storage capacity for perishable foods, could further improve the reach and impact of the nonprofit sector.

Conclusion

Inadequate, unstable income harms a range of downstream outcomes, from children's educational achievement to health outcomes and neighborhood characteristics. It also reduces wealth accumulation—for example, data demonstrate that homeownership rates increase with household income (see Figure 3-8)—and harms families' abilities to weather economic shocks. Racial and ethnic inequities in wealth will be discussed in the next section of this chapter.

> Conclusion 3-3: Federal social benefit programs, such as the Supplemental Nutrition Assistance Program, Special Supplemental Nutrition Program for Women, Infants, and Children, and the Earned Income Tax Credit, significantly alleviate poverty and reduce the negative health consequences of poverty; however, there are barriers that prevent participation among many people who would otherwise qualify for these programs. Some racial, ethnic, and tribal populations have lower

---

[9] The Personal Responsibility and Work Opportunity Reconciliation Act, Pub. L. 104–193, 110 Stat. 2105 (Aug. 22, 1996).

participation rates in these programs, contributing to racial and ethnic health inequity. Therefore, policies that address administrative barriers, hold programs accountable for participation rates, and improve administrative capacity can improve participation rates and reduce racial and ethnic health inequity.

Conclusion 3-4: Federal social benefit programs, such as the Supplemental Nutrition Assistance Program, Special Supplemental Nutrition Program for Women, Infants, and Children, and the Earned Income Tax Credit, significantly alleviate poverty and reduce the negative health consequences of poverty. In some cases, eligibility for these and similar programs has been restricted for some groups, including childless adults, formerly incarcerated individuals, and immigrants. Because these groups disproportionately represent racially and ethnically minoritized populations, these restrictive policies contribute to racial and ethnic health inequity.

Conclusion 3-5: Nonprofit sector partnerships play an important role in poverty alleviation and emergency food assistance that can influence racial and ethnic health inequities. Federal programs, such as the Emergency Food Assistance Program, help the nonprofit sector more effectively serve those in need by providing food for distribution and grants for infrastructure and capacity building.

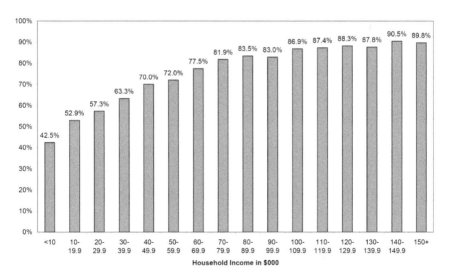

FIGURE 3-8 Homeownership rate by household income in 2001.
SOURCE: Herbert et al., 2005.

WEALTH

Wealth, which is typically defined as what you own minus what you owe, is responsible for a significant component of economic inequality (Oliver and Shapiro, 2006; Sherraden, 2005). Race (along with education and age) increasingly determines whether and to what extent one is able to accumulate wealth (Boshara et al., 2015a,b,c). Many experts attribute a substantial component of wealth disparities to the U.S. legacy of slavery and racist economic policies (Siripurapu, 2022). For example, homeownership is the primary route through which people in the United States amass wealth, and for decades, Black people's ability to participate was severely limited by federal policies. The Home Owners' Loan Corporation (HOLC), a federal agency established in the 1930s, mandated redlining, a discriminatory practice that denied mortgages to residents of certain areas based on their race or ethnicity. The Federal Housing Administration (FHA) and HOLC, in tandem with real estate organizations and developers, are widely considered to be responsible for the discriminatory practices that shaped housing markets for decades (Rothstein, 2017). Freund (2010) found that "following the rules that governed FHA practice nationwide, the Detroit area office focused almost exclusively on promoting the construction, purchase, and repair of privately owned homes by *certain* White people. There is no evidence that Black people qualified for FHA-insured loans before World War II" (pp. 134–135). Other research shows similar situations in Peoria, Illinois, Greensboro, North Carolina, and Baltimore, Maryland (Fishback et al., 2022). Land is a similar form of wealth. The 1887 Dawes Act[10] authorized the federal government to break up tribal lands and allowed American Indians who accepted the division to become citizens. Through this process, 90 million acres of land were seized and sold to non-AIAN people. Only about one-half of the AIAN population received citizenship through the Dawes Act (Rollings, 2004). As discussed in Chapter 7, territorial dispossession resulted in a "near total" reduction in tribal land (Farrell et al., 2021).

Policies such as the mortgage tax deduction and the GI Bill[11] were designed to create opportunities for asset accumulation. However, these opportunities have not been equally accessible to all. They enabled wealth generation for (mostly) White people but effectively left Black and other minoritized families even further behind. The 1944 GI Bill, which provided U.S. veterans with funds for education, housing, and unemployment insurance, disproportionately aided wealth building for White veterans. Turner and Bound (2003), for example, show that, among men limited to

---

[10] Also known as the Indian General Allotment Act, Feb. 8, 1887, ch. 119, 24 Stat. 388.

[11] Also known as the Servicemen's Readjustment Act of 1944, June 22, 1944, ch. 268, 58 Stat. 284.

educational opportunities in the South, where segregation restricted opportunities for Black people, "the GI Bill exacerbated rather than narrowed the economic and educational differences between blacks and whites." Black veterans were also largely shut out of the homeownership opportunities that the GI Bill granted to White veterans because the bill only provided veterans with a cosigner for loans. They had to first secure a loan from a bank or other lending agency, which was more difficult for Black veterans due to discrimination. They also had to offer collateral for the loan (Onkst, 1998). Similarly, by not accounting for existing inequities, other policies such as the mortgage tax deduction, which rewards existing wealth in the form of homeownership, can exacerbate rather than close gaps.

Today, Black households score consistently lower than White households in nearly every national metric of wealth—asset ownership, intergenerational wealth transfers, and home value (Addo and Darity, 2022; Bhutta et al., 2020; Thompson and Suarez, 2019). Black and Latino/a families are five times less likely to receive a significant inheritance than White families (McKernan et al., 2012). AIAN people living on trust lands (reservations) have very specific probate laws (Trust and Will, n.d.). It is very difficult to know inheritance rates for AIAN people off reservations (87 percent of the AIAN population) (OMH, 2023), as these data are not gathered or reported. Figure 3-9, from the Hamilton Project's 2020 report, illustrates the income and wealth gaps between Black and White households (Hardy and Logan, 2020). Research that centers the systemic barriers to asset accumulation is necessary to understand the factors that contribute to the gap and devise strategies to close it. Additionally, although economic factors play a large role in the existence and growth of racial economic inequality, political and cultural aspects also have an effect (Piketty, 2013). Research also needs to consider the nuanced role of such political and cultural aspects in perpetuating the racial wealth gap.

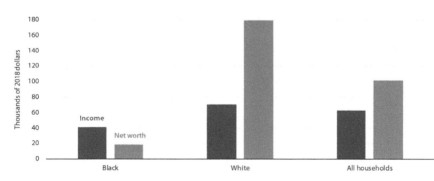

FIGURE 3-9 Median family income and net worth in 2018, by race.
SOURCE: Hardy and Logan, 2020.

The Connection Between Health and Wealth

The connection between income and health has been firmly established, as the preceding sections discuss. The link between wealth and health has been less intensively studied, partly because data on wealth are more complex and inconsistent than data on income. However, a growing body of research illustrates that higher wealth predicts better health outcomes (Braveman et al., 2018). A 2007 review of studies examining the connection found that, in most of the studies examined, greater wealth was associated with better health (Pollack et al., 2007). Wealth operates in tandem with income to enable healthier living conditions, access to quality health care, and amelioration of stress. A 2018 report from the Robert Wood Johnson Foundation argues that wealth affects health in three ways:

1. Wealth and income can lead to better health by providing material benefits, including healthier living conditions and access to health care.
2. Wealth and income can promote health by providing psychosocial benefits, including protection from chronic stress.
3. Parents' wealth shapes their children's educational, economic, and social opportunities, which in turn shapes their children's health throughout life (Braveman et al., 2018, pp. 6–8) (see Figure 3-10).

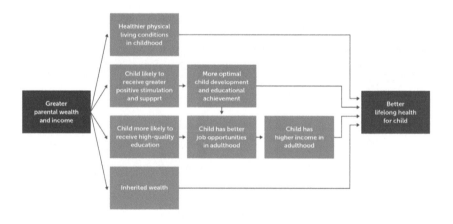

Health is transmitted across generations, along with wealth, through material and psychosocial advantages.

FIGURE 3-10 Intergenerational transmission of wealth and health.
SOURCE: Braveman et al., 2018.

The COVID-19 pandemic has further revealed the way in which wealth and health interact. Black people already had poorer health conditions than White people when the pandemic struck, as other chapters of this report document. Black families' lack of assets, including emergency funds, bank accounts, and homeownership, made them less able to cope with unanticipated expenses, such as medical emergencies, job loss, and transportation issues. They were more likely to fall behind on their mortgage payments than White families and less likely to be able to retire or plan for retirement. In addition to exposing the vulnerability of Black households from a health and wealth perspective, the pandemic has likely also laid the foundation for widening the racial wealth gap (Weller and Figueroa, 2021).

Baby Bonds

Wealth begets wealth. One policy that could help close wealth differences across groups, increase economic stability, and improve health and well-being outcomes is for the federal government to create savings accounts for children at birth. Pilot programs and initiatives across a range of states and localities and international experience offer evidence on the effects of subsidized savings accounts. The amount of the initial deposit, and whether the government makes later deposits to supplement family contributions, varies by program or proposal. For example, through the Keystone Scholars program, Pennsylvania creates education savings accounts with $100 for every child born in the state on or after January 1, 2019 (PA 529, n.d.).

Sherraden first proposed such an idea (Child Development Accounts) in his 1991 book *Assets and the Poor: A New American Welfare Policy* (Sherraden, 1991). His idea, which he noted can build on the 529 college-savings plan, was adopted by several U.S. cities and states, as well as Singapore and Israel (Miller, 2018). The SEED for Oklahoma Kids (SEED OK) experiment is a large-scale, longitudinal study on the impact of Child Development Accounts on children and families (Huang et al., 2021). At its launch in 2007, SEED OK opened OK 529 accounts for every newborn child in the experimental group with an initial $1,000 deposit and added an additional $600 for low-income children and $200 for others in 2019. SEED OK data from 2019, when the 2,704 enrolled children were about 12 years old, reveal "very large" positive impacts on financial outcomes and "some" positive impacts on nonfinancial outcomes (such as social-emotional development of children and parenting practices). At the end of 2019, the experimental group had more than three times the OK 529 assets of the control group (Huang et al., 2021). In the control group, children with OK 529 assets were primarily very high-income (over half), had mothers with college degrees (three-quarters), and were White (over three-quarters). In the control group, only 1 percent of low-income children and 2 percent of racially and ethnically minoritized children had any OK 529 assets (Clancy et al., 2021). Since SEED OK provided OK 529 assets to children "across the socioeconomic and geographic spectrum of the state," the program increased the likelihood of holding such assets by 99 and 98 percentage points for low-income and racially and ethnically minoritized children, respectively (Clancy et al., 2021, p. 5). The characteristics of children in the experimental group (i.e., household income, mother's education, and race/ethnicity) "mirror the diversity of the state population" (Clancy et al., 2021, p. 6). These data suggest that baby bonds, Child Development Accounts, and similar policies designed to increase asset accumulation can both improve wealth overall and address racial and ethnic inequities.

A bill proposed in Congress in 2023,[12] building on the work of economist Darrick Hamilton, proposed the creation of American Opportunity Accounts that would establish an account with $1,000 in it for every U.S. newborn and would continue to contribute up to $2,000 annually (Hamilton and Darity, 2010). Using an annual compound interest rate of 2 percent, researchers at the Urban Institute estimated that those accounts would grow to up to $42,253 by the time the child turned 18 (Kijakazi and Carther, 2020). The family could also choose to add funds, setting the child up for greater economic stability as they emerge into adulthood, with savings that could be used for homeownership, entrepreneurship, or higher education. Zewde (2020) found that the creation of these accounts could reduce the gap in wealth held by White and Black young adults to a factor of 1.4 instead of 16, while increasing wealth for both groups.

In addition to government subsidies of savings accounts for children, other policies to support savings and wealth accumulation could also have important implications for racial and ethnic inequities in wealth. For example, tax refunds, often seen as "surplus or bonus funds," provide a unique opportunity for saving. Data from H&R Block and Volunteer Income Tax Assistance tax preparation sites suggest that access to savings products, such as U.S. savings bonds, individual retirement accounts, and savings accounts, during the tax preparation process results in use of this saving opportunity by low-income and unbanked tax filers. The IRS's 2007 expansion of direct deposit options for refunds, which allowed filers to divide their refund into up to three accounts, supported the use of such savings programs (IRS, 2006; Tufano and Schneider, 2008).

---

[12] American Opportunity Accounts Act, H.R. 1041, S.411, 118th Congress (2023).

Affordable Higher Education

Given the relationship between education, income, and wealth, the affordability of higher education is relevant to the connection between racial and ethnic inequities in wealth, health, and well-being (Wolla and Sullivan, 2017). This topic is discussed in detail in Chapter 4, which addresses education as an SDOH and its role in racial and ethnic health equity.

Financialization of the Criminal Legal System

Individuals involved with the criminal legal system and their families face significant barriers to asset accumulation, a situation linked to the financialization of this system. The financialization of the criminal legal system refers to the increasing financial burden associated with criminal legal system involvement, including fines/penalties, fees, and other costs, such as markups of commissary store items. It has left a disproportionate number of Black, Latino/a, and low-income individuals with a financial "second sentence," as these burdens are effectively additional penalties for individuals already facing disciplinary action through incarceration or other nonmonetary conditions of their probation or parole (The Financial Justice Project, n.d.; Huebner and Giuffre, 2022; Pacewicz and Robinson, 2021; Pattillo and Kirk, 2021; Servon and Esquier, 2022; Servon et al., 2021). Since 2008, almost every state has increased monetary sanctions (e.g., costs, restitution, surcharges, and other penalties imposed from encounters with the criminal legal system) or added new ones, and the categories that trigger fines have expanded (Bannon et al., 2010; Harris et al., 2010; Menendez et al., 2019; Sobol, 2016). Furthermore, these costs perpetuate inequity because they disproportionately burden Black, Latino/a, and economically disadvantaged individuals through the debt accrued and the time required to address the penalties (Bannon et al., 2010; Bing et al., 2022; Harris, 2016; Harris et al., 2010; U.S. Commission on Civil Rights, 2017). The consequences of nonpayment include greater debt from accrued interest, prolonged contact with the criminal legal system, disenfranchisement, and reincarceration.

Harris et al. (2010) estimate that 66 percent of incarcerated individuals have financial sanctions. In 1995, 84.3 percent of adults on probation had monetary conditions associated with that probation (Bonczar, 1995). Research also shows that the imposition of these fines and fees is predatory and rooted in racial capitalism (Harris et al., 2022; Page and Soss, 2021). The cost is often borne not by the person who is directly involved but by their families.

The Financial Justice Project in San Francisco, housed in the Office of the Treasurer and Tax Collector, has pioneered a range of reforms aimed at reducing the financial harm created by the criminal legal system

(The Financial Justice Project, n.d.), including making phone calls from county jails free, eliminating the practice of marking up items in the commissary store, and waiving $33 million in criminal legal debt and administrative fees. Supporters of programs and proposals that aim to reduce or eliminate criminal legal debt recognize that the system is unfair and at cross purposes to efforts to reintegrate those who are justice involved into society. Those who oppose these reforms express concern about how to replace the government revenue these programs contribute. Given the disproportionate incarceration of Black, Latino/a, AIAN, and NHPI people and data demonstrating that Black and Latino/a people are disproportionately impacted by these fines and fees, pursuing similar reforms at the federal level is another option to address racial and ethnic inequities in wealth, health, and well-being (Prison Policy Initiative, n.d.).

Conclusion 3-6: Gaps in wealth for many racially and ethnically minoritized populations are linked to past and current federal policies, including redlining, disparate access to benefits of the 1944 GI Bill, and the financialization of the criminal legal system. Furthermore, policies that reward existing wealth, like the mortgage tax deduction, can exacerbate these gaps. Since wealth operates in tandem with income to enable access to healthier living conditions, quality health care, and amelioration of stress, these racial and ethnic inequities in wealth produce racial and ethnic inequities in health and well-being.

Conclusion 3-7: Policies to support savings and wealth accumulation, for example, government subsidies of savings accounts for children, can increase wealth and narrow racial and ethnic differences in savings rates and wealth holding.

FINANCIAL SERVICES

Banking

The ability to save, spend, borrow and plan—one definition of financial well-being—is enabled by access to safe and effective financial services. Many people lack this access, relying on unsafe or expensive alternatives to manage their money (Servon, 2017). The FDIC (Federal Deposit Insurance Corporation) 2021 Survey of Unbanked and Underbanked Households found that for nearly 6 million U.S. households, no one in the household had a bank account. Those 6 million make up approximately 4.5 percent of total U.S. households, with significant differences across racial and ethnic groups. Among White households the unbanked rate was 2.1 percent, while for Asian, AIAN, Hispanic, and Black households, it was 2.9, 6.9, 9.3, and 11.3 percent, respectively. Black households are more than five times as likely as White households to be unbanked (FDIC, 2021). In 2019, these rates were 1.7, 16.3, 12.2, and 13.8 percent for Asian, AIAN, Hispanic, and Black households, respectively (FDIC, 2019). Rural households were more likely to be unbanked than people living in metro areas (6.2 versus 4.2 percent). In addition, people with disabilities (age 25–64) are significantly more likely to be unbanked; 14.8 percent of these households are unbanked, highlighting another link between health and banking status (FDIC, 2021). Of all depository institutions owned by minoritized groups, AIAN-owned banks are the smallest single group (other than the one multiracial owned bank). Even considering credit unions, there are fewer AIAN-owned banks than Black- or Asian American-owned banks (NICOA, 2021).

In approximately 18.7 million households, individuals had bank accounts but also relied on "alternative" financial services, such as check cashers, pawn shops, and payday lenders (FDIC, 2021). Even controlling for income and education, high-cost credit products and financial services are more likely to be located in areas with higher shares of racially and ethnically minoritized populations (Wherry and Chakrabarti, 2022). The most commonly cited reasons for not having a bank account were cost, specifically the inability to afford the minimum balance required for a free account and variable and unexpected fees (such as overdraft fees), consumer trust of banks, and the inability to produce identification needed to open an account (FDIC, 2021). There are several methods by which the federal government could eliminate or substantially reduce these barriers. One is to directly provide free checking and savings accounts to everyone. Another is to require banks and credit unions, all of which have governmental charters and regulation, to offer basic accounts.

The federal government could directly provide basic accounts through several governmentally backed entities, such as the Post Office. Postal banking has been implemented in multiple countries, including the United Kingdom and Japan (Australian Citizens Party, n.d.). The U.S. Postal Service (USPS) already provides various forms of financial access, including postal money orders. The USPS Inspector General has studied the potential for broader provision of financial services (USPS Office of the Inspector General, 2014). Advocates of postal banking highlight USPS's broad physical presence, particularly in underserved areas, including heavily minority and rural areas (Baradaran, 2014). They also argue that USPS can structurally offer credit at lower rates due to the federal government's funding advantage in private markets (Baradaran, 2014). USPS enjoys significant public support, which could enable it to overcome the lack of trust that causes some to not enter the commercial banking system (DiVito, 2022). Some have raised concerns about whether USPS's comparative advantages offer the correct solution. A large physical presence is not useful, as financial services continues a long-term trend of going digital (Conti-Brown, 2018). A lack of bank branches and hours is a not a main reason cited by the unbanked, with only 4.4 percent citing location issues as the main reason they do not have an account (FDIC, 2021). Additionally, concerns about how USPS would allocate credit, deciding who gets a loan and who does not, and how borrowers are treated if they do default could undermine its popularity and trust (Conti-Brown, 2018).

The Federal Reserve (Fed) system could also provide direct accounts, known as "Fed accounts." This idea builds upon the Fed's system of providing access for financial institutions and expands it directly to individuals (Crawford et al., 2021). Unlike USPS, which is required to be self-funded, the Fed generally generates a profit from its central bank functions, allowing it to more easily subsidize these accounts. As operator of a substantial portion of the U.S. payment system, including the automated clearinghouse (ACH) system (The Federal Reserve, 2020), Fedwire Funds Service (The Federal Reserve, 2021a), and National Settlement Service (The Federal Reserve, 2021b), the Fed could integrate these accounts into the system, allowing users easier access to higher-quality services that they need (Crawford et al., 2021). Fed accounts (and likely USPS accounts as well) would also be able to quickly disburse government assistance during times of need, such as the COVID-19 pandemic.

Economic impact payments (EIPs) made during the pandemic were significantly delayed to those who did not file taxes and who were outside of the formal banking system, which were disproportionately racially and ethnically minoritized populations. One in ten people ended up receiving a paper check from the first federal relief bill, even though 95 percent of U.S. families have a bank account capable of receiving a direct deposit (Murphy, 2021). Over 3 million of those checks were cashed at high-cost check cashing stores. Vulnerable consumers, even those with bank accounts, may use such services if they need quick access to their funds. For example, consumers may need access to their paycheck or EIP more quickly than it could clear over the ACH system. Consumers with outstanding overdrafts or garnishment orders may have chosen to use high-cost check cashing stores "for fear that some of the funds would be reclaimed by their bank or garnished by a creditor" (Murphy, 2021, p. 14). Estimates of check cashing fees for first round COVID-19 stimulus payments reached $66 million (Murphy, 2021), despite 70 percent of check cashing customers having commercial bank accounts (Klein, 2021b).

The Fed has taken the position, however, that it is not allowed to offer consumer accounts. Chair Powell has stated that it is "not equipped to service individual commercial and retail accounts. . . That's never been our role and it's really not been the role of other central banks" (ABA Banking Journal, 2021). Concerns have also been raised over the impact of retail access to Fed accounts and correspondingly, the impact that

Fed liabilities (as opposed to commercial bank liabilities) would have on the stability of the commercial banking system. During periods of financial systemic stress, consumers may move money out of commercial banks and into Fed accounts, as in a "run on the bank" (Baer, 2021).

As an alternative to the creation of Fed or USPS accounts, commercial banks and credit unions could do a better job of reaching those who do not have bank accounts. Roughly half (about 49 percent) of unbanked households reported previously having a bank account, according to 2021 data from FDIC, indicating that a substantial share of the unbanked may be willing to have an account, but perhaps for reasons related to cost, did not maintain ownership (FDIC, 2021). FDIC developed a set of criteria for low-cost, high-quality accounts known as "Safe Accounts" under a pilot program. Implementation of this pilot was functionally transferred to Bank On, an arm of Cities for Financial Empowerment Fund that certifies banks that offer compliant accounts. The 2023–2024 Bank On National Account Standards include a low minimum opening deposit, low or waivable monthly maintenance fee, and no fees for overdrafts, insufficient funds, account activation, closure, dormancy, inactivity, or low balance (Cities for Financial Empowerment Fund, n.d.). Bank On accounts are considered a best-practice offering by the American Bankers Association (FindCRA Learning Center, 2020) but are not required.

In addition to benefiting individuals who could otherwise not afford to maintain a bank account, these low-cost accounts also have benefits for financial institutions. First, Bank On accounts enable institutions to meet regulations for community reinvestment. Additionally, access to a basic account is a critical first step that allows unbanked individuals to enter the mainstream financial system and potentially build savings and use credit in the future. According to data from the Federal Reserve Bank of St. Louis, Bank On accounts brought nearly 1.8 million new customers to 17 reporting institutions in 2020. Overall, in 2020, there were 3.8 million open and active Bank On accounts across these institutions (Briggs et al., 2021; Cities for Financial Empowerment Fund, 2018). Banks also stand to profit off debit usage from these accounts. Bank On account holders across reporting institutions had over 767 million debit transactions in 2020, which totaled nearly $29 billion (Briggs et al., 2021; Cities for Financial Empowerment Fund, 2018).

Some have argued that if the federal government were to require all banks to offer Bank On accounts, potentially as the default basic account for lower-income consumers, financial inclusion[13] would be greatly

---

[13] Financial inclusion is part of the broader goal of economic inclusion, defined by the FDIC as "all consumers have access to safe, secure, and affordable financial products and services" (FDIC, 2022).

enhanced (Klein, 2021a). Furthermore, as these accounts do not contain costly products, such as overdraft fees (which were estimated to cost consumers $15–35 billion a year), they would produce substantial savings to those already in the banking system but struggling to afford the cost of operating their accounts (Klein, 2021a,b). Finally, these accounts could be used to more effectively distribute financial assistance for emergency and standard government benefits, given the interlinking between the U.S. government and commercial banks and credit unions (Klein and Karaflos, 2021).

However, relying on the commercial systems to market these accounts and reach consumers who may not be profitable to bank could result in a failure to fully solve the problem, unlike accounts offered directly by the government. Commercial banks (but not credit unions) are required under the Community Reinvestment Act of 1977 (CRA)[14] to "help meet the credit needs of communities in which they do business, including low- and moderate-income neighborhoods" (The Federal Reserve, 2022). Federal bank regulators are required to assess commercial banks and provide CRA ratings, a process that is undergoing substantial revision. The extent to which regulators implement the new CRA system and hold banks accountable may impact the ability of low- and moderate-income families to have better access to lower-cost and higher-quality financial services.

As described above, banking status is highly correlated to race, with Hispanic and Black households about 4.4 and 5.4 times more likely to be unbanked than White households (FDIC, 2021). Racial discrimination past and present helped to drive what have been termed "banking and credit deserts" in racially and ethnically minoritized and underserved rural communities (Broady et al., 2021), including tribal communities. Underlying causes for these inequities are concentrated in gaps in health, wealth, and cultural hurdles, not citizenship status or desire for privacy (Blanco et al., 2019). Black and Hispanic checking account holders are estimated to pay up to twice as much as White account holders in bank fees, resulting in substantially high costs for services (CNBC, 2021). This gap leaves racially and ethnically minoritized households more vulnerable to negative economic outcomes (Moss et al., 2020). Thus, policies that reduce the cost of having an account, such as providing low-cost bank accounts through governmentally backed entities, requiring banks and credit unions to offer Bank On accounts, or holding banks accountable to the CRA, would have important implications for racial and ethnic inequities in economic stability and, consequently, health and well-being.

---

[14] 12 U.S.C. § 2901 *et seq.*

Credit Scoring

A related barrier to financial health is credit scoring, which privileges those who already possess assets. A credit score is intended to reflect how creditworthy a person is. Scores below about 620 are considered subprime; those above are prime. A minority of people are "prime credits," with most considered subprime or credit invisible (they have insufficient information from which to create a credit score) (Meni, 2016). Consumers with lower scores are deemed less able to take on and repay debt. As a result, they pay more for credit (in interest and fees). Credit scores are imperfect measures of creditworthiness, especially for certain groups. The data used to compute the scores are limited and often inaccurate. For example, monthly payments for utilities are generally not reflected on credit reports, but mortgage payments are (Chase, n.d.). Credit scores are also based on a relatively narrow definition of what "creditworthy" means. Just as having too much debt can make it harder to get a loan, so can having no debt at all. Using historical information to predict future behavior also has drawbacks. For example, discrimination in access to financial products can result in shorter credit histories for racially and ethnically minoritized people (Rice and Swesnik, 2012). Because the number of years of credit history is one of the largest factors in credit score, scores can remain depressed for minoritized communities for lengthy periods using this backward-looking system (Rice and Swesnik, 2012). Over the past decade or so, credit scores have increasingly been used more broadly. Landlords and employers often use credit scores to screen prospective renters and employees (Servon, 2017). Auto insurance companies use them to determine insurance premiums, sparking a debate about whether they are a proxy for driving risk or being used to screen for income or race (Steeg Morris et al., 2017). This broader use of credit scores, and higher insurance premiums and interest rates on credit cards, auto loans, and mortgages for those with lower scores, amplify challenges for those already disadvantaged by the current system (Consumer Financial Protection Bureau, 2022).

For several years, fintech companies and others have been exploring the use of alternative data to create more accurate pictures of creditworthiness. Those who support this idea argue that including data such as rent, utility, mobile phone, and bank account payments will enable improved assessments of consumers' risk profiles, more timely information, and increased access to lower-cost credit (Kreiswirth et al., 2017). Research has shown alternative data can be as or more predictive than the current system (Berg et al., 2018). Opponents express concern that the kinds of alternative data that have been proposed may be more prone to inaccuracy than the data that are currently used. A fear of discrimination has also been expressed, in the event that a new type of data is closely linked to a factor such as race, gender, or ethnicity (Akinwumi et al., 2021).

Existing credit scores "reflect the social economic disparities that are out there" (Lee, 2022). Many argue that, "although credit scores never formally take race into account, they draw on data about personal borrowing and payment history that is profoundly shaped by generations of discriminatory public policies and corporate practices that limited access to wealth for Black and Latinx families" (Traub, 2021). Differences in credit score by race are substantial; Black people have an average score 57 points lower than White people (see Figure 3-11) (Broady et al., 2021).

One potential solution is to underwrite credit on the basis of a consumer's cash flow, which could replace credit scoring and credit reporting with information on the daily balance of a person's primary bank account. Measuring bank account balance has been shown to be as or in many cases more predictive than credit scores (FinRegLab, 2019). Because cash flow underwriting uses a more current view of a consumer's economic situation, it can be more financially inclusive, providing credit to individuals who would not qualify on the basis of their traditional score (PYMNTS, 2018). There are many impediments to using cash flow or any alternative to credit scoring, including the reliance on credit scores for a variety of regulatory and market functions. Some have described credit scores as the out-of-tune oboe the financial orchestra has tuned into (Klein, 2020).

The Office of Comptroller of the Currency (OCC) has created Project REACh in part to examine disadvantages caused by the credit scoring

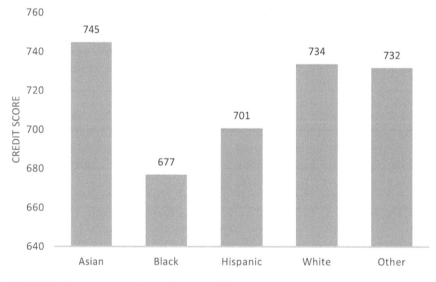

FIGURE 3-11 Average credit score by race, 2021.
SOURCE: Data from Shift Credit Card Processing, 2021.

system, which it estimates impact nearly 50 million people, and identify alternatives and solutions (OCC, n.d.). Other regulators could work similarly or in conjunction with the OCC to identify specific regulatory barriers and remove or alter them to enhance financial inclusion. Congress could help regulators prioritize improvement of the credit scoring system via oversight hearings, letters, or by requesting the Government Accountability Office identify regulatory barriers to alternatives and propose solutions. These and other efforts to use alternative credit scoring methods could enhance financial inclusion and increase economic well-being and health outcomes for low-income individuals and racially and ethnically minoritized populations. Action on this issue could also come from the Consumer Financial Protection Bureau, which supervises credit reporting agencies (USAGov, n.d.).

Conclusion 3-8: Unequal access to safe and affordable financial services, including bank accounts and low-cost credit, is a driver of inequities. Enabling the provision of financial services that allow all Americans to spend, save, borrow, and plan will enable greater economic stability and increase health equity for low-income and racially and ethnically minoritized populations.

CONCLUDING OBSERVATIONS

This chapter outlined numerous examples of how federal policy contributes to inequities in economic stability for racially and ethnically minoritized populations and tribal communities. Rather than proposing recommendations for changes to these specific federal policies and programs, the committee offers mainly crosscutting recommendations. However, many existing National Academies reports have evidence-based and promising recommendations for federal action to advance health equity in the area of economic stability (including and beyond the federal policies reviewed in this chapter) that have not been implemented and are still relevant today (see Box 3-1 for examples) (NASEM, 2019a,b).

Several crosscutting themes the committee identified provide promising strategies to improve economic stability via federal policies so that all communities can thrive. For economic stability, the policy examples discussed highlight the importance of access, eligibility, and accountability to existing legislation. For example, broadening access to programs such as SNAP, WIC, and EITC by addressing administrative barriers, holding programs accountable for participation rates, and improving administrative capacity can reduce racial and ethnic health inequities. Eligibility restrictions for such programs, such as for childless adults, formerly incarcerated individuals, and immigrants, contribute to health inequities because these groups disproportionately represent racially and ethnically minoritized

BOX 3-1
Example Recommendations from National Academies Reports

Vibrant and Healthy Kids: Aligning Science, Practice, and Policy to Advance Health Equity (NASEM, 2019b)

Recommendation 6-1: Federal, state, local, tribal, and territorial policy makers should implement paid parental leave. In partnership with researchers, policy makers should model variations in the level of benefits, length of leave, and funding mechanisms to determine alternatives that will have the largest impacts on improving child health outcomes and reducing health disparities.

Recommendation 6-2: Federal, state, local, territorial, and tribal agencies should reduce barriers to participation in the Special Supplemental Nutrition Program for Women, Infants, and Children (WIC) and Supplemental Nutrition Assistance Program (SNAP) benefits. Receipt of WIC and SNAP benefits should not be tied to parent employment for families with young children or for pregnant women, as work requirements are likely to reduce participation rates.

Recommendation 6-6: Federal, state, tribal, and territorial policy makers should address the critical gaps between family resources and family needs through a combination of benefits that have the best evidence of advancing health equity, such as increased Supplemental Nutrition Assistance Program benefits, increased housing assistance, and a basic income allowance for young children.

A Roadmap to Reducing Child Poverty (NASEM, 2019a)

Recommendation 9-1: Relevant federal departments and agencies, especially those granting waivers to state and local governments to test new work-related programs, should prioritize high-quality, methodologically rigorous research and experimentation to identify ways to boost the job skills and employment of parents of low-income families receiving public assistance. Congress should ensure that sufficient funding is made available to conduct these evaluations.

Recommendation 9-2: Relevant federal departments and agencies should prioritize research and experimentation aimed at finding ways to reduce the financial instability of low-income families participating in assistance programs. Program features that may contribute to this goal and merit evaluation include streamlined program administration, more convenient access to the benefits that families are eligible to receive, provisions for emergency assistance, and flexibility in the frequency of benefit payments.

Recommendation 9-3: Relevant federal departments and agencies should prioritize research and experimentation designed to improve the administration of assistance programs, especially to facilitate full and equitable access to the benefits to which low-income families are entitled. Such research should focus not only on streamlining program processes but also on making outreach about programs more effective, enhancing the communication skills of program staff, and strengthening program staff's ability to interact with all population groups.

> ### BOX 3-1 Continued
>
> The committee for this consensus study also developed four program and policy packages aimed at reducing child poverty by 50 percent and assessed the predicted impact of these packages.

populations. Ensuring accountability to existing legislation, such as CRA, could improve racial and ethnic inequities in income and banking. A lack of data for NHPI and AIAN populations was also a crosscutting theme identified by the committee. The lack of data for NHPI populations in this chapter makes this issue especially apparent.

REFERENCES

ABA Banking Journal. 2021. *Powell: Fed 'Not Equipped' to Service Individual Accounts.* https://bankingjournal.aba.com/2021/03/powell-fed-not-equipped-to-service-individual-accounts/ (accessed March 17, 2023).

Addo, F. R., and W. A. Darity, Jr. 2022. *Racial disparities in household wealth following the Great Recession.* Madison, WI: University of Wisconsin—Madison, Institute for Research on Poverty.

Agan, A., and S. Starr. 2018. Ban the box, criminal records, and racial discrimination: A field experiment. *The Quarterly Journal of Economics* 133(1):191–235.

Akee, R. 2019. *How Does Measuring Poverty and Welfare Affect American Indian Children?* https://www.brookings.edu/blog/up-front/2019/03/12/how-does-measuring-poverty-and-welfare-affect-american-indian-children/ (accessed March 7, 2023).

Akee, R., W. Copeland, E. J. Costello, and E. Simeonova. 2018. How does household income affect child personality traits and behaviors? *American Economic Review* 108(3):775–827.

Akinwumi, M., J. Merrill, L. Rice, K. Saleh, and M. Yap. 2021. *An AI fair lending policy agenda for the federal financial regulators.* Washington, DC: The Brookings Institution.

Almond, D., H. W. Hoynes, and D. Schanzenbach. 2008. *NBER working paper series: Inside the war on poverty: The impact of food stamps on birth outcomes.* Cambridge, MA: National Bureau of Economic Research.

Almond, D., J. Currie, and V. Duque. 2018. Childhood circumstances and adult outcomes: Act II. *Journal of Economic Literature* 56(4):1360–1446.

Altonji, J. G., and R. M. Blank. 1999. Race and gender in the labor market. In *Handbook of labor economics,* Vol. 3, edited by O. C. Ashenfelter and D. Card. Amsterdam, Netherlands: Elsevier Science B.V. Pp. 3143–3259.

Australian Citizens Party. n.d. *International Examples of Post Office Banking.* https://citizensparty.org.au/campaigns/public-post-office-bank/int-examples-post-office-bank (accessed March 15, 2023).

Averett, S., and Y. Wang. 2013. The effects of Earned Income Tax Credit payment expansion on maternal smoking. *Health Economics* 22(11):1344-1359.

Baer, G. 2021. *Staff working paper: Central bank digital currencies: Costs, benefits and major implications for the U.S. economic system.* Washington, DC: Bank Policy Institute.

Baker, K. 2008. *Do cash transfer programs improve infant health: Evidence from the 1993 expansion of the Earned Income Tax Credit.* Notre Dame, IN: University of Notre Dame.

Bannon, A., M. Nagrecha, and R. Diller. 2010. *Criminal justice debt: A barrier to reentry.* New York, NY: Brennan Center for Justice.

Baradaran, M. 2014. It's time for postal banking. *Harvard Law Review* 127(4):165–175.

Bastian, J., and K. Michelmore. 2018. The long-term impact of the Earned Income Tax Credit on children's education and employment outcomes. *Journal of Labor Economics* 36(4):1127–1163.

Bayer, P., and K. K. Charles. 2016. *NBER working paper series: Divergent paths: Structural change, economic rank, and the evolution of Black–White earnings differences, 1940–2014.* Cambridge, MA: National Bureau of Economic Research.

Berg, T., A. Gombovic, V. Berg, and M. Puri. 2018. *Working paper series: On the rise of the fintechs—credit scoring using digital footprints.* Washington, DC: Federal Deposit Insurance Corporation.

Bernstein, H., D. Gonzalez, M. Karpman, and S. Zuckerman. 2020. *Amid confusion over the public charge rule, immigrant families continued avoiding public benefits in 2019.* Washington, DC: Urban Institute.

Bernstein, H., D. Gonzalez, M. Karpman, and S. Zuckerman. 2021. *Immigrant families continued avoiding the safety net during the COVID-19 crisis.* Washington, DC: Urban Institute.

Bertrand, M., and S. Mullainathan. 2004. Are Emily and Greg more employable than Lakisha and Jamal? A field experiment on labor market discrimination. *American Economic Review* 94(4):991–1013.

Bhutta, N., A. C. Chang, L. J. Dettling, and J. W. Hsu. 2020. *Feds Notes: Disparities in Wealth by Race and Ethnicity in the 2019 Survey of Consumer Finances.* https://www.federalreserve.gov/econres/notes/feds-notes/disparities-in-wealth-by-race-and-ethnicity-in-the-2019-survey-of-consumer-finances-20200928.html (accessed June 2, 2023).

Bing, L., B. Pettit, and I. Slavinski. 2022. Incomparable punishments: How economic inequality contributes to the disparate impact of legal fines and fees. *The Russell Sage Foundation Journal of the Social Sciences* 8(2):118–136.

Bitler, M., H. W. Hoynes, and D. Schanzenbach. 2020. *NBER working paper series: The social safety net in the wake of COVID-19.* Cambridge, MA: National Bureau of Economic Research.

Bitler, M., H. W. Hoynes, and D. Schanzenbach. 2023. Suffering, the safety net, and disparities during COVID-19. *The Russell Sage Foundation Journal of the Social Sciences* 9(3):32–59.

Black, S. E., D. Schanzenbach, and A. Breitwieser. 2017. *The recent decline in women's labor force participation.* Washington, DC: The Hamilton Project.

Blanco, L. R., M. Angrisani, E. Aguila, and M. Leng. 2019. Understanding the racial/ethnic gap in bank account ownership among older adults. *The Journal of Consumer Affairs* 53(2):324–354.

Bleich, S. N., A. J. Moran, K. A. Vercammen, J. M. Frelier, C. G. Dunn, A. Zhong, and S. E. Fleischhacker. 2020. Strengthening the public health impacts of the Supplemental Nutrition Assistance Program through policy. *Annual Review of Public Health* 41(1):453–480.

BLS (Bureau of Labor Statistics). 2023. *Labor Force Statistics from the Current Population Survey: Employed Persons by Occupation, Race, Hispanic or Latino Ethnicity, and Sex.* https://www.bls.gov/cps/cpsaat10.htm (accessed March 11, 2023).

Bolen, E. 2021. *Restore SNAP for People with Drug-Related Convictions.* https://www.cbpp.org/blog/restore-snap-for-people-with-drug-related-convictions (accessed March 17, 2023).

Bonczar, T. B. 1995. *Bureau of Justice Statistics special report: Characteristics of adults on probation, 1995.* Washington, DC: U.S. Department of Justice, Office of Justice Programs.

Boshara, R., W. R. Emmons, and B. J. Noeth. 2015a. *The demographics of wealth: How age, education and race separate thrivers from strugglers in today's economy: Essay no. 1: Race, ethnicity and wealth.* St. Louis, MO: Federal Reserve Bank of St. Louis.

Boshara, R., W. R. Emmons, and B. J. Noeth. 2015b. *The demographics of wealth: How age, education and race separate thrivers from strugglers in today's economy: Essay no. 2: Education and wealth.* St. Louis, MO: Federal Reserve Bank of St. Louis.

Boshara, R., W. R. Emmons, and B. J. Noeth. 2015c. *The demographics of wealth: How age, education and race separate thrivers from strugglers in today's economy: Essay no. 3: Age, birth year and wealth.* St. Louis, MO: Federal Reserve Bank of St. Louis.

Braveman, P., J. Acker, E. Arkin, D. Proctor, A. Gillman, K. A. McGeary, and G. Mallya. 2018. *Wealth matters for health equity.* Princeton, NJ: Robert Wood Johnson Foundation.

Briggs, M. L., N. Chalise, and V. Gutkowski. 2021. *The Bank On national data hub: Findings from 2020.* St. Louis, MO: Federal Reserve Bank of St. Louis.

Broady, K., M. McComas, and A. Ouazad. 2021. *An analysis of financial institutions in Black-majority communities: Black borrowers and depositors face considerable challenges in accessing banking services.* Washington, DC: The Brookings Institution.

Cabili, C., E. Eslami, and R. Briefel. 2013. *White paper on the Emergency Food Assistance Program (TEFAP).* Alexandria, VA: USDA, Food and Nutrition Service, Office of Policy Support.

Cajner, T., T. Radler, D. Ratner, and I. Vidangos. 2017. *Finance and economics discussion series: Racial gaps in labor market outcomes in the last four decades and over the business cycle.* Washington, DC: The Federal Reserve.

CBO (Congressional Budget Office). 2022. *How Increasing the Federal Minimum Wage Could Affect Employment and Family Income.* https://www.cbo.gov/publication/55681 (accessed March 7, 2023).

CBPP (Center on Budget and Policy Priorities). 2023a. *Policy Basics: The Earned Income Tax Credit.* https://www.cbpp.org/research/federal-tax/the-earned-income-tax-credit (accessed June 1, 2023).

CBPP. 2023b. *States Are Using Much-Needed Temporary Flexibility in SNAP to Respond to COVID-19 Challenges.* https://www.cbpp.org/research/food-assistance/states-are-using-much-needed-temporary-flexibility-in-snap-to-respond-to (accessed March 8, 2023).

Census Bureau. 2022. *America's Families and Living Arrangements: 2022: Table H3. Households, by Race and Hispanic Origin of Household Reference Person and Detailed Type.* https://www.census.gov/data/tables/2022/demo/families/cps-2022.html (accessed March 6, 2023).

Chase. n.d. *Does Paying Monthly Bills Build Your Credit History?* https://www.chase.com/personal/credit-cards/education/build-credit/does-paying-monthly-bills-build-credit-history (accessed March 17, 2023).

Chetty, R., J. N. Friedman, and J. Rockoff. 2011. *SOI working paper: New evidence on the long-term impacts of tax credits.* Washington, DC: IRS.

Chetty, R., N. Hendren, M. R. Jones, and S. R. Porter. 2020. Race and economic opportunity in the United States: An intergenerational perspective. *The Quarterly Journal of Economics* 135(2):711–783.

Chorniy, A. V., J. Currie, and L. Sonchak. 2020. *NBER working paper series: Does prenatal WIC participation improve child outcomes?* Cambridge, MA: National Bureau of Economic Research.

Cities for Financial Empowerment Fund. 2018. *The present and future of Bank On account data: Pilot results and prospective data collection.* New York, NY: Cities for Financial Empowerment Fund.

Cities for Financial Empowerment Fund. n.d. *Bank On National Account Standards (2023–2024).* https://joinbankon.org/wp-content/uploads/2022/08/Bank-On-National-Account-Standards-2023-2024.pdf (accessed June 2, 2023).

Clancy, M. M., S. G. Beverly, M. Schreiner, J. Huang, and M. Sherraden. 2021. *CSD research summary 21-06: Financial outcomes in a child development account experiment: Full inclusion, success regardless of race or income, and investment growth for all.* St. Louis, MO: Washington University, Center for Social Development.

CNBC. 2021. *Black and Hispanic Americans Pay Twice as Much in Bank Fees as Whites, Survey Finds.* https://www.cnbc.com/2021/01/13/black-and-hispanics-paying-twice-amount-banking-fees-than-whites-survey.html (accessed March 11, 2023).

Coleman-Jensen, A., M. P. Rabbitt, C. A. Gregory, and A. Singh. 2022. *Household food security in the United States in 2021.* Washington, DC: USDA, Economic Research Service.

Consumer Financial Protection Bureau. 2022. *What Is a Credit Score?* https://www.consumerfinance.gov/ask-cfpb/what-is-a-credit-score-en-315/ (accessed June 12, 2023).

Conti-Brown, P. 2018. *Why the next big bank shouldn't be the USPS.* Washington, DC: The Brookings Institution.

Cooper, D., S. Martinez Hickey, and B. Zipperer. 2022. *The Value of the Federal Minimum Wage Is at Its Lowest Point in 66 Years.* https://www.epi.org/blog/the-value-of-the-federal-minimum-wage-is-at-its-lowest-point-in-66-years/ (accessed March 7, 2023).

Council of Economic Advisers. 2016. *The long-term decline in prime-age male labor force participation.* Washington, DC: Executive Office of the President of the United States.

Craigie, T. A., A. Grawert, and C. Kimble. 2020. *Conviction, imprisonment, and lost earnings: How involvement with the criminal justice system deepens inequality.* New York, NY: Brennan Center for Justice.

Crawford, J., L. Menand, and M. Ricks. 2021. Fedaccounts: Digital dollars. *The George Washington Law Review* 89(1):113–172.

Creamer, J., E. A. Shrider, K. Burns, and F. Chen. 2022. *Poverty in the United States: 2021.* Washington, DC: United States Census Bureau.

Currie, J., and I. Rajani. 2015. Within-mother estimates of the effects of WIC on birth outcomes in New York City. *Economic Inquiry* 53(4):1691–1701.

Dahl, G. B., and L. Lochner. 2012. The impact of family income on child achievement: Evidence from the Earned Income Tax Credit. *American Economic Review* 102(5):1927–1956.

Dahl, G.B., and L. Lochner. 2017. The impact of family income on child achievement: Evidence from the Earned Income Tax Credit: Reply. *American Economic Review* 107(2):629–631.

Daly, M. C., B. Hobijn, and J. H. Pedtke. 2017. *FRBSF Economic Letter: Disappointing Facts About the Black–White Wage Gap.* https://www.frbsf.org/economic-research/publications/economic-letter/2017/september/disappointing-facts-about-black-white-wage-gap/ (accessed March 3, 2023).

DiVito, E. 2022. *Banking for All: How the USPS Could Provide Public Banking.* https://rooseveltinstitute.org/2022/06/30/banking-for-all/ (accessed March 10, 2023).

Dobbie, W., and C. Yang. 2021. *The economic costs of pretrial detention.* Washington, DC: The Brookings Institution.

DOL (Department of Labor). 2023. *State Minimum Wage Laws.* https://www.dol.gov/agencies/whd/minimum-wage/state (accessed May 29, 2023).

Dube, A. 2014. *Proposal 13: Designing thoughtful minimum wage policy at the state and local levels.* Washington, DC: The Hamilton Project.

East, C. N. 2020. The effect of food stamps on children's health: Evidence from immigrants' changing eligibility. *Journal of Human Resources* 55(2):387–427.

East, C. N., and A. J. Friedson. 2020. An apple a day? Adult food stamp eligibility and health care utilization among immigrants. *American Journal of Health Economics* 6(3):289–323.

Economic Development Administration. n.d. *Economic Resilience.* https://www.eda.gov/grant-resources/comprehensive-economic-development-strategy/content/economic-resilience (accessed May 30, 2023).

Evans, W. N., and C. L. Garthwaite. 2014. Giving mom a break: The impact of higher EITC payments on maternal health. *American Economic Journal: Economic Policy* 6(2):258–290.

Farrell, J., P. B. Burow, K. McConnell, J. Bayham, K. Whyte, and G. Koss. 2021. Effects of land dispossession and forced migration on Indigenous peoples in North America. *Science* 374(6567):eabe4943.

FDIC (Federal Deposit Insurance Corporation). 2019. *How America banks: Household use of banking and financial services.* Washington, DC: Federal Deposit Insurance Corporation.

FDIC. 2021. *FDIC national survey of unbanked and underbanked households.* Washington, DC: Federal Deposit Insurance Corporation.

FDIC. 2022. *What Is Economic Inclusion?* https://www.fdic.gov/analysis/household-survey/economic-inclusion/index.html (accessed March 17, 2023).

The Federal Reserve. 2020. *Automated Clearinghouse Services.* https://www.federalreserve.gov/paymentsystems/fedach_about.htm (accessed May 31, 2023).

The Federal Reserve. 2021a. *Fedwire Funds Services.* https://www.federalreserve.gov/paymentsystems/fedfunds_about.htm (accessed May 31, 2023).

The Federal Reserve. 2021b. *National Settlement Service.* https://www.federalreserve.gov/paymentsystems/natl_about.htm (accessed May 31, 2023).

The Federal Reserve. 2022. *Community Reinvestment Act (CRA).* https://www.federalreserve.gov/consumerscommunities/cra_about.htm (accessed June 20, 2023).

Federal Reserve Bank of St. Louis. n.d. *Current Population Survey (household survey).* https://fred.stlouisfed.org/categories/12 (accessed March 3, 2023).

Figlio, D., S. Hamersma, and J. Roth. 2009. Does prenatal WIC participation improve birth outcomes? New evidence from Florida. *Journal of Public Economics* 93(1-2):235–245.

Figlio, D., J. Guryan, K. Karbownik, and J. Roth. 2014. The effects of poor neonatal health on children's cognitive development. *American Economic Review* 104(12):3921–3955.

The Financial Justice Project. n.d. *The Financial Justice Project.* https://sfgov.org/financialjustice/ (accessed March 15, 2023).

FindCRA Learning Center. 2020. *ABA: America's Banks Urged to Offer Bank On-Certified Accounts.* https://www.learncra.com/aba-americas-banks-urged-to-offer-bank-on-certified-accounts/ (accessed March 17, 2023).

Finkelstein, A., and M. J. Notowidigdo. 2018. *NBER working paper series: Take-up and targeting: Experimental evidence from SNAP.* Cambridge, MA: National Bureau of Economic Research.

Finkelstein, D. M., J. F. Harding, D. Paulsell, B. English, G. R. Hijjawi, and J. Ng'andu. 2022. Economic well-being and health: The role of income support programs in promoting health and advancing health equity. *Health Affairs* 41(12):1700–1706.

FinRegLab. 2019. *The use of cash-flow data in underwriting credit: Empirical research findings.* Washington, DC: FinRegLab.

Fishback, P. V., J. Rose, K. A. Snowden, and T. Storrs. 2022. *NBER working paper series: New evidence on redlining by federal housing programs in the 1930s.* Cambridge, MA: National Bureau of Economic Research.

Fox, D. L., C. D. Hansen, and A. M. Miller. 2023. *Over-incarceration of Native Americans: Roots, inequities, and solutions.* Chicago, IL: Safety + Justice Challange.

Freund, D. M. P. 2010. *Colored property: State policy and White racial politics in suburban America.* Chicago, IL: The University of Chicago Press.

Garfield, R., K. Orgera, and A. Damico. 2020. *Issue Brief: The Coverage Gap: Uninsured Poor Adults in States That Do Not Expand Medicaid.* https://files.kff.org/attachment/Issue-Brief-The-Coverage-Gap-Uninsured-Poor-Adults-in-States-that-Do-Not-Expand-Medicaid (accessed March 7, 2023).

Gleckman, H., and E. Maag. 2020. *Free File Is an Easy Way for Government to Get Coronavirus Payments to Non-Filers.* https://www.taxpolicycenter.org/taxvox/free-file-easy-way-government-get-coronavirus-payments-non-filers (accessed June 20, 2023).

Global Social Development Innovations. n.d. *Economic Security.* https://gsdi.unc.edu/our-work/economic-security/ (accessed May 30, 2023).

Goldin, J., T. Homonoff, R. Javaid, and B. Schafer. 2022. Tax filing and take-up: Experimental evidence on tax preparation outreach and benefit claiming. *Journal of Public Economics* 206:104550.

Gorman, K. S., A. M. Smith, M. E. Cimini, K. M. Halloran, and A. G. Lubiner. 2013. Reaching the hard to reach: Lessons learned from a statewide outreach initiative. *Journal of Community Practice* 21(1–2):105–123.

Gothro, A., K. Chesnut, M. Hu, and R. Briefel. 2020. *ESAP state enrollment data collection project.* Washington, DC: Mathematica Policy Research.

Gould, E. 2020. *State of working America wages 2019: A story of slow, uneven, and unequal wage growth over the last 40 years.* Washington, DC: Economic Policy Institute.

Gray, C. 2019. Leaving benefits on the table: Evidence from SNAP. *Journal of Public Economics* 179:104054.

Gray, K., C. Trippe, C. Tadler, C. Perry, P. Johnson, and D. Betson. 2019. *National- and state-level estimates of WIC eligibility and WIC program reach in 2017.* Arlington, VA: Insight Policy Research, Inc.

Grodsky, E., and D. Pager. 2001. The structure of disadvantage: Individual and occupational determinants of the Black–White wage gap. *American Sociological Review* 66(4):542–567.

Hamilton, C., C. Wimer, S. Collyer, and L. Sariscsany. 2022. *Monthly cash payments reduce spells of poverty across the year.* New York, NY: Columbia University, Center on Poverty and Social Policy.

Hamilton, D., and W. Darity, Jr. 2010. Can "baby bonds" eliminate the racial wealth gap in putative post-racial America? *The Review of Black Political Economy* 37:207–216.

Hardy, B. L., and T. D. Logan. 2020. *Racial economic inequality amid the COVID-19 crisis.* Washington, DC: The Hamilton Project.

Hardy, B.L., H. D. Hill, and J. Romich. 2019. Strengthening social programs to promote economic stability during childhood. *Social Policy Report* 32(2):1–36.

Hardy, B. L., S. M. Collyer, and C. T. Wimer. 2023. *The antipoverty effects of the expanded Child Tax Credit across states: Where were the historic reductions felt?* Washington, DC: The Hamilton Project.

Harris, A. 2016. *A pound of flesh: Monetary sanctions as punishment for the poor.* New York, NY: Russell Sage Foundation.

Harris, A., H. Evans, and K. Beckett. 2010. Drawing blood from stones: Legal debt and social inequality in the contemporary United States. *American Journal of Sociology* 115(6):1753–1799.

Harris, A., M. Pattillo, and B. L. Sykes. 2022. Studying the system of monetary sanctions. *The Russell Sage Foundation Journal of the Social Sciences* 8(1):1–33.

Herbert, C. E., D. R. Haurin, S. S. Rosenthal, and M. Duda. 2005. *Homeownership gaps among low-income and minority borrowers and neighborhood.* Cambridge, MA: Abt Associates, Inc.

HHS. 2020. *Healthy People 2030: Economic Stability.* https://health.gov/healthypeople/objectives-and-data/browse-objectives/economic-stability (accessed March 22, 2023).

Homonoff, T., and J. Somerville. 2021. Program recertification costs: Evidence from SNAP. *American Economic Journal: Economic Policy* 13(4):271–298.

Horowitz, J. M., R. Igielnik, and R. Kochhar. 2020. *Most Americans say there is too much economic inequality in the U.S., but fewer than half call it a top priority.* Washington, DC: Pew Research Center.

Hoynes, H., D. Miller, and D. Simon. 2015. Income, the Earned Income Tax Credit, and infant health. *American Economic Journal: Economic Policy* 7(1):172–211.

Hoynes, H., M. Page, and A. H. Stevens. 2011. Can targeted transfers improve birth outcomes?: Evidence from the introduction of the WIC program. *Journal of Public Economics* 95(7–8):813–827.

Hoynes, H., and A. J. Patel. 2015. *NBER working paper series: Effective policy for reducing inequality? The Earned Income Tax Credit and the distribution of income.* Cambridge, MA: National Bureau of Economic Research.

Hoynes, H., D. Schanzenbach, and D. Almond. 2016. Long-run impacts of childhood access to the safety net. *American Economic Review* 106(4):903–934.

Huang, J., S. G. Beverly, M. M. Clancy, M. Schreiner, and M. Sherraden. 2021. *CSD research report no. 21-07: A long-term experiment on child development accounts: Update and impacts of SEED for Oklahoma Kids.* St. Louis, MO: Washington University, Center for Social Development.

Huebner, B. M., and A. Giuffre. 2022. Reinforcing the web of municipal courts: Evidence and implications post-Ferguson. *The Russell Sage Foundation Journal of the Social Sciences* 8(1):108–127.

IRS (Internal Revenue Service). 2006. *News Release: IRS Expands Taxpayers' Options for Direct Deposit of Refunds.* https://www.irs.gov/pub/irs-news/ir-06-085.pdf (accessed March 9, 2023).

IRS. 2023. *How the Expanded 2021 Child Tax Credit Can Help Your Family.* https://www.irs.gov/newsroom/how-the-expanded-2021-child-tax-credit-can-help-your-family (accessed May 25, 2023).

Kennedy-Moulton, K., S. Miller, P. Persson, M. Rossin-Slater, L. Wherry, and G. Aldana. 2022. *NBER working paper series: Maternal and infant health inequality: New evidence from linked administrative data.* Cambridge, MA: National Bureau of Economic Research.

KFF (Kaiser Family Foundation). n.d. *Poverty Rate by Race/Ethnicity.* https://www.kff.org/other/state-indicator/poverty-rate-by-raceethnicity/?currentTimeframe=0&sortModel=%7B%22colId%22:%22Location%22,%22sort%22:%22asc%22%7D# (accessed March 2, 2023).

Kijakazi, K., and A. Carther. 2020. *How Baby Bonds Could Help Americans Start Adulthood Strong and Narrow the Racial Wealth Gap.* https://www.urban.org/urban-wire/how-baby-bonds-could-help-americans-start-adulthood-strong-and-narrow-racial-wealth-gap#:~:text=Would%20baby%20bonds%20close%20the,These%20results%20are%20very%20promising (accessed March 9, 2023).

Klein, A. 2020. *Reducing bias in AI-based financial services.* Washington, DC: The Brookings Institution.

Klein, A. 2021a. *Can fintech improve health?* Washington, DC: The Brookings Institution.

Klein, A. 2021b. *Opening Statement of Aaron Klein at Roundtable on America's Unbanked and Underbanked.* https://www.brookings.edu/opinions/opening-statement-of-aaron-klein-at-roundtable-on-americas-unbanked-and-underbanked/ (accessed March 17, 2023).

Klein, A., and M. Karaflos. 2021. *Universal Bank Accounts Necessary for Families to Bank On Child Tax Credit.* https://www.brookings.edu/opinions/universal-bank-accounts-necessary-for-families-to-bank-on-child-tax-credit/ (accessed March 17, 2023).

Kline, P., E. K. Rose, and C. R. Walters. 2022. Systemic discrimination among large U.S. employers. *The Quarterly Journal of Economics* 137(4):1963–2036.

Kreiswirth, B., P. Schoenrock, and P. Singh. 2017. *Using Alternative Data to Evaluate Creditworthiness.* https://www.consumerfinance.gov/about-us/blog/using-alternative-data-evaluate-creditworthiness (accessed March 10, 2023).

Krogstad, J. M. 2014. *One-in-Four Native Americans and Alaska Natives Are Living in Poverty.* https://www.pewresearch.org/fact-tank/2014/06/13/1-in-4-native-americans-and-alaska-natives-are-living-in-poverty/ (accessed March 2, 2023).

Lee, D. S. 1999. Wage inequality in the United States during the 1980s: Rising dispersion or falling minimum wage? *The Quarterly Journal of Economics* 114(3):977–1023.

Lee, J. 2022. *How Structural Racism Plays a Role in Lowering Credit Scores.* https://www.cnbc.com/2022/10/11/how-structural-racism-plays-a-role-in-lowering-credit-scores.html (accessed March 9, 2023).

Looney, A., and N. Turner. 2018. *Work and opportunity before and after incarceration.* Washington, DC: The Brookings Institution.

Mabli, J. 2015. Supplemental Nutrition Assistance Program participation and local program outreach and eligibility services. *Agricultural and Resource Economics Review* 44(3):291–314.

Maxim, R., R. Akee, and G. R. Sanchez. 2022. *For the First Time, the Government Published Monthly Unemployment Data on Native Americans, and the Picture Is Stark.* https://www.brookings.edu/blog/the-avenue/2022/02/09/despite-an-optimistic-jobs-report-new-data-shows-native-american-unemployment-remains-staggeringly-high/ (accessed March 3, 2023).

McKernan, S. M., C. Ratcliffe, M. Simms, and S. Zhang. 2012. *Do financial support and inheritance contribute to the racial wealth gap?* Washington, DC: Urban Institute.

Meckel, K. 2020. Is the cure worse than the disease? Unintended effects of payment reform in a quantity-based transfer program. *American Economic Review* 110(6):1821–1865.

Menendez, M., M. F. Crowley, L. B. Eisen, and N. Atchison. 2019. *The steep costs of criminal justice fees and fines: A fiscal analysis of three states and ten counties.* New York, NY: Brennan Center for Justice.

Meni, D. 2016. *Fact file: The Importance of Credit Reports and Credit Scores for Building Financial Security.* https://prosperitynow.org/files/PDFs/Credit_Fact_File_07-2016.pdf (accessed March 17, 2023).

Miller, J. 2018. *Michael Sherraden: We Already Have "Baby Bonds."* https://csd.wustl.edu/michael-sherraden-we-already-have-baby-bonds/ (accessed March 9, 2023).

Mora, M. T., and A. Dávila. 2018. *The Hispanic–White wage gap has remained wide and relatively steady: Examining Hispanic–White gaps in wages, unemployment, labor force participation, and education by gender, immigrant status, and other subpopulations.* Washington, DC: The Economic Policy Institute.

Moss, E., K. McIntosh, W. Edelberg, and K. Broady. 2020. *The Black–White Wealth Gap Left Black Households More Vulnerable.* https://www.brookings.edu/blog/up-front/2020/12/08/the-black-white-wealth-gap-left-black-households-more-vulnerable/ (accessed March 17, 2023).

Murphy, D. 2021. *Economic Impact Payments: Uses, payment methods, and costs to recipients.* Washington, DC: The Brookings Institution.

NASEM (National Academies of Sciences, Engineering, and Medicine). 2015. *The growing gap in life expectancy by income: Implications for federal programs and policy responses.* Washington, DC: The National Academies Press.

NASEM. 2017. *Communities in action: Pathways to health equity.* Washington, DC: The National Academies Press.

NASEM. 2019a. *A roadmap to reducing child poverty.* Washington, DC: The National Academies Press.

NASEM. 2019b. *Vibrant and healthy kids: Aligning science, practice, and policy to advance health equity.* Washington, DC: The National Academies Press.

National Academy of Social Insurance. 2021. *Social Security benefits, finances, and policy options: A primer.* Washington, DC: National Academy of Social Insurance.

National Association of Counties. 2013. *Strategies to bolster economic resilience: County leadership in action.* Washington, DC: National Association of Counties.

NCOA (National Council on Aging). 2023. *American Indians and Alaska Natives: Key Demographics and Characteristics.* https://www.ncoa.org/article/american-indians-and-alaska-natives-key-demographics-and-characteristics (accessed March 17, 2023).

NCSL (National Conference of State Legislatures). 2022. *State Minimum Wages.* https://www.ncsl.org/labor-and-employment/state-minimum-wages (accessed March 7, 2023).

Neal, D. A., and W. R. Johnson. 1995. *NBER working paper series: The role of premarket factors in Black–White wage differences*. Cambridge, MA: National Bureau of Economic Research.

NICOA (National Indian Council on Aging, Inc.). 2021. *Native Households Have Highest Unbanked Percentage*. https://www.nicoa.org/native-households-have-highest-unbanked-percentage/ (accessed March 17, 2023).

Northwestern Institute for Policy Research. 2017. *Policy research brief: SNAP's short- and long-term benefits*. Evanston, IL: Northwestern University.

OCC (Office of the Comptroller of the Currency). n.d. *Project Reach: Removing Barriers to Financial Inclusion*. https://www.occ.treas.gov/topics/consumers-and-communities/project-reach/project-reach.html (accessed March 9, 2023).

Oliver, M., and T. Shapiro. 2006. *Black wealth/White wealth: A new perspective on racial inequality. 10th anniversary edition*. New York, NY: Routledge.

OMH (Office of Minority Health). 2023. *Profile: American Indian/Alaska Native*. https://minorityhealth.hhs.gov/omh/browse.aspx?lvl=3&lvlid=62 (accessed May 25, 2023).

Onkst, D. H. 1998. "First a negro. . . Incidentally a veteran": Black World War Two veterans and the G.I. Bill of Rights in the Deep South, 1944–1948. *Journal of Social History* 31(3):517–543.

PA 529. n.d. *Keystone Scholars*. https://www.pa529.com/keystone/ (accessed March 9, 2023).

Pacewicz, J., and J. N. Robinson, III. 2021. Pocketbook policing: How race shapes municipal reliance on punitive fines and fees in the Chicago suburbs. *Socio-Economic Review* 19(3):975–1003.

Page, J., and J. Soss. 2021. The predatory dimensions of criminal justice. *Science* 374(6565):291–294.

Pathak, A. 2021. *How the government can end poverty for Native American women*. Washington, DC: Center for American Progress.

Pattillo, M., and G. Kirk. 2021. Layaway freedom: Coercive financialization in the criminal legal system. *American Journal of Sociology* 126(4):889–930.

The Pew Charitable Trusts. 2010. *Collateral costs: Incarceration's effect on economic mobility*. Washington, DC: The Pew Charitable Trusts.

Piketty, T. 2013. *Capital in the twenty-first century*. Cambridge, MA: The Belknap Press of Harvard University Press.

Pollack, C. E., S. Chideya, C. Cubbin, B. Williams, M. Dekker, and P. Braveman. 2007. Should health studies measure wealth? *American Journal of Preventive Medicine* 33(3):250–264.

Prison Policy Initiative. n.d. *U.S. Incarceration Rates by Race and Ethnicity, 2010*. https://www.prisonpolicy.org/graphs/raceinc.html (accessed March 10, 2023).

PYMNTS. 2018. *Petal CEO: Using Cashflow—Not FICO—to Issue Credit Cards*. https://www.pymnts.com/news/financial-inclusion/2018/credit-cards-petal-webbank-financial-inclusion/ (accessed March 9, 2023).

Rice, L., and D. Swesnik. 2012. *Discriminatory effects of credit scoring on communities of color*. Washington, DC: National Fair Housing Alliance.

Rollings, W. H. 2004. Citizenship and suffrage: The Native American struggle for civil rights in the American West, 1830–1965. *Nevada Law Journal* 5:126–140.

Rossin-Slater, M. 2013. *Department of Economics discussion paper series: WIC in your neighborhood: New evidence on the impacts of geographic access to clinics*. New York, NY: Columbia University.

Rothstein, R. 2017. *The color of law: A forgotten history of how our government segregated America*. New York, NY: Liveright Publishing Corporation.

Schanzenbach, D., and A. Pitts. 2020. *IPR rapid research report: Food insecurity during COVID-19 in households with children: Results by racial and ethnic groups*. Evanston, IL: Northwestern Institute for Policy Research.

Schanzenbach, D., and M. R. Strain. 2020. *NBER working paper series: Employment effects of the Earned Income Tax Credit: Taking the long view.* Cambridge, MA: National Bureau of Economic Research.

Schanzenbach, D., and B. Thorn. 2020. Supporting development through child nutrition. *The Future of Children* 30(2):115–141.

Schanzenbach, D., L. Bauer, and G. Nantz. 2016a. *Twelve facts about food insecurity and SNAP.* Washington, DC: The Hamilton Project.

Schanzenbach, D., M. Mumford, R. Nunn, and L. Bauer. 2016b. *Money lightens the load.* Washington, DC: The Hamilton Project.

Scherer, Z., and Y. Mayol-García. 2022. *Half of People of Dominican and Salvadoran Origin Experienced Material Hardship in 2020.* https://www.census.gov/library/stories/2022/09/hardships-wealth-disparities-across-hispanic-groups.html (accessed March 3, 2023).

Semega, J., and M. Kollar. 2022. *Income in the United States: 2021.* Washington, DC: United States Census Bureau.

Servon, L. 2017. *The unbanking of America: How the new middle class survives.* New York, NY: Houghton Mifflin Harcourt Publishing Company.

Servon, L., and A. Esquier. 2022. Women, reentry, and the financialization of the criminal justice system. *Federal Sentencing Reporter* 34(2–3):193–195.

Servon, L., A. Esquier, and G. Tiley. 2021. Gender and financialization of the criminal justice system. *Social Sciences* 10(11):1–14.

Shambaugh, J., R. Nunn, P. Liu, and G. Nantz. 2017. *Thirteen facts about wage growth.* Washington, DC: The Hamilton Project.

Sherraden, M. 1991. *Assets and the poor: A new American welfare policy.* Armonk, NY: M. E. Sharpe, Inc.

Sherraden, M. 2005. *Inclusion in the American dream: Assets, poverty, and public policy.* New York, NY: Oxford University Press, Inc.

Shift Credit Card Processing. 2021. *Credit Score Statistics.* https://shiftprocessing.com/credit-score/#race (accessed June 9, 2023).

Siripurapu, A. 2022. *Backgrounder: The U.S. Inequality Debate.* https://www.cfr.org/backgrounder/us-inequality-debate (accessed March 6, 2023).

Sobol, N. L. 2016. Charging the poor: Criminal justice debt & modern-day debtors' prisons. *Maryland Law Review* 75(2):485–540.

Steeg Morris, D., D. Schwarcz, and J. C. Teitelbaum. 2017. Do credit-based insurance scores proxy for income in predicting auto claim risk? *Journal of Empirical Legal Studies* 14(2):397–423.

Strully, K. W., D. H. Rehkopf, and Z. Xuan. 2010. Effects of prenatal poverty on infant health: State Earned Income Tax Credits and birth weight. *American Sociology Review* 75(4):534–562.

Thompson, J. P., and G. A. Suarez. 2019. *Accounting for racial wealth disparities in the United States.* Boston, MA: Federal Reserve Bank of Boston.

Thomson, D., R. Ryberg, K. Harper, J. Fuller, K. Paschall, J. Franklin, and L. Guzman. 2022. *Lessons from a historic decline in child poverty.* Bethesda, MD: Child Trends.

Tiehen, L. 2002. *Private provision of food aid: The emergency food assistance system.* Washington, DC: USDA, Economic Research Service.

Tilly, Z. 2022. *Families Deserve a Robust, Permanent Simplified Tax Filing Option.* https://www.childrensdefense.org/blog/permanent-simplified-tax-filing-option/ (accessed March 17, 2023).

Traub, A. 2021. *A biased, broken system: Examining Proposals to Overhaul Credit Reporting to Achieve Equity: Written Testimony of Demos Associate Director of Policy Research, Amy Traub Before the U.S. House of Representatives Committee on Financial Services.* https://www.demos.org/testimony-and-public-comment/biased-broken-system-examining-proposals-overhaul-credit-reporting#footnote3_xe5tcuc (accessed March 9, 2023).

Trust and Will. n.d. *5 Things You Didn't Know About Tribal Law & Estate Planning.* https://trustandwill.com/learn/native-american-estate-planning (accessed March 17, 2023).

Tufano, P., and D. Schneider. 2008. *Harvard Business School finance working paper no. 08-075: Using financial innovation to support savers: From coercion to excitement.* Boston, MA: Harvard Business School.

Turner, S., and J. Bound. 2003. Closing the gap or widening the divide: The effects of the GI Bill and World War II on the educational outcomes of Black Americans. *The Journal of Economic History* 63(1):145–177.

Tuttle, C. 2019. Snapping back: Food stamp bans and criminal recidivism. *American Economic Journal: Economic Policy* 11(2):301–327.

USAGov. n.d. *Consumer Financial Protection Bureau.* https://www.usa.gov/agencies/consumer-financial-protection-bureau (accessed May 30, 2023).

U.S. Commission on Civil Rights. 2017. *Targeted fines and fees against communities of color: Civil rights and constitutional implications.* Washington, DC: U.S. Commission on Civil Rights.

USDA (U.S. Department of Agriculture). 2020a. *Elderly Simplified Application Project.* https://www.fns.usda.gov/snap/elderly-simplified-application-project (accessed March 7, 2023).

USDA. 2020b. *TEFAP Fact Sheet: What Is the Emergency Food Assistance Program?* https://www.fns.usda.gov/tefap/tefap-fact-sheet (accessed June 20, 2023).

USPS Office of the Inspector General. 2014. *White paper: Providing non-bank financial services for the underserved.* Washington, DC: United States Postal Service.

Wang, L. 2021. *The U.S. Criminal Justice System Disproportionately Hurts Native People: The Data, Visualized.* https://www.prisonpolicy.org/blog/2021/10/08/indigenouspeoplesday/ (accessed March 3, 2023).

Waxman, E. 2021. *Statement before the Committee on Rules, United States House of Representatives: Tackling Food Insecurity Among Older Adults and Multigenerational Families.* https://www.urban.org/research/publication/tackling-food-insecurity-among-older-adults-and-multigenerational-families (accessed March 7, 2023).

Weller, C. E., and R. Figueroa. 2021. *Wealth matters: The Black–White wealth gap before and during the pandemic.* Washington, DC: Center for American Progress.

Wherry, F. F., and P. Chakrabarti. 2022. Accounting for credit. *Annual Review of Sociology* 48(1):131–147.

Wimer, C., L. Fox, I. Garfinkel, N. Kaushal, J. Laird, J. Nam, L. Nolan, J. Pac, and J. Waldfogel. 2022. *Historical Supplemental Poverty Measure data 1967–2020.* New York, NY: Center on Poverty and Social Policy, Columbia University.

Wolla, S. A., and J. Sullivan. 2017. *Education, Income, and Wealth.* https://research.stlouisfed.org/publications/page1-econ/2017/01/03/education-income-and-wealth (accessed March 21, 2023).

Wursten, J., and M. Reich. 2022. *IRLE working paper #101-21: Racial inequality and minimum wages in frictional labor markets.* Berkeley, CA: Institute for Research on Labor and Employment.

Zewde, N. 2020. Universal baby bonds reduce Black–White wealth inequality, progressively raise net worth of all young adults. *The Review of Black Political Economy* 47(1):3–19.

4

Education Access and Quality

This chapter discusses key issues in education access and quality, beginning with an overview of how federal laws and policies shape U.S. education and especially reflecting on the linkages between equity and quality. Key policies include the Elementary and Secondary Education Act (ESEA), as amended by the Every Student Succeeds Act (ESSA), the Individuals with Disabilities Education Act (IDEA), the Higher Education Act (HEA), Section 504 of the Americans with Disabilities Act, and Title VI of the Civil Rights Act. The history of racism and social and educational segregation have affected the quality of education afforded to children who have been racially and ethnically minoritized. Chapters 2 and 7 discuss the federal government boarding schools that mistreated and traumatized American Indian and Alaska Native (AIAN) and Native Hawaiian children who were forcibly removed from their families, and this chapter discusses racially segregated schools separated by stark gaps in all kinds of resources. Unfortunately, education inequities persist. A 2013 report from the Equity and Excellence Commission, a federal advisory committee of the U.S. Department of Education (DOE), succinctly summarized the state of U.S. education in a way that still resonates a decade later (DOE, 2013):

> Our education system, legally desegregated more than a half century ago, is ever more segregated by wealth and income, and often again by race. Ten million students in America's poorest communities—and millions more African American, Latino, Asian American, Pacific Islander, American Indian and Alaska Native students who are not poor—are having their lives unjustly and irredeemably blighted by a system that consigns

them to the lowest-performing teachers, the most run-down facilities, and academic expectations and opportunities considerably lower than what we expect of other students. These vestiges of segregation, discrimination and inequality are unfinished business for our nation.

In addition to reviewing key policies, this chapter discusses the evidence on federal approaches and the interface with states on issues of funding, teacher quality, social supports and social context, and other key aspects of the educational experience, with additional discussion of aspects relevant to higher education. Although the federal government plays a large role in constructing frameworks for equitable treatment of all students and equitable access to educational opportunities, the role of states is preeminent and may outweigh federal policies and guidance, including on matters of education equity, such as in funding. The federal role also has fluctuated over time, with periods of robust engagement followed by times of more limited guidance to or engagement with states and local school districts. Although a great deal of flexibility and responsiveness to unique local circumstances is needed, furthering education equity (and by extension, health equity) undoubtedly requires federal leadership.

INTRODUCTION

The National Academies report *Monitoring Educational Equity* found that

The history of constitutional amendments, U.S. Supreme Court decisions, and federal, state, and local legislation and policies indicates: (1) a recognition that population groups—such as racial and ethnic minorities, children living in low-income families, children who are not proficient in English, and children with disabilities—have experienced significant barriers to educational attainment; and (2) an expressed intent to remove barriers to education for all students. (NASEM, 2019b, p. 2)

That report's authoring committee concluded that "educational equity requires that educational opportunity be calibrated to need, which may include additional and tailored resources and supports to create conditions of true educational opportunity" (NASEM, 2019b, p. 2).

Federal law, including case law, shapes several important aspects of education, with broad consideration of equity, but in practice, the limitations are evident. In 1954, the milestone Supreme Court decision in *Brown v. Board of Education of Topeka*[1] found state-sanctioned segregation of public schools unconstitutional because it violated the 14th amendment (equal protection

---

[1] 347 U.S. 483 (1954).

under the law). However, the practice of "separate but equal" endorsed by *Plessy v. Ferguson*[2] in 1896 persisted in many settings and policies (The Century Foundation, 2018; The Equity Collaborative, n.d.).

Brown was followed by enactment of some state laws that aimed to prolong educational segregation (see, for example, the Massive Resistance effort organized by Southern lawmakers) (NAACP Legal Defense Fund, 2023). The 1964 Civil Rights Act provided an even more expansive framework for prohibiting discrimination and was followed 2 years later by the Equality of Educational Opportunity Study (the Coleman Report), which concluded that Black students benefited from attending integrated schools and introduced busing as a strategy for desegregation (The Equity Collaborative, n.d.).

> In 1965, when the federal government stepped in with direct investments to the states via Title I of the Elementary and Secondary Education Act (ESEA) to provide compensatory funding to states with a high proportion of poor children, it was due to a lack of states' attention or willingness to address the unequal experiences poor and minority students faced in state public education systems. (The Century Foundation, 2018)

School segregation is not a relic of the past; it has continued to produce unequal learning opportunities (Orfield et al., 2014) and is still being addressed in case law and state ballot measures (e.g., in California during the 1990s) (The Equity Collaborative, n.d.).

Two major amendments of the ESEA focused on closing achievement gaps. The No Child Left Behind (NCLB) Act (2001) considerably expanded the federal role in education; it included provisions that focused on state and local strategies to support "students from economically disadvantaged families, students from racial and ethnic minority groups, and students with disabilities" (20 U.S.C. 6623) (Congress.gov, 2001) and "support of local educational agencies that are implementing court-ordered desegregation plans and local educational agencies that are voluntarily seeking to foster meaningful interaction among students of different racial and ethnic backgrounds, beginning at the earliest stage of such students' education" (20 U.S.C. 7231) (Congress.gov, 2001). NCLB also called for disaggregating student performance data by race, disability, English proficiency, and income level (NASEM, 2019b; The Century Foundation, 2018).

In 2015, ESSA reauthorized the 50-year-old ESEA and added provisions that required a new set of high academic standards, protections for high-need students, and the nurturing of local, evidence-based

---

[2] 163 U.S. 537 (1896).

interventions, while allowing flexibility for states (DOE, n.d.-b). Unfortunately, although ESSA provided an opportunity for states and school districts to include racial and socioeconomic diversity in their improvement plans, the emphasis on flexibility also allowed states to avoid more robust efforts to further equity. In the initial round of ESSA plans, only one state included a diversity component (The National Coalition on School Diversity, 2020).

The repercussions from an education policy aimed at AIAN people—assimilation in federal Indian Law—are still felt today. During this period, children were removed from their homes, families, and cultures to attend schools far from home (Newland, 2022). The first and most infamous was the Carlisle Indian School in Pennsylvania; from 1879 until 1918, over 10,000 children from 140 tribes attended and were forced to assimilate (National Park Service, 2020). Children were often emotionally, physically, and sexually abused, and many died as a result (National Park Service, 2020; Newland, 2022). Many never saw their families again, and mass graves have recently been identified at these "school" sites (Newland, 2022). Studies show that survivors of these schools are more likely to have cancer, tuberculosis, high cholesterol, diabetes, anemia, arthritis, gallbladder disease, and negative mental health outcomes compared to adult nonattendees (Evans-Campbell et al., 2012; Running Bear et al., 2018, 2019) (see Chapter 7).

The Linkages Between Education and Health

Education is a powerful force for advancing health equity. The quantity and quality of education interacts in important ways with other social determinants of health as well. The skills developed in schools—whether measured by standardized tests or a broader range of social and emotional skills that can be nurtured and taught in schools, such as persistence, sociability, creativity, and motivation—influence educational attainment, economic outcomes, residential neighborhood characteristics, and even the quality of interpersonal relationships (NASEM, 2019d; Schrag, 2014). Each of these in turn impact health status. An extensive body of evidence links education and health outcomes, such as self-rated health, infant mortality, and life expectancy (Schrag, 2014).

Educational attainment impacts communities across generations as well—parental attainment is linked to child health and well-being (Evans et al., 2021). Although the literature linking education and health is robust, some debate exists about to what extent the relationship is causal (Baker et al., 2011; Fujiwara and Kawachi, 2009; Grossman, 2015). In addition, it is bidirectional: education impacts health and health influences educational outcomes (NASEM, 2017).

Education can affect health through many pathways. Those with higher levels of educational attainment, on average, have higher incomes and better employment characteristics, such as employment that is more stable, have healthier working conditions, and are more likely to be offered employment-based benefits, such as paid leave and health insurance (Egerter et al., 2008). Higher attainment also predicts greater financial wealth (Wolla and Sullivan, 2017).

Education can also improve health knowledge, influence adoption of healthy behaviors, and enable people to make better-informed choices about receiving and managing medical care (Egerter et al., 2009). Education is also associated with psychological and social factors, including sense of control and social support, that affect health. A strong education system that works for everyone is fundamental to achieving health and social equity.

Responsibility for education policy rests largely with state and local governments, with the federal government primarily filling gaps in state and local funding, disseminating emerging knowledge, and helping to strengthen the effectiveness of education for all students (DOE, 2021a). Although its role in education is somewhat indirect, it has some powerful levers for influencing the educational inequities that characterize the U.S. educational systems. One of the most powerful is DOE's Civil Rights mandates, which charge it with enforcing civil rights law across multiple dimensions of the educational system, including through data collection. Box 4-1 discusses key aspects of the department's civil rights functions addressing discrimination on the basis of race and ethnicity and disability status.

Addressing racial and ethnic education inequities will have economic effects as well (and that also shapes health status). A McKinsey report noted that achievement gaps between demographic groups present "unrealized economic gains" and "underutilized human potential" (Auguste et al., 2009). For example, the gap between White students and Black and Hispanic students deprived the U.S. economy of $310 billion to $525 billion a year in productivity, equivalent to 2 to 4 percent of gross domestic product (GDP) (Auguste et al., 2009).

This chapter examines levers for federal engagement in early childhood, K–12, and higher education. Many policies and issues could be reviewed, but four areas particularly warrant attention and improvement (see Chapter 1 for an overview of the committee's process for selecting the policies reviewed in this report). The first is the *quantity* of schooling. Starting with access to high-quality early education, so that children from all backgrounds start kindergarten on track and ready to learn, and continuing through high school graduation and equitable opportunities for higher education, the number of years in school is an important determinant of a range of outcomes. The second is the *quality* of those years of schooling— that is, making sure that time spent in school is used productively so that

BOX 4-1
Protecting Civil Rights and
Addressing Disabilities in Education

The Office of Civil Rights (OCR) in the Department of Education enforces the Rehabilitation Act of 1973 and Section 504 of the Americans with Disabilities Act Title II (DOE, n.d.-a). The OCR has authority under section 203(c)(1) of the Department of Education Organization Act (20 U.S.C. 3413(c)(1)) to collect data that are necessary to ensure compliance with civil rights laws and regulations OCR enforces. These laws include Title VI of the Civil Rights Act of 1964, which prohibits discrimination based on race, color, or national origin; Title IX of the Education Amendments of 1972, which prohibits discrimination based on sex, including sexual orientation and gender identity; and Section 504 of the Rehabilitation Act of 1973, which prohibits discrimination on the basis of disability. The regulations for these laws require recipients of DOE's federal financial assistance to submit to OCR "complete and accurate compliance reports at such times, and in such form and containing such information" as OCR "may determine to be necessary to enable [OCR] to ascertain these laws and implementing regulations" (Office for Civil Rights, n.d.).

The data collection has been performed approximately every other school year since 1968 and includes leading civil rights indicators related to access and barriers to educational opportunity from preschool through 12th grade. It gathers information about student enrollment; access to courses, programs and school staff; and school climate factors, such as bullying, harassment, and student discipline. Most data collected are disaggregated by race, ethnicity, sex, disability, and English Learners (Office for Civil Rights, n.d.).

Before 1975, U.S. public schools were not required to educate children with disabilities, and many states had laws that banned children with physical and intellectual disabilities from attending school. It took changes to state and federal laws to secure a right to education for children with disabilities. As with many calls for equity, this movement started with a group of determined parents and advocates who organized, marched, and appealed to local, state, and federal leaders to draft legislation that would change the trajectory of the lives of children and youth with disabilities (Littleton, n.d.).

Two seminal cases in the District of Columbia and Pennsylvania set the stage for what would become the predecessor to the Individuals with Disabilities Education Act (IDEA). In 1971, the Public Interest Law Center brought the lawsuit *Pennsylvania Association for Retarded Children v. Commonwealth of Pennsylvania* (334 F. Supp. 1257), the first right-to-education suit in the country, to overturn the Pennsylvania law that denied educational services to children "who have not attained a mental age of five years" by the start of first grade (The Public Interest Law Center, n.d.). The case settlement in the U.S. District Court for the Eastern District of Pennsylvania resulted in a consent decree in which the state agreed to provide a free public education for children with intellectual or developmental disabilities (The Public Interest Law Center, n.d.). In 1972, *Mills v. Board of Education of the District of Columbia* (348 F. Supp. 866) found that the public school board could not exclude from receiving a free public education students it deemed to be "exceptional" (those who had "behavioral problems [or] were mentally handicapped, emotionally disturbed or hyperactive").

BOX 4-1 Continued

Quoting *Brown v. Board of Education*, the presiding judge stated that public education is "a right which must be made available to all on equal terms" (Civil Rights Litigation Clearinghouse, 2021).

The Education for All Handicapped Children Act (Pub. L. 94–142) was enacted in 1975, renamed IDEA in the 1990 reauthorization, and again reauthorized in 2004. IDEA provides access to equitable education for over 7.5 million students, with Part B covering children 3–21 years and Part C covering children 0–2 years. Its key tool is the Individualized Education Program, which ensures "that an appropriate program and curriculum is developed to meet each child's unique needs" (U.S. Commission on Civil Rights, 2002). IDEA includes formula grants for both special education and related services and early intervention and discretionary grants that fund research, technical assistance, workforce training, parent training and information, and other services (DOE, n.d.-a). New or revised regulations have added changes to further integrate children with disabilities into neighborhood schools and the regular curriculum (DOE, 2023a).

---

society's investments in education pay off for individuals and communities. Third, schools often provide services that directly influence health, from medical services at health clinics to prepared meals. The best evidence needs to be used to ensure those services are delivered in a health-promoting, equitable manner. Fourth, schools are based in communities, with noteworthy efforts across the nation to create environments that link students and families with community services and social supports.

This chapter is, for the most part, unable to report data on the Native Hawaiian and Pacific Islander (NHPI) population specifically due to data aggregation with the Asian population or lack of data. This renders the population invisible in this discussion and masks differences between NHPI and Asian people (see Chapter 2 for more details). The chapter begins with a discussion of the link between education and health, including an overview of racial, ethnic, and tribal inequities, followed by examples of federal policies that impact health equity organized by early care and education, K–12 education, higher education, and direct health provision via the education system.

Education and Health Inequity

Much of the association between education, health, and economic outcomes is mediated through the total years of education completed; most racial and ethnic groups have seen steady progress. Figure 4-1 shows high school graduation rates, as measured by the DOE adjusted cohort graduation rate, which is the percentage of first-time ninth-graders in public high schools who graduate with a regular diploma within 4 years,

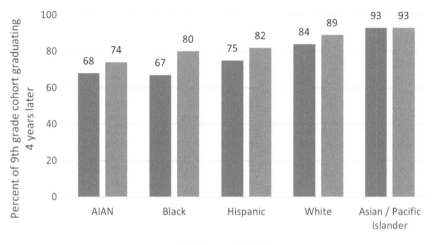

FIGURE 4-1 High school graduation rate, by race and ethnicity.
NOTES: AIAN = American Indian or Alaska Native. States have the option of reporting data for either a combined "Asian/Pacific Islander" group or the "Asian" and "Pacific Islander" groups separately. This table aggregates the "Asian/Pacific Islander" data and the separate "Asian" and "Pacific Islander" data to compute the "Asian/Pacific Islander" adjusted cohort graduation rate. This represents an inaccurate representation of the Native Hawaiian and Pacific Islander and Asian populations as distinct racial Office of Management and Budget minimum categories.
SOURCES: Data from NCES, 2021, n.d.

for graduation years 2011 and 2019. Graduation rates have increased overall, from 80 percent in 2011 to 86 percent in 2019, and the differences across racial and ethnic groups have narrowed. For example, Black students' rates were 80 percent as high as White students' in 2011 but 90 percent as high in 2019; that ratio for Hispanic students increased from 84 percent to 92 percent, and AIAN students' rates increased from 81 percent to 83 percent. The differences by race and ethnicity, albeit at historic lows, are large and meaningful.

Educational attainment is an important determinant of outcomes such as earnings levels, the likelihood of living above the poverty line and being food secure, neighborhood quality, and marital status (Creamer et al., 2022; Parker and Stepler, 2017). Furthermore, in some domains, its importance is growing over time (see the following section for more information). Some worry that the increase in graduation rates reflect schools making it easier to graduate in response to accountability pressures (e.g. through lowered grading standards or increased use of "credit-recovery" programs). Recent research finds that relatively little of the increase is due to changed graduation standards but instead reflects a substantial increase in human capital (Harris, 2020; Harris et al., 2023; NASEM, 2023b).

Educational attainment is also highly correlated with a range of health outcomes (Campbell et al., 2014; Cutler and Lleras-Muney, 2006). Adults with lower attainment are more likely to report worse health status, more chronic disease burden, a higher likelihood of obesity, and higher rates of smoking and substance abuse (Egerter et al., 2009; Ogden et al., 2017). Ultimately, life expectancy is strongly correlated with attainment; those with a college degree or more gained years of life expectancy over the last two decades, but those without a college degree experienced a decline (Case and Deaton, 2021).

The relationship between education and health spans across generations as well. Babies of mothers who did not graduate high school experience increased infant mortality and have lower birthweights than those born to mothers with a college degree or more (Gage et al., 2013; Sosnaud, 2019). Mothers' education predicts children's likelihood of being in fair or poor health (Monheit and Grafova, 2018). These health characteristics in turn influence children's education (Figlio et al., 2014), setting up a cycle that repeats across multiple generations.

The relationship between education and earnings varies by race and ethnicity. Figure 4-2 shows median earnings among 25–34-year-old adults

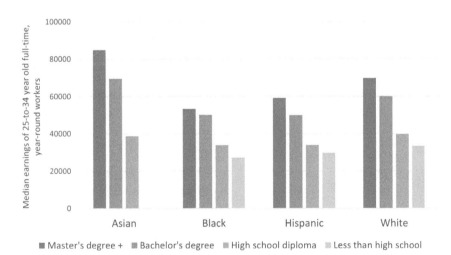

FIGURE 4-2 Median earnings of young adults by education, race, and ethnicity.
NOTE: Data source includes other racial and ethnic groups not separately shown, including Native Hawaiian or Pacific Islander and American Indian or Alaska Native (AIAN); however, annual earnings by educational attainment for Pacific Islander young adults and AIAN young adults are not available because these data did not meet reporting standards.
SOURCE: NCES, 2022a.

who work full time and year round, with no statistical difference across race and ethnicity among those with less than a high school diploma. Differences between White and Asian people on one hand, and Black and Hispanic people on the other hand, become statistically significant and larger as educational attainment is higher. Within each race and ethnicity category, median earnings among those with more education are higher than for those with less education.

Education policy has no panaceas. Nonetheless, strong evidence shows that some policy changes and investments will improve outcomes and narrow differences in educational attainment and quality across racial and ethnic groups. Although the best mix of changes to policy and practice to improve outcomes will vary by state, district, school, or student group, research can guide policy makers on which choices are likely to have a strong return on investment.

Conclusion 4-1: There remain large differences in educational achievement and attainment between White and Asian students, on one hand, and Black, Latino/a, and American Indian and Alaska Native students, on the other. The empirical evidence that education is associated with health is strong. The causal evidence that more education can improve health is compelling given the many pathways through which education can affect health.

The Intersection of Race, Ethnicity, and Disability Status in Education

Health and health care access in education settings have ramifications for children with disabilities, especially at the intersection with race and ethnicity. Inequitable diagnosis of autism may reflect disparities in access to health care, underscoring the importance of offering early developmental screenings in education settings, and "research shows that among Medicaid-eligible children with autism diagnoses, White children are diagnosed over a year earlier than Black children" (Gordon, 2017).

Individuals with disability have been denied equitable educational opportunities (see Box 4-1). The intersection of disability and race and ethnicity in education also has sparked intense debates about measures and methodology to ascertain whether racially and ethnically minoritized children, particularly Black children, have been over- or underrepresented in special education. IDEA requires states to regularly collect and review district-level data to assess variation across racial and ethnic groups by disability category and educational setting without adjusting for variables that correlate with need for services (Gordon, 2017). The 2002 NRC report *Minority Students in Special and Gifted Education* "cautioned against using unadjusted aggregate group-level identification rates to guide public policy" because of the difficulty of interpreting differences and ascertaining their proportionality (NRC, 2002). Identifying students for special education varies widely across school districts and states, but "forcing states to establish uniform standards is dangerously inconsistent with the IDEA mandate of a free and appropriate public education for all. When identifying another student pushes a district over a risk ratio threshold, the district faces a clear incentive to under identify—that is, to withhold services from—children who already face a broad array of systemic disadvantages" (Gordon, 2017).

Data reported by DOE under the IDEA indicate that "Black or African American students with disabilities are more likely to be identified with intellectual disability or emotional disturbance than all students with disabilities and more likely to receive a disciplinary removal than all students with disabilities" and "White students with disabilities are more likely to be served inside a regular class 80% or more of the day than all students with disabilities" (DOE, 2021b). Moreover, "Black students have been overrepresented in special education since the U.S. Office of Civil Rights first started to sample school districts in 1968. Disparities in identification are greatest for more subjective disabilities, such as specific learning disabilities (SLD), intellectual disabilities (ID), and emotional disturbances (ED)" (National Center for Learning Disabilities, 2020).

The National Academies report *Closing the Opportunity Gap for Young Children* (NASEM, 2023b) provides additional detailed discussion about the intersection of race, ethnicity, and disability and examines the policies and practices that can create opportunity gaps for children from racially and ethnically minoritized groups. It recommends that DOE fully integrate IDEA programming with general early childhood and K–12 education. The recommendation includes specific strategies to address uneven access; quality and dosage of interventions; inclusion; nonbiased and accurate disability identification that specifically considers over- and underidentification of specific groups, such as children of color; and prohibiting punitive and harsh forms of discipline, with special attention to students of color "who are disproportionately subject to those practices" (NASEM, 2023b, p. 8).

EARLY CHILDHOOD EDUCATION

Inequality in education starts early, with sizable differences across race and ethnicity groups in average math and reading scores when children enter kindergarten (Fryer and Levitt, 2004; Reardon and Portilla, 2016). These gaps tend to stay constant or increase as students age (NASEM, 2023b; Reardon and Portilla, 2016). Evidence shows that preschool attendance can help improve kindergarten readiness, increase school achievement, and provide a range of other benefits.

Many lower-income children attend preschool through the Head Start program,[3] which has been shown to have substantial long-term impacts, including raising high school graduation rates and college attendance (Bauer and Schanzenbach, 2016; Deming, 2009; Garces et al., 2002). More recently, a randomized controlled trial demonstrated that Head Start improves language skills and literacy, especially in children who would not attend preschool without Head Start (Kline and Walters, 2016; Puma et al., 2010). Impacts of early childhood education (ECE) programs vary across settings and program characteristics (Cascio, 2021). Evaluations of some ECE programs demonstrate little or no positive impact on child health outcomes or even negative impacts (Durkin et al., 2022). For example, a recent randomized controlled trial suggests the initial test score gains from Head Start dissipate over time. Other studies, though, have indicated that even when effects on test scores fade, interventions, especially in early childhood, can affect outcomes over the long term, perhaps due to how Head Start influences social, behavioral, and emotional skills (Chetty et al., 2011; Heckman, 2006). As discussed in the National Academies report *Vibrant and Healthy Kids* (NASEM, 2019d), the mixed findings in the literature may result from lack of program quality, poor fidelity to program models, or limited program duration.

Despite promising evidence of impacts, especially in high-quality preschool programs, many children do not attend school in early childhood (Cabrera et al., 2022). Figure 4-3 shows school enrollment rates by age, race, and ethnicity. A majority of 3- and 4-year-olds do not attend school across all groups; for both age groups, enrollment was lower in 2020 than in 2019, before the COVID-19 pandemic. Between 2019 and 2020, overall school enrollment dropped from 91 to 84 percent for 5-year-olds and 54 to 40 percent for 3- and 4-year-olds.

Government policies can improve access to high-quality ECE programs with investments in expanding coverage directly, through programs such as Head Start, or by supporting state and local area investments in expanding affordable early childhood care and education. At the same time, it is important to ensure the high quality of ECE through supports including low child–teacher ratios, teacher training and coaching, and evidence-based curricula (Weiland et al., 2022). *Closing the Opportunity Gap for Young Children* has recommended that the federal government partner with the states to "fully implement a voluntary universal high-quality public early care and education system using a targeted universal approach (i.e., setting universal goals that are pursued using processes and strategies targeted to the needs of different groups). Such programs should

---

[3] Head Start is a Department of Health and Human Services program that provides comprehensive early childhood education, health, nutrition, and parent involvement services to low-income children and families.

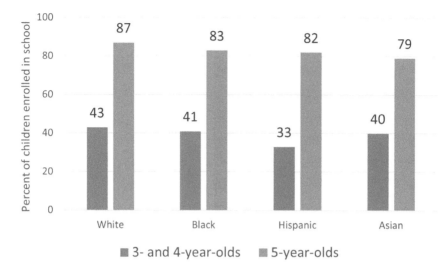

FIGURE 4-3 Percentage of young children enrolled in school in 2020, by age, race, and ethnicity.
NOTE: Reporting standards were not met for the American Indian or Alaska Native and Native Hawaiian and Pacific Islander populations—either too few cases were available for a reliable estimate or the coefficient of variation is 50 percent or greater. Data exclude children living in institutions. Race categories exclude persons of Hispanic ethnicity.
SOURCE: Data from NCES, 2022b.

be responsive to community needs, reflect the true cost of quality, and have strong monitoring and accountability systems that specifically address gaps in opportunity" (NASEM, 2023b, p. 6).

One example of how to address racial and ethnic inequities in ECE through federal policy levers include expanding Early Head Start-Child Care Partnerships (HHS, 2020). These were first established in 2014 to increase access to high-quality care for infants and toddlers. The model supports Early Head Start grantees to partner with licensed family and center-based child care providers who agree to meet Early Head Start standards (ACF, n.d.). It increases resources to infant and toddler providers to use the Early Head Start model and so enables a greater number of children and families access to its services, including low ratios and group sizes, credentialed and supported teachers, research-based curriculum and assessment, and comprehensive services (HHS, 2020). Early Head Start is an evidence-based program and among the models approved for the states to support through the Maternal, Infant, and Early Childhood Home Visiting Program (Hoffman and Ewen, 2011). Furthermore, unlike Head Start, the program permits states to serve as grantees, allowing for states to braid any Early Head Start funding with their block grant funding to take a statewide approach to serving infants and toddlers with high-quality, evidence-based programming (Matthews and Schmit, 2014; Wallen and Hubbard, 2013). These partnerships could be replicated and expanded by increasing appropriations for the program.

K–12 EDUCATION

Educational achievement as measured by test scores is linked to a host of outcomes, ranging from educational attainment and earnings to risky behaviors, such as smoking, teen pregnancy, and criminal activity (Heckman et al., 2006). Racial and ethnic groups have substantial differences in achievement that likely contribute to differences in attainment and health outcomes. A nationally representative metric of math and reading skills comes from the Nation's Report Card (National Assessment of Education Progress) tests, which are given to a sample of students in grades 4 and 8 approximately every other year. One way to examine test score data is the share of students who score above the threshold for "proficiency." Overall, 41 percent of students scored proficient or above in fourth grade math in 2019, and 34 percent of eighth grade students did (NAEP, 2019).

Achievement inequities—which are important in part because they translate into disparate later-life outcomes—are stark across racial and ethnic groups, as shown in Figure 4-4. Although differences in proficiency rates have been narrowing across groups over time, they remain large, and some groups also show declines in proficiency between grades 4 and 8. Over 60 percent of Asian students are proficient in math in both fourth and eighth grade, and 52 and 44 percent of White 4th and 8th graders, respectively, are proficient. Math proficiency among Hispanic students is 28 percent in grade 4 and 20 percent in grade 8; estimates for Native Hawaiian and "other Pacific Islander" students are nearly identical (NAEP, 2022). In fourth grade, approximately one in four AIAN students is proficient in math, and the rate among Black students is one in five. In eighth grade, 15 percent of AIAN students and 14 percent of Black students score proficient in math (NAEP, 2022).

School Spending

Increases in per-pupil school spending have been shown to improve a range of student outcomes in the short run, including test scores, graduation rates, and earnings. These results have been shown in the "modern school finance" literature (see for example, Jackson et al., 2016; Jackson and Mackevicius, 2021; Lafortune et al., 2018; Rothstein and Schanzenbach, 2022), which is able to separate correlation from causality and demonstrate strong returns to increased spending (Deming, 2022).

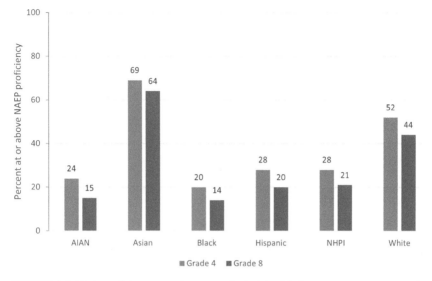

FIGURE 4-4 Math proficiency rates by race and ethnicity, 2019.
NOTE: AIAN = American Indian or Alaska Native; NAEP = National Assessment of Educational Progress; NHPI = Native Hawaiian or Pacific Islander.
SOURCE: Adapted from NAEP, 2022.

Consistent with this, decreases in spending, such as those due to economic recessions that result in states cutting education budgets, lead to worse test performance and college attendance, especially for Black students and those in low-income neighborhoods (Jackson et al., 2021).

Although the modern school finance literature has not tested the impact of school spending on health outcomes directly, it has shown that school spending improves educational attainment. Because of the established relationship between increased educational attainment and better health, it is reasonable to infer that higher school spending will lead to improved health (Buckles et al., 2016; Lleras-Muney, 2005).

Most school spending comes from states and localities, with less than 10 percent from federal sources (Urban Institute, n.d.). Local governments generally raise funds via property taxes, setting up a system in which areas with low property values, which disproportionately serve low-income children and racial and ethnic minorities, can raise and spend less money on their schools. Data also show that a majority of U.S. public-school students attend high-poverty schools, which experience high teacher attrition, larger class sizes, and lower-quality facilities (Schanzenbach et al., 2016). In 2021, 38 percent of Hispanic students attended high-poverty schools, as did 37 percent of Black, 30 percent of AIAN, and 23 percent of Pacific Islander students (NCES, 2023a).

In recent decades, state school finance reforms have increased the share of school spending from the state relative to local governments, increasing funding overall and reducing the relationship with local property values. But because state funding was often targeted based on district-level characteristics, such as property wealth, and not student-level characteristics, such as race or family income, on average, these reforms failed to close spending gaps between students of different income levels, races, or ethnicities (Lafortune et al., 2018). There are differences in national averages in education spending across race and ethnicity (Rubinton and Isaacson, 2022). Total spending is roughly twice the amount spent on instruction alone, and it includes capital expenditures for property and buildings, as well as salaries and benefits, supplies, and purchased services (NCES, 2023b).

Many differences in funding across racial and ethnic groups are driven by cross-state differences in spending. Some costs, such as salaries, are lower in low-spending states as well, but even adjusting for differences in costs of living, variation in education spending is substantial across states (Schanzenbach et al., 2016). Black students disproportionately live in states (often in the South) that spend less per pupil. As a result, even when the within-state spending is the same for all racial and ethnic groups, overall, Black students will have less spending than White students because of the different composition of states represented (NCES, 2022c, Schanzenbach et al., 2016).

Federal policy can offset differences in cross-state spending and close spending gaps, which will be expected to improve educational outcomes and health. This is an indirect route, and policy levers may give a larger return in terms of reducing health inequities. However, increasing educational spending would also be expected to improve a range of economic and social outcomes that are not directly health related.

One approach to improvement in low-spending states could be to increase funding for Title I, a federal block grant program that earmarks extra funding to school districts serving low-income children. As Black and Hispanic students and students from other racial and ethnic groups that are minoritized are more likely than White students to be low income, providing more resources through this program could also reduce racial and ethnic differences in spending. Title I is underfunded relative to what the federal formula implies, and its allocation is complicated by rules such as small state minimum provisions (that is, setting a minimum funding threshold for less populous—and less racially and ethnically diverse—states, such as Wyoming and Vermont, offsets some of its ability to reduce differences in spending) (NCES, 2016). As a result, Title I sends less money per low-income student to states with a higher share of such students (Gordon, 2016), including states with high concentrations of the racial and ethnic groups considered in this report. Increasing Title I funding to states with higher shares of low-income students would reduce funding disparities. Another approach could be to provide federal funds outside of the Title I program; it has many inefficiencies, and it may be more effective to use a different mechanism.

Closing the Opportunity Gap for Young Children provides additional detailed discussion of the effects of funding on educational outcomes and highlights specific areas where federal funding is inadequate, such as for individuals with disabilities (NASEM, 2023b). Most notably, it indicates that federal funding is not adequate to close gaps in state and local funding, and the federal government "has never fully funded its share of IDEA, leaving an outsized burden on state and local governments and families" (NASEM, 2023b, p. 142). Although IDEA's enactment in 1974 "authorized federal funding for up to 40% of average per-pupil spending nationwide" to pay for some of the costs of providing special education services to students with disabilities, funding never reached that target (Kolbe et al., 2022). Congress approved a 20 percent increase in IDEA appropriations in the fiscal year (FY) 2023 budget, but there is concern that even so, the formula for allocating funding systematically advantages some states, such that "states with larger shares of children experiencing poverty, children receiving special education, and non-White and Black children would on average receive smaller IDEA grants per child" (Kolbe et al., 2022).

Other Policies to Improve School Quality

Other ways to improve educational outcomes could be promoted by federal policies. One important factor is high-quality school personnel. Research shows that standardized test scores also improve when teachers can successfully improve a range of other student outcomes, such as teen pregnancy, college attendance, and their eventual earnings (Chetty et al., 2014a,b). Even after accounting for impacts on test scores, teachers who are good at improving behaviors on outcomes such as absence and suspension rates and grades also raise the likelihood of graduating from high school and going on to college (Jackson, 2018). Additional evidence shows that Black students benefit in both the short and long run from Black teachers (Dee, 2004; Gershenson et al., 2022). Improving the proportion of diverse teachers requires diversifying the pipeline, and research indicates that begins with supporting Black and Hispanic youth to succeed in and complete high school and college (Urban Institute, 2017). Quality school leadership is an important factor as well. Research shows that principals, especially those skilled at management, improve student achievement and teacher instructional practices and well-being (Branch et al., 2013; Grissom and Loeb, 2011; Liebowitz and Porter, 2019).

Evidence exists on policies and practices to adopt to improve students' access to high-quality classroom teaching and school leadership. For example, professional evaluation of mid-career teachers can improve teacher skill, effort, or both, in enduring ways that improve long-run performance (Taylor and Tyler, 2012). Highly skilled teachers also influence their peers' performance—research shows that a teacher's ability to increase students' test scores improves when working in the same schools with high-performing teachers (Jackson and Bruegmann, 2009). Recognizing the importance of teachers, research and experimentation is needed to improve tools to recruit, train, and retain excellent classroom teachers and administrators.

Other promising methods include providing individualized, small-group tutoring to students who are behind grade level in math, which has been shown to improve math achievement and reduce the number of classes failed (Ander et al., 2016; Guryan et al., 2023). Extra instruction during school vacations, from a classroom teacher and in small groups of roughly 10 students, also yields strong achievement gains in the subject (Schueler, 2020; Schueler et al., 2017). Computer-assisted learning programs designed to meet students at their skill level and teach targeted skill development have also been shown to be successful, particularly for mathematics (Escueta et al., 2020).

Federal school accountability policies, such as provisions of NCLB and the ESSA, may improve achievement and narrow racial and ethnic gaps (Dee and Jacob, 2011; NASEM, 2017). For example, ESSA requires that "states establish student performance goals, hold schools accountable for student achievement, and include a broader measure of student performance in their accountability systems beyond test scores" (ASCD, 2016).

School choice may also improve education through several avenues, including allowing parents to find schools that may better meet their children's needs than their neighborhood public school (Whitehurst, 2017). One approach to increasing choice is to expand charter schools, which are available in most states and enroll nearly 7 percent of public-school students (Snyder et al., 2019). Although average student performance is no different in charter schools compared to public schools, differences in impacts are wide across schools and students, with generally stronger evidence of positive effects among urban and low-income students (for recent reviews see Cohodes and Parham, 2021; Kho et al., 2020). A study of the relationship between racial segregation and school choice (including charter schools) found a positive correlation between them and urged that decision makers implementing school choice policies incentivize schools to implement concrete actions to improve diversity (Whitehurst, 2017).

Conclusion 4-2: There is strong evidence some federal policy changes and investments can improve educational outcomes and narrow differences in educational attainment and quality across racial and ethnic groups. However, the best mix of changes to policy and practice to improve student outcomes will vary across states, districts, schools, or groups of students. Thus, evidence-based policy, accountability, and community engagement play a critical role in improving federal policy for education as it relates to equity.

Conclusion 4-3: Increases in per-pupil school spending have been shown to improve a range of student outcomes in the short and long run, including test scores, educational attainment, and earnings—all of which in turn are correlated with better health outcomes. Decreases in school spending lead to worse student outcomes, especially for children living in low-income neighborhoods and Black students. Federal policy could play a role to offset differences in cross-state spending and close spending gaps across racial and ethnic groups.

The Role of Communities

Communities are both the places and the organizations and social networks that help to shape the conditions for health and well-being, including education. Chapter 7 of this report discusses important dimensions of the community role in health equity and federal approaches that value the voice and priorities of and help to build the power of communities, and Recommendation 4 (Chapter 8) calls on the federal government to prioritize community input and expertise when changing or developing federal policies to advance health equity—including by assessing the placement, composition, and role of community advisory boards. This recommendation has clear applications to the community role in shaping public education, and the discussion that follows explores the existing context for community–school collaboration.

Schools can partner with communities and community organizations in ways that are mutually beneficial and can further both educational and social outcomes (see, for example, Gross et al., 2015). Community schools are public schools that provide services and support that fit a specific school's/neighborhood's need—educators, local community members, families, and students work together to strengthen conditions for student learning and healthy development. The concept of a community school and its variants across the country can be traced back to John Dewey's description of schools as "social centers" that could be responsive to students' needs in a comprehensive way (Annie E. Casey Foundation, 2021;

Kimner et al., 2022). In recent years, the work of community schools has been shown to not only improve student outcomes but also further educational equity (Maier et al., 2017; Quinn and Blank, n.d.).

The movement to strengthen ties between education and community building reflects a belief in benefits that accrue to not only individual students and families (i.e., wraparound supports to keep students in school and help them succeed) but also the community by providing an important hub for civic life.

Education also has an important role in civic and social engagement (Campbell, 2006)—throughout their education, individuals develop their identities, along with their associates, which influences their future via social connectedness and critical thinking (NASEM, 2019c). Education in the aspect of social and self-identity is beneficial for student health, as it plays a role in the student discovering their own confidence, self-motivation, independence, and decision making, which are all needed to shape their life and create career goals (NASEM, 2019c).

Different models or approaches for community schools exist, all of which recognize that schools are a core component of civic infrastructure in communities—they train the next generation of citizens, and many serve as community centers and voting locations—and that school success is dependent on access to a range of community and social supports, especially in communities affected by past and continuing social and economic inequities. The COVID-19 pandemic underscored the evidence on the important school and community bond and especially its effectiveness in closing education equity gaps (Task Force on Next Generation Community Schools, 2021). The Communities in Schools model implemented nationwide and the Coalition for Community Schools have yielded improvement on certain measures, ranging from attendance rates to passing standardized state tests (Maier et al., 2017; MDRC, 2017). A related framework, the Whole School, Whole Community, Whole Child Model developed by the Centers for Disease Control and Prevention (CDC) with the Association for Supervision and Curriculum, is student centered and comprises 10 components that the community can use to support the school (CDC, 2022). These range from physical activity to social and emotional climate and include community involvement.

In 2020, the Brookings Institution, Child Trends, and community school leaders launched a task force on Next Generation Community Schools (Harper et al., 2020), which outlined seven ways community schools can close inequities and transform education and provided an overview of the impact of community schools on educational outcomes (Task Force on Next Generation Community Schools, 2021). A follow-up to the Task Force on Next Generation Schools, the Community Schools Forward Project launched in 2021–22; in early 2023, it co-convened a second community schools task force focused on implementation guidance to education systems and their partners (Kimner et al., 2022). The Biden Administration announced in 2023 that it provided $63 million in grants to 42 grantees under its Full-Service Community Schools program (OESE, 2023).

HIGHER EDUCATION

Background

Brown v. Board of Education shaped school integration and provided a foundation for education equity in K–12 education; along with several statutes (e.g., Title VI of the Civil Rights Act of 1964, Title IX of the Education Amendments of 1972, and Title II of the Americans with Disabilities Act of 1990), it has also served as a foundation for affirmative action in higher education (Cornell Law School, n.d.). Affirmative action refers to procedures intended to "eliminate unlawful discrimination among applicants, remedy the results of such prior discrimination, and prevent such discrimination in the future" (Cornell Law School, n.d.). The 2003 Supreme Court decision *Grutter v. Bollinger*[4] upheld the status quo, asserting that consideration of race was just one dimension of a holistic approach to weighing all aspects of an applicant's background (Reichmann, 2022). Affirmative action in higher education has bearing on both the ability of racially and ethnically minoritized students to be accepted to competitive schools and programs (and thus on their future trajectories) and the diversity of those institutions and the effect that has on talent and innovation across various fields of study (NASEM, 2023a).

A 2023 National Academies report concluded that so called race-neutral or color-blind admissions criteria, which are advocated by the plaintiffs in *Students for Fair Admissions, Inc. v. President & Fellows of Harvard College*[5] and *Students for Fair Admissions, Inc. v. University of North Carolina*[6]—two cases that were heard by the Supreme Court in 2023— overlook inequities that "may produce racially disparate outcomes. These differential outcomes reflect—and can reinforce—the broader race-related history of access and barriers, wealth accumulation, and discrimination in the United States. A neutral policy or standard cannot erase this history and ignoring the impacts of race can perpetuate cumulative and inequitable outcomes" (NASEM, 2023a, p. 220).

---

[4] *Grutter v. Bollinger*, 539 U.S. 306 (2003).
[5] *Students for Fair Admissions, Inc. v. President & Fellows of Harvard College*, 600 U.S. ___ (2023).
[6] *Students for Fair Admissions, Inc. v. University of North Carolina*, 600 U.S. ___ (2023).

The Linkages Between Health and Higher Education

As noted, research shows that quantity of education is important to health outcomes, with college graduates expected to live at least five years longer than individuals who have not completed high school (Egerter et al., 2009). College enrollment and completion rates generally have also risen in recent years, with increasing convergence across racial and ethnic groups. Between 2010 and 2021, the share of young adults ages 25–29 with a bachelor's degree or higher rose from 32 percent to 39 percent; rates rose among White people by 15 percent, Asian people by 29 percent, Black people by 37 percent, Pacific Islander people by 40 percent, and Hispanic people by 77 percent (see Figure 4-5) (NCES, 2020). Estimated rates among AIAN people fell from 19 to 11 percent, in contrast with their increase in high school graduation rates over nearly the same period.

Improving Outcomes in Higher Education

Even though the cost of tuition and fees for a college education has increased in inflation-adjusted terms, the benefits in increased earnings still outweigh the up-front investment cost on average (Barrow and Malamud, 2015). Like other investments, college comes with some risk of not paying off, such as if students pay tuition but do not complete their degree

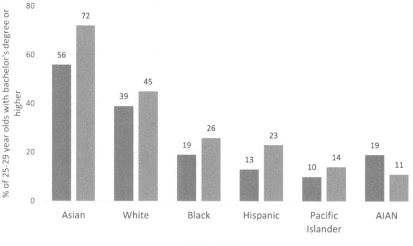

FIGURE 4-5 Bachelor's degree or higher, 25–29-year-olds.
NOTE: AIAN = American Indian or Alaska Native.
SOURCE: Data from Digest of Education Statistics, Table 104.20 in NCES, 2020.

(Athreya and Eberly, 2021). Policies that reduce financial barriers to higher education can improve the enrollment and graduation rates, especially among low-income students. Notably, the federal–state balance of funding for higher education has shifted since the 2008 recession, with state funding declining and federal funding increasing, especially through Pell Grants and Veterans' Education Benefits (Pew Research Center, 2019).

Information about financial assistance and help navigating the complex system may improve student outcomes. For example, a recent large-scale experiment tested the impact of providing simplified information about high-achieving, low-income students' eligibility for free tuition at an elite public university. Providing clear information but not actually changing the amount of aid offered substantially increased both application and enrollment (Dynarski et al., 2021). Another randomized experiment provided student aid application assistance to low-income individuals while they were receiving help with tax preparation. Students whose families received this assistance were 28 percent more likely to complete 2 years of college during the subsequent 3 years (Bettinger et al., 2012).

Support to address potential barriers to student success has also been shown to improve graduation rates. The City University of New York's Accelerated Study in Associate Programs program offered a range of supports to students: financial supports, including a tuition waiver that covered any gap between financial aid and college costs, and free access to textbooks and public transportation. Students were required to attend college full time and had access to blocked courses and consolidated schedules along with support services, such as academic planning, accessing campus services, balancing school with other responsibilities, and staying on track to graduate. The program substantially increased graduation rates (Weiss et al., 2019). It was replicated in Ohio, with similar effects (Miller and Weiss, 2022). A similar intensive case-management program in Texas also substantially increased degree completion among low-income women attending community colleges (Evans et al., 2020).

Pell Grants

The Federal Pell Grant[7] Program marked its 50th anniversary in 2022, and it has played a crucial role in helping approximately 80 million students from low-income families, many from Black and Hispanic communities (Biden, 2022) attend college. In the 2022–2023 academic year, the Congressional Budget Office projects that 5.9 million people will receive

---

[7]The Pell Grant is awarded to eligible undergraduate students who have not earned a bachelor's or professional degree. In some cases, individuals may receive a grant if enrolled in a postbaccalaureate teacher certificate program.

Pell Grants, with a maximum award of $6,895 and an average of $4,640; total federal spending is $27.4 billion in 2022–2023 (Koestner, 2022). With more than $28 billion aid in the 2017–2018 award year, Pell Grants are the second-largest source of need-based aid for postsecondary education, after federal student loans (College Board, 2022). Eligibility for additional need-based grant aid increases students' attendance, bachelor's degree completion, and earnings (Castleman and Long, 2016; Denning et al., 2019). But the Pell Grant has not kept up with inflation and covers a shrinking portion of tuition (Protopsaltis and Parrott, 2017). Some researchers argue that increasing it will increase college affordability in an efficient, targeted manner (Levine, 2021). Estimates suggest that doubling the Pell Grant would substantially reduce education debt for recipients receiving the maximum award, by approximately 85, 83, and 80 percent for AIAN, Latino/a, and Black students, respectively (GEPI, 2021).

Pell Grants for incarcerated people Postsecondary education in prison has been shown to contribute to successful re-entry. Participants are more likely to be employed after release and have decreased recidivism (Bozick et al., 2018; Davis et al., 2013). In 1994, Congress disqualified incarcerated people from Pell Grant eligibility (before that time, eligibility had few legislative restrictions) (Oakford et al., 2019).

In 2015, DOE announced the Second Chance Pell experiment under the Experimental Sites Initiative, which allows incarcerated students who would be eligible for Pell Grants if they were not incarcerated to access them (DOE, n.d.-c). It allows a limited number of college programs to accept Pell Grants for incarcerated students. These programs enrolled 28,000 students between 2016 and 2021, 32 percent of whom obtained either a certificate or an associate's or bachelor's degree (Chesnut et al., 2022). However, several barriers that kept incarcerated people from being able to take advantage of the program were documented, including meeting Pell Grant eligibility standards and applying for the Free Application for Federal Student Aid (FAFSA) (GAO, 2019).

In December 2020, Congress restored the law to give incarcerated people the opportunity to obtain a college education by making changes to the Higher Education Act of 1965 and FAFSA (FSA, 2022). This change allows any public or private nonprofit college to start a prison education program, following a set of guidelines and an approval process, and will provide Pell Grants to those in prison starting in July 2023. No eligibility restrictions related to conviction type or sentence length were included, and Congress eliminated FAFSA questions about selective service registration and drug convictions—common barriers to Pell Grant access. According to one estimate, as many as 463,000 Pell Grant–eligible incarcerated people stand to benefit (Oakford et al., 2019). To ensure high-quality programs, Congress designed the approval process to control for program quality with up-front vetting and ongoing evaluation (Custer, 2022). Lifting the Pell Grant restriction for incarcerated people will further the goal of health equity.

> *Conclusion 4-4: In 1994, the federal government disqualified incarcerated people from Pell Grant eligibility, and in 2020, lawmakers reinstated Pell Grant access for incarcerated people enrolled in qualifying prison education programs. This is a promising example of how removing erected barriers to access for specific populations, such as incarcerated people, can address unequal access to federal programs that are linked to social determinants of health and health inequities.*

Financial aid can help incarcerated students gain access to postsecondary education; however, both colleges and students need to understand the complexities of administering Pell Grants in the corrections environment.

Student Loans and Repayment

Student loans have received considerable attention, and high repayment burdens cause financial struggles for some borrowers. Figure 4-6 shows characteristics of federal student loans for the cohort of students receiving a bachelor's degree in 2015 to 2016. As shown in the panel on the left, 86 percent of Black recipients borrowed federal loans, compared with

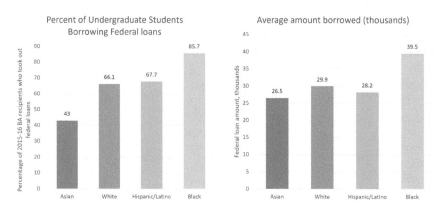

FIGURE 4-6 Characteristics of federal loans among bachelor's degree recipients, 2015–2016.
NOTE: "Black" refers to not Hispanic or Latino and also includes African American; "Other or Two or more races, not Hispanic or Latino" (not reported in the graph) includes American Indian or Alaska Native (AIAN), Native Hawaiian or Pacific Islander (NHPI), and respondents who identify as more than one race. This masks inequities for AIAN and NHPI people.
SOURCE: Data from Thomsen et al., 2020.

70 percent of Hispanic or Latino, 68 percent of White, and 44 percent of Asian recipients. On average, Black students borrowed a higher amount than other groups, at nearly $40,000, compared with $26,000–30,000 for other racial and ethnic groups, as shown in the right panel.

Certain federal policies can reduce the burden of student debt, especially for those in low-earning jobs. For example, programs such as income-driven repayment plans tie repayment amounts to incomes. Similarly, programs forgive outstanding balances under certain conditions. However, the program that forgives student loans after 10 years of employment in the nonprofit sector (and after making 120 qualifying monthly payments) has administrative burdens (Link et.al, 2022). This is an active area of policy discussion, and reasonable people can disagree about the best manner to structure these policies (Chingos, 2023; DOE, 2023b; Knott, 2023; Looney, 2022; Oakford et al., 2019). It is clear that targeted student debt relief will disproportionately impact Black and Latino borrowers and potentially also borrowers from other groups discussed in this report.

Minority Serving Institutions

Minority serving institutions (MSIs) were established in response racism and the exclusion of racially and ethnically minoritized people from institutions of higher education. The first MSIs were the 108 Historically Black colleges and universities founded before the 1964 Civil Rights Act (DOI, n.d.). The first tribal college and university (TCU) was Diné College, founded in 1968 on tribal land and under the control of Navajo Nation (Diné College, n.d.). Federally run schools and colleges also exist for AIAN people. These fall under the Bureau of Indian Education (BIE) (Bureau of Indian Education, n.d.). The Indian Self-Determination and Education Assistance Act of 1975[8] gave authority to federally recognized tribes to contract with the Bureau of Indian Affairs to operate Bureau-funded schools. BIE operates 58 of the 183 tribal schools that it funds. BIE also directly operates two postsecondary institutions: the Haskell Indian Nations University in Lawrence, Kansas, and the Southwest Indian Polytechnic Institute in Albuquerque, New Mexico (Bureau of Indian Education, n.d.). MSIs also include Hispanic serving institutions (HSIs) and Asian American, Native American, and Pacific Islander serving institutions. MSIs in the states and territories are heterogeneous in their histories, formation, resources, geographies, and challenges but do participate in MSI programs.

Institutions of higher learning that have an explicit mission to educate Black, Hispanic, tribal or sovereign nations, or other minoritized students provide many of the elements needed to support educational success, including cultural competence and relevance, a profound recognition of the

---

[8] Pub. L. 93–638, 25 U.S.C. 450 (1975).

legacies, contemporary currents, and catastrophic harms of racism, exclusion, and othering (NASEM, 2019a). But due to those legacies and their ramifications, these institutions are generally underresourced compared to those that do not have that mission and serve predominantly White students (CMSI, n.d.; Flores and Park, 2013).

The high level of diversity at most MSIs creates considerable heterogeneity within specific institutions; for example, a historically Black college or university may also be an HSI (NASEM, 2019a). These designations make these institutions eligible for certain federal programs and research grants. The categorical funding opportunities were meant to level the playing field and target resources to these institutions; however, this has not been fully realized (NASEM, 2019a).

Research on the state of and gaps in MSI funding reveals several structural and systemic inequities. MSIs receive less support in grants and contracts from federal and state governments, have much smaller endowments, and must rely more on tuition—but are more likely to serve students with higher financial need (see, for example, Toldson, 2016; Williams and Davis, 2019). At the state level, outcomes-based funding can affect education inequities, because these institutions "serve larger percentages of students who are traditionally underserved in [the] K–12 system, they require more resources and supports to best serve these students" (Li et al., 2017).

A 2019 National Academies study of the role of MSIs in strengthening STEM education reviewed data on the educational outcomes to evaluate student success and found that some measures are flawed because they fail to appropriately incorporate context (NASEM, 2019a). For example, measures of graduation rates do not consider complex student pathways (e.g., moving to another MSI, part-time study) or a richer set of characteristics, such as disability status, or first-generation college attendance. Gasman and colleagues (2017) found that benefits of education, such as leadership and critical thinking skills, are not included in data collection on MSI educational outcomes and noted that TCUs prioritize some hard-to-quantify outcomes, such as "community engagement, language revitalization, leadership, and cultural appreciation" (p. 3).

Economic outcomes of MSI-educated students are promising, according to research from Espinosa and colleagues (2018), who found that "MSIs propel their students from the bottom to the top of the income distribution at higher rates than do non-MSIs" and that the data make a strong case for "increased investment in institutions that are meeting students where they are, and making good on the value of higher education for individuals, families, and communities" (p. iii and iv).

Despite the recognition that measuring the outcomes and demonstrating the value of the MSI education requires better and more expansive types of data, state funding approaches continue to be premised on narrow and inadequate metrics. The federal government can be important in strengthening the flow of research and other funding to MSIs, and a long list of federal agencies provide opportunities targeting MSIs (see, for example, Lewis-Burke Associates LLC, 2021).

> *Conclusion 4-5: Minority serving institutions have demonstrated value on investment in economic outcomes for their students, and their effects on the racially and ethnically minoritized communities they serve merit research and measurement.*

SCHOOL OPPORTUNITIES TO DIRECTLY PROMOTE HEALTH, INSURANCE COVERAGE, AND ACCESS TO CARE

Schools have unique opportunities to advance health. For example, they can assist in outreach and enrollment of eligible children in Medicaid and the Children's Health Insurance Program (CHIP). In turn, through school-based services and school-based health centers (SBHCs), they can provide Medicaid-covered services, including through Individualized Education Programs under IDEA,[9] and behavioral health services to eligible children. They can also help children enrolled in Medicaid access needed services (CMCS Informational Bulletin, 2022), including children who are not served by IDEA. In 2014, CMS allowed schools to use Medicaid for school-based free health care services, but uptake of this policy has been slow for a variety of reasons, including schools' administrative burdens and costs (CMS, 2014; Healthy Students, n.d.; Wilkinson et al., 2020).

Ensuring that eligible students are enrolled in Medicaid can have positive budgetary implications for schools, because Medicaid may cover services and evaluation required for an individualized education plan (MACPAC, 2018). In addition, Medicaid and CHIP can directly improve children's health, enabling them to do better in school, miss fewer days due to illness or injury, finish high school, graduate from college, and earn more as adults (Cohodes et al., 2016; Levine and Schanzenbach, 2009). Oregon has innovated in connecting health care reform with educational outcomes through its Healthy Kids Learn Better Partnership, which brought together schools and the state's coordinated care organizations to collaborate on public health interventions at the local and state levels. A health system leader from Oregon described Medicaid as "the scaffolding that helps families receive the services they need to get out of poverty," helping to "improve kindergarten readiness and help the next generation to avoid

---

[9]This law makes a free appropriate public education available to eligible children with disabilities throughout the nation and ensures special education and related services. It governs how states and public agencies provide early intervention, special education, and related services to more than 7.5 million (as of school year 2020–21) eligible infants, toddlers, children, and youth (DOE, n.d.-a).

poverty and become high users of Medicaid services" (NASEM, 2020). In a recent communication, CMS reminds states that the federal government can match state and local expenditures for administrative activities, including outreach and enrollment (CMCS Informational Bulletin, 2022). It specifically mentions "that local education agencies can use school registration processes and other regular contacts they have with families to help children (and their family members) enroll in Medicaid or CHIP. Obtaining Medicaid reimbursement for outreach and enrollment allows schools to expand health care services and programs" (Orris and Wagner, 2022). School partnerships may be particularly helpful as the COVID-era prohibition against terminating Medicaid coverage is sunset, and many children are expected to experience "churn"—loss of coverage and quick reenrollment. Such coverage disruptions often reflect administrative burdens, which disproportionately impact racially and ethnically minoritized people, and can be both economically costly and harmful, such as resulting in interrupted treatment or medication access (Wikle et al., 2022).

School-Based Health Centers

SBHCs play a unique, direct role in health promotion. An estimated 20.3 million children suffer from insufficient access to health care, with 3.3 million uninsured, 10.3 million without primary care, and 6.7 million with unmet specialty care needs (Children's Health Fund, 2016). Increasingly, students can directly receive medical care at school through SBHCs, which have doubled over the past 20 years, with nearly 2,600 in the 2016–2017 school year (Love et al., 2019). SBHCs use a variety of models, including a single clinician providing primary care, a team of staff providing primary care and mental health care, and a larger staff of clinical and other staff (e.g., social worker, health educator, dental providers) (Kjolhede et al., 2021). Their range of services vary, including treatment from a school nurse, immunizations, behavioral health care, and asthma treatment (MACPAC, 2018). Almost half of the centers employ an expanded care team, often including providers of dental and eye care, helping resolve common problems that interfere with student learning (Conley and Schanzenbach, 2020).

SBHCs are funded by a range of public and private sources, from local and state funding to federal block grants (e.g., Maternal and Child Health Block Grant) and project grants and school districts billing the federal Medicaid program (APHA, 2017; PATH, 2020). Both CDC's Community Guide and the Community Preventive Services Task Force recommended SBHCs as an effective approach to furthering health equity because of their impact on health, educational, and other student outcomes (Kjolhede et al., 2021).

A recent study found that SBHCs reduce teen pregnancy rates (Lovenheim et al., 2016). Other studies have found that SBHCs reduced students' depressive episodes and suicide risks and improved academic measures, such as GPAs, attendance rates, and suspensions (Conley and Schanzenbach, 2020; Knopf et al., 2016; Paschall and Bersamin, 2018). Only 6.3 million students have access to an SBHC—about 13 percent of total students (Love et al., 2019). Expanding the number of centers will help more kids get the care they need, promoting both academic and health equity in the process.

School Meals Programs

The National School Lunch Program (NSLP), established in 1946, is a federally assisted program administered by the Department of Agriculture (USDA) Food and Nutrition Service (USDA, n.d.). NSLP is usually administered through state agencies that operate through agreements with school authorities. Participating schools receive cash reimbursement for each lunch or snack served and USDA commodity food donations for lunches.

Although the program was originally created out of concern that malnourishment affected national security and welfare, school meals (including lunch, breakfast, and snacks) now help combat child hunger and can encourage healthy eating (Ralston et al., 2008). NSLP provides nutritionally balanced meals at low or no cost to students attending public schools, nonprofit private schools, and residential child care institutions. Under the traditional rules, students with a household income at or below 130 percent of the federal poverty guidelines receive free meals, and those with household incomes above 130 percent and at or below 185 percent receive meals at reduced price (USDA, 2019b). Many schools and districts offer free meals to all students through the Community Eligibility Provision (CEP), which reimburses schools using a formula based on the share of students who are categorically eligible for free meals due to participation in other programs, such as the Supplemental Nutrition Assistance Program (SNAP) (USDA, 2019a). In 2019–20, nearly 15 million children attended schools that have CEP (FRAC, 2020). Overall, in 2022 approximately 30 million children participate in the NSLP and 15 million in the School Breakfast Program (SBP) (USDA, 2023).

Similar to schools' incentives to help families enroll in Medicaid, they have incentives to help eligible families learn about SNAP, because students who are in a household receiving SNAP are directly certified for free school meals. Medicaid coverage also conveys direct certification for free school meals in most states (Bauer et al., 2023).

Alleviating hunger and providing improved nutrition to schoolchildren likely has a range of positive spillover effects. Behavioral, emotional, and mental health and academic problems are more prevalent among children and adolescents struggling with hunger (FRAC, n.d.), who have lower math scores (Jyoti et al., 2005). Cotti et al. (2018) find that students' test score performance is worse when the test is given a longer time after their families' monthly SNAP payments are made, when food consumption tends to be lower. Hoynes et al. (2016) found that children with more years of access to SNAP benefits in the 1960s and 1970s were substantially more likely to graduate high school.

Low-income students in both SBP and NSLP tend to consume a significantly better diet compared to low-income nonparticipants. Studies also show that rates of food insecurity among children are higher in the summer when these programs are not available (FRAC, n.d.).

Evidence suggests that free access to NSLP among schools and districts with high poverty rates improves academic achievement and related outcomes. Schwartz and Rothbart (2020) found that providing free meals to all students in New York City middle schools substantially increased participation in school lunch and improved math and reading performance for both low- and higher-income students. Similarly, Ruffini (2022) found sizable increases in meal participation and some evidence of improved performance in mathematics, and Gordon and Ruffini (2021) found reduced rates of suspension in elementary schools when schools offer CEP.

There are several routes to increasing students' access to universal free meals. Raising CEP reimbursement rates would likely increase participation among schools with high shares of low-income children. Some support offering free meals to all students, regardless of the level of poverty in the school or district. During the COVID-19 pandemic, the federal government made lunch free to all 50 million public-school students nationwide (Hayes and FitzSimons, 2022). Since then, California, Colorado, and Maine passed bills ensuring all students had free school meals; 21 other states are considering similar policies (Hunter College, 2023).

Summer Feeding Programs

Before 2020, federal policy addressed the summer food gap by offering prepared meals through the Seamless Summer Option and the Summer Food Service Program (SFSP). However, many children lacked access to SFSP sites. For example, Bauer and Parsons (2020) find that in 2018, only 43 percent of children lived in a census tract with a meal site; only about one child for every seven who participated in school lunch programs in the 2017–2019 school year participated in the summer lunch program (FRAC, 2019).

During the COVID-19 pandemic, Congress authorized pandemic electronic benefits transfer (EBT) payments, similar to SNAP benefits, to families of children who lost their access to free or reduced-price school meals. Providing vouchers for grocery purchases instead of prepared meals increased participation rates and substantially reduced food hardship among low-income populations (Bauer et al., 2020, 2021). This program had its roots in a series of randomized controlled trials for summer EBT payments that had been conducted in conjunction with USDA and shown to substantially reduce food insecurity and very low food security among children (Collins et al., 2014). In December 2022, Congress permanently authorized summer EBT at a level of $40 per child per month (Neuberger, 2022; USDA, 2022). Evidence suggests this will reduce food hardship and improve children's summer outcomes. Success of this important new program will require states to invest in capacity, expertise, relationships, and data systems to increase the reach of the program and reduce excessive administrative costs and burdens to families.

> *Conclusion 4-6: Schools have unique opportunities to advance health, ranging from assisting in outreach and enrollment of eligible children in public health insurance programs and income support programs, to offering direct care through school-based health centers, to reducing food insecurity and improving dietary quality through school meals programs. Evidence shows that when schools adopt or improve these opportunities, both health and educational outcomes can be improved.*

CONCLUDING OBSERVATIONS

This report examines the broad effect of federal policies on health equity, and rather than proposing recommendations for changes to specific federal programs reviewed in each chapter, the committee mainly offers crosscutting recommendations (see Chapter 8). However, many National Academies reports list evidence-based and promising recommendations for federal action specific to education access and quality to advance health equity and the factors that affect it (including and beyond the federal policies reviewed in this chapter). Most of those recommendations have not been implemented, and are still relevant today (see Box 4-2 for examples).

The key themes of accountability, community voice, data equity, coordination, and eligibility figure in important ways in federal education policy effects on health equity. For example, and as noted, federal education policy can call on states and local school districts to assess and report on measures of educational achievement by racial and ethnic group, English language proficiency, and disability status. The 2001 reauthorization of the ESEA, NCLB, required that states provide disaggregated data to show education performance by race and ethnicity along with other important dimensions. Community voice arises in the context of school-community

---

BOX 4-2
Example Recommendations from National Academies Reports

The National Academies has published numerous reports on the intersection of education and health (see, for example, NASEM, 2017, 2019c,d). Three specific recommendations that are still relevant:

The Promise of Adolescence: Realizing Opportunity for All Youth (NASEM, 2019c) called on federal (and state) governments to investigate opportunities to rectify disparities across racial and ethnic groups in resources, school quality, and other factors that influence student achievement and attainment in grades K–12. The report also recommended that in coordination with states and localities, the federal government should develop "NextStep," a program targeting underprivileged adolescents to promote both their academic and non-academic development (Recommendation 6-1).

Vibrant and Healthy Kids: Aligning Science, Practice, and Policy to Advance Health Equity (NASEM, 2019d) recommended that federal agencies investigate opportunities to increase participation in high-quality preschool overall for all racial and ethnic groups (Recommendation 7-1).

Communities in Action: Pathways to Health Equity (NASEM, 2017) recommended that the U.S. Department of Education Institute for Educational Science and other divisions in the department should support states, localities, and their community partners with evidence and technical assistance on the impact of quality early childhood education programs, on interventions that reduce disparities in learning outcomes, and on the keys to success in school transitions (i.e., pre-K and K–12 or K–12 postsecondary; Recommendation 7-6).

---

interactions, and recent federal policy has supported the community school models that have been shown to yield shared benefits to schools (through improved student achievement) and to communities. There are promising examples of coordination among federal agencies on education equity, but more could be done, and examples may be found in innovative local and state partnerships (e.g., between school districts and public health departments). Examples of cross-sector partnerships to support student health include the Vision for Baltimore effort, involving Johns Hopkins University, Baltimore City Schools, and other public and private sector partners; the partnership supporting 29 SBHCs in Alameda County, California; and the Arkansas departments of education and of health providing yearly influenza immunization in school, which has had measurable impact on the absenteeism rate (NASEM, 2020).

REFERENCES

ACF (Administration for Children and Families). n.d. *Exploring the Head Start Program Performance Standards.* https://eclkc.ohs.acf.hhs.gov/sites/default/files/docs/pdf/hs-prog-pstandards-final-rule-factsheet_0.pdf (accessed March 21, 2023).

Ander, R., J. Guryan, and J. Ludwig. 2016. *Improving academic outcomes for disadvantaged students: Scaling up individualized tutorials.* Washington, DC: The Hamilton Project—Brookings.

Annie E. Casey Foundation. 2021. *What Are Community Schools?* https://www.aecf.org/blog/what-are-community-schools-baltimore (accessed March 22, 2023).

APHA (American Public Health Association). 2017. *Federal policies and opportunities for school-based health centers: For policy makers.* Washington, DC: American Public Health Association.

ASCD (Association for Supervision and Curriculum Development). 2016. *ESSA and accountability: Frequently asked questions.* Arlington, VA: Association for Supervision and Curriculum Development.

Athreya, K., and J. Eberly. 2021. Risk, the college premium, and aggregate human capital investment. *American Economic Journal: Macroeconomics* 13(2):168–213.

Auguste, B. G., B. Hancock, and M. Laboissiere. 2009. *The Economic Cost of the U.S. Education Gap.* https://www.mckinsey.com/industries/education/our-insights/the-economic-cost-of-the-us-education-gap (accessed February 8, 2023).

Baker, D. P., J. Leon, E. G. Smith Greenaway, J. Collins, and M. Movit. 2011. The education effect on population health: A reassessment. *Population and Development Review* 37(2):307–332.

Barrow, L., and O. Malamud. 2015. Is college a worthwhile investment? *Annual Review of Economics* 7(1):519–555.

Bauer, L., and J. Parsons. 2020. *Why Extend Pandemic EBT? When Schools Are Closed, Many Fewer Eligible Children Receive Meals.* https://www.brookings.edu/blog/up-front/2020/09/21/why-extend-pandemic-ebt-when-schools-are-closed-many-fewer-eligible-children-receive-meals/ (accessed February 21, 2023).

Bauer, L., A. Pitts, K. Ruffini, and D. Schanzenbach. 2020. *The effect of pandemic EBT on measures of food hardship.* Washington, DC: The Brookings Institution.

Bauer, L., K. Ruffini, and D. W. Schanzenbach. 2021. *An Update on the Effect of Pandemic EBT on Measures of Food Hardship.* https://www.hamiltonproject.org/blog/an_update_on_the_effect_of_pandemic_ebt_on_measures_of_food_hardship (accessed February 21, 2023).

Bauer, L., K. Ruffini, and D. Whitmore Schanzenbach. 2023. *The case for and challenges of delivering in-kind nutrition assistance to children.* Washington, DC: The Hamilton Project—Brookings.

Bauer, L., and D. W. Schanzenbach. 2016. *The long-term impact of the Head Start program.* Washington, DC: The Hamilton Project—Brookings.

Bettinger, E. P., B. T. Long, P. Oreopoulos, and L. Sanbonmatsu. 2012. The role of application assistance and information in college decisions: Results from the H&R Block FAFSA experiment*. *The Quarterly Journal of Economics* 127(3):1205–1242.

Biden, J. 2022. *A Proclamation on the 50th Anniversary of the Federal Pell Grant Program.* https://www.whitehouse.gov/briefing-room/presidential-actions/2022/06/22/a-proclamation-on-the-50th-anniversary-of-the-federal-pell-grant-program/ (accessed June 15, 2023).

Bozick, R., J. Steele, L. Davis, and S. Turner. 2018. Does providing inmates with education improve postrelease outcomes? A meta-analysis of correctional education programs in the United States. *Journal of Experimental Criminology* 14(3):389–428.

Branch, G. F., E. A. Hanushek, and S. G. Rivkin. 2013. School leaders matter: Measuring the impact of effective principals. *Education Next* 13(1):62–69.

Buckles, K., A. Hagemann, O. Malamud, and M. Morrill. 2016. The effect of college education on mortality. *Journal of Health Economics* 50:99–114.

Bureau of Indian Education. n.d. *Bureau of Indian education (BIE)*. https://www.bia.gov/bie (accessed March 17, 2023).

Cabrera, N., D. Deming, V. de Rugy, L. A. Gennetian, R. Haskins, D. B. Matthew, R. V. Reeves, I. V. Sawhill, D. W. Schanzenbach, K. Simon, K. B. Stevens, M. R. Strain, R. Streeter, J. Sullivan, W. B. Wilcox, and L. Bauer. 2022. *Rebalancing: Children first.* Washington, DC: AEI—Brookings.

Campbell, D. 2006. 3. What is education's impact on civic and social engagement? In *Measuring the effects of education on health and civic engagement: Proceedings of the Copenhagen Symposium.* Paris, France: OECD. Pp. 25–126.

Campbell, F., G. Conti, J. Heckman, S. Moon, R. Pinto, L. Pungello, and Y. Pan. 2014. Abecedarian & health: Improve adult health outcomes with quality early childhood programs that include health and nutrition. *Science* 343:1478–1485.

Cascio, E. 2021. *Early childhood education in the United States: What, when, where, who, how, and why: Working paper 28722.* Cambridge, MA: National Bureau of Economic Research.

Case, A., and A. Deaton. 2021. Life expectancy in adulthood is falling for those without a BA degree, but as educational gaps have widened, racial gaps have narrowed. *Proceedings of the National Academy of Sciences* 118(11):e2024777118.

Castleman, B. L., and B. T. Long. 2016. Looking beyond enrollment: The causal effect of need-based grants on college access, persistence, and graduation. *Journal of Labor Economics* 34(4):1023–1073.

CDC (Centers for Disease Control and Prevention). 2022. *Whole School, Whole Community, Whole Child (WSCC).* https://www.cdc.gov/healthyschools/wscc/index.htm#print (accessed February 8, 2023).

The Century Foundation. 2018. *Under ESSA, Achieving Equity in Education Is Still Challenging.* https://tcf.org/content/commentary/essa-achieving-equity-education-still-challenging/ (accessed March 12, 2023).

Chesnut, K., N. Taber, and J. Quintana. 2022. *Second chance Pell: Five years of expanding higher education programs in prisons, 2016–2021.* New York, NY: Vera Institute of Justice.

Chetty, R., J. N. Friedman, N. Hilger, E. Saez, D. W. Schanzenbach, and D. Yagan. 2011. How does your kindergarten classroom affect your earnings? Evidence from Project Star. *Quarterly Journal of Economics* 126(4):1593–1660.

Chetty, R., J. N. Friedman, and J. E. Rockoff. 2014a. Measuring the impacts of teachers I: Evaluating bias in teacher value-added estimates. *American Economic Review* 104(9):2593–2632.

Chetty, R., J. N. Friedman, and J. E. Rockoff. 2014b. Measuring the impacts of teachers II: Teacher value-added and student outcomes in adulthood. *American Economic Review* 104(9):2633–2679.

Children's Health Fund. 2016. *Unfinished business: More than 20 million children in U.S. still lack sufficient access to essential health care.* New York, NY: Children's Health Fund.

Chingos, M. 2023. *Comment letter on the Department of Education's proposed rule on income-driven repayment.* Washington, DC: Urban Institute.

Civil Rights Litigation Clearinghouse. 2021. *Case: Mills v. Board of Education of the District of Columbia.* https://clearinghouse.net/case/11084/ (accessed June 1, 2023).

CMCS (Center for Medicaid and CHIP Services) 2022. *Informational Bulletin: Information on School-Based Services in Medicaid: Funding, Documentation and Expanding Services.* https://www.medicaid.gov/federal-policy-guidance/downloads/sbscib081820222.pdf (accessed March 1, 2023).

CMS (Centers for Medicare and Medicaid Services). 2014. *SMD# 14-006: Medicaid payment for services provided without charge (free care).* https://www.medicaid.gov/federal-policy-guidance/downloads/smd-medicaid-payment-for-services-provided-without-charge-free-care.pdf (accessed February 21, 2023).

CMSI (Center for Minority Serving Institutions). n.d. *2016–2017: National campaign on the return on investment of minority serving institutions.* Philadelphia, PA: University of Pennsylvania Graduate School of Education and Center for MSIs.

Cohodes, S. R., and K. S. Parham. 2021. *Charter schools' effectiveness, mechanisms, and competitive influence: Blueprint labs discussion paper #2021.12.* Cambridge, MA: National Bureau of Economic Research.

Cohodes, S. R., D. S. Grossman, S. A. Kleiner, and M. F. Lovenheim. 2016. The effect of child health insurance access on schooling: Evidence from public insurance expansions. *The Journal of Human Resources* 51(3):727–759.

College Board. 2022. *Table 5. Number of Recipients, Total Awards and Aid per Recipient for Federal Aid Programs in Current Dollars and in 2021 dollars, 1976–77 to 2021–22.* https://research.collegeboard.org/media/xlsx/trends-student-aid-excel-data-2021-0.xlsx (accessed June 15, 2023).

Collins, A., R. Briefel, J. A. Klerman, A. Wolf, G. Rowe, A. Enver, C. W. Logan, S. Fatima, M. Komarovsky, J. Lyskawa, and S. Bell. 2014. *Summer electronic benefits transfer for children (SEBTC) demonstration: 2013 final report.* Alexandria, VA: Office of Research and Analysis.

Congress.gov. 2001. *H.R.1—No Child Left Behind Act of 2001.* https://www.congress.gov/bill/107th-congress/house-bill/1/text (accessed March 11, 2023).

Conley, D., and D. W. Schanzenbach. 2020. *Invest in school-based health centers to improve child health.* https://www.milbank.org/quarterly/opinions/invest-in-school-based-health-centers-to-improve-child-health/ (accessed February 28, 2023).

Cornell Law School. n.d. *Affirmative Action.* https://www.law.cornell.edu/wex/affirmative_action (accessed March 15, 2023).

Cotti, C., J. Gordanier, and O. Ozturk. 2018. When does it count? The timing of food stamp receipt and educational performance. *Economics of Education Review* 66:40–50.

Creamer, J., E. A. Shrider, K. Burns, and F. Chen. 2022. *Poverty in the United States: 2021.* Washington, DC: United States Census Bureau.

Custer, B. D. 2022. *How colleges and universities can bring Pell grant–funded programs back to prisons.* Washington, DC: Center for American Progress.

Cutler, D. M., and A. Lleras-Muney. 2006. *Education and health: Evaluating theories and evidence.* Cambridge, MA: National Bureau of Economic Research.

Davis, L. M., R. Bozick, J. L. Steele, J. Saunders, and J. N. V. Miles. 2013. *Evaluating the effectiveness of correctional education: A meta-analysis of programs that provide education to incarcerated adults.* Santa Monica, CA: RAND Corporation.

Dee, T. S. 2004. Teachers, race, and student achievement in a randomized experiment. *The Review of Economics and Statistics* 86(1):195–210.

Dee, T. S., and B. Jacob. 2011. The impact of No Child Left Behind on student achievement. *Journal of Policy Analysis and Management* 30(3):418–446.

Deming, D. 2009. Early childhood intervention and life-cycle skill development: Evidence from Head Start. *American Economic Journal: Applied Economics* 1(3):111–134.

Deming, D. 2022. *Four facts about human capital.* Cambridge, MA: National Bureau of Economic Research.

Denning, J. T., B. M. Marx, and L. J. Turner. 2019. Propelled: The effects of grants on graduation, earnings, and welfare. *American Economic Journal: Applied Economics* 11(3):193–224.

Diné College. n.d. *Diné College History*. https://www.dinecollege.edu/about_dc/history/ (accessed March 11, 2023).

DOE (Department of Education). 2013. *For each and every child—a strategy for education equity and excellence*. Washington, DC: Department of Education.

DOE. 2021a. *The Federal Role in Education*. https://www2.ed.gov/about/overview/fed/role. html (accessed February 8, 2023).

DOE. 2021b. *OSEP Fast Facts Looks at Race and Ethnicity of Children with Disabilities Served Under IDEA*. https://sites.ed.gov/idea/osep-fast-facts-looks-at-race-and-ethnicity-of-children-with-disabilities-served-under-idea/ (accessed June 1, 2023).

DOE. 2023a. *A History of the Individuals with Disabilities Education Act*. https://sites.ed.gov/idea/IDEA-History (accessed June 1, 2023).

DOE. 2023b. *New proposed regulations would transform income-driven repayment by cutting undergraduate loan payments in half and preventing unpaid interest accumulation*. https://www.ed.gov/news/press-releases/new-proposed-regulations-would-transform-income-driven-repayment-cutting-undergraduate-loan-payments-half-and-preventing-unpaid-interest-accumulation (accessed February 28, 2023).

DOE. n.d.-a. *About IDEA*. https://sites.ed.gov/idea/about-idea/ (accessed February 15, 2023).

DOE. n.d.-b. *Every Student Succeeds Act (ESSA)*. https://www.ed.gov/essa?src=rn (accessed March 15, 2023).

DOE. n.d.-c. *Second Chance Pell Fact Sheet*. https://www2.ed.gov/about/offices/list/ope/pell-secondchance.pdf (accessed June 15, 2023).

DOI (Department of the Interior). n.d. *Minority Serving Institutions Program*. https://www.doi.gov/pmb/eeo/doi-minority-serving-institutions-program (accessed March 11, 2023).

Durkin, K., M. W. Lipsey, D. C. Farran, and S. E. Wiesen. 2022. Effects of a state wide pre-kindergarten program on children's achievement and behavior through sixth grade. *American Psychological Association* 58(3):470–484.

Dynarski, S., C. Libassi, K. Michelmore, and S. Owen. 2021. Closing the gap: The effect of reducing complexity and uncertainty in college pricing on the choices of low-income students. *American Economic Review* 111(6):1721–1756.

Egerter, S., M. Dekker, J. An, R. Grossman-Kahn, and P. Braveman. 2008. *Issue Brief 4: Work and Health*. http://www.commissiononhealth.org/PDF/0e8ca13d-6fb8-451d-bac8-7d15343aacff/Issue%20Brief%204%20Dec%2008%20-%20Work%20and%20Health. pdf (accessed June 15, 2023).

Egerter, S., P. Braveman, T. Sadegh-Nobari, R. Grossman-Kahn, and M. Dekker. 2009. *Issue Brief 6: Education and Health*. http://www.commissiononhealth.org/PDF/c270deb3-ba42-4fbd-baeb-2cd65956f00e/Issue%20Brief%206%20Sept%2009%20-%20Education%20 and%20Health.pdf#page=3&zoom=auto,-226,767 (accessed June 15, 2023).

The Equity Collaborative. n.d. *A Partial Timeline of Educational Oppression in the U.S.* http://www.theequitycollaborative.com/wp-content/uploads/2017/09/Education-Timeline-Handout.pdf (accessed March 11, 2023).

Escueta, M., A. J. Nickow, P. Oreopoulos, and V. Quan. 2020. Upgrading education with technology: Insights from experimental research. *Journal of Economic Literature* 58(4):897–996.

Espinosa, L. L., R. Kelchen, and M. Taylor. 2018. *Minority serving institutions as engines of upward mobility*. Washington, DC: American Council on Education.

Evans-Campbell, T., K. L. Walters, C. R. Pearson, and C. D. Campbell. 2012. Indian boarding school experience, substance use, and mental health among urban two-spirit American Indian/Alaska Natives. *The American Journal of Drug and Alcohol Abuse* 38(5):421–427.

Evans, M., J. Daw, and S. M. Gaddis. 2021. The generational boundaries of educational advantage: Does great-grandparent educational attainment predict great-grandchild early academic achievement? *Socius* 7:23780231211060573.

Evans, W. N., M. S. Kearney, B. Perry, and J. X. Sullivan. 2020. Increasing community college completion rates among low-income students: Evidence from a randomized controlled trial evaluation of a case-management intervention. *Journal of Policy Analysis and Management* 39(4):930–965.

Figlio, D., J. Guryan, K. Karbownik, and J. Roth. 2014. The effects of poor neonatal health on children's cognitive development. *American Economic Review* 104(12):3921–3955.

Flores, S. M., and T. J. Park. 2013. Race, ethnicity, and college success: Examining the continued significance of the minority-serving institution. *Educational Researcher* 42(3):115–128.

FRAC (Food Research & Action Center). 2019. *Hunger doesn't take a vacation: Summer nutrition status report.* Washington, DC: Food Research & Action Center.

FRAC. 2020. *Community Eligibility Report 2020.* https://frac.org/cep-report-2020 (accessed June 15, 2023).

FRAC. n.d. *Benefits of School Lunch.* https://frac.org/programs/national-school-lunch-program/benefits-school-lunch#:~:text=School%20lunch%20is%20critical%20to,obesity%20rates%2C%20and%20poor%20health (accessed February 21, 2023).

Fryer, R. G., and S. D. Levitt. 2004. Understanding the Black–White test score gap in the first two years of school. *The Review of Economics and Statistics* 86(2):447–464.

FSA (Federal Student Aid). 2022. *Prison Education Programs.* https://fsapartners.ed.gov/knowledge-center/topics/prison-education-programs# (accessed February 28, 2023).

Fujiwara, T., and I. Kawachi. 2009. Is education causally related to better health? A twin fixed-effect study in the USA. *International Journal of Epidemiology* 38(5):1310–1322.

Gage, T. B., F. Fang, E. O'Neill, and G. Dirienzo. 2013. Maternal education, birth weight, and infant mortality in the United States. *Demography* 50(2):615–635.

GAO (Government Accountability Office). 2019. *Federal student aid: Actions needed to evaluate Pell grant pilot for incarcerated students.* Washington, DC: GAO.

Garces, E., D. Thomas, and J. Currie. 2002. Longer-term effects of Head Start. *American Economic Review* 92(4):999–1012.

Gasman, M., A. C. Samayoa, W. C. Boland, A. Washington, C. D. Jimenez, P. Esmieu, T. J. Park, S. M. Flores, C. J. Ryan, S. Carroll Rainie, G. C. Stull, T. L. Strayhorn, C. M. Alcantar, M. Martin, B. M. D. Nguyen, R. T. Teranishi, and J. Muño. 2017. *Investing in student success: Examining the return on investment for minority-serving institutions.* Princeton, NJ: Policy Information Center.

GEPI (Gender Equity Policy Institute). 2021. *Tackling the student debt crisis: An analysis of congressional proposals to increase Pell grants.* Los Angeles, CA: Gender Equity Policy Institute.

Gershenson, S., C. M. D. Hart, J. Hyman, C. A. Lindsay, and N. W. Papageorge. 2022. The long-run impacts of same-race teachers. *American Economic Journal: Economic Policy* 14(4):300–342.

Gordon, C. 2017. *Race, poverty, and interpreting overrepresentation in special education.* Washington, DC: The Brookings Institution.

Gordon, N. 2016. *Increasing targeting, flexibility, and transparency in Title I of the Elementary and Secondary Education Act to help disadvantaged students.* Washington, DC: The Hamilton Project—Brookings.

Gordon, N., and K. Ruffini. 2021. Schoolwide free meals and student discipline: Effects of the community eligibility provision. *Education Finance and Policy* 16(3):418–442.

Grissom, J. A., and S. Loeb. 2011. Triangulating principal effectiveness: How perspectives of parents, teachers, and assistant principals identify the central importance of managerial skills. *American Educational Research Journal* 48(5):1091–1123.

Gross, M. S. J., J. S. Haines, J. Hill, L. G. Francis, M. Blue-Banning, and P. A. Turnbull. 2015. Strong school–community partnerships in inclusive schools are "part of the fabric of the school . . . . we count on them." *School Community Journal* 25(2).

Grossman, M. 2015. The relationship between health and schooling: What's new? *Nordic Journal of Health Economics* 3(1):7–17.

Guryan, J., J. Ludwig, M. P. Bhatt, P. J. Cook, J. M. V. Davis, K. Dodge, G. Farkas, R. G. Fryer, S. Mayer, H. Pollack, L. Steinberg, and G. Stoddard. 2023. Not too late: Improving academic outcomes among adolescents. *American Economic Review* 113(3):738–765.

Harper, K., S. Jonas, and R. Winthrop. 2020. *Education Inequality, Community Schools, and System Transformation: Launching the Task Force on Next Generation Community Schools.* https://www.brookings.edu/blog/education-plus-development/2020/11/10/education-inequality-community-schools-and-system-transformation-launching-the-task-force-on-next-generation-community-schools/ (accessed February 21, 2023).

Harris, D. 2020. *Are America's rising high school graduation rates real—or just an account-ability-fueled mirage.* Washington, DC: The Brookings Institution.

Harris, D. N., L. Liu, N. Barrett, and R. Li. 2023. Is the rise in high school graduation rates real? High-stakes school accountability and strategic behavior. *Labour Economics* 82:102355.

Hayes, C., and C. FitzSimons. 2022. *The reach of breakfast and lunch: A look at pandemic and pre-pandemic participation.* Washington, DC: Food, Research, and Action Council.

Healthy Students, P. F. n.d. *"Free Care" Rule.* https://healthystudentspromisingfutures.org/free-care-rule/ (accessed June 2, 2023).

Heckman, J. J. 2006. Skill formation and the economics of investing in disadvantaged children. *Science* 312(5782):1900–1902.

Heckman, J. J., J. Stixrud, and S. Urzua. 2006. The effects of cognitive and noncognitive abilities on labor market outcomes and social behavior. *Journal of Labor Economics* 24(3).

HHS (Department of Health and Human Services) 2020. *Early Head Start–Child Care Partnerships.* https://www.acf.hhs.gov/ecd/early-learning/ehs-cc-partnerships (accessed March 8, 2023).

Hoffman, E., and D. Ewen. 2011. *What State Leaders Should Know About Early Head Start.* https://files.eric.ed.gov/fulltext/ED538030.pdf (accessed March 8, 2023).

Hoynes, H., D. W. Schanzenbach, and D. Almond. 2016. Long-run impacts of childhood access to the safety net. *American Economic Review* 106(4):903-934.

Hunter College. 2023. *States That Have Passed Universal Free School Meals (So Far).* https://www.nycfoodpolicy.org/states-that-have-passed-universal-free-school-meals/ (accessed March 21, 2023).

Jackson, C. K. 2018. What do test scores miss? The importance of teacher effects on non–test score outcomes. *Journal of Political Economy* 126(5):2072–2107.

Jackson, C. K., and E. Bruegmann. 2009. Teaching students and teaching each other: The importance of peer learning for teachers. *American Economic Journal: Applied Economics* 1(4):85–108.

Jackson, C. K., and C. Mackevicius. 2021. *The distribution of school spending impacts: Working paper 28517.* Cambridge, MA: National Bureau of Economic Research.

Jackson, C. K., R. C. Johnson, and C. Persico. 2016. The effects of school spending on educational and economic outcomes: Evidence from school finance reforms. *The Quarterly Journal of Economics* 131(1):157–218.

Jackson, C. K., C. Wigger, and H. Xiong. 2021. Do school spending cuts matter? Evidence from the great recession. *American Economic Journal: Economic Policy* 13(2):304–335.

Jyoti, D. F., E. A. Frongillo, and S. J. Jones. 2005. Food insecurity affects school children's academic performance, weight gain, and social skills. *The Journal of Nutrition* 135(12):2831–2839.

Kho, A., R. Zimmer, and R. Buddin. 2020. The economics of charter schools. In *The economics of education*, 2nd ed., edited by S. Bradley and C. Green. Amsterdam, NL: Elsevier Ltd. Pp. 531–542.

Kimner, H., L. Maysonet, and R. Winthrop. 2022. *Community Schools and a Critical Moment in the Fight Against Education Inequality.* https://www.brookings.edu/blog/education-plus-development/2022/03/08/community-schools-and-a-critical-moment-in-the-fight-against-education-inequality/ (accessed February 15, 2023).

Kjolhede, C., A. C. Lee, and Council on School Health. 2021. School-based health centers and pediatric practice. *Pediatrics* 148(4):e2021053758.

Kline, P., and C. Walters. 2016. Evaluating public programs with close substitutes: The case of Head Start. *The Quarterly Journal of Economics* 131(4):1795–1848.

Knopf, J. A., R. K. C. Finnie, Y. Peng, R. A. Hahn, B. I. Truman, M. Vernon-Smiley, V. C. Johnson, R. L. Johnson, J. E. Fielding, C. Muntaner, P. C. Hunt, C. Phyllis Jones, and M. T. Fullilove. 2016. School-based health centers to advance health equity. *American Journal of Preventive Medicine* 51(1):114–126.

Knott, K. 2023. *Income-Driven Repayment Overhaul 'a Step Forward.'* https://www.insidehighered.com/news/2023/02/13/income-driven-repayment-overhaul-step-forward (accessed February 28, 2023).

Koestner, L. 2022. *The Pell Grant Program.* https://www.cbo.gov/system/files/2022-06/58152-Pell%20Grant.pdf (accessed June 15, 2023).

Kolbe, T., E. Dhuey, and S. M. Doutre. 2022. *More money is not enough: The case for reconsidering federal special education funding formulas.* Washington, DC: The Brookings Institution.

Lafortune, J., J. Rothstein, and D. W. Schanzenbach. 2018. School finance reform and the distribution of student achievement. *American Economic Journal: Applied Economics* 10(2):1–26.

Levine, P. 2021. *The economic case for doubling the Pell grant.* Washington, DC: The Brookings Institution.

Levine, P. B., and D. Schanzenbach. 2009. The impact of children's public health insurance expansions on educational outcomes. *Forum for Health Economics & Policy* 12(1).

Lewis-Burke Associates LLC. 2021. *Federal Opportunities for Minority Serving Institutions.* https://diversity.ucf.edu/document/federal-opportunities-for-minority-serving-institutions/ (accessed June 15, 2023).

Li, A., D. Gándara, and A. Assalone. 2017. *Can Equity Be Bought? Minority-Serving Institutions and Outcomes-Based Funding.* https://edtrust.org/the-equity-line/minority-serving-institutions-outcomes-based-funding/ (accessed February 21, 2023).

Liebowitz, D. D., and L. Porter. 2019. The effect of principal behaviors on student, teacher, and school outcomes: A systematic review and meta-analysis of the empirical literature. *Review of Educational Research* 89(5):785–827.

Link, E., J. Romero, and S. Turner. 2022. *The potential impact of public service student loan forgiveness in the fifth district.* Washington, DC: Federal Bank Reserve of Richmond.

Littleton, K. n.d. *A Milestone for Civil Rights: Celebrating 45 Years of IDEA.* https://sites.ed.gov/osers/2020/12/idea45-a-milestone-for-civil-rights/ (accessed June 1, 2023).

Lleras-Muney, A. 2005. The relationship between education and adult mortality in the United States. *The Review of Economic Studies* 72(1):189-221.

Looney, A. 2022. *Does Biden's Student Debt Forgiveness Achieve His Stated Goals?* https://www.brookings.edu/blog/up-front/2022/09/26/does-bidens-student-debt-forgiveness-achieve-his-stated-goals/ (accessed February 21, 2023).

Love, H. E., J. Schlitt, S. Soleimanpour, N. Panchal, and C. Behr. 2019. Twenty years of school-based health care growth and expansion. *Health Affairs* 38(5):755–764.

Lovenheim, M. F., R. Reback, and L. Wedenoja. 2016. *How does access to health care affect teen fertility and high school dropout rates? Evidence from school-based health centers: Working paper 22030.* Cambridge, MA: National Bureau of Economic Research.

MACPAC (Medicaid and CHIP Payment and Access Commission). 2018. *Medicaid in Schools.* https://www.macpac.gov/wp-content/uploads/2018/04/Medicaid-in-Schools.pdf (accessed June 15, 2023).

Maier, A., J. Daniel, and J. Oakes. 2017. *Community schools as an effective school improvement strategy: A review of the evidence (research brief)*. Palo Alto, CA: Learning Policy Institute.

Matthews, H., and S. Schmit. 2014. *What State Leaders Should Know About Early Head Start*. https://files.eric.ed.gov/fulltext/ED561734.pdf (accessed March 21, 2023).

MDRC. 2017. *MDRC's Evaluations of Communities in Schools*. https://www.mdrc.org/publication/mdrc-s-evaluations-communities-schools (accessed June 15, 2023).

Miller, C., and M. J. Weiss. 2022. Increasing community college graduation rates: A synthesis of findings on the ASAP model from six colleges across two states. *Educational Evaluation and Policy Analysis* 44(2):210-233.

Monheit, A. C., and I. B. Grafova. 2018. Education and family health care spending. *Southern Economic Journal* 85(1):71–92.

NAACP (National Association for the Advancement of Colored People) Legal Defense Fund. 2023. *The Southern Manifesto and "Massive Resistance" to Brown*. https://www.naacpldf.org/brown-vs-board/southern-manifesto-massive-resistance-brown/ (accessed June 1, 2023).

NAEP (National Assessment of Educational Progress). 2019. *NAEP Report Card: Mathematics*. https://www.nationsreportcard.gov/highlights/mathematics/2019/ (accessed June 15, 2023).

NAEP. 2022. *NAEP Report Card: Mathematics*. https://www.nationsreportcard.gov/mathematics/?grade=4 (accessed June 15, 2023).

NASEM (National Academies of Sciences, Engineering, and Medicine) 2017. *Communities in action: Pathways to health equity*. Washington, DC: The National Academies Press.

NASEM. 2019a. *Minority serving institutions: America's underutilized resource for strengthening the stem workforce*. Washington, DC: The National Academies Press.

NASEM. 2019b. *Monitoring educational equity*. Washington, DC: The National Academies Press.

NASEM. 2019c. *The promise of adolescence: Realizing opportunity for all youth*. Washington, DC: The National Academies Press.

NASEM. 2019d. *Vibrant and healthy kids: Aligning science, practice, and policy to advance health equity*. Washington, DC: The National Academies Press.

NASEM. 2020. *School success: An opportunity for population health: Proceedings of a workshop*. Washington, DC: The National Academies Press.

NASEM. 2023a. *Advancing antiracism, diversity, equity, and inclusion in STEMM organizations: Beyond broadening participation*. Washington, DC: The National Academies Press.

NASEM. 2023b. *Closing the opportunity gap for young children*. Washington, DC: The National Academies Press.

National Center for Learning Disabilities. 2020. *Significant disproportionality in special education: Trends among Black students*. Washington, DC: National Center for Learning Disabilities.

The National Coalition on School Diversity. 2020. *Including Racial and Socioeconomic Diversity in ESSA District Plans*. https://files.eric.ed.gov/fulltext/ED607737.pdf (accessed March 15, 2023).

National Park Service. 2020. *The Carlisle Indian Industrial School: Assimilation with Education After the Indian Wars (Teaching with Historic Places)*. https://www.nps.gov/articles/the-carlisle-indian-industrial-school-assimilation-with-education-after-the-indian-wars-teaching-with-historic-places.htm (accessed March 17, 2023).

NCES (National Center for Education Statistics). 2016. *Allocating Grants for Title I*. https://nces.ed.gov/surveys/annualreports/pdf/titlei20160111.pdf (accessed June 1, 2023).

NCES. 2020. *Table 104.20. Percentage of Persons 25 to 29 Years Old with Selected Levels of Educational Attainment, by Race/Ethnicity and Sex: Selected Years, 1920 Through 2020*. https://nces.ed.gov/programs/digest/d20/tables/dt20_104.20.asp (accessed March 21, 2023).

NCES. 2021. *Digest of Education Statistics: Table 219.47 Public High School 4-Year Adjusted Cohort Graduation Rate (ACGR), by Selected Student Characteristics and Locale: 2018–2019*. https://nces.ed.gov/programs/digest/d20/tables/dt20_219.47.asp (accessed June 2, 2023).

NCES. 2022a. *Annual Earnings by Educational Attainment.* https://nces.ed.gov/programs/coe/indicator/cba/annual-earnings#suggested-citation (accessed June 15, 2023).

NCES. 2022b. *Enrollment Rates of Young Children.* https://nces.ed.gov/programs/coe/indicator/cfa/enrollment-of-young-children (accessed March 21, 2023).

NCES. 2022c. *Table 203.50. Enrollment and Percentage Distribution of Enrollment in Public Elementary and Secondary Schools, by Race/Ethnicity and Region: Selected Years, Fall 1995 Through Fall 2031.* https://nces.ed.gov/programs/digest/d22/tables/dt22_203.50.asp (accessed June 2, 2023).

NCES. 2023a. *Concentration of Public School Students Eligible for Free or Reduced-Price Lunch.* https://nces.ed.gov/programs/coe/indicator/clb/free-or-reduced-price-lunch (accessed June 1, 2023).

NCES. 2023b. *Public School Expenditures.* https://nces.ed.gov/programs/coe/indicator/cmb/public-school-expenditure (accessed June 1, 2023).

NCES. n.d. *Common Core of Data: Annual Diploma Counts and the Averaged Freshman Graduation Rate (AFGR) in the United States by Race/Ethnicity: School Years 2007–08 Through 2011–12.* https://nces.ed.gov/ccd/tables/AFGR0812.asp (accessed June 2, 2023).

Neuberger, Z. 2022. *Permanent summer grocery benefits are a big win for children in low-income families, despite disappointing tradeoffs.* Washington, DC: Center on Budget and Policy Priorities.

Newland, B. 2022. *Federal Indian Boarding School Initiative investigative report.* Washington, DC: The Office of the Assistant Secretary—Indian Affairs.

NRC (National Research Council). 2002. *Minority students in special and gifted education.* Washington, DC: The National Academies Press.

Oakford, P., C. Brumfield, G. Goldvale, L. Tatum, M. diZerega, and F. Patrick. 2019. *Investing in futures: Economic and fiscal benefits of postsecondary education in prison.* New York, NY: Vera Institute of Justice.

OESE (Office of Elementary and Secondary Education). 2023. *Full-Service Community Schools Program (FSCS).* https://oese.ed.gov/offices/office-of-discretionary-grants-support-services/school-choice-improvement-programs/full-service-community-schools-program-fscs/ (accessed February 21, 2023).

Office for Civil Rights. n.d. *Civil Rights Data Collection (CRDC).* https://www2.ed.gov/about/offices/list/ocr/frontpage/faq/crdc.html (accessed June 1, 2023).

Ogden, C. L., T. H. Fakhouri, M. D. Carroll, C. M. Hales, C. D. Fryar, X. Li, and D. S. Freedman. 2017. Prevalence of obesity among adults, by household income and education—United States, 2011–2014. *Morbidity and Mortality Weekly Report* 66(50):1369–1373.

Orfield, G., E. Frankenberg, J. Ee, and J. Kuscera. 2014. *Brown at 60: Great progress, a long retreat and an uncertain future.* Los Angeles, CA: The Civil Rights Project.

Orris, A., and J. Wagner. 2022. *Medicaid School-Based Services Can Help Prevent "Unwinding" Coverage Losses.* https://www.cbpp.org/blog/medicaid-school-based-services-can-help-prevent-unwinding-coverage-losses (accessed February 21, 2023).

Parker, K., and R. Stepler. 2017. *As U.S. Marriage Rate Hovers at 50%, Education Gap in Marital Status Widens.* https://www.pewresearch.org/fact-tank/2017/09/14/as-u-s-marriage-rate-hovers-at-50-education-gap-in-marital-status-widens/ (accessed June 15, 2023).

Paschall, M. J., and M. Bersamin. 2018. School-based health centers, depression, and suicide risk among adolescents. *American Journal of Preventive Medicine* 54(1):44–50.

PATH Team (Policy Advancing Transformation and Healing). 2020. *Memorandum: Re: School-Based Health Centers.* https://www.clasp.org/wp-content/uploads/2022/04/Memorandum20on20SBHCs_final-2.pdf (accessed June 15, 2023).

Pew Research Center. 2019. *Two decades of change in federal and state higher education funding.* Washington, DC: Pew Research Center.

Protopsaltis, S., and S. Parrott. 2017. *Pell grants—a key tool for expanding college access and economic opportunity—need strengthening, not cuts.* Washington, DC: Center on Budget and Policy Priorities.

The Public Interest Law Center. n.d. *Pennsylvania Association for Retarded Citizens (PARC) v. Commonwealth of Pennsylvania.* https://pubintlaw.org/cases-and-projects/pennsylvania-association-for-retarded-citizens-parc-v-commonwealth-of-pennsylvania/ (accessed June 1, 2023).

Puma, M., S. Bell, R. Cook, C. Heid, G. Shapiro, P. Broene, F. Jenkins, P. Fletcher, L. Quinn, J. Friedman, J. Ciarico, M. Rohacek, G. Adams, and E. Spier. 2010. *Head Start Impact Study: Final report.* Washington, DC: Head Start Impact Study.

Quinn, J., and J. M. Blank. n.d. *Twenty Years, Ten Lessons: Community Schools as an Equitable School Improvement Strategy.* https://steinhardt.nyu.edu/metrocenter/vue/twenty-years-ten-lessons (accessed March 21, 2023).

Ralston, K., C. Newman, A. Clauson, J. Guthrie, and J. Buzby. 2008. *The National School Lunch Program: Background, trends, and issues.* Washington, DC: U.S. Department of Agriculture.

Reardon, S. F., and X. A. Portilla. 2016. Recent trends in income, racial, and ethnic school readiness gaps at kindergarten entry. *AERA Open* 2(3):233285841665734.

Reichmann, K. 2022. *Affirmative Action Case Puts Equality in Education Back Before the Justices.* https://www.courthousenews.com/affirmative-action-case-puts-equality-in-education-back-before-the-justices/ (accessed March 15, 2023).

Rothstein, J., and D. W. Schanzenbach. 2022. Does money still matter? Attainment and earnings effects of post-1990 school finance reforms. *Journal of Labor Economics* 40(S1):S141–S178.

Rubinton, H., and M. Isaacson. 2022. *School District Expenditures and Race.* https://research.stlouisfed.org/publications/economic-synopses/2022/02/16/school-district-expenditures-and-race (accessed June 15, 2023).

Ruffini, K. 2022. Universal access to free school meals and student achievement: Evidence from the community eligibility provision. *Journal of Human Resources* 57(3):776–820.

Running Bear, U., C. D. Croy, C. E. Kaufman, Z. M. Thayer, and S. M. Manson. 2018. The relationship of five boarding school experiences and physical health status among Northern Plains Tribes. *Quality of Life Research* 27(1):153–157.

Running Bear, U., Z. M. Thayer, C. D. Croy, C. E. Kaufman, and S. M. Manson. 2019. The impact of individual and parental American Indian boarding school attendance on chronic physical health of northern plains tribes. *Family & Community Health* 42(1):1–7.

Schanzenbach, D. W., D. Boddy, M. Mumford, and G. Nantz. 2016. *Fourteen economic facts on education and economic opportunity.* Washington, DC: The Hamilton Project.

Schrag, J. 2014. *Social Determinants of Health: Education.* https://essentialhospitals.org/quality/social-determinants-of-health-education/ (accessed February 8, 2023).

Schueler, B. 2020. *Summer "Vacation Academies" Can Narrow Coronavirus Learning Gaps.* https://www.educationnext.org/summer-vacation-academies-narrow-coronavirus-learning-gaps-springfield/ (accessed February 15, 2023).

Schueler, B. E., J. S. Goodman, and D. J. Deming. 2017. Can states take over and turn around school districts? Evidence from Lawrence, Massachusetts. *Educational Evaluation and Policy Analysis* 39(2):311–332.

Schwartz, A. E., and M. W. Rothbart. 2020. Let them eat lunch: The impact of universal free meals on student performance. *Journal of Policy Analysis and Management* 39(2):376–410.

Snyder, T. D., C. de Brey, and S. A. Dillow. 2019. *Digest of education statistics 2017 (NCES 2018070).* Washington, DC: Institute of Education Sciences.

Sosnaud, B. 2019. Inequality in infant mortality: Cross-state variation and medical system institutions. *Social Problems* 66(1):108–127.

Task Force on Next Generation Community Schools. 2021. *Addressing education inequality with a next generation of community schools.* Washington, DC: The Brookings Institution.

Taylor, E. S., and J. H. Tyler. 2012. The effect of evaluation on teacher performance. *American Economic Review* 102(7):3628–3651.

Thomsen, E., C. Peterson, E. D. Velez, and RTI International. 2020. *One year after a bachelor's degree: A profile of 2015–16 graduates.* Washington, DC: Institute for Educational Sciences.

Toldson, I. A. 2016. The funding gap between historically Black colleges and universities and traditionally White institutions needs to be addressed. *Journal of Negro Education* 85(2):97–100.

Urban Institute. 2017. *Diversifying the Classroom: Examining the Teacher Pipeline.* https:// www.urban.org/features/diversifying-classroom-examining-teacher-pipeline (accessed June 15, 2023).

Urban Institute. n.d. *Elementary and Secondary Education Expenditures.* https://www.urban. org/policy-centers/cross-center-initiatives/state-and-local-finance-initiative/state-and-local-backgrounders/elementary-and-secondary-education-expenditures (accessed March 1, 2023).

U.S. Commission on Civil Rights. 2002. *Making a good IDEA better: The reauthorization of the Individuals with Disabilities Education Act.* Washington, DC: U.S. Commission on Civil Rights.

USDA (U.S. Department of Agriculture). 2019a. *Community Eligibility Provision.* https://www. fns.usda.gov/cn/community-eligibility-provision (accessed Februray 21, 2023).

USDA. 2019b. *School Meals FAQS.* https://www.fns.usda.gov/cn/school-meals-faqs#:~:text= Schools%20are%20required%20to%20serve,185%20percent%20of%20these%20 guidelines (accessed February 21, 2023).

USDA. 2022. *Summer Electronic Benefit Transfer for Children (SEBTC).* https://www.fns. usda.gov/ops/summer-electronic-benefit-transfer-children-sebtc (accessed June 2, 2023).

USDA. 2023. *Child Nutrition Tables.* https://www.fns.usda.gov/pd/child-nutrition-tables (accessed February 21, 2023).

USDA. n.d. *National School Lunch Program.* https://www.fns.usda.gov/nslp (accessed February 28, 2023).

Wallen, M., and A. Hubbard. 2013. *Blending and Braiding Early Childhood Program Funding Streams Toolkit: Enhancing Financing for High-Quality Early Learning Programs.* https://www.startearly.org/app/uploads/pdf/NPT-Blended-Funding-Toolkit.pdf (accessed March 1, 2023).

Weiland, C., D. Bassok, D. A. Phillips, E. U. Cascio, C. Gibbs, and D. Stipek. 2022. *What Does the Tennessee Pre-K Study Really Tell Us About Public Preschool Programs?* https:// www.brookings.edu/blog/brown-center-chalkboard/2022/02/10/what-does-the-tennessee-pre-k-study-really-tell-us-about-public-preschool-programs/ (accessed June 15, 2023).

Weiss, M. J., A. Ratledge, C. Sommo, and H. Gupta. 2019. Supporting community college students from start to degree completion: Long-term evidence from a randomized trial of CUNY's ASAP. *American Economic Journal: Applied Economics* 11(3):253–297.

Whitehurst, G. J. 2017. *New evidence on school choice and racially segregated schools.* Washington, DC: The Brookings Institution.

Wikle, S., J. Wagner, F. Erzouki, and J. Sullivan. 2022. *States can reduce Medicaid's administrative burdens to advance health and racial equity.* Washington, DC: Center on Budget and Policy Priorities.

Wilkinson, A., A. Gabriel, B. Stratford, M. Carter, Y. Rodriguez, O. Okogbue, S. Somers, D. Young, and K. Harper. 2020. *Early evidence of Medicaid's important role in school-based health services.* Bethesda, MD: Child Trends.

Williams, K. L., and B. L. Davis. 2019. *Public and Private Investments and Divestments in Historically Black Colleges and Universities.* https://www.acenet.edu/Documents/public-and-private-investments-and-divestments-in-hbcus.pdf (accessed June 15, 2023).

Wolla, S. A., and J. Sullivan. 2017. *Education, Income, and Wealth.* https://research.stlouisfed.org/ publications/page1-econ/2017/01/03/education-income-and-wealth (accessed March 21, 2023).

5

Health Care Access and Quality

INTRODUCTION

As described throughout this report, racial, ethnic, and tribal health inequities are created and sustained by factors both inside and outside of the health care system. However, health is strongly tied to the health care system—a healthy population requires access to high-quality, comprehensive, affordable, timely, respectful, and culturally appropriate health care. The health care system serves as an important setting for delivery of care and treatment, individual- and population-level prevention and health improvement interventions, and clinical research and as an important source of data needed to measure health outcomes and health inequities. Some health inequities are created and sustained in the health care system—these are often referred to as "*health care* inequities," due to their direct tie to the health care system, as distinguished from "health inequities," which describe the outcomes related to factors both in and outside the system. This distinction becomes important when focusing on the federal health care policies that contribute to health and health care inequities to identify policy-level intervention points.

This chapter summarizes the role of federal policy across the U.S. health care system, followed by an overview of health inequities within (created and propagated by) it. It also

- reviews a selection of federal health care policies that either contribute to racial, ethnic, and tribal health inequities or advance equity;
- is organized around access, quality, and inclusion; and

- concludes with a section outlining impacts of the system on a few specific populations that were selected to provide a broadly illustrative, but not comprehensive or exhaustive, perspective on the interactions between populations and health care policies and systems.

Numerous policies could be reviewed along with their effects on every racially and ethnically minoritized population and in different geographic settings (e.g., urban, rural, U.S. territory); see Chapter 1 for an overview of the committee's process for selecting policies. As it has done in other chapters, however, the committee identified a limited set of salient examples that contribute to or promote racial, ethnic, and tribal health inequities in a number of different areas (e.g., Medicaid and the Children's Health Insurance Program [CHIP] and policies and practices related to health literacy and language access, value-based payment, inclusion in clinical trials and the workforce, the Indian Health Service [IHS], and maternal, territorial, and immigrant health). This approach does not mean that policies that were not reviewed, or not discussed in detail, are less important—rather, the goal of this and other chapters is to illustrate the different ways federal policies contribute to inequities and can further health equity.

FEDERAL HEALTH CARE POLICY OVERVIEW

Federal policies drive all aspects of the U.S. health care system. Congress legislates many aspects of health care finance, delivery, access, and quality; the Department of Health and Human Services (HHS) is the principal executive agency serving as the primary regulator/administrator of these laws, and it includes several subagencies responsible for specific policies and programs. Due to the substantial role of the federal government in health care policy, HHS accounts for the largest percent of federal budget resources at nearly 25 percent, largely because of public health insurance programs (CBPP, 2022). HHS has agencies that finance and regulate public insurance programs (Centers for Medicare & Medicaid Services [CMS]), health care access (Health Resources and Services Administration [HRSA]), medical devices, pharmaceuticals, and clinical trials (Food and Drug Administration [FDA]), public health (Centers for Disease Control and Prevention [CDC]), research (National Institutes of Health [NIH] and Office for Human Research Protections), and the IHS, among others related to health and health care.

HHS also has the Office of Minority Health (OMH), which was created in 1986, following the Secretary's Task Force Report on Black and Minority Health (also known as the "Heckler report" (Heckler, 1985)), the first federal report to acknowledge racial and ethnic health disparities. OMH is intended to "improve the health of racial and ethnic minority populations through the development of health policies and programs that will help eliminate health disparities" (OMH, 2019). In 2010, as part of the Patient Protection and Affordable Care Act (ACA)[1], Offices of Minority Health were established in six agencies at HHS (Agency for Healthcare Research and Quality [AHRQ], CDC, CMS, FDA, HRSA, and Substance Abuse and Mental Health Services Administration), which, in partnership with the NIH National Institute on Minority Health and Health Disparities, are responsible for leading and coordinating activities across the agency. However, as noted in the HHS Equity Action Plan, "HHS currently lacks the data and equity assessment capacity to consistently identify and address inequities in health and human services" (HHS, 2022c, p. 12). HHS' lack of capacity, ability to coordinate, and limited authority contributes to racial and ethnic health inequities.

In the United States, access to health care is largely dependent on insurance coverage; federal policy drives that and many other aspects of health care, including how it is delivered, the data collected, the health care workforce, use of technology, and innovation; examples of such policies include the Emergency Medical Treatment and Active Labor Act,[2] the Health Information Technology for Economic and Clinical Health Act,[3] and FDA regulation of the process of developing, testing, and marketing pharmaceuticals. Federal policies have created the health care safety net, designating medically underserved areas and health professional shortage areas, and authorizing federally qualified health centers, critical access hospitals, and other safety net settings in these areas, many of which serve a disproportionate share of racially and ethnically minoritized populations.

Mistrust in Health Care and Looking to the Future

The federal government has had an active role in major events that created racial, ethnic, and tribal health inequities and severely harmed trust in the health system. This includes, for example, the Tuskegee Syphilis Study, which the U.S. Public Health Service conducted from 1932 through 1972

---

[1] Pub. L. 111–148, 124 Stat. 119 (Mar. 23, 2010).

[2] Largely codified in 42 U.S.C. § 1395dd, this requires hospitals to stabilize emergency conditions regardless of a patient's ability to pay. This improved access to emergency services but created a system of universal access for those with disease at the most severe stage or an emergency medical condition (as opposed to preventing illness and treating diseases early); patients are still required to bear the cost of treatment.

[3] Pub. L. 111–5, 123 Stat. 226. This regulates the adoption and use of electronic health records, health information exchanges, and other technology by clinicians and health care settings. It created the Office of the National Coordinator for Health Information Technology with an explicit goal of reducing health disparities, yet inequities remain in clinician access to and use of technology for underserved communities and patients (Lee, 2015; Washington et al., 2017).

and withheld available treatment from Black men with syphilis, and the involuntary sterilization of American Indian women by IHS in the 1970s, of Puerto Rican women through Law 116, and of Mexican women in California using federal funds through the 1970s (Arce, 2021; Carpio, 2004; Krase, 1996; Lawrence, 2000; Reyes, 2016; Torpy, 2000). These and many other examples of intentional harm to racially and ethnically minoritized people and communities have eroded trust in the federal government and the U.S. health care system generally (see Chapter 7 for more information on this and on trauma and healing). The landmark study of how the behavior of Black men changed after the revelation of Tuskegee in 1972 found increases in medical mistrust and mortality and declining physician interactions with greater proximity to the victims (Alsan and Wanamaker, 2018). The closure of Black hospitals is also part of the landscape of medical mistrust—people lack access to health care institutions and providers who are from and center their communities. Before the Civil Rights Movement, hospitals outright refused to admit Black patients or treated them in segregated wards in undesirable locations, and Black doctors were excluded from working in many hospitals. Black-run hospitals opened in the late 1890s, though many were underresourced (Jordan, 2022; McBride, 2022). The Freedman's Hospital was the only federally funded health care facility for Black people when it was established in 1862 to provide care for formerly enslaved people (Duke University Medical Center Library, 2022; Howard University Hospital, n.d.). It is now Howard University Hospital, one of the few remaining traditional Black hospitals. Title VI[4] of the 1964 Civil Rights Act outlawed segregation and discrimination based on race, color, or national origin in any program or activity receiving federal funds or financial assistance. Passed 1 year later, Medicare made hospital funding contingent on desegregation (Duff-Brown, 2021; Yearby et al., 2022). See the sections later in this chapter on implicit bias and racism and the health care workforce.

Federal policies related to health care are generally intended to improve health, with some explicitly meant to address health inequities. Yet racial and ethnic health inequities can be identified across most, if not all, federal health care programs. Federal policies continue to contribute to health and health care inequities but also serve as a powerful tool to mitigate and eliminate inequities and advance health equity.

Federal policies have also reduced inequities. In recognition of the role the federal government plays in advancing health equity, HHS released the *CMS Framework for Health Equity 2022–2032*, which outlines in five domains its strategy to advance health equity through CMS policy: improving data collection; identifying and adopting policies that can advance health equity; building appropriate health care organizations and workforce; advancing language

---

[4] 42 U.S.C. § 2000d *et seq.*

access, health literacy, and cultural humility; and improving all forms of access regardless of ability (CMS, 2022a). This document identifies health equity as a national priority and is broadly inclusive in defining underserved populations as identified in Executive Order 13985[5] *Advancing Racial Equity and Support for Underserved Communities Through the Federal Government.*

HEALTH CARE ACCESS AND HEALTH CARE INEQUITY

Health care access and quality, one of the five broad categories of social determinants of health (SDOH), is directly tied to health outcomes (AHRQ, 2022; HHS, n.d.-b; University of Wisconsin Population Health Institute, 2023). Understanding different domains of access and quality can help clarify the impact federal policies have on health care inequities and identify opportunities to reduce these.

Health Insurance Coverage

Health insurance coverage is critical for accessing health care in the United States; it is a combination of insurance segments, all of which are a result of federal policy. Those with insurance have dramatically lower financial barriers to care, and providers are more likely to provide care to those with health insurance (Glied et al., 2020; Tolbert et al., 2022). Insurance is provided through private insurance markets and the public sector. The private sector includes employer-sponsored, individual, and other nongovernmental plans. Public-sector insurance includes Medicare, Medicaid, (CHIP), TRICARE, and several other programs, as detailed below. According to the Census Bureau, employer-sponsored health insurance covered 54.3 percent, Medicare 18.4 percent, and Medicaid 18.9 percent of the U.S. population in 2021 (Keisler-Starkey and Bunch, 2022) (see Figure 5-1). The racial distribution for the under 65 population varies by insurance segment (see Figures 5-2 and 5-3). About three-quarters of White and Asian nonelderly adults ages 19–64 have employer or other private coverage, as do about 60 percent of Native Hawaiian and Pacific Islander (NHPI) and Black people, but about half of Hispanic and 42 percent of American Indian and Alaska Native (AIAN) adults do (Artiga et al., 2022b). Gaps in rates of public coverage and uninsured are reversed: they are relatively lower for White and Asian adults. The gaps in uninsured are most consequential, with 25 percent of Hispanic and AIAN adults uninsured compared to 8 percent of White adults. Fourteen percent of Black adults and 12 percent of NHPI adults are uninsured (Artiga et al., 2022b). Similar trends by race and ethnicity are seen among children ages 0–18, but higher percentages in general have Medicaid and other public insurance and lower

[5] Exec. Order No. 13985, 86 FR 7009 (January 2021).

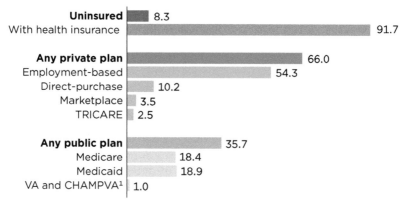

Type of Coverage in 2021

Uninsured	8.3
With health insurance	91.7
Any private plan	66.0
Employment-based	54.3
Direct-purchase	10.2
Marketplace	3.5
TRICARE	2.5
Any public plan	35.7
Medicare	18.4
Medicaid	18.9
VA and CHAMPVA¹	1.0

FIGURE 5-1 Percentage of people by type of health insurance coverage, 2021.
NOTES: The estimates by type of coverage are not mutually exclusive; people can have more than one type during the year. Information on confidentiality protection, sampling error, nonsampling error, and definitions is available at https://www2.census.gov/programs-surveys/cps/techdocs/cpsmar22.pdf. CHAMPVA = Civilian Medical Program of the Department of Veterans Affairs; VA = Department of Veterans Affairs.
¹ Includes CHAMPVA and care provided by VA and the military.
SOURCE: Keisler-Starkey and Bunch, 2022.

Legend: Employer/Other Private ▓ Medicaid/Other Public ■ Uninsured

White
	Employer/Other Private	Medicaid/Other Public	Uninsured
2019	68%	28%	4%
2021	66%	30%	4%

Black
2019	37%	59%	5%
2021	35%	60%	5%

Hispanic
2019	37%	54%	9%
2021	37%	55%	9%

Asian
2019	71%	25%	4%
2021	68%	29%	

AIAN
2019	32%	54%	14%
2021	28%	59%	13%

NHOPI
2019	43%	48%	9%
2021	41%	52%	7%

FIGURE 5-2 Health care coverage of children by race and ethnicity, 2019 and 2021 (ages 0–18).
NOTES: Persons of Hispanic origin may be of any race but are categorized as Hispanic for this analysis; other groups are non-Hispanic. Totals may not sum to 100 percent due to rounding. AIAN = American Indian or Alaska Native; NHOPI = Native Hawaiian or Other Pacific Islander.
SOURCE: Artiga et al., 2022b; licensed under CC BY-NC-ND 4.0 (https://creativecommons.org/licenses/by-nc-nd/4.0/).

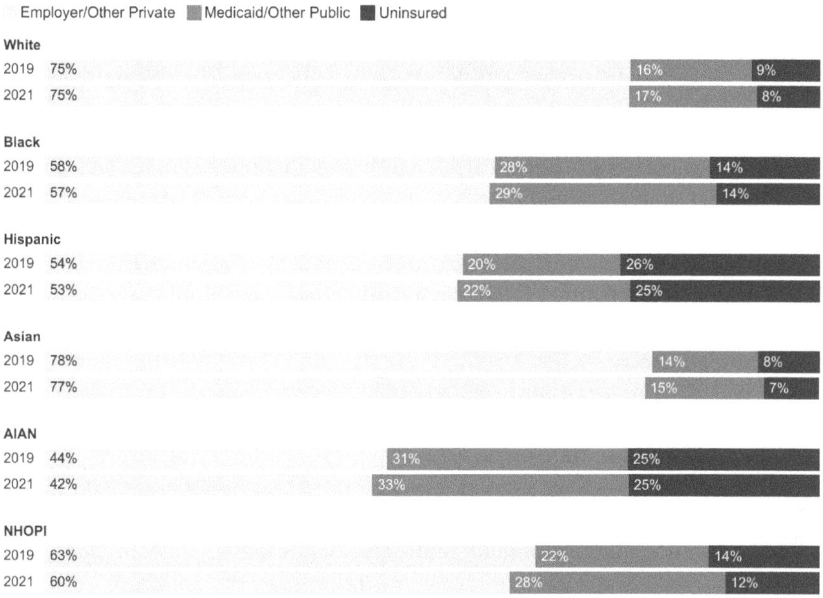

FIGURE 5-3 Health care coverage of nonelderly population by race and ethnicity, 2019 and 2021 (ages 19–64).
NOTES: Persons of Hispanic origin may be of any race but are categorized as Hispanic for this analysis; other groups are non-Hispanic. Totals may not sum to 100 percent due to rounding. AIAN = American Indian or Alaska Native; NHOPI = Native Hawaiian or Other Pacific Islander.
SOURCE: Artiga et al., 2022b; licensed under CC BY-NC-ND 4.0 (https://creativecommons.org/licenses/by-nc-nd/4.0/).

percentages are uninsured than adults. More than half of Black, AIAN, Hispanic, and NHPI children have Medicaid or other public insurance. Uninsured rates are highest among AIAN (13 percent), Hispanic (9 percent), and NHPI (7 percent) children (Artiga et al., 2022b). This system of insurance as the gateway to services is derived directly from employment status, age, income, and/or other social factors. This results in many individuals who are uninsured or underinsured and contributes to inequities in access that disproportionately affect Black, Latino, AIAN, NHPI, and other minoritized populations.

Health insurance coverage is highly fragmented largely because the system was designed around private employer-sponsored health insurance with federal programs developed to address groups not covered by their employers. Employer-sponsored health insurance is supported by a federal tax exclusion that has been in place since the 1940s (Carpenter, 2019); these insured do not pay federal (or state) taxes for this part of their compensation. This policy creates tax inequity, as it benefits those with employment and provides greater subsidies to those with higher incomes (CRS, 2011). The fiscal year (FY) 2023 income tax expenditure for the exclusion of employer contributions for medical insurance premiums and care is estimated at more than $200 billion (Department of the Treasury, 2023; Tax Policy Center, 2020). Nongroup insurance covers a relatively small segment of the population, and these individuals do not benefit from this tax exclusion. ACA added subsidies scaled by income and regulations to make it easier for those outside of the employer-based system and other public programs to obtain insurance. This nongroup private market has expanded since 2014, when these rules went into effect. In addition to creating subsidies for individuals and businesses to purchase private insurance market products, federal policy also regulates many other aspects of the private market, such as mandating coverage for certain types of services and regulating industry policies and practices. For example, the Mental Health Parity and Addiction Equity Act[6] required private plans that cover treatment for behavioral health conditions to do so in the same way as for other medical conditions. The Employee Retirement Income Security Act[7] sets minimum standards for employer-sponsored private health insurance and retirement plans. ACA mandated that all public and private plans cover preventive services at no cost to the patient.[8]

Government-sponsored health programs include Medicare, Medicaid and CHIP, military health programs, such as TRICARE and the Veterans Health Administration (VHA), IHS, and the Native Hawaiian Health Care Systems. Medicare has eligibility based on age (65 years and older), some disabilities and conditions, and other factors, with over 63 million enrolled in 2021 (CMS, 2021a). Medicaid is the federal and state program for eligible low-income children, adults, pregnant people, elderly adults, and people with disabilities (Medicaid.gov, n.d.-b). More than 86 million people were enrolled in Medicaid and CHIP in 2021, including 35.9 percent of children (Keisler-Starkey and Bunch, 2022; Medicaid.gov, 2022; Mykyta et al., 2022). The national health expenditures in 2021 were $900 billion for Medicare and $734 billion for Medicaid ($513 billion federal, $221 billion state and local) (CMS, 2023d). The federal government pays for more than one-third of total national health expenditures through Medicare and Medicaid, providing insurance coverage to approximately one-third of the population (CMS, 2023d; Keisler-Starkey and Bunch, 2022). In 2014, through ACA, federal law allowed[9] states to

---

[6]Pub. L. 110–343, 122 Stat. 3881 (Oct. 3, 2008).

[7]29 U.S.C. § 1001 *et seq.*

[8]As of May 2023, ACA's requirement of private plans to cover preventive services without cost sharing was in litigation (KFF, 2023a).

[9]ACA required states to expand Medicaid or lose federal funding for the program; the Supreme Court ruled this unconstitutional in *National Federation of Independent Business v. Sebelius*, 567 U.S. 519 (2012) (Cornell Law School, n.d.).

expand their Medicaid eligibility criteria to cover all adults with incomes below 138 percent of the federal poverty level. Medicaid and CHIP enrollment also increased after 2020 in part because of the continuous enrollment provision of the Families First Coronavirus Response Act[10] (Tolbert and Ammula, 2023).

TRICARE provides insurance for 9.6 million active-duty and retired service members, members of the National Guard and Reserve, and eligible family; it costs about $50 billion annually (DHA, 2022; Schaettle et al., 2021). VHA is the country's largest integrated health care system, serving 9 million veterans annually; Department of Veterans Affairs (VA) medical services receive about $120 billion in discretionary funding (Shane, 2022; VA, 2022; The White House, 2023). IHS is the health care system for AIAN people from federally recognized tribes, serving around 2.7 million persons, with a FY2022 budget of $6.8 billion (ASPE, 2022a). The Native Hawaiian Health Care Improvement Act[11] established Papa Ola Lōkahi and five Native Hawaiian Health Care Systems that serve Native Hawaiians in Hawaii and provide culturally responsive, community-based health promotion, disease prevention, and primary care services; the majority of funding is federal grant money from HRSA (HRSA, 2023; Hui No Ke Ola Pono, n.d.). The program received $22 million in 2022 (Hiraishi, 2022; Office of Senator Schatz, 2022). See sections later in this chapter for more information on Medicaid and IHS.

Even with all of these programs, 27.2 million people, or about 8 percent of the population, were uninsured in 2021; 5 percent of children were uninsured (Keisler-Starkey and Bunch, 2022). Although disparities in rates of uninsured between racial and ethnic groups have declined as a result of ACA expansions, gaps remain (Artiga et al., 2022b; Keisler-Starkey and Bunch, 2022; Lee et al., 2021). Racially and ethnically minoritized and low-income people, including children, continue to be more likely be uninsured. More specifically, individuals living in the 11[12] states that have not expanded Medicaid were two times more likely to be uninsured (Artiga et al., 2022b; KFF, 2023c; Lee et al., 2021; Tolbert et al., 2022; Yearby et al., 2022). Yet it is not just a gap in federal and state policy; it is also a function of implementation, including availability and affordability of health insurance options, which affect an individual's decision to enroll. Approximately 63 percent of these 27 million uninsured individuals were eligible for some type of subsidized insurance coverage (see Figure 5-4).

---

[10] Pub. L. 116–127, 134 Stat. 178 (Mar. 18, 2020).

[11] 42 U.S.C. § 11701 *et seq.*

[12] As of February 2023: Alabama, Florida, Georgia, Kansas, Mississippi, North Carolina, South Carolina, Tennessee, Texas, Wisconsin, and Wyoming.

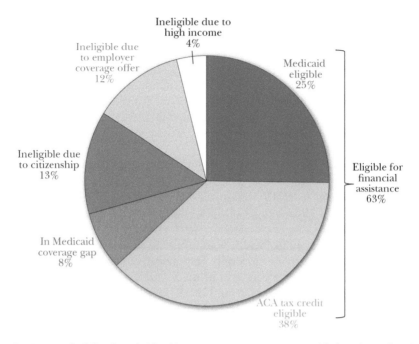

FIGURE 5-4 Eligibility for subsidized insurance coverage among nonelderly uninsured, 2021. NOTES: The graph shows the share of uninsured Americans under age 65 who are already eligible for subsidized insurance via Medicaid or ACA tax credits to purchase coverage on state insurance exchanges. Overall, 63 percent of the uninsured are eligible for financial assistance, while 37 percent are not. The "Medicaid coverage gap" refers to low-income individuals living in states that have not expanded Medicaid under ACA. ACA = Patient Protection and Affordable Care Act.
SOURCE: Baicker et al., 2023 [Copyright American Economic Association; reproduced with permission of the *Journal of Economic Perspectives*].

Access to Health Care Services

In addition to inequities in health care coverage, access to health care services, including a regular primary care provider, is also inequitable. Having a regular source of care is associated with better health outcomes, fewer disparities, and lower costs (AHRQ, 2016). Health care quality and use can be affected by discrimination, bias, and racism in health care settings (Bailey et al., 2017; Williams et al., 2019). The landmark Institute of Medicine report, *Unequal Treatment: Confronting Racial and Ethnic Disparities in Health Care*, describes the solid evidence base indicating Black, Latino/a, AIAN, and other minoritized people receive lower-quality care compared to White people; this remains true after adjusting for income and insurance coverage (AHRQ, 2022; IOM, 2003; Yearby et al., 2022). These populations are also more likely than White people to live in areas with shortages of primary care physicians, mental health professionals, and surgeons. Public and rural hospital closures contribute to this, in part because hospitals can be a base for some primary care physicians' practices (Bailey et al., 2017; Yearby et al., 2022). Rural communities with larger proportions of Black and AIAN residents are farther from many hospital services, such as emergency and trauma services, than those with a high proportion of White residents (Eberth et al., 2022).

One mechanism by which poor access to providers may affect health is suggested by the literature on the effects of lacking a regular primary care provider. It is associated with delayed or no consistent care (HHS, n.d.-c). According to a Kaiser Family Foundation analysis, 34 percent of Hispanic adults reported not having a provider in 2021 (Hill et al., 2023). Percentages for other racially and ethnically minoritized people were similarly higher than for White adults (16 percent): 24 percent of AIAN and 21 percent of NHPI people reported lacking a provider, as did 19 and 18 percent of Asian and Black people, respectively (Hill et al., 2023). The same analysis found more Hispanic and Black children (9 and 7 percent, respectively) without a usual source of care than White children (4 percent) (Hill et al., 2023). Access to specialty care is also inequitable among racially and ethnically minoritized children (Flores and The Committee on Pediatric Research, 2010).

The relationship between access to care and health also plays out in differential rates of early detection of disease that result from differential engagement in clinical preventive services can help prevent or slow disease progression. Based on 2018 data, differences among racial and ethnic groups exist for preventive care (HHS, n.d.-d). For example, whereas 7.8 percent of White adults ages 35 years or over report receiving appropriate clinical preventive services, only 5.4 percent of Black and 4.2 percent of Hispanic or Latino/a people did so (HHS, n.d.-d).

MEDICAID

Given the high cost of health care, affordability is an important element of access, and health insurance is the primary policy lever. The committee focused on Medicaid (including Medicaid structure, eligibility, enrollment and administrative burden, and innovation) because Medicaid is a major source of health care coverage for people with low income, racially and ethnically minoritized populations, people with disabilities, and other underserved groups. Medicaid and CHIP are also critical sources of insurance for children; more than one-third of U.S. children are covered by Medicaid or CHIP (Keisler-Starkey and Bunch, 2022; Mykyta et al., 2022).

Medicaid, enacted in 1965 alongside Medicare, was designed to provide health insurance for individuals with limited income; that focus makes it a key policy lever for addressing health equity. An analysis by Kaiser Family Foundation found more than half of nonelderly enrollees identify as Black, Hispanic, Asian, or another minoritized race or ethnicity (KFF, n.d.-e). As a more specific example, Medicaid paid for 41 percent of U.S. births in 2021, including 58 and 64 percent of births to Latina and Black women, respectively (Osterman et al., 2023). Medicaid is a critically important program and has improved health access and some health outcomes and reduced racial inequities, financial burden, and mortality rates (Baicker et al., 2013; Flores et al., 2017; Guth and Artiga, 2022; Lee et al., 2021; Miller et al., 2021; NASEM, 2017b).

The Oregon Health Insurance Experiment was a significant study of the effect of expanding health insurance through a Medicaid lottery. Oregon initiated an experimental limited expansion of its Medicaid program in 2008 by filling spots on a waiting list with a lottery system. About 90,000 adults signed up for the waiting list; approximately one-third of these names were drawn for 10,000 spots. The limited number of spots created a natural opportunity to randomize Medicaid coverage to understand its effects on health care use and outcomes, financial hardship, and well-being in the first 1–2 years of coverage (NBER, n.d.-a). Research found that it resulted in significantly more outpatient and emergency department visits, hospitalizations, and prescriptions (Baicker et al., 2017; Finkelstein et al., 2016). It also reduced prevalence of depression but did not significantly change cardiovascular risk or cholesterol and blood pressure levels (Baicker et al., 2013, 2018; NBER, n.d.-b). The likelihood of experiencing a catastrophic medical expenditure dramatically reduced and medical debt was significantly lowered (Baicker et al., 2013; Finkelstein et al., 2012; NBER, n.d.-b). Additionally, several studies have examined changes in health disparities resulting from the ACA Medicaid expansions that were not implemented in all states (Donohue et al., 2022). Lee and colleagues (2021) found "Medicaid expansion was associated with significant decreases in uninsured rates and increases in Medicaid coverage among all racial and ethnic groups." Decreases in racial and ethnic disparities in delayed and unmet need for care were also observed. See Box 5-1 for information on the recent expansions of public health insurance and benefits to children.

However, Medicaid-relevant inequities remain. Within Medicaid, one cross-sectional study found Black enrollees generated lower spending and used fewer primary care and recommended care services than White enrollees but had more emergency department visits (Wallace et al., 2022). This important study suggests that additional steps to ensure equity are needed within this critical program that reduces health inequity in important ways (Wallace et al., 2022). The following sections highlight those program

BOX 5-1
Benefits of Recent Expansions in Children's
Health Insurance Coverage

Improvements in children's health insurance coverage rates in recent decades have improved a range of outcomes, including children's health, human capital, and future outcomes. In 2021, 95 percent of those under age 19 were covered by health insurance: 61.9 and 36.4 percent by private and public health insurance, respectively (private and public coverage are not mutually exclusive) (Keisler-Starkey and Bunch, 2022). From its inception in 1965, Medicaid has extended eligibility to children incrementally (Gruber and Simon, 2008). The Children's Health Insurance Program (CHIP), enacted in 1997, is operated by the federal government in partnership with state governments to provide health insurance to those under 19 in families with incomes too high to qualify for Medicaid (Medicaid.gov, n.d.-a). Like Medicaid, states have flexibility in designing and implementing CHIP, including setting income eligibility rules. States may elect to allow legally present immigrants, refugees, and asylees who are children to receive CHIP with a waiting period. The program is jointly financed by the federal government and states; the federal government provides an enhanced federal medical assistance percentage. Unlike Medicaid, CHIP is a block grant program requiring reauthorization, putting children's coverage at risk if the funding lapses. CHIP funding was extended in 2018 through fiscal year 2027 (MACPAC, 2018).

As shown in Figure 5-5, the percentage of children without health insurance substantially declined between 2007 and 2021. Overall, the rate of uninsurance dropped, from 11.0 percent in 2007 to 5.0 percent in 2021. Among White, Asian, and Hispanic children, the rate of uninsurance in 2021 was 39–47 percent of the 2007 rates for each group. Among Black children, the rate of uninsurance in 2021 was 35 percent as large as it was in 2007.

Many studies have quantified the benefit of the expansions in public health insurance coverage to children on access to care and health outcomes. For example, Medicaid expansions to children and CHIP have improved access to care, overall health, and parental satisfaction, increased visits to physicians and dentists, and decreased unmet health needs, out-of-pocket expenses, and mortality among children and teenagers (Currie and Gruber, 1996a; Flores et al., 2017; Lykens and Jargowsky, 2002; Paradise, 2014; Park et al., 2020; Wherry and Meyer, 2016); expansions to pregnant people reduced infant mortality and the rate of low-birthweight infants (Currie and Gruber, 1996b; Park et al., 2020).

Public health insurance for children has spillover benefits onto other areas. For example, studies have shown that Medicaid coverage improves children's education outcomes, ranging from test scores to high school graduation and college attendance (Cohodes et al., 2016; Levine and Schanzenbach, 2009; Paradise, 2014; Park et al., 2020). Even as adults, benefits to Medicaid coverage during childhood continued to pay off, with those insured as children more likely to work and less likely to be hospitalized or receive disability insurance (Park et al., 2020). Calculations suggest that the additional revenue of their increased earnings (and thus higher tax payments) is enough to recoup more than half of public expenditures on their childhood Medicaid (Brown et al., 2020; Park et al., 2020).

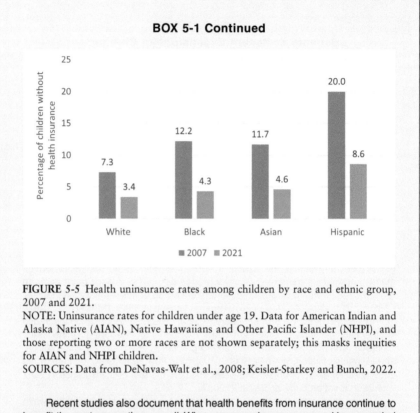

BOX 5-1 Continued

FIGURE 5-5 Health uninsurance rates among children by race and ethnic group, 2007 and 2021.
NOTE: Uninsurance rates for children under age 19. Data for American Indian and Alaska Native (AIAN), Native Hawaiians and Other Pacific Islander (NHPI), and those reporting two or more races are not shown separately; this masks inequities for AIAN and NHPI children.
SOURCES: Data from DeNavas-Walt et al., 2008; Keisler-Starkey and Bunch, 2022.

Recent studies also document that health benefits from insurance continue to benefit the next generation as well. When women who were covered by expanded Medicaid as infants—and thus were born with improved health—go on to have their own children, those children have better birth outcomes than children born to mothers who were not covered by expanded Medicaid coverage (East et al., 2023; Park et al., 2020).

aspects that contribute to inequities and identify how improvements to Medicaid can further advance health equity.

Medicaid Structure

As Medicaid is a federal–state partnership, both governments are jointly responsible for its many aspects, including financing, eligibility, implementation, and delivery. Medicaid is financed based on the federal medical assistance percentage (FMAP) formula (which considers each state's average per capita income relative to the national average) (KFF, n.d.-b).

The FMAP formula favors state investments—the more a state spends, the more it receives in matching federal funds.[13] FMAP ranges from 50.0 percent in several states to 77.3 percent in Mississippi in FY2024 (KFF, n.d.-b). Furthermore, additional federal subsidies incentivize state participation, program requirements, and implementation policies and procedures.[14]

This financing structure also provides states with financial flexibility to tailor programs to align with state budgetary priorities, political preferences, and population health needs. Federal policy offers states substantial flexibility to design and implement their Medicaid programs. States can use waivers, innovation awards, and other program mechanisms to support innovations, provide services to specific populations, and test strategies for improving efficiency and effectiveness (see the Innovation section in this chapter). Many states have leveraged these flexibilities to focus on health equity, but these have also contributed to health inequities, as discussed later.

Medicaid and CHIP coverage in U.S. territories has some similarities and important differences compared to the 50 states and DC. The territories use different eligibility criteria, and Puerto Rico's CHIP program covers additional children who exceed the federal poverty level for Medicaid eligibility (MACPAC, 2021b). Due to differences in economic status and determining eligibility, the five territories vary widely in the proportion of the population enrolled in Medicaid and CHIP, from 68.4 percent in American Samoa to 21.2 percent in Guam (MACPAC, 2021b). Some of the requirement differences in the states and DC compared to the territories create inequities in health care coverage and access to health care for U.S. citizens (those born in the Commonwealth of the Northern Mariana Islands, Guam, Puerto Rico, and U.S. Virgin Islands) and U.S. nationals (those born in American Samoa) residing in the territories. The most high-profile example is that the territories' FMAP has been capped[15] at 55 percent (with occasional increases by Congress), and the territories have been responsible for costs beyond that federal match limit (MACPAC, 2021b). In 2023, the Consolidated Appropriations Act[16] increased the FMAP to 83 percent for American Samoa, the Commonwealth of the Northern Mariana Islands, Guam, and the U.S. Virgin Islands, along with a 5-year extension of the 76 percent FMAP for Puerto Rico (McCoy and Wheatley, 2023).

---

[13] For example, in a state with an FMAP of 50 percent, the federal government contributes one dollar for every dollar spent by the state on Medicaid, or 50 percent of the combined total. In a state with an FMAP of 75 percent, the federal government would contribute three dollars for each state dollar (Provost Peters, 2008).

[14] ACA included an enhanced FMAP rate for the Medicaid expansion population, with 100 percent federal financing from 2014 to 2016 and a decrease to 90 percent by 2020 (Snyder and Rudowitz, 2015).

[15] In accordance with Section 1108 of the Social Security Act.

[16] Pub. L. 117–328, 136 Stat. 4459 (Dec. 29, 2022).

In discussing the contributions of Medicaid to racial and ethnic health inequities, it is important to recognize the context and historical origins of its creation. Medicaid and Medicare were adopted on the same day (July 30, 1965) in the same piece of legislation, yet researchers have attributed fundamental differences in the programs to the influence of racism and compromise tied to federalism (see Chapter 2 for more on federalism) (Katznelson, 2013; Katznelson and Mulroy, 2012; Lieberman, 2001; Pearson, 2019; Skocpol, 1995). In 1935, when President Franklin Roosevelt proposed a universal social security program, Southern White people feared disruption of the racial hierarchy and financial dependence of Southern Black people, resulting in a compromise that excluded domestic workers and agricultural laborers (both groups were predominantly Black) from the Social Security Act.[17] Medicare passed in 1965 as a program fully administered by the federal government, based generally on reaching age 65. However, because of the concurrent civil rights legislation (the Voting Rights Act[18] and Civil Rights Act[19]) and immense changes it brought about, Southern states were generally resistant to federal involvement (Nolen et al., 2020; Pearson, 2019). Therefore, unlike Medicare, Medicaid was determined to be a state-run program, as it limited federal involvement and allowed states to administer health programs for low-income people (Nolen et al., 2020). Medicaid was created on the foundation of public assistance programs, including means and asset eligibility requirements, and a federal–state partnership, which allowed states to opt out entirely and determine many important aspects of eligibility and coverage. Under this shared authority, Southern states were generally slower to participate, but 49 states implemented the program by 1970 (Kaiser Commission on Medicaid and the Uninsured, 2012). Slow uptake by some states of the original program (CHCS, 2019; Paradise et al., 2015) and rejection of Medicaid expansion by Southern states, with disproportionately large racially and ethnically minoritized populations, contributed to inequities since the program's inception and continue today.

Medicaid Eligibility

The federal–state structure of Medicaid contributes to inequities in eligibility because states have substantial discretion to decide who is eligible and the process for enrollment. To be eligible, individuals and families must be either U.S. citizens or qualified noncitizens and meet specific financial and nonfinancial criteria. Federal law requires states to cover specific

---

[17] 42 U.S.C. §301 *et seq.*
[18] Pub. L. 89–110, 79 Stat. 437 (Aug. 6, 1965).
[19] Pub. L. 88–352, 78 Stat. 241 (July 2, 1964).

groups, including low-income families, pregnant people, children, and individuals receiving Supplemental Security Income (SSI) based on a disability determination (Rudowitz et al., 2019). Financial eligibility is determined based on an individual or family's modified adjusted gross income and other assets. Although the process and frequency vary by state, Medicaid agencies generally require applicants to provide proof of their monthly income to qualify and remain enrolled. The monthly income of working individuals and families, especially those with irregular working hours, seasonal employment, and/or multiple jobs, is more likely to fluctuate, resulting in changes in eligibility and gaps in coverage.

States can expand their Medicaid program to include individuals and additional groups based on financial and/or medical need, and income eligibility criteria vary highly by state. Individuals and families living in the states that expanded Medicaid under ACA are eligible if their incomes are 138 percent of the federal poverty level, or $31,781 for families and $18,754 for individuals (KFF, n.d.-c). The 11 states that have declined to expand their Medicaid programs have much lower income-based eligibility criteria. For example, Georgia families (parents in a family of three) are eligible if their income is just 33 percent of the federal poverty level, or $7,600, and childless adults are not eligible at all (CBPP, 2021).

Many eligible individuals and families are not enrolled. Of the approximately 27 million uninsured people in the United States in 2021, 25 percent were eligible for Medicaid (Baicker et al., 2023). In 2020, 60 percent of those uninsured and eligible were adults, nearly two-thirds were racially and ethnically minoritized people, and nearly three out of four were working families (Orgera et al., 2021). Additionally, more than half of uninsured children are eligible for but not enrolled in Medicaid or CHIP (Whitener and Alker, 2020). Participation among eligible children and parents varies highly by state. In 2015, 14 states and DC had child participation rates above 95 percent, 12 states had rates of 85–89 percent, and 2 states were below 85 percent (Kenney et al., 2017). Participation rates among eligible parents were much lower, with only 3 states and DC having more than 90 percent, 19 states having 80–89 percent, and 27 states with less than 79 percent (Kenney et al., 2017). Barriers to enrollment include lack of awareness, uncertainty regarding eligibility, and administrative hurdles in application. Simple and inexpensive efforts, such as mailing reminders about enrollment deadlines, increase enrollment, especially among low-income individuals (Domurat et al., 2021).

Medicaid Enrollment and Administrative Burden

Administrative burden as a barrier to Medicaid and CHIP participation is not a new problem; it has been recognized as an issue for decades

(Camillo, 2021; Flores et al., 2005) and is not unique to Medicaid. In 2021, the Office of Management and Budget found that administrative burden exacerbates inequity, leading to disproportionate underuse and unequal access costs (OMB, 2021). It includes activities such as excessive paperwork and documentation for initial and continued enrollment, frequent "proof of eligibility" requirements, time and method for enrollment (for example, websites with limited enrollment hours, state enrollment agency working hours, language barriers), transportation to enrollment sites, Internet access, face-to-face interviews, and pending decisions and long waits (Flores et al., 2005; Fox et al., 2020). Frequent renewal processes, eligibility checks, and documentation requirements can result in temporary loss of coverage, causing people to be disenrolled and then re-enroll within a short period, or "churn" (loss of coverage can also occur because of income fluctuations, for example, that result in Medicaid ineligibility). In 2018, it was estimated that approximately 10 percent of enrollees experienced churn, defined by a gap in coverage for less than 1 year (Corallo et al., 2021). Churn affects children as well; one study found churn rates increased more than two times following annual renewal and increased the most among Hispanic children (Williams et al., 2022). Furthermore, the burden of collecting proof of income documentation and submitting it to the state generally falls on the applicant/enrollee. Challenges with providing required documentation results in delays in eligibility determinations and terminated coverage. Administrative burden in Medicaid is costly to individuals, including learning costs associated with navigating eligibility and application processes, psychological costs associated with stigma and stress, and compliance costs associated with time and effort required to fill out forms, collect required documents, and complete application and renewal processes (Wikle et al., 2022).

During the COVID-19 public health emergency, states were required to ensure continuous Medicaid enrollment and were compensated with temporarily increased FMAP rates (Tolbert and Ammula, 2023). In December 2022, Congress separated that requirement from the public emergency; as part of the Consolidated Appropriations Act of 2023, continuous enrollment ended on March 31, 2023, potentially leaving a sizable number of former recipients without health care coverage and necessitating alternative insurance options, such as employer-sponsored insurance or marketplace coverage, for those determined to be ineligible for Medicaid or CHIP (ASPE, 2022b; Tolbert and Ammula, 2023). One major impact of this decision is the potential increase in the number of individuals who are no longer with Medicaid or health insurance and the inequitable impact on children, those with limited English proficiency, and people with disabilities, all of whom are more impacted by the administrative burden (ASPE, 2022b; Tolbert and Ammula, 2023). Resuming eligibility determinations places coverage for eligible individuals and families at risk due to administrative challenges that must be met to retain coverage. Although the continuous enrollment policy change was temporary and necessitated by the pandemic, its end has serious implications for health equity. Medicaid enrollment increased by about 20 percent in the first 2 years of the pandemic (Tolbert and Ammula, 2023), largely attributed to that policy. Minoritized populations are disproportionately affected by the pandemic and also at higher risk of losing Medicaid coverage once the continuous enrollment requirement ends.

A range of solutions to address the problem of administrative burden have been tested and evaluated. Reductions in administrative burden are associated with increased Medicaid enrollment (Baicker et al., 2023; Fox et al., 2020). Even small steps, such as outreach, enrollment reminders, and autoenrollment and retention practices, can have significant positive effects (Domurat et al., 2021; McIntyre et al., 2021; Shepard and Wagner, 2022; Wright et al., 2017). Continuous enrollment is associated with better cancer survival rates, increased postpartum care visits, and improved child health outcomes (Brantley and Ku, 2021; Dawes et al., 2014; Desisto et al., 2020). Parent mentors (parents of at least one child covered by Medicaid or CHIP for at least 1 year who underwent additional training about the two programs and application processes) have also been found to be cost-effective and significantly more effective than traditional outreach and enrollment methods in insuring children, achieving faster coverage, and renewing coverage among Black and Latino/a study participants (Flores et al., 2016, 2018). Parental satisfaction was higher and children were less likely to have no primary care provider and unmet medical or dental needs if they had a parent mentor. Children who benefited from the parent mentor program had higher coverage rates 2 years after the intervention ended (Flores et al., 2016, 2018). Box 5-2 describes presumptive eligibility for pregnancy, an example of a policy option that reduces administrative burden. Box 5-3 describes the Medicaid inmate exclusion policy, which contributes to administrative burden for a specific vulnerable population. Both examples highlight flexibility in Medicaid policy implementation.

Finding: Non-expansion Medicaid states have the highest uninsured rates and disproportionately large racially and ethnically minoritized populations compared with states that have expanded Medicaid.

Conclusion 5-1: Medicaid and the Children's Health Insurance Program are the most important federal policies that address the racial and ethnic inequities in access to affordable health care. The Medicaid expansions in eligibility incentivized in the 2010 Affordable Care Act have increased insurance coverage, improved health outcomes, and reduced racial and ethnic health inequities in access to preventive services, delayed care, and unmet health care needs.

BOX 5-2
Presumptive Eligibility for Pregnancy

Medicaid is an important source of health insurance coverage for pregnant people; states have been able to opt in to offer presumptive eligibility since the 1980s. This policy option presumes that a low-income pregnant person seeking medical services is eligible for Medicaid; therefore, a provider can offer necessary prenatal care immediately and be reimbursed, even if the patient is later deemed ineligible. The presumptive eligibility period lasts up to 60 days, while eligibility for full benefits is determined. However, some states do not allow this option, leading to delayed initiation of prenatal care. The Affordable Care Act expanded the policy to allow hospitals to make presumptive eligibility determinations in every state. This policy disproportionately affects Black and other racial and ethnic groups without pre-existing insurance; some states with a large percentage of Black residents have not opted into the policy option (such as Alabama, Louisiana, Maryland, and Mississippi (KFF, n.d.-d)). Presumptive eligibility increases the likelihood that pregnant people will enroll in prenatal care and receive care in the first trimester (Boozang et al., 2020). Early prenatal care can result in better maternal and infant outcomes (NICHD, 2017; Partridge et al., 2012; Taylor et al., 2005). Political will and adverse views of Medicaid expansion can be barriers to policy change. State flexibility and the varied implementation inherent to Medicaid's structure are both barriers and opportunities in changing the presumptive eligibility policy to improve maternal and child health; a federal requirement for presumptive eligibility would also be an opportunity to advance health equity.

SOURCES: Caucci, n.d.; Center for Mississippi Health Policy, 2020; MACPAC, 2023a.

Strong evidence suggests that Medicaid expansion under ACA substantially decreased racial and ethnic health inequities by dramatically increasing insurance coverage and decreasing uninsured rates, improving access to care, preventive care rates, and treatment, and decreasing rates of unmet need across racially and ethnically minoritized groups. Medicaid expansion also decreased inequities in preventable hospitalizations and emergency department visits and improved treatment and outcomes for cancer, diabetes, maternal and child health, and behavioral health (Crocker et al., 2019; Gasoyan et al., 2022; Moriya and Chakravarty, 2023; Solomon, 2021; Steenland and Wherry, 2023).

Despite this evidence, 11 states have declined expansion (South Dakota adopted expansion in 2022, with planned implementation in July 2023). If all of these states expanded coverage to adults with incomes up to 138 percent of the federal poverty level, an estimated 3.8 million additional nonelderly adults would be eligible, increasing eligible Black and Hispanic adults fivefold and sixfold, respectively (Rudich et al., 2022). Box 5-4

BOX 5-3
Medicaid Inmate Exclusion Policy

Medicaid is not permitted to pay for health care services for people who are incarcerated, including adults in jails or prison and youth in state or local juvenile facilities, except for inpatient care outside of a carceral setting (Gates et al., 2014). The policy does not bar being enrolled in Medicaid while incarcerated. State policy on suspended versus terminated Medicaid coverage while incarcerated varies. The majority of states suspend coverage for enrollees in jail (41 states and DC) and prison (42 states and DC), and 23 have automated data exchange processes to aid enrollment suspension and reinstatement (KFF, n.d.-f). Suspension, rather than termination, of Medicaid enrollment makes receiving Medicaid-covered care in inpatient settings while incarcerated easier and allows coverage to be active when the individual is released, which helps improve access to health care providers in the community (Haldar and Guth, 2021).

The incarcerated population is majority racially and ethnically minoritized male adults, particularly Black, Latino, and AIAN men. People involved in the criminal legal system are disproportionately uninsured and low-income, have significant mental and physical health conditions (for example, chronic diseases, such as hepatitis C and diabetes, and mental health disorders and alcohol or substance use disorder), and face challenges such as poverty and housing instability (Camhi et al., 2020; Gates et al., 2014). Therefore, this policy disproportionately affects racially and ethnically minoritized men with complex medical needs and the lack of means to access and pay for care. It also creates barriers to care once released and challenges successful re-entry. Modifying or repealing it would improve coordination and continuity of care. Furthermore, treatment of behavioral health disorders has been associated with reduced recidivism rates (Wallace and Wang, 2020). Removing the policy would also result in states receiving federal funds to help provide health care to incarcerated populations, rather than shouldering the entire costs.

See the section on innovation later in this chapter for more information. States can seek Section 1115 waivers to provide Medicaid coverage before release; pending waivers of the policy vary by state in eligibility criteria, services provided before release, and timing of coverage initiation (Haldar and Guth, 2021). See Chapter 7 for more information on the criminal legal system.

---

describes another way to expand Medicaid coverage for a vulnerable population, postpartum people.

Conclusion 5-2: Among those eligible for Medicaid under the current federal eligibility criteria, racial and ethnic inequities in enrollment and participation remain. While acknowledging the important role of states, the federal government can play a role in addressing these issues, such as by reducing administrative burden and examining the racial and ethnic health equity implications of policies that exclude specific populations, such as immigrants and people involved with the criminal legal system.

BOX 5-4
Medicaid Postpartum Coverage

The postpartum period is essential to the continuum of perinatal care to address pregnancy complications (e.g., preeclampsia, fetal anomalies, gestational diabetes mellitus) and chronic medical comorbidities that may impact overall health during pregnancy, both mentally and physically, over the life course (ACOG, 2018, 2019b). More than half (52 percent) of maternal deaths occur between 1 day and 1 year postpartum, with more than two-thirds of these in the first 6 weeks after delivery (Tikkanen et al., 2020). However, 12 percent of these deaths occur between 6 weeks and 12 months postpartum. Medicaid continuous coverage is central to addressing the rising rate of maternal mortality.

Under current law, people eligible for Medicaid based on their pregnancy become ineligible 60 days after the end of pregnancy. Although some can transition to other coverage after 60 days, many are left vulnerable to being uninsured and with reduced access to postpartum care (Daw et al., 2019; McMorrow and Kenney, 2018).

Coverage disruptions disproportionately affect racially and ethnically minoritized people. Based on data from the Centers for Disease Control and Prevention's Pregnancy Risk Assessment and Monitoring System, about half of non-Hispanic Black and AIAN pregnant people had continuous insurance from prepregnancy to postpartum, while only 20 percent of Spanish-speaking Hispanic pregnant persons had continuous insurance (Daw et al., 2020). Additionally, about one in five of those who became uninsured postpartum had gestational diabetes or pregnancy-related hypertension, more than one-quarter reported postpartum depression, and one-third were recovering from a Cesarean section (McMorrow et al., 2020). These health risks could be diminished if Medicaid coverage was maintained.

The current law, though, makes it difficult for providers to offer the care needed for the full 12-month postpartum period. The 60-day limit increases risk of poor health outcomes, including maternal mortality. These data have led multiple state maternal mortality review committees to recommend extending coverage to 12 months postpartum (including Alabama, Arizona, Georgia, Illinois, Iowa, Louisiana, Maryland, Mississippi, New Mexico, Oklahoma, Tennessee, Texas, Utah, and Washington); they see this as a way to reduce preventable maternal deaths. In 2021, Congress amended Medicaid policy to provide states with the option to increase eligibility to up to 12 months following delivery. As of April 2023, 33 states and DC had done so (KFF, 2023b), including several states that declined ACA expansion.

Innovation in Medicaid

Despite the federal Medicaid program requirements, states have substantial flexibility to develop and tailor their programs and can use several mechanisms to increase coverage and access, improve efficiency, and deliver services, including Medicaid waivers that support Section 1115 demonstration projects and innovation, allowing states to "waive" certain statutory provisions of the federal law, as long as the alternative approach achieves federal objectives and is budget neutral. Waivers require federal approval, often following negotiations between state and federal officials. Through waivers and other innovation mechanisms, Medicaid allows for a range of strategies and tools to specifically address racial and ethnic health inequities; in 2022, 35 states reported Medicaid initiatives to do so (Guth and Artiga, 2022).

Medicaid and SDOH

Federal Medicaid policies generally prohibit using Medicaid funds for nonmedical services. However, 33 states report addressing SDOH through contractual provisions with Medicaid managed care organizations. These requirements aimed at reducing inequities range in focus and include screening for behavioral health and social needs, improving data collection, partnering with community-based organizations, employing community health workers (CHWs), and offering social services referrals (Guth and Artiga, 2022). Another way to leverage managed care organizations to reduce health inequities is to allow them to pay for "in-lieu-of" services; California has used this strategy to address SDOH such as housing, food, and behavioral health needs. Additionally, 12 states include reducing racial and ethnic health inequities as performance metrics in quality incentive programs (Guth and Artiga, 2022).

Moreover, states can use Section 1115 demonstration waivers to experiment with new approaches to reducing racial, ethnic, and tribal health inequities. For example, Massachusetts' 1115 waiver was approved and includes a Hospital Quality and Equity Initiative, which will incentivize data collection, performance-based equity metrics, and programs to improve workforce competence, capacity, and diversity (HHS, 2022b; MassHealth, 2022). Section 1115 waivers can be used to target SDOH and allow states to provide high-need enrollees with health-related social needs services, including housing and nutrition support and linkage to other benefit programs. California received first-in-the-nation approval in 2023 for a Section 1115 demonstration amendment to provide people returning from jails and prisons with certain prerelease services to increase health care coverage, improve care transitions, and maximize successful re-entry into the community by connecting them to Medicaid providers in their communities (CMS, 2023b). Substance use treatment and behavioral health services can be paid for 90 days before release. Soon after California received its waiver, the federal government encouraged additional states to seek waivers to cover substance use treatment for incarcerated people (Han, 2023).

In 2022, a 1332 waiver[20] was approved for Washington State to expand health insurance access for all residents by exempting it from ACA requirements and allowing the state to offer undocumented people access to qualified health plans (Choi, 2022; CMS, 2022c).

Medicaid and Substance Use Disorders

Residential treatment for substance use disorders is not a covered service under Medicaid in 13 states, but states can apply for Section 1115 waivers to permit this service coverage. Thirty-seven states and DC have sought Section 1115 waivers to provide residential substance use treatment in institutions for mental diseases. CMS guidance describes criteria for states to obtain such a waiver. There is variation in execution, as states need to request and receive a Section 1115 waiver to provide access to residential treatment services. The policy impacts a disproportionate proportion of Black and other racial and ethnic groups dependent on Medicaid; some states with a large percentage of Black residents have not applied for the Section 1115 waiver (such as Alabama, Georgia, Mississippi, and South Carolina) (MACPAC, 2023b).

> *Conclusion 5-3: State variation in implementation of the federal Medicaid law, most notably the state variation in the implementation of ACA Medicaid expansions, creates barriers to enrollment and differences in program eligibility and accessibility that have widened the gap in insurance coverage and access to care. The barriers disproportionately affect racially and ethnically minoritized populations, thus contributing to place-based racial and ethnic health inequities. While federal policies can address these barriers by limiting restrictive use of Medicaid flexibilities and effectively incentivize increasing access, these policy changes will require overcoming political and philosophical barriers related to Medicaid, federalism, and the role of government to ensure universal access to health care.*

Summary

This section reviewed how Medicaid has both hindered and advanced racial and ethnic health equity and additional tools states can use. Other aspects of Medicaid policy promote inequities in other areas, such as Medicaid

---

[20] "Section 1332 of the Affordable Care Act (ACA) permits a state to apply for a State Innovation Waiver (also referred to as section 1332 waiver) to pursue innovative strategies for providing residents with access to high quality, affordable health insurance while retaining the basic protections of the ACA" (CMS, n.d.).

BOX 5-5
Medicaid Estate Recovery

Federal law mandates that states pursue the assets from the estates, including the homes, of deceased beneficiaries who used long-term care services funded by Medicaid. These services include nursing facility services, home and community-based services, and hospital and prescription drug services related to care from either source. Under federal law, this recoupment was optional before 1993. Given the low income and wealth requirements needed to qualify for long-term care services under Medicaid, most families affected are lower income. This liquidation of assets adversely affects the intergenerational transfer of wealth disproportionately among historically disadvantaged communities. Families of wealthier beneficiaries have access to estate planning tools that can shield assets from estate recovery. These efforts recoup only a small fraction of Medicaid expenditures and require significant effort and cost (MACPAC, 2021a).

Despite the federal requirement, states are afforded broad latitude in enforcement, with great variability in implementation. A survey identified great variation in the number of estates recovered ranging from 9 in Alaska to 6,005 in Wisconsin for 2020 (MACPAC, 2021a). Although hardship waivers are permissible in principle, they are rarely granted in practice, and criteria vary by state. The report made recommendations to Congress to mitigate the inequitable effects of the rule (MACPAC, 2021a). These included changing the law to make the recovery policy optional to states, as before 1993; limiting the recovery to a value that is consistent with the cost of services used; and setting minimum standards for the implementation of hardship waiver.

States can incorporate mechanisms to limit estate recovery so as to maximize the potential for the transfer of wealth among lower-income populations, such as limiting it to the minimum number of services enumerated under federal law; excluding homes of modest value (as defined by the state); maximizing access to hardship exemptions; limiting asset definition to only those qualifying for probate estate; and identifying cost-effectiveness thresholds and not pursuing recovery below a certain threshold.

estate recovery (see Box 5-5). However, addressing issues such as eligibility and implementation (including administrative burden) can help Medicaid meet its full potential to advance health equity.

HEALTH LITERACY AND LANGUAGE ACCESS

Access to health care is multifaceted, and health literacy and language access are key components of successfully accessing care (IOM, 2004, 2015; NASEM, 2017c, 2020, 2021a, 2023a,b,c).

The health care system is complex and challenging for most to understand. For millions of consumers from diverse racial and ethnic backgrounds, the pervasive lack of forms, descriptions of insurance coverage and benefits, health education materials, and instructions for hospital discharge and prescription medications in plain language, languages in addition to English (and sometime Spanish), and alternative formats are a stark example of how federal policies can perpetuate racial inequities. On one hand, HHS recognizes the importance of health literacy in all health-related communications and has funded and made available vital resources on addressing health literacy and numeracy.[21] For example, HHS includes language access as a major focus of its 2022 department-wide equity action plan (see Box 5-6), and its Office of Disease Prevention and Health Promotion issued a National Action Plan to Improve Health Literacy in 2010 (OASH, 2010). In addition, the CMS Framework for Health Equity 2022–2032 identifies improved language access, health literacy, and culturally appropriate care as a key pillar to improve health equity (CMS, 2022a). CDC has numerous resources on addressing health literacy and numeracy (CDC, 2022c) and its own Action Plan on Health Literacy (CDC, 2022a). AHRQ has developed a Health Literacy Universal Precautions Toolkit that compiles best practices for addressing health literacy (AHRQ, n.d.). The National Academies have also published a significant body of research and numerous recommendations on how to create systems of care and health care organizations that are responsive to health literacy and numeracy (Brach et al., 2012; Hudson and Rikard, 2018; IOM, 2004; Logan et al., 2015; NASEM, n.d.; Simon et al., 2020). Moreover, the HHS OMH National Standards for Culturally and Linguistically Appropriate Services (CLAS) highlight the importance of language access, with 4 of the 15 standards for health care organizations focused on ensuring language access (standards 5–8) to improve quality and advance health equity (HHS, n.d.-e; OMH, 2023):

- "Offer language assistance to individuals who have limited English proficiency and/or other communication needs, at no cost to them, to facilitate timely access to all health care and services.
- Inform all individuals of the availability of language assistance services clearly and in their preferred language, verbally and in writing.
- Ensure the competence of individuals providing language assistance, recognizing that the use of untrained individuals and/or minors as interpreters should be avoided.
- Provide easy-to-understand print and multimedia materials and signage in the languages commonly used by the populations in the service area."

---

[21] "In the context of health literacy, numeracy describes a person's ability to understand clinical and public health data. We use numeracy to make decisions about screening and treatment options" (CDC, 2022d).

BOX 5-6
HHS Equity Action Plan: Language Access

HHS noted in its health equity plan that, although some federal health and human services programs produce substantial translated material, others do not and instead rely primarily on telephonic interpretation. However, the plan notes that all programs struggle with providing material in languages that are less common. HHS has identified several goals in its equity plan to address these needs:

- HHS will focus on addressing barriers that individuals with [limited English proficiency] face in obtaining information, services and/or benefits from HHS federally conducted programs (e.g., the 1-800-MEDICARE number where the services are provided directly by CMS) and federally assisted programs (e.g., Medicaid, where CMS funding allows a beneficiary to receive health care services from a private provider). HHS will address the following items:
  - o Access to in-language content through webpages, listserv announcements, and public outreach material;
  - o Telephonic interpreter services;
  - o Program and benefit information in other languages; and
  - o Federal funding for recipients of HHS funds to provide language access services.

The plan includes medium and long-term indicators to track progress, including the following mid-term (2–4 years):

- Establish how funding for language access services can be distributed in compliance with federal law;
- Establish HHS-wide procedures for providing telephonic interpreter services;
- Establish website accessibility guidance for HHS Staff Divisions and Operating Divisions;
- Establish an action plan for pushing out in-language program and benefit information; and
- Establish goals for funding language access services internally and externally.

SOURCE: Excerpts from HHS, 2022a,c.

OMH has developed free, online trainings on implementing the CLAS standards and commissioned RAND to compile resources for evaluating effective implementation (HHS, n.d.-a; Williams et al., 2018).

The HHS Office for Civil Rights (OCR) is charged with enforcing Title VI of the Civil Rights Act of 1964 and Section 1557 of ACA, requiring meaningful access to federally funded health care programs and services for individuals with limited English proficiency (HHS, 2020, 2023b). However, OCR's enforcement capabilities and effectiveness are limited by its resources, competing enforcement priorities, such as protecting the privacy of personal health information, and lack of accessible complaint processes (HHS, 2013a; Lo, 2011; Office for Civil Rights, 2013; U.S. Commission on Civil Rights, 2019). Increasing OCR staffing and enforcement capabilities, community education about the right to language assistance services, and availability and training of health care interpreters are potential approaches to advancing health equity (Chen et al., 2007). Other changes in federal policies, such as expanding reimbursement for health care interpreters and other language assistance services through Medicare and Medicaid, would also increase language access (Khanijou, 2005; Office of Inspector General, 2010a,b). Furthermore, the Biden Administration has proposed restoring the original regulation implementing the protections against discrimination in ACA Section 1557 under the Obama Administration, rescinding their rollback by the Trump Administration (HHS, 2023b). HHS also has developed a Language Access Plan in compliance with Executive Order 13166[22] *Improving Access to Services for Persons with Limited English Proficiency*, which applies the language access requirements of Title VI of the 1964 Civil Rights Act to the federal government itself (HHS, 2013b). However, the plan has not been updated since 2013 and therefore does not address the continued and growing use of technology in health care—including electronic patient portals to access health information and telehealth and other trends that impact language access; HHS released an annual progress report on language access in 2023 and acknowledged that the 2013 plan needs to be updated (HHS, 2023a; HHS OCR, 2023).

Although HHS clearly recognizes the importance of addressing health literacy and numeracy and ensuring language access, these action plans and standards are not legally binding or enforceable. For example, federal contracts do not require contractors to comply with the National CLAS Standards, or address health literacy and numeracy if there are direct communications with patients, health care consumers, or members of the public. With no requirements, monitoring, or enforcement of these "best practices" for effective communication with racially and ethnically diverse people, inequities will be perpetuated because vital information will simply not be available or understandable. The literature is extensive on how applying the standards discussed in this section and health literacy interventions and ensuring language access can advance health literacy and therefore improve both access to health care and health outcomes (Berkman et al., 2011; Diamond et al., 2019; Flores, 2005; Flores et al., 2003, 2012; IOM, 2004; Karliner et al., 2007; Miller, 2016; Sheridan et al., 2011).

In 2016, HHS OMH published a compendium on CLAS in health and health care; although it provided a state-by-state review of standards,

---

[22] Exec. Order No. 13166, 65 FR 50121 (August 2000).

planning, policies, and collaboration on CLAS, it found U.S. territories "did not have information online about their National CLAS Standards implementation activities at the time this research was conducted" (OMH, 2016, p. 1).

HEALTH EQUITY IN VALUE-BASED CARE
AND QUALITY PROGRAMS

Access to health care alone will not advance health equity—quality of care is essential. Although efforts to improve quality have increased, racial and ethnic inequities remain. For example, AHRQ Annual Quality and Disparities Reports show that although quality has improved for the general population, racial and ethnic inequities have decreased only minimally in those same measures (AHRQ, 2022).

In the last several years, federal health care financing policies have shifted from paying for quantity, through a fee-for-service model, to paying for quality, primarily through alternative payment models, including value-based payment. ACA included several provisions that advance value-based payment. Congress passed the bipartisan Medicare Access and CHIP Reauthorization Act[23] in 2015, which introduced a complete overhaul of how CMS pays physicians through Medicare and created the Quality Payment Program. It includes two tracks: (1) the Merit-Based Incentive Payment System, which adjusts payment based on quality, cost, interoperability, and improvement activities; and (2) Advanced Alternative Payment Models, which include several accountable care organization (ACO)-style programs involving shared risk. CMS has encouraged value-based payment in state Medicaid programs, primarily through demonstration programs (Section 1115 waivers) and alternative payment methodologies, with high levels of variation in adoption and implementation by state (CMS, 2020). CMS has also implemented alternative payment models that hold providers accountable for both quality and cost (Liao et al., 2020). This shift to value-based payment is occurring across all aspects of the health care system, including private and public programs, and has gained traction as a response to rising costs.

In general, CMS alternative payment model programs reflect two types: population-based payment models that target specific populations (e.g., ACOs, Medicare Shared Savings Program, Comprehensive Care Model) and episode-based payment models (Acute Care Episode, Bundled Payments for Care Improvement Initiative, Comprehensive Care for Joint Replacement). These models have demonstrated some spending reductions, without impacting quality (Liao et al., 2020). However, unintended consequences

---

[23]Pub. L. 114–10, 129 Stat. 87 (Apr. 16, 2015).

on health inequities have been raised (Werner, 2005; Werner et al., 2005), including the following:

- Population-based payment models dissuade providers from joining to avoid higher risk and/or costly patients (Yasaitis et al., 2016).
- Population-based payment models encourage providers to have a patient pool that is at lower risk or less costly (Lee et al., 2020).
- Episodic payment models, such as bundled payments for lower extremity joint replacement, may have differential receipt by racial and ethnic groups due to providers avoiding financial penalties of caring for complex patients (Kim et al., 2021).
- Geographic variation may occur for participating providers, which may be correlated to those areas deemed as medically underserved.
- Value-based payment models that do not adjust for social risk may exacerbate health disparities by penalizing providers who care for a higher fraction of these patients.

For example, Liao and colleagues (2021) suggests that areas with higher rates of chronic health conditions and socioeconomic deprivation were less likely to have access to providers in episodic payment models. In addition, CMS uses value-based reimbursements to reward or penalize hospitals for key performance measures, such as readmissions. These performance measures, however, do not account for SDOH. For example, the Hospital Care Compare, helps rate U.S. hospitals on care quality (CMS, 2023c). Fahrenbach and colleagues (2020) found that hospitals with a poorer rating were more likely to be in neighborhoods with a higher level of social risk.

Considerable discussion and experimentation have addressed whether, and how to, make adjustments in value-based payment arrangements for the varying social risks experienced by diverse patients that negatively impact health (Alberti et al., 2020; ASPE, 2021b; Jaffery and Gelb Safran, 2021; NASEM, 2016; NQF, 2014). Most current health care payment arrangements do adjust based on *clinical risk factors*, usually by age (for example, higher use and costs among older patients) and by some measure of the number, severity, and complexity of diagnosed diseases and conditions (for example, the hierarchical condition category coding) (Watson, 2018). The Assistant Secretary for Planning and Evaluation has listed poverty, race and ethnicity, social isolation, and limited community resources as among the *social risks* that impact health (ASPE, 2021a). The National Academies has defined social risks as including socioeconomic position; race, ethnicity, and cultural context; gender; social relationships; and residential and community context (NASEM, 2016). As noted, value-based payment models generally do not account for social risk and its contribution to exacerbating racial and ethnic inequities. Not accounting for social risk results in adverse consequences, such as underpaying providers who care for a disproportionately higher number of complex and socially at-risk patients and disincentivizing health insurance companies and payers from paying for services for the sickest of the sick (i.e., cherry-picking) (NASEM, 2017a). Accounting for social risk factors in value-based payment can help reduce health inequities by aligning incentives to improve quality, improve accuracy of reporting and monitoring health care and quality inequities, and adequately compensate providers with a higher number of complex patients.

Given the adverse consequences in the current value-based payment models, efforts to include social risk factors are warranted to reduce racial and ethnic inequities more effectively. Jaffery and Gelb Safran (2021) recommend two approaches. One includes up-front, additional payments based on social risk much like CMS reimburses hospital and Medicare Advantage plans based on diagnosis and severity of illness (Jaffery and Gelb Safran, 2021). The Health Care Payment Learning and Action Network Health Equity Advisory Team also recommends up-front payments and adjustments for social risk to advance equity in value-based payments (HCPLAN, 2021, 2022, n.d.); this includes up-front infrastructure payments to support the participation of providers who have served a higher number of patients with increased social risks and generally have less capacity and experience with value-based payment (HCPLAN, 2022). The second includes incentives for improvements that incorporate social risk in a way that drives overall improvement but with added incentives for improvements in groups with higher social risks (an approach with demonstrated success) (Jaffery and Gelb Safran, 2021). The National Quality Forum recommends adjustments for social risks in quality measurement when there is a conceptual or methodological basis for doing so, such as qualitative or empirical evidence documenting the impact of social risk factors on care delivery, health outcomes, or costs (NQF, n.d.). Most recently and based on the findings from a National Academies (2017a) report, CMS proposes[24] to incorporate social risk factors through the "health equity index reward" as part of its 2027 STARS Ratings. The objective is to incentivize Medicare Advantage plans to provide high-quality care to populations with specific social risk factors (CMS, 2022b).

Awareness is increasing that optimal health is not solely the result of health insurance or use of health care services. Similar to Medicaid innovations related to SDOH described earlier in this chapter, incremental efforts

---

[24] Medicare program; contract year 2024 policy and technical changes to the Medicare Advantage program, Medicare Prescription Drug Benefit program, Medicare cost plan program, Medicare Parts A, B, C, and D overpayment provisions of the Affordable Care Act and programs of all-inclusive care for the elderly; health information technology standards and implementation specifications, 87 FR 79452 (December 2022).

to address SDOH in some Medicare alternative payment models are also underway. HHS has highlighted the importance of addressing the SDOH and more proximate health-related social needs, such as housing insecurity and food insecurity. For example, CMS developed a tool and required screening for these needs in its Accountable Health Communities innovation model, based on work by the National Academies (ASPE, 2021b; CMMI, n.d.; CMS, 2023a; NASEM, 2016). More recently, CMS' ACO Realizing Equity, Access, and Community Health model requires collecting health-related social needs and demographic data and payment adjustments for ACOs serving Medicare beneficiaries who have historically been underserved (CMS. gov, 2023a; Corner et al., 2023). Other ACO models also have incorporated addressing health-related social needs in their design and implementation (Fraze et al., 2016). As described, CMS has issued guidance for states to use Medicaid and CHIP funding to address health-related social needs, and states are increasingly incorporating strategies to do so in their Medicaid programs (CMS, 2021b; Guth, 2022). CMS also has issued specific guidance for Medicare Advantage health plans to address food insecurity and transportation as part of the Health Equity Incubation Program in the Medicare Advantage Value-Based Insurance Design model for calendar year 2023 (CMS.gov, 2023b). More recently, CMS has begun requiring screening for health-related social needs by hospitals as part of the Inpatient Prospective Payment System and encouraging such screening by physicians as part of the Medicare Merit-Based Incentive Payment Program.[25]

Conclusion 5-4: Value-based payment and other programs intended to improve quality have, to date, not prioritized health equity. For example, such programs do not measure and incentivize reduction of racial and ethnic health inequities.

REPRESENTATION AND INCLUSION IN HEALTH CARE

As discussed earlier in this chapter, access to quality care requires more than insurance. Care needs to be appropriate—for example, representation matters in clinical trials. Care needs to be unbiased and culturally responsive and include a workforce that represents a diverse population. Critically, community voice and expertise are needed to inform federal policies

---

[25] Medicare program; hospital inpatient prospective payment systems for acute care hospitals and the long-term care hospital prospective payment system and policy changes and fiscal year 2023 rates; quality programs and Medicare Promoting Interoperability Program requirements for eligible hospitals and critical access hospitals; costs incurred for qualified and non-qualified deferred compensation plans; and changes to hospital and critical access hospital conditions of participation, 87 FR 48780 (August 2022).

to ensure that care is accessible and tailored to the needs of racially and ethnically minoritized populations.

Clinical Trial Inclusion

Health care innovation is largely driven by the development of new medical treatments and devices. Clinical trials and FDA approval of medical treatments and devices are the pathways through which these advances are made available to the public. Although racially and ethnically minoritized people comprise approximately 40 percent of the U.S. population, over the past 25 years, they have accounted for only around 4 percent of trial participants (Ma et al., 2021). Additionally, about 8 percent of the U.S. population has limited English proficiency (Census Bureau, 2020). A 1996 survey of researchers with publications on provider–patient communication found that three-quarters excluded study participants with limited English proficiency (Frayne et al., 1996). A 2021 systematic analysis of clinical trials identified from ClinicalTrials.gov found that approximately 29 percent of federally funded clinical trials excluded such participants and only about 5 percent identified specific accommodations for other languages (Muthukumar et al., 2021). It is important to include diverse populations in clinical trials, as many diseases under study disproportionately affect minoritized communities, and it is well documented that a large proportion of therapeutics affect participants of different racial and ethnic backgrounds differently (Ramamoorthy et al., 2015); a diverse study population also broadens study generalizability (for a detailed overview, see NASEM, 2022).

NIH and FDA have sponsored several directives and guidelines aimed at improving inclusion and representation of minoritized populations and women in clinical trials, including the NIH Revitalization Act of 1993[26] (NASEM, 2022; OASH, 2020). FDA also requires reporting of data on race, age, and gender in clinical trials. Despite these efforts, inclusion of minoritized populations remains largely unimproved (Kozlov, 2023; Ma et al., 2021; NASEM, 2022). That NIH-sponsored trials have a far higher inclusion rate compared to non-NIH-sponsored trials (about 11 percent and 3 percent, respectively, in one study) offers insight that, although the rate is still unacceptably low, targeted approaches can help (Ma et al., 2021).

In 2022, HHS and FDA published new industry guidance for enrolling underrepresented racial and ethnic groups in clinical trials (FDA, 2022; Kozlov, 2023). These guidelines support creating a Racial and Ethnicity Diversity Plan that includes developing clinical trials with an appreciation of the populations most affected by a disease, goal setting to include racial and ethnic minorities, and plans of action to enroll and retain these populations.

---

[26] Pub. L. 103–43, 107 Stat. 122 (June 10, 1993).

Recommended strategies for enrollment and retention include improving access, community engagement, and reducing barriers to participation (for example, considering the lived realities of participants in the research design and not excluding people with limited English proficiency and providing language assistance for them).

This guidance also outlines recommendations for improved data collection for subsets of minority populations to include race, ethnicity, sex, gender identity, age, and pregnancy and lactation status. Greater diversity in clinical trials is possible; for example, SARS-CoV-2 vaccine trials were completed under time pressure but were more diverse than other clinical trials have been (although racially and ethnically minoritized communities were still underrepresented) (Artiga et al., 2021; Khalil et al., 2022). The National Academies also released a report with 17 recommendations on how to improve representation (NASEM, 2022); implementing these would advance this area. See Box 5-9 at the end of the chapter for a selection of relevant recommendations from that report.

The new FDA guidance is a welcome step forward in promoting fair representation of racially and ethnically minoritized populations in clinical trials. However, these recommendations are nonbinding and will not ensure improvements in trial inclusion. HHS and FDA will need to closely monitor progress on this and report regularly and investigate the inclusion of required elements in future iterations to include both process measures (e.g., investment in barrier reduction) and outcome measure (i.e., proportion of trial participants from racial/ethnic minorities).

Including racially and ethnically minoritized populations, including people with limited English proficiency, is key to understanding the differential effectiveness and toxicity of preventive or therapeutic interventions and expanding study generalizability. Inclusion rates are woefully inadequate, which perpetuates racial inequities. Federal agencies will need to continue efforts to improve clinical trial participation in racially and ethnically minoritized populations and develop concrete steps to ensure improvement in inclusion rates.

In addition to improving clinical trial inclusion, it is incumbent on the NIH, "the largest public funder of biomedical and behavioral research in the world" (NIH, n.d.), to address structural inequality and racism within its policies and programs and reflect on how that affects whose and what kind of research is funded, for which disparities exist. For example, diseases that primarily affect men received more NIH funding than those that affect mainly women (Mirin, 2021; Pierson, 2021), and White researchers are more likely to be funded than Black researchers (Ginther et al., 2011; Hoppe et al., 2019; Pierson, 2021; Taffe and Gilpin, 2021). In 2021, NIH acknowledged "structural racism has significantly disadvantaged the lives of many people of color across our society, including those who conduct or support the science funded by NIH" (Collins et al., 2021, p. 3075). Its new framework for beginning to address this issue "includes understanding barriers; developing robust health disparities/equity research; improving its internal culture; being transparent and accountable; and changing the extramural ecosystem so that diversity, equity, and inclusion are reflected in funded research and the biomedical workforce" (Collins et al., 2021, p. 3075). As part of this plan, NIH announced $60 million for projects focused on reducing health disparities and inequalities and up to $30 million for studying the effect of structural racism and discrimination on health and health disparities (Collins et al., 2021).

Community Voice

Due to the substantial federal investment in health care and the ubiquitous nature of federal policy making related to health care, health care policy is of particular interest to many powerful industries, including pharmaceuticals, insurance, hospitals, and care professionals. These industries are represented by organizations with strong relationships and resources, which are used to inform and influence federal policy making. Large interest groups (for example, Pharmaceutical Research and Manufacturers of America, America's Health Insurance Plans, and AARP) are equipped to participate in all aspects of federal policy making, including the public comment process, the judicial process, and lobbying. Patients and communities, by contrast, are often unheard and unrepresented, resulting in a power imbalance between the industries and those being cared for.

This power imbalance trickles down to state, local, organizational, and individual health care decisions. Increasingly, federal efforts to level the playing field are underway. For example, federal agencies are undertaking listening sessions, roundtables, and other methods to hear from communities and community-based organizations. Patient-reported data are included in value-based payment programs and made publicly available as hospital and physician quality ratings. Federally qualified health centers are required to have patient advisory boards/patient governing boards/patient representation to guide organizational policies and practices. The Patient Centered Outcomes Research Institute, with substantial funding from the federal government, is developing, testing, and implementing patient-centered research and clinical practices. Efforts to include meaningful community involvement and community voice in health research and federal health policy making, such as Medicaid, are promising and could be strengthened by increased investment and standardization across all federal policy-making activities, as called for in Executive Order 13985 (Adkins-Jackson et al., 2022; Etchegary et al., 2022; Goold et al., 2018, 2019; Manafò et al., 2018; Myers et al., 2020; NAM, 2022; Race Forward and PolicyLink, 2023).

Implicit Bias and Racism

As described, race and ethnicity are predictors of the quality of health care received, in part because of health care professionals' and systems' biases (IOM, 2003). Racism in health care operates at the individual (in the form of implicit and explicit bias and internalized racism), interpersonal, institutional, and structural levels (AMA, 2021; Jones, 2000). At the individual level, health care workers are not immune to biases and prejudices that contribute to disparities (IOM, 2003). In studies, implicit biases have been reported by race, ethnicity, age, gender, and body mass index, among other characteristics (Chapman et al., 2013; Coyte et al., 1996; Green et al., 2007; Hawker et al., 2000; Schwartz et al., 2003; Wright et al., 1995). Such biases are associated with worse health outcomes, likely due to a combination of factors, such as impaired patient–clinician relationship, lack of trust, poor communication, and racism (Feagin and Bennefield, 2014; IOM, 2003; Van Ryn et al., 2011). For example, Black patients are more likely to die after being diagnosed with breast or endometrial cancer and are less likely to receive prostate cancer treatments like chemotherapy and radiation therapy (IOM, 2003; The Joint Commission, 2016). Racially and ethnically minoritized patients are less likely to be prescribed pain medicines and more likely to be blamed for being passive about their health care and receive fewer cardiovascular interventions and renal transplants (The Joint Commission, 2016). As individuals, developing awareness of one's implicit biases; developing skills in partnership, empathy, and trust-building; undertaking bystander trainings; and modifying written and oral communication to eliminate derisive terminology are key to mitigating individual-level impacts of implicit and explicit biases (The Joint Commission, 2016; Sabin, 2022).

However, individual-level solutions cannot mitigate what is fundamentally a structural problem (Gee and Ford, 2011; Smedley, 2012). At the larger levels, racism has been institutionalized in medicine. Although race is a social construct,[27] it was manufactured within medicine and science as a proxy for genetic ancestry and hierarchy and used to explain relative differences in form and function (Menand, 2001; Smedley and Smedley, 2005; Wallis, 1995). This has been used to legitimize preferential treatment of White patients and has been institutionalized in medical practice in the form of inclusion into clinical algorithms (Chokshi et al., 2022; Tong and Artiga, 2021; Vyas et al., 2020). This is problematic for two reasons. First, it incorrectly attributes race as a biologically relevant variable rather than

---

[27] Genetic ancestry affects human health; however, this is distinct from the impact of race, which is a social construct that has its foundations in systemic racism.

accounting for the social and structural determinants of health; racism is a risk factor (Chokshi et al., 2022). For example, race was previously part of the clinical calculator for success rate for a vaginal birth after a previous Cesarean delivery (Vyas et al., 2019). However, there is no genetic basis for such differences. Rather, given that calculators are often based on cohort data, disparate results when race is changed in the calculator simply illustrate racial disparities in health outcomes in the study population upon which the algorithm was developed. In this case, this trend is likely due to the higher rate of primary Cesarean delivery for Black patients, decreased access to obstetrical care, implicit and explicit bias on the part of health care workers, differences in diet, and other differences that may impact fetal growth and pregnancy health. Thus, genetic, epigenetic, and physiologic differences in individuals are conflated with social and structural factors that impact care.

Second, including race in clinical calculators only perpetuates and exacerbates ongoing disparities in health care access and outcomes. For example, using race in the calculator described above leads to a lower predicted likelihood of success for a Black patient with the same clinical characteristics as a White patient. A clinician may alter their practice based on this prediction (ACOG, 2021; Vyas et al., 2019). Recognizing that including race reinforced inequities rather than supporting patient-centered care, the original investigators developed a new calculator for trial of labor after Cesarean without the variables of race and ethnicity, which has been recommended by the American College of Obstetricians and Gynecologists for use rather than the prior version (ACOG, 2021; Vyas et al., 2019). A positive step in redressing racially biased algorithms is the recent recommendation by the American Society of Nephrology and the National Kidney Foundation to use race-free equations in estimating kidney function, and the decision by the Organ Procurement and Transplantation Network to modify kidney transplant wait time for Black patients who have been delayed in receiving a transplant (Mohottige et al., 2023).

Addressing implicit bias and racism requires system-wide reforms, and the federal government plays an important role in eliminating harmful policies, practices, and programs and supporting wide-scale implementation of equitable solutions. For example, it could require that health systems receiving federal funding report outcomes stratified by race and ethnicity (which it already does for some programs). It could also expand the use of patient-reported outcomes to include experiences of bias, discrimination, and/or mistreatment. However, given the opportunities to misuse these data, it is critical that federal policies account for unintended consequences that could exacerbate existing inequities (see Chapter 2 for more information on data challenges and opportunities). Furthermore, identification of inequities is only the first step; it needs to be followed by action to make progress.

Workforce

Health care outcomes are dependent not only on *what* care is delivered but *where* it is delivered and *who* is delivering it. Compounding the severe nursing shortage (NASEM, 2021b) is a significant shortage of physicians and other professionals. By 2034, a shortage of almost 38,000–124,000 physicians is estimated (AAMC, 2021). In one study, half of women in rural areas had to drive more than 30 minutes to reach an obstetrician-gynecologist (ACOG, 2019c). Health professional shortage areas are designated by HRSA as geographic areas or populations with shortages in professionals in primary care, mental health, or dental care; in 2023, approximately 100 million people lived in primary care health professional shortage areas (HRSA, n.d.). In one study in Philadelphia, census tracts with a high proportion of Black Americans were 28 times more likely to be a low-access area than those with a low proportion of Black Americans (Brown et al., 2016). In another study, states with residents who had higher aggregate racial bias against Black Americans had fewer federally qualified community health centers serving health professional shortage areas (Snowden and Michaels, 2023).

The United States also lacks a diverse and inclusive health care workforce. In 2018, most active physicians were White and male (AAMC, n.d.-a); less than 12 percent were Hispanic (5.8 percent) or Black (5.0 percent), and the percentage of Black male physicians in particular remains small (AAMC, n.d.-b; NASEM, 2018a; Poll-Hunter et al., 2023). AIAN and NHPI people are also underrepresented in medicine relative to their proportion of the overall population (Morris et al., 2021). The consistently low proportion of Black physicians is related to systemic barriers and SDOH, as discussed in other chapters, and to the consequences of the Flexner Report (NASEM, 2018a; Poll-Hunter et al., 2023). Released in 1910, the Flexner Report changed the medical education system in the United States; it also resulted in permanently closing five of the seven operating Black medical colleges in 1914. Howard University in DC and Meharry Medical College in Nashville, Tennessee, survived (and only two more have opened since) (Dent et al., 2021; Harley, 2006). A 2020 modeling study estimated that, had these five schools not been closed, they could have hypothetically trained an additional 27,000–35,000 total graduates by 2019 (Campbell et al., 2020). Furthermore, over the last 10 years, more Black physicians have graduated from the 4 historically Black medical schools than from a combination of the top 10 predominantly White medical schools (Montgomery Rice, 2021). The diversity of the pediatric workforce has also not kept pace with the ongoing demographic shift in the racial and ethnic composition of U.S. children. By 2060, about two-thirds of children under age 18 are projected to be a race other than non-Hispanic White (Jones et al., 2021; Saenz and Poston, 2020; Vespa et al., 2020). However, less than 20 percent of certified general pediatricians, pediatric subspecialists, and pediatric trainees are AIAN, NHPI, Black, or Hispanic or Latino/a (The American Board of Pediatrics, 2023). Cultural congruency between patient and health care professional has been shown to improve patient satisfaction and affect outcomes such as improved access to care and reduced maternal and infant mortality (Diamond et al., 2019; Jones et al., 2017; Ku and Vichare, 2023). Thus, investing in and cultivating a workforce that reflects patients' and communities' lived experiences and languages help to build trust, improve access to and quality of care, and advance health equity. For example, a diverse nursing workforce is associated with a reduced risk of severe adverse outcomes, like eclampsia and blood transfusion, during delivery (Guglielminotti et al., 2022).

Additionally, doulas are an evidence-based and cost-effective way to improve birth support and mitigate some racial and ethnic health inequities in maternal morbidity and mortality. Doula care is increasingly recommended to support high-risk racially and ethnically minoritized people during labor (ACOG, 2019a). Doulas are nonclinical support paraprofessionals who provide physical, informational, and emotional support to people before, during, and just after labor (Gruber et al., 2013); such personnel provide continuous one-to-one emotional support (ACOG, 2019a). Their presence is associated with shortened labor, fewer reports of dissatisfaction with the labor experience, and fewer Cesarean and preterm births and low-birthweight babies (Bohren et al., 2017; Boozang et al., 2020; Kennell et al., 1991). It is posited that doulas may mitigate the effects of racism and other SDOH in underserved populations (Hardeman and Kozhimannil, 2016; Wint et al., 2019). They have been used to help initiate breastfeeding among Medicaid beneficiaries in Minnesota: about 98 percent of those with doulas did so compared to about 81 percent of the general population (Kozhimannil et al., 2013).

As with other positions in the health care workforce, the cost associated with training, certification, and registration across states limits the doula workforce and therefore its diversity and patient access to doula care during pregnancy, highlighting the need to improve doula recruitment, payment, and career advancement (Kozhimannil et al., 2015; Van Eijk et al., 2022a,b). Additionally, no national certification standard exists, and reimbursement and funding remain a challenge. However, states can cover doula care through Medicaid; as of 2023, at least 17 states have or are planning to do so (Guarnizo, 2022). Reimbursement and requirements vary by state. For example, Minnesota allows for certified doula care if the doula is supervised by a physician, nurse practitioner, or certified midwife. In 2022, the payment rate was $47 per pre- and postpartum visits (up to six visits) with assistance at the birth billable for $488. Oregon provides reimbursement for two prenatal and two postpartum visits and labor and delivery coverage up to $350 for state-registered doulas (Platt and Kaye, 2020). New Jersey also started using Medicaid funding for doula care, reimbursing up to eight visits and $900 per birth (Robles-Fradet, 2021). Indiana and Nebraska use federal block grant funds for doula care (Platt and Kaye, 2020).

Like doulas, CHWs and patient navigators (PNs) have long been deployed to reach patients, build trust, and address health disparities in underserved areas. CHWs and PNs are able to connect with patients through shared culture and language, similar life experiences, and an understanding of their community members' barriers to health care access. They can identify SDOH issues, suggest referrals to resources, and help patients develop a better understanding of their needs, where to access services, and how to advocate for their health care needs. They have been associated with improved access to health care services, communication with providers, and adherence to health recommendations for racially and ethnically minoritized people (Allgood et al., 2018; Feinglass et al., 2019; Gilmore and McAuliffe, 2013; Simon et al., 2015, 2019). Additionally, several published randomized controlled trials document that parent mentors are highly effective in improving insurance coverage, asthma outcomes, care access and quality, and patient satisfaction, while reducing or eliminating insurance disparities, saving money, and creating jobs in minoritized communities (Flores et al., 2009, 2016, 2018). The *Unequal Treatment* report (IOM, 2003) also recommended supporting the use of CHWs, and in response to the COVID-19 pandemic, several states reported plans to add CHWs as a Medicaid-covered service and/or a Medicaid provider type or integrate them into care coordination improvement work (Gifford et al., 2021).

Taken together, the roles of doulas, CHWs, PNs, and parent mentors in support of racially and ethnically minoritized patients are meaningful to mitigating disparities that stem from factors such as lack of support, racism, discrimination, and socioeconomic factors (e.g., poverty). Thus, research is needed that examines policies that promote scaling and extending the benefits that doulas, CHWs, and PNs confer to these patients.

> *Conclusion 5-5: A lack of inclusion and representation in clinical research may perpetuate health inequities because it limits the ability to identify issues of safety or effectiveness that might be specific to the populations that are not well represented. A lack of inclusion and representation in the health care workforce may perpetuate health inequities, given the evidence that suggests better health outcomes when there is identity concordance between patients and providers.*

HEALTH CARE ACCESS, QUALITY, AND INCLUSION FOR SPECIFIC POPULATIONS

Federal policies uniquely contribute to health and health care inequities, but as noted throughout this report, not all populations are impacted in the same way. For example, the health care system looks very different for AIAN people than it does for the population as a whole due to the unique treaty relationship. The immigrant population and people living in U.S. territories have unique barriers to access, and some populations have specific needs along their life course, such as maternal health, where racial and ethnic inequities are striking. The following sections describe these populations, inequities, and the role of federal policy.

American Indian and Alaska Native Health

It is necessary here to restate that the long-standing history of detrimental federal Indian-related policies has played an important role in the health inequities seen today in AIAN populations (see Chapter 2 for an overview of that history and how it permeates all parts of AIAN life; see Chapter 7 for a review of federal policies that have led to generational trauma). By just about any measure of health, AIAN people are worse off than other racial and ethnic groups; this includes life expectancy, suicide, homicide, and chronic diseases resulting in earlier and increased functional disability and death (see Box 5-7 for these and other health outcomes) (IHS, 2014). As explained throughout this report, the structures, funding, oversight, and data are inadequate to ensure adequate SDOH (i.e., shelter, safety, water, food, education, transportation) to reverse these poor outcomes. This section provides evidence that this is also true for access to quality health care.

As described in Chapter 2, Tribal Nations have a legal relationship with the federal government that originated in the 1700s and has shaped the conditions that affect their health. The government is obligated to protect tribal lands, assets, and resources, as well as treaty rights and health care, among other responsibilities required by the federal trust relationship (NASEM, 2017b). Yet, the United States severed the government-to-government relationship during the Termination Era[28] (see Chapter 2 for more information) and more than 100 tribes lost federal recognition, affecting who were considered Indians in the eyes of Congress and the federal government. For example, they could no longer access IHS hospitals for care, nor could their descendants. No other U.S. population can have its racial or ethnic status legislated, highlighting the unique status of AIAN people. These events

---

[28]This period ended the federal government's recognition of sovereignty of tribes, trusteeship over Indian reservations, and the exclusion of state law's applicability to Native persons.

BOX 5-7
2014 Report: Comparison of 2007–2009 American Indian or
Alaska Native Death Rates to 2008 U.S. All Races Death Rates

- Alcohol related—520 percent greater;
- Tuberculosis—450 percent greater;
- Chronic liver disease and cirrhosis—368 percent greater
- Motor vehicle crashes—207 percent greater;
- Diabetes mellitus—177 percent greater;
- Unintentional injuries—141 percent greater;
- Poisoning—118 percent greater;
- Homicide—86 percent greater;
- Suicide—60 percent greater;
- Pneumonia and influenza—37 percent greater; and
- Firearm injury—16 percent greater.

NOTE: More recent data are not available because HHS has not released updated data since the 2014 *Trends in Indian Health* report.
SOURCE: Excerpt from IHS, 2014.

---

constitute a unique source of trauma—the almost complete invisibility of both this history and present circumstances outside of Indian Country. Therefore, it is important that health care providers know whether their patients are members of federally recognized tribes and about their ability to use IHS for care. It can affect referrals and resources available. This and other issues related to access to care for AIAN people are discussed below.

The Indian Health System

The Indian health system is composed of three parts: IHS, tribal health services, and urban Indian health programs (see Box 5-8 regarding the founding and structure of IHS). The population(s) served are members of the 574 federally recognized tribes found in 37 states with a patient population of 2.56 million AIAN (2015–2020 data) (IHS, 2020).

Great strides were made through IHS largely coinciding with progress made in health care nationally, such as the development and availability of antibiotics and improved nutrition. However, the health status of the AIAN population still lags on many indicators compared to all other U.S. racial groups. The official report on IHS is *Trends in Indian Health*, but it has not been updated since 2014. Data for the AIAN population are lagging, misreported and undercounted, and characterized by myriad other difficulties (see Chapter 2 for more on data barriers).

BOX 5-8
History of Indian Health Service (IHS)

Unlike other racially and ethnically minoritized groups in the United States, American Indian/Alaska Native (AIAN) people have legal rights to federal health care services. That federal responsibility was codified in the Snyder Act of 1921[1] and the Indian Health Care Improvement Act (IHCIA) of 1976,[2] which form the legislative authority for the federal agency known today as IHS (U.S. Commission on Civil Rights, 2004). The Snyder Act authorized funding for health care services to federally recognized tribes, and the IHCIA defined the structure for service delivery and authorized constructing and maintaining health care and sanitation facilities on reservations (U.S. Commission on Civil Rights, 2004). Although these pieces of legislation marked significant progress, the Snyder Act has been criticized for its broad and vague language, which does not facilitate long-term planning or provide resources based on need. This is considered to have influenced the piecemeal approach that has shaped the funding and distribution of health care resources (IOM, 2003).

IHS is the federal agency responsible for fulfilling the trust obligation to provide health services to AIAN people. When the federal responsibility for health care services was transferred from the Department of the Interior to the Department of Health, Education, and Welfare in 1955, IHS was established under the Public Health Service. This transfer resulted in doubling appropriations for IHS. Currently, IHS operates within the HHS, consists of a network of hospitals, clinics, field stations, and other programs, and is divided into three major branches: the federally operated direct health care services (IHS), tribally operated health care services (tribal health services), and Urban Indian Health Programs. Those who are eligible can receive services at any IHS facility; however, complex rules restrict contract medical care that is not available in IHS facilities (Jim et al., 2014).

Since the passage and amendments of the Indian Self-Determination and Education Assistance Act (ISDEAA),[3] there has been an increasing trend toward tribal self-governance with respect to all domains of life, including health care. As a result, tribes can receive direct services from IHS, assume responsibility for health care with the option to contract with IHS, or fund the establishment of their own programs or supplementation of ISDEAA programs (IHS, 2020). The self-governance option allows tribes to tailor services to their communities. IHS operates from the understanding that tribal leaders are in the best position to assess and address the needs of their communities. Over 60 percent of the IHS appropriation is administered by tribes, through self-determination contracts, or self-governance compacts (IHS, 2020).

---

[1] 25 U.S.C. § 13.
[2] Pub. L. 94–437, 90 Stat. 1400 (Sept. 30, 1976).
[3] 25 U.S.C. § 5301 et seq.

SOURCE: Adapted excerpt from NASEM, 2017b.

Several challenges keep IHS from reaching its full potential of providing high-quality, efficient health care services and advancing health equity. One major barrier is how it is funded—IHS has not received advance appropriations or mandatory funding.[29] Instead, Congress appropriates funds annually to IHS to fulfill the trust responsibility. Per capita spending is far below need at $4,078 (2019 data) (IHS, 2020) versus even the 2019 per capita spending of $11,456 in national health expenditures (CMS.gov, 2022). Funding per person for IHS is much less than Medicaid ($8,109), VA ($10,692), and Medicare patients ($13,815) (see Figure 5-6)—this forces IHS to do more with less and essentially values some lives below others (GAO, 2018). IHS spent $6.68 billion in total in 2017; this is less than 10 percent of the VHA's spending and approximately 1 percent of spending by either Medicare or Medicaid (GAO, 2018). It is important to note that these programs do differ in many ways—such as design, structure, and services—making a direct comparison difficult. However, scholarship on this topic reflects a broad consensus that IHS is underfunded (GAO, 2018; Heisler and McClanahan, 2020; Lofthouse, 2022; Tribal Budget Formulation Workgroup, 2022).

AIAN people can purchase private health insurance for expenses that IHS does not cover. However, high rates of poverty and low employment rates and free IHS services—even if inadequate—lead to high rates of uninsurance in the AIAN population (Lofthouse, 2022). In 2021, 38 percent of nonelderly AIAN people had employer or other private insurance and 41 percent were covered by Medicaid or other public insurance, leaving the remaining 21 percent to rely completely on IHS services or pay out of pocket (Artiga et al., 2022b).

IHS receives funding through congressional appropriations (mainly discretionary) and a smaller share via collections from reimbursement, including Medicare, Medicaid, CHIP, VA, and private insurance. IHS appropriations have increased gradually from $4.8 billion in FY2016 to $6.0 billion in FY2020 (Lofthouse, 2022) and to $6.8 billion in FY2022 for all its operations (this includes facility maintenance, clinical services, and preventive health measures but not COVID-19 supplemental funding) (ASPE, 2022a). Tribal consultation and priorities (e.g., mental health, alcohol/substance use, and health care facility construction)

---

[29] "Advance appropriations become available for obligation one or more fiscal years after the budget year covered by the appropriations act. Although advance appropriations are provided in order to manage specific planning concerns, they also have implications for the prevention of funding gaps and the avoidance continuing appropriations" (Tollestrup and McClanahan, 2019). Mandatory spending, also known as "direct spending," is mandated by existing authorization laws. This type of spending includes funding for entitlement programs, such as Medicare and Social Security, and other payments to people, businesses, and state and local governments (Tollestrup, 2021).

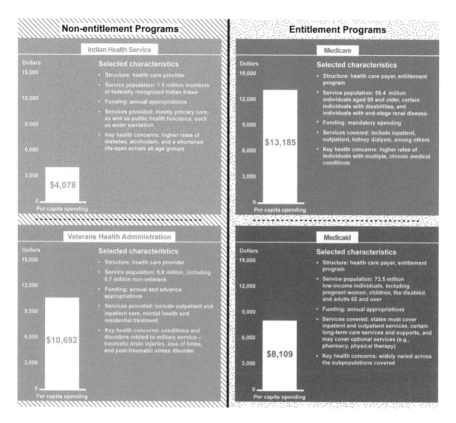

FIGURE 5-6 2017 per capita spending levels and selected program characteristics for four federal health programs: Indian Health Service, Veterans Health Administration, Medicaid, and Medicare.
NOTE: Some individuals may receive or have services covered through more than one program; however, the reported per capita spending amounts do not account for spending across multiple programs. While Indian Health Service and Veterans Health Administration receive most of their funding from annual appropriations, they also received mandatory amounts for specific purposes. For Indian Health Service the report calculated per capita spending as total obligations divided by the number of individuals served. Indian Health Service defines individuals served as those who have accessed a federally or tribally operated facility at least once over the past 3 years. For Veterans Health Administration, the per capita spending represents obligations per unique patient (uniquely identified individuals treated by VHA or whose treatment is paid for by Veterans Health Administration). For Medicare and Medicaid, the figure reports on expenditures (including those by states for Medicaid) by the number of individuals served. Spending for Medicare represents total expenditures from the Medicare trust funds and does not include beneficiary cost-sharing spending. The data for Indian Health Service, Veterans Health Administration, and Medicaid are for fiscal year 2017, and the Medicare data are for calendar year 2017. The Medicaid data are based on estimates published by Centers for Medicaid & Medicaid Services' Office of the Actuary, as actual data were not yet available at the time of the report.
SOURCE: GAO, 2018.

inform the annual HHS and IHS budget formulation processes. The Tribal Budget Formulation Workgroup concluded that $49.8 billion was needed to fully fund IHS in FY2023 (National Indian Health Board, 2021); the FY2023 President's Budget proposed increased funding from $9.3 billion in FY2023 to $36.7 billion in FY2032, including advance appropriations (ASPE, 2022a). The 2023 omnibus spending package provided IHS with $6.96 billion for FY2023, and, in a historic change, also included advance appropriations totaling $5.13 billion for FY2024 (NCUIH, 2023a). However, it is not clear if advance appropriations will continue past 2024.

Without advance appropriations, IHS is always waiting for the next budget, which is dependent on politics and competing priorities in the House and Senate. Advance appropriations would allow IHS to plan and strategize and avoid gaps in funding. For example, during government shutdowns, funding largely becomes unavailable. This leads to uncertainties for planning, disruptions in operations, and loss of IHS employees. This has greatly impacted the ability of IHS to provide care and leaves the population with the lowest health statistics in many domains and the lowest life expectancy in the United States. Fully funding IHS would help advance health equity among AIAN people. Other large programs that pay for health services receive mandatory funding (such as most Medicare funding) or receive discretionary advance appropriations, allowing for the provided or paid-for services to continue across fiscal years without disruption. Congress could grant IHS advance appropriation authority, as is done for VA. In 2020, the Congressional Research Service released a detailed report reviewing IHS funding and shortfalls and how its funding structure is inadequate (Heisler and McClanahan, 2020). For example, "IHS often runs out of funding for specialty services that are contracted out within its fiscal year, leaving many patients to pay fully out of pocket, use health insurance, or go without care" (Lofthouse, 2022). Indian Country has a saying: better get sick by June (when the money runs out), and only life or limb will be authorized out of direct care (by Contact Health Services or indirect care).

This lack of resources leads to other shortcomings within IHS as well. A 2007 physician survey found that inadequate access to necessary health services such as high-quality specialists and outpatient mental health services, nonemergency hospital admission, and diagnostic imaging services were barriers for quality improvement; physicians reported a lack of funding from IHS for subspecialist care as a critical obstacle (Sequist et al., 2011). The COVID-19 pandemic hit this population exceptionally hard and highlights additional barriers to care, including weather, long distances to obtain health services, unavailability of water, and transporting providers to the care areas in adequate numbers (Arrazola et al., 2020; Hatcher et al., 2020).

Funding shortages have led to long patient wait times for routine services and gaps in care because of lack of staff or equipment for onsite services (Lofthouse, 2022). A GAO study concluded that IHS "has not conducted any systematic, agency-wide oversight of the timeliness of primary care provided in its federally operated facilities and, as a result, cannot ensure that patients have access to timely primary care" (GAO, 2016, p. 13).

IHS facilities operate out of 12 physical areas: Alaska, Albuquerque, Bemidji, Billings, California, Great Plains, Nashville, Navajo, Oklahoma, Phoenix, Portland, and Tucson (IHS, n.d.). Notably, all but Nashville are west of the Mississippi River. All but two hospitals and most other facilities (such as clinics) are west as well (see Figure 5-7). This leads to many AIAN people not being able to access IHS care. For example, New York City is the city with the most AIAN people, due in large part to the relocation programs of the Termination Era. About 194,000 New Yorkers identify as AIAN (Khurshid, 2020; USAFacts, 2022), yet they have no direct

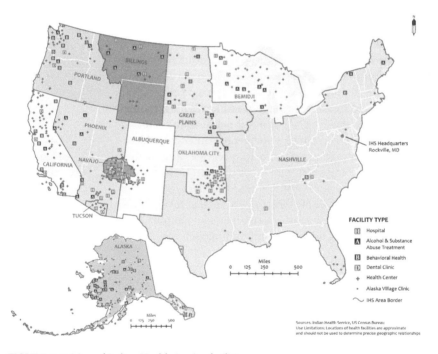

FIGURE 5-7 Map of Indian Health Service facilities.
NOTE: Colors represent the 12 Indian Health Service Areas (regions): Alaska, Albuquerque, Bemidji, Billings, California, Great Plains, Nashville, Navajo, Oklahoma City, Phoenix, Portland, and Tucson.
SOURCE: ASPE, 2022a.

service IHS facilities, including hospitals, in New York City, Washington, DC (where IHS headquarters is located), or any other major eastern city. Therefore, to access IHS hospitals, a member of a federally recognized tribe would have to travel to the west to seek care (direct) or try to get authorized for care (indirect) in the east.

IHS funding for urban health has been around 1 percent of an already inadequate budget (NCUIH, 2023b). Yet 70 percent of AIAN live in urban areas (ASPE, 2022a). Therefore, an eligible patient who lives in the east faces an undue burden. Access is affected geographically, financially, by setting (urban or rural), and by allowances for direct or indirect care.

It is important to understand that as people in a unique situation as sovereign nations, AIAN individuals are highly regulated, as is their health system. A federal trust responsibility has been in place since the turn of the 19th century (see Box 5-8). That is, tribes ceded land under treaties, and in return, the federal government owed a trust responsibility to acknowledge their sovereignty and provide for their well-being. However, the responsibility has not been upheld. The implications of this are far reaching. Senator Daniel Inouye (D-HI) famously noted, "Over 100 years ago, the Indian people of this nation purchased the first pre-paid health care plan, a plan that was paid for by the cession of millions of acres of land to the United States" (Inouye, 1993). Land for federal services was in effect "a prepaid health care plan in perpetuity" (Bergman et al., 1999, p. 588).

Increased funding alone will not solve all IHS institutional problems—for example, the AIAN population has many socioeconomic factors that also contribute greatly to poor health outcomes. However, increased funding would improve access to health services and medical equipment and address the shortage of trained medical staff. Until funding levels for IHS meet parity to other federal government health care programs (such as Medicaid and VA), no persistent, strategic, and structural change in this agency and for the AIAN population is possible (see Chapter 8 for a recommendation to increase IHS funding and related needs).

Conclusion 5-6: The Indian Health Service is the primary source of health care for many American Indian and Alaska Native people. The current structure and inadequate funding level of the Indian Health Service contributes to health inequities for American Indian and Alaska Native people.

Maternal Health

There are profound racial, ethnic, and tribal inequities in maternal health. Maternal deaths are on the rise in the United States, with approximately 1,200 in 2021 (versus about 806 in 2020 and 750 in 2019) (Hoyert,

2023). Furthermore, a staggering 84 percent of pregnancy-related deaths in 36 states from 2017 to 2019 were preventable (CDC, 2022b). There are stark racial inequities in maternal mortality due to differences in access to prenatal care, quality care, and other factors, such as unconscious bias in health care professionals. Black and AIAN women are more likely to suffer serious pregnancy-related complications than non-Hispanic White women; Black women are three times more likely to die from pregnancy-related causes and AIAN women are more than two times more likely to die from pregnancy-related causes than non-Hispanic White women (Hill et al., 2022; Petersen et al., 2019; Radley et al., 2021). One access issue for racially and ethnically minoritized populations is lack of maternity care, especially in rural areas, where many labor and delivery units are closing in part because of staffing and financial challenges and stringent abortion restrictions (March of Dimes, 2020; Musa and Bonifield, 2023; Sonenberg and Mason, 2023; Varney and Lenei Buhre, 2023; The White House, 2022). For example, a report found that approximately 7 million women of childbearing age lived in a county with limited or no access to maternity health care services (March of Dimes, 2020). Access to permanent contraception after delivery also varies by race and ethnicity (Grady et al., 2015); the inability to access the desired method can result in unintended, short-interval pregnancies, which increases the risk of maternal and neonatal/pediatric morbidity and mortality (Arizona MMRC, 2020; Potter et al., 2017).

Many federal policies are relevant; not all could be included here. See, for example, Chapter 3 for information on the Special Supplemental Nutrition Program for Women, Infants, and Children, a national program created to ensure that women, infants, and children under 5 years who are from low-income backgrounds can access food and information on healthy eating practices (Marchi et al., 2013); it provides breastfeeding support and promotion and health care referrals. See also the previous sections in this chapter on Medicaid presumptive eligibility for pregnant people and postpartum coverage. This section discusses the Black Maternal Health Momnibus Act of 2021 (Momnibus),[30] a comprehensive bill aimed to address multiple aspects of maternal health, and the lack of a federal policy protecting access to abortion.

Momnibus

Given the complex interplay of SDOH that contribute to women's health, perinatal health, and racial and ethnic health inequities, needed policies are transectoral, requiring multiple sets of bills bundled as a collective

---

[30] H.R. 959, 117th Congress (2021) and S. 346, 117th Congress (2021).

approach that seeks to improve health inequities. Evidence-based, equitable, and patient-centered health policy change that accounts for the multilevel causes of disparities is needed to improve health outcomes. One such example is Momnibus, proposed by the Black Maternal Health Caucus (Black Maternal Health Caucus, n.d.). It is a set of 12 individual bills, each of which was orchestrated around an identified lead contributor to maternal mortality inequities, including addressing SDOH, such as housing, nutrition, and employment; funding equity-promoting community-based organizations that work to improve maternal outcomes; and expanding and diversifying the perinatal care workforce. A Momnibus bill addressed the compelling need for improvement in data collection and related processes and quality measures to better understand and track improvements in maternal health care delivery and related inequities. Investment in maternal mental health care and women who are incarcerated were also specific foci for these bills. Digital tools to improve telehealth delivery were included along with a call for novel payment models to incentivize high-quality care. Investment for veterans' maternity care coordination was the one piece of legislation of the 12 that was signed into law (Maternal Health Learning & Innovation Center, 2022). Many other components were included in the House-passed Build Back Better Act[31] but excluded from the Inflation Reduction Act[32]; additional pieces were enacted in the FY2022 appropriations bill and included in the FY2023 budget proposal, but Congress has not acted on many bills from the Momnibus package aimed specifically at the Black maternal health crisis (Clark, 2023; Clark and Johnson, 2022; Georgetown University, 2022). Momnibus is a good example of comprehensively acknowledging the many factors that contribute to health inequities and the comprehensive legislation needed to address such complexity.

Medical Care Access for Unintended Pregnancies

Unintended pregnancy is an important problem in the United States that is associated with health risks to a pregnant person, their family, and society. About half of all U.S. pregnancies are unintended (CDC, 2021; Guttmacher Institute, 2019). An integral factor underlying this rate is a lack of access to effective family planning services (Dehlendorf et al., 2010; Finer and Henshaw, 2006; Frost et al., 2008). Unintended pregnancy is also associated with poor outcomes like low-birthweight infants, infant mortality, and maternal morbidity and mortality (Dehlendorf et al., 2010). Empowering people to plan when they want to have children is essential, and thus access to abortion is an important part of reproductive care.

---

[31] H.R. 5376, 117th Congress (2021).
[32] Pub. L. 117–169, 136 Stat. 1818 (Aug. 16, 2022).

Pregnancy is not easy or safe for everyone and it can affect the physical, emotional, social, and economic health of individuals and families. Additionally, pre-existing and co-occurring medical conditions can present additional risks in carrying a pregnancy to term. Pregnancy takes a mental toll as well; mental health conditions are one of the most frequent underlying causes of pregnancy-related deaths in the United States (Trost et al., 2022). Abortion restriction has economic effects as well; people can be confronted with numerous financial challenges in carrying a pregnancy to term while supporting their children and families (Bahn et al., 2020; Banerjee, 2023; Foster et al., 2022).

Relevant policy change affecting reproductive care is the overturning of *Roe v. Wade*;[33] the Supreme Court overturned the Roe precedent in June 2022 with its decision in the *Dobbs v. Jackson Women's Health Organization*[34] case, invalidating the basic Constitutional right to abortion and leaving its legality to states. Legal abortions are safe and effective and are an evidence-based, standard-of-care option within comprehensive medical care (NASEM, 2018c). The procedure is highly prevalent; the Guttmacher Institute estimates that about 25 percent of U.S. women have had an abortion by age 45 (Guttmacher Institute, 2017). Adolescent, lower-income, minoritized, and single women who have poverty rates twice that of other groups have higher rates of unintended pregnancies, exacerbating the financial effect (Artiga et al., 2022a; Troutman et al., 2020). CDC data report that in 2019, Black women accounted for 38 percent of abortions, White women 33 percent, Hispanic women 21 percent, and 7 percent were among other racial and ethnic groups. The abortion rate was highest among Black (23.8 per 1,000 women) and Hispanic (11.7) women compared to 6.6 among White women (data for other racial and ethnic groups were not available) (Artiga et al., 2022a). Estimates from 2021 suggest that a nationwide abortion ban would increase maternal mortality by 21 percent overall and 33 percent among Black people (Stevenson, 2021). Overturning the Roe precedent and subsequent state laws will likely have the most serious consequences for patients, clinicians, clinics, and communities in states with the largest racial inequities in maternal and reproductive health, the highest maternal mortality rates, and fewer government resources, such as expanded Medicaid (Declercq et al., 2022; Kozhimannil et al., 2022; Redd et al., 2021; Rosenbaum, 2022); providers and specialists may be reluctant to practice in abortion-restriction states, contributing to racial, ethnic, and tribal maternal health inequities (Musa and Bonifield, 2023; Nirappil and Stead Sellers, 2023;

---

[33] *Roe v. Wade*, 410 U.S. 113 (1973).
[34] *Dobbs v. Jackson Women's Health Organization*, 597 U.S. ___ (2022).

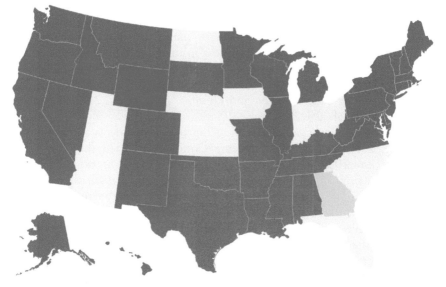

FIGURE 5-8 Status of abortion bans in the United States as of March 20, 2023.
NOTES: Since the Dobbs decision, 23 states (Alabama, Arizona, Arkansas, Florida, Georgia, Idaho, Indiana, Iowa, Kentucky, Louisiana, Mississippi, Missouri, North Dakota, Ohio, Oklahoma, South Carolina, South Dakota, Tennessee, Texas, Utah, West Virginia, Wisconsin, and Wyoming) have tried to implement a complete or previability ban. In six states, these laws are blocked by courts. LMP = Last menstrual period.
SOURCE: KFF, n.d.-a; licensed under CC BY-NC-ND 4.0 (https://creativecommons.org/licenses/by-nc-nd/4.0/).

Varney and Lenei Buhre, 2023) (see Figure 5-8 for a summary of state abortion bans as of early 2023). Research describing the consequences of this ruling is critical.

Territorial Health

The five U.S. territories, the U.S. Virgin Islands, American Samoa, Guam, the Commonwealth of the Northern Mariana Islands, and Puerto Rico represent unique confluences of historical legacies and contemporary challenges, including inequitable policies (Stolyar et al., 2021). Territorial populations represent U.S. citizens and U.S. nationals (the latter are the residents of American Samoa) whose way of life has been profoundly affected by federal policies that used the territories' land for military purposes and agricultural exports. Those living in the territories—approximately 3.5 million people, 98 percent of whom are racially and ethnically minoritized—experience deep poverty, and a high proportion are dependent on Medicaid and CHIP, but Medicaid financing in the territories has hampered the ability to provide the necessary health care due to limited funds (O'Rourke, 2019; Stolyar et al., 2021). Health centers are an important part of the health care infrastructure and also a good source of information about health in the territories (Stolyar et al., 2021). According to territorial data from the HRSA Uniform Data System, the most prevalent conditions are heart disease, diabetes, obesity, and mental health disorders. In 2020, the economic effects of the pandemic and endemic poverty were cited as the most significant social issues. To illustrate the disparity in poverty rates, 87 percent of health center patients in the territories "had incomes at or below the federal poverty level (FPL) and 98 [percent] had incomes at or below 200 [percent] FPL in 2020. In comparison, 68 [percent] of health center patients in the 50 states and DC had incomes at or below poverty and 91 [percent] had incomes at or below 200 [percent] FPL" (Stolyar et al., 2021). Territories' health centers are funded by Medicaid reimbursement and federal Section 330 grants.

Immigrant Health

In 2019, approximately 45 million individuals, or 14 percent of the U.S. population, were immigrants (i.e., born outside of the United States; "foreign-born"); however, over half of those immigrants (23 million) are now citizens ("naturalized"), and another 8 million are eligible for citizenship. In 2019, the United States had an estimated 10.3 million undocumented immigrants, or 3 percent of the population (American Immigration Council, n.d.).

Immigration status is an SDOH, impacting access to health insurance, health care and services, quality of care, and ultimately, health outcomes (Asad and Clair, 2018; KFF, 2022a; NASEM, 2018b). Evidence identifies disparities in health care access and outcomes based on immigration status (Cabral and Cuevas, 2020; Hacker et al., 2015; Misra et al., 2021; Morey, 2018; Ornelas et al., 2020; Philbin et al., 2018; Sudhinaraset et al., 2017; Wilson et al., 2018). Immigrants experience differences in health care access and outcomes because of unique and common factors. Many are explicitly ineligible and excluded from health and other resources that other U.S. residents receive because of their immigration status. Moreover, immigrants also experience challenges that impact their health and well-being similar to other low-income racially and ethnically minoritized communities (e.g., inadequate employment opportunities and low wages, lack of employer-based health insurance, poor quality and insecure housing, lack of equitable educational opportunities, community-level violence, and threats to safety). An additional factor for immigrants is the fear of accessing government programs and services because of real and perceived consequences to immigration status, including denial of permanent immigration status, deportation, or family separation (Cabral and Cuevas, 2020; Castañeda et al., 2015; Martinez et al., 2015; Saadi et al., 2020).

In 1996, Congress enacted legislation[35] that restricted Medicaid eligibility for 5 years for immigrants granted legal permanent residence (commonly known as getting a "green card"); this is now known as the "5-year bar" (Broder et al., 2022) (see Chapter 8 and Recommendation 11 for more information). Under the 1996 legislation, states could extend eligibility for Medicaid and CHIP to immigrants during the 5-year bar, using state-only funds. In 2009, the CHIP Reauthorization Act[36] authorized federal matching funds for such expansion (KFF, 2009). As of January 2022, 35 states have extended Medicaid and/or CHIP eligibility to immigrant children (KFF, 2022b). However, only 24 states have extended Medicaid eligibility to immigrant pregnant persons and only four states have extended CHIP eligibility to immigrant pregnant persons. HHS can do more to facilitate and incentivize states to extend Medicaid and CHIP coverage to immigrant children and pregnant people (KFF, 2022b; Medicaid.gov, 2021; Whitner, 2022).

In 2019, the Department of Homeland Security finalized the "public charge" regulation[37] that would have significantly expanded the types of public benefits received that could disqualify an individual from obtaining permanent legal residence status. Prior to this re-interpretation, immigrants would only be potentially disqualified for receipt of SSI, Temporary Assistance for Needy Families (TANF), local General Assistance, and government support for long-term institutional care. The 2019 regulation added receipt of Medicaid, Supplemental Nutrition Assistance Program (SNAP), and federal housing assistance to the list of potentially disqualifying benefits. Multiple federal courts initially blocked implementation, but the Supreme Court overturned those preliminary injunctions while the

---

[35] Personal Responsibility and Work Opportunity Reconciliation Act of 1996, Pub. L. 104–193, 110 Stat. 2105 (Aug. 22, 1996) and Illegal Immigration Reform and Immigrant Responsibility Act of 1996, enacted as Division C of the Defense Department Appropriations Act, 1997, Pub. L. 104–208, 110 Stat. 3008 (Sept. 30, 1996).

[36] Pub. L. 111–3, 123 Stat. 8 (Feb. 7, 2009).

[37] Inadmissibility on Public Charge Grounds, 84 FR 41292 (August 2019).

litigation continued, and the regulation became effective in all states in February 2020 (CIS, 2022b; ILRC, 2021). Significant evidence indicates that it had a chilling effect on immigrants accessing public benefits, including Medicaid and SNAP (Bernstein et al., 2022; Capps et al., 2020; Haley et al., 2020, 2021; Nguyen et al., 2023). The public charge rule has been rescinded and the long-standing interpretation limiting potential disqualifications to receipt of SSI, TANF, local General Assistance, and public support for long-term institutional care has been restored; the regulation went into effect in late 2022.[38] In addition, the fate of over 594,000 immigrants (CIS, 2022a) who have been granted Deferred Action for Childhood Arrivals (DACA)[39] status since 2012 remains in active litigation, as of 2022. The Biden Administration issued a final regulation[40] codifying the program in August 2022, but federal courts enjoined implementation (CIS, n.d.). DACA recipients are not eligible to purchase health coverage through ACA marketplaces because they are excluded from the ACA definition of "lawfully present" (NILC, 2013). Based on a 2021 survey of over 1,000 DACA recipients administered by the University of California, San Diego, United We Dream, National Immigration Law Center, and Center for American Progress, one-third of DACA recipients are uninsured (with 18 percent of respondents losing employer-based health insurance coverage during the COVID–19 pandemic). Nearly half reported a time that they had delayed medical care because of their immigration status, and two-thirds reported that they or a family member had been unable to pay their medical bills or expenses (Lundie et al., 2022). Advocacy efforts are underway to extend eligibility for federally funded health insurance, including Medicaid and state health insurance marketplaces established by ACA (Castro, 2022; NILC, 2013). Finally, efforts to provide a pathway for DACA immigrants to permanent legal residence and eventual citizenship have stalled in Congress (Martínez Rosas, 2022).

CONCLUDING OBSERVATIONS

Improving health care access and quality through federal policies so that all communities can thrive will require collaboration among federal agencies, prioritizing the needs of communities, and removing barriers to accessing care, which are among the crosscutting themes identified by the

---

[38] Public Charge Ground of Inadmissibility, 87 FR 55472 (September 2022).

[39] Immigration policy that provides temporary protection from deportation, as well as work authorization, to eligible undocumented immigrants who came to the United States as children.

[40] Deferred Action for Childhood Arrivals, 87 FR 53152 (August 2022).

committee (see Chapter 8). Many federal health care policies contribute to racial, ethnic, and tribal health inequities. Although the committee could not review all such policies in this report, federal health care policy does provide powerful tools to advance health equity for all people. The examples in this chapter illustrate the importance of access, eligibility, and accountability to existing legislation. For example, removing administrative burden, improving participation rates (e.g., through Medicaid expansion or state innovation waivers), and reducing Medicaid churn could improve coverage and therefore racial and ethnic health equity. Reversing policies that exclude immigrants and people involved with the criminal legal system is also a promising strategy. Changes to the funding level and structure of IHS could improve health equity for the AIAN population. Finally, coordination across HHS could lead to more efficient and higher-quality health programs.

> *Conclusion 5-7: A lack of coordination, measurement, and prioritization of equity activities across the Department of Health and Human Services contributes to racial, ethnic, and tribal health inequities.*

> *Conclusion 5-8: Increasing access to high-quality, comprehensive, affordable, accessible, timely, respectful, and culturally appropriate health care would advance racial and ethnic health equity. Progress toward universal health care access can be achieved through many federal policy avenues, including but not limited to increasing access to public and private insurance coverage.*

Many National Academies reports have evidence-based and promising recommendations for federal action to advance health equity for health care access and quality (including and beyond the federal policies reviewed in this chapter) that have not been implemented and are still relevant (see Box 5-9 for examples on a broad range of health care topics for federal action). In addition, there is more to come. Additionally, a consensus study charged with revisiting the 2003 *Unequal Treatment* report (IOM, 2003) is underway (Unequal Treatment Revisited: The Current State of Racial and Ethnic Disparities in Health Care).[41]

---

[41] See https://www.nationalacademies.org/our-work/unequal-treatment-revisited-the-current-state-of-racial-and-ethnic-disparities-in-healthcare (accessed July 6, 2023).

BOX 5-9
Example Recommendations from
National Academies Reports

Unequal Treatment: Confronting Racial and Ethnic Disparities in Health Care
(IOM, 2003)
Recommendation 5-2: Strengthen the stability of patient-provider relationships in publicly funded health plans.

Recommendation 5-3: Increase the proportion of underrepresented U.S. racial and ethnic minorities among health professionals.

Vibrant and Healthy Kids: Aligning Science, Practice, and Policy to Advance Health Equity (NASEM, 2019b)
Recommendation 5-1: The U.S. Department of Health and Human Services, state, tribal, and territorial Medicaid agencies, public and private payers, and state and federal policy makers should adopt policies and practices that ensure universal access to high-quality health care across the life course. This includes

- Increasing access to patient- and family-centered care,
- Ensuring access to preventive services and essential health benefits, and
- Increasing culturally and linguistically appropriate outreach and services.

Integrating Social Care into the Delivery of Health Care: Moving Upstream to Improve the Nation's Health (NASEM, 2019a)
Recommendation 5d: The Centers for Medicare & Medicaid Services, the U.S. Department of Health and Human Services, state Medicaid agencies, the National Quality Forum, and the National Committee for Quality Assurance should establish mechanisms that ensure that research on effective demonstrations informs more permanent health care reforms, including the development of accountability measures and payment models.

Implementing High-Quality Primary Care: Rebuilding the Foundation of Health Care (NASEM, 2021c)
Action 2.1: To facilitate an ongoing primary care relationship, all individuals should have the opportunity to have a usual source of primary care.

- a. Payers—Medicaid, Medicare, commercial insurers, and self-insured employers—should ask all covered individuals to declare a usual source of primary care annually and should assign non-responding enrollees using established methods, track this information, and use it for payment and accountability measures.
- b. Health centers, hospitals, and primary care practices should assume and document an ongoing clinical relationship with the uninsured people they are treating.

BOX 5-9 Continued

The Future of Nursing 2020-2030: Charting a Path to Achieve Health Equity
(NASEM, 2021b)
Recommendation 2: By 2023, state and federal government agencies, health care and public health organizations, payers, and foundations should initiate substantive actions to enable the nursing workforce to address social determinants of health and health equity more comprehensively, regardless of practice setting.

Recommendation 4: All organizations, including state and federal entities and employing organizations, should enable nurses to practice to the full extent of their education and training by removing barriers that prevent them from more fully addressing social needs and social determinants of health and improving health care access, quality, and value. These barriers include regulatory and public and private payment limitations; restrictive policies and practices; and other legal, professional, and commercial impediments.

Improving Representation in Clinical Trials and Research: Building Research Equity for Women and Underrepresented Groups (NASEM, 2022)
Recommendation 1: HHS should establish an intradepartmental task force on research equity charged with coordinating data collection and developing better accrual tracking systems across federal agencies to:

a. Produce an annual report to Congress on the status of clinical trial and clinical research enrollment in the United States, including the number of patients recruited into clinical studies by phase and condition; their age, sex, gender, race, ethnicity, and trial location (i.e., where participants are recruited); their representativeness of the conditions under investigation; and the research sponsors.
b. Make data more accessible and transparent throughout the year, such as through a data dashboard that is updated in real time.
c. Determine what "representativeness" means for protocols and product development plans.
d. Develop explicit guidance on equitable compensation to research participants and their caregivers, including differential compensation for those who will bear a financial burden to participate.

Recommendation 17: HHS should substantially invest in community research infrastructure that will improve representation in clinical trials and clinical research. This funding should go to agencies such as the HRSA, NIH, AHRQ, CDC, and IHS to expand the capacity of community health centers and safety-net hospitals to participate in and initiate clinical research focused on conditions that disproportionately affect the patient populations they serve.

REFERENCES

AAMC (Association of American Medical Colleges). 2021. *The complexities of physician supply and demand: Projections from 2019 to 2034.* Washington, DC: Association of American Medical Colleges.

AAMC. n.d.-a. *Diversity in Medicine: Facts and Figures 2019.* https://www.aamc.org/data-reports/workforce/report/diversity-medicine-facts-and-figures-2019 (accessed March 17, 2023).

AAMC. n.d.-b. *Diversity in Medicine: Facts and Figures 2019: Figure 18.* https://www.aamc.org/data-reports/workforce/interactive-data/figure-18-percentage-all-active-physicians-race/ethnicity-2018 (accessed March 17, 2023).

ACOG (American College of Obstetricians and Gynecologists). 2018. ACOG Committee Opinion No. 736: Optimizing postpartum care. *Obstetrics & Gynecology* 131(5):e140–e150.

ACOG. 2019a. ACOG Committee Opinion No. 766: Approaches to limit intervention during labor and birth. *Obstetrics & Gynecology* 133(2):e164–e173.

ACOG. 2019b. Obstetric care consensus no. 8: Interpregnancy care. *Obstetrics & Gynecology* 133(1):e51–e72.

ACOG. 2019c. *Why OB-Gyns Are Burning Out.* https://www.acog.org/news/news-articles/2019/10/why-ob-gyns-are-burning-out (accessed March 17, 2023).

ACOG. 2021. *Counseling Regarding Approach to Delivery After Cesarean and the Use of a Vaginal Birth After Cesarean Calculator.* https://www.acog.org/clinical/clinical-guidance/practice-advisory/articles/2021/12/counseling-regarding-approach-to-delivery-after-cesarean-and-the-use-of-a-vaginal-birth-after-cesarean-calculator (accessed March 17, 2023).

Adkins-Jackson, P. B., N. J. Burke, P. R. Espinosa, J. M. Ison, S. D. Goold, L. G. Rosas, C. A. Doubeni, and A. F. Brown. 2022. Inclusionary trials: A review of lessons not learned. *Epidemiologic Reviews* 44(1):78–86.

AHRQ (Agency for Healthcare Research and Quality). 2016. *Chartbook on Access to Health Care.* https://www.ahrq.gov/research/findings/nhqrdr/chartbooks/access/elements2.html (accessed March 13, 2023).

AHRQ. 2022. *2021 national healthcare quality and disparities report.* Rockville, MD: Agency for Healthcare Research and Quality.

AHRQ. n.d. *AHRQ Health Literacy Universal Precautions Toolkit, Second Edition.* https://www.ahrq.gov/health-literacy/improve/precautions/index.html (accessed March 15, 2023).

Alberti, P. M., C. Teigland, and D. R. Nerenz. 2020. *To Design Equitable Value-Based Payment Systems, We Must Adjust for Social Risk.* https://www.healthaffairs.org/content/forefront/design-equitable-value-based-payment-systems-we-must-adjust-social-risk (accessed May 30, 2023).

Allgood, K. L., B. Hunt, J. M. Kanoon, and M. A. Simon. 2018. Evaluation of mammogram parties as an effective community navigation method. *Journal of Cancer Education* 33(5):1061–1068.

Alsan, M., and M. Wanamaker. 2018. Tuskegee and the health of Black men. *The Quarterly Journal of Economics* 133(1):407–455.

AMA (American Medical Association). 2021. *Organizational strategic plan to embed racial justice and advance health equity: 2021–2023.* Washington, DC: American Medical Association.

The American Board of Pediatrics. 2023. *Latest Race and Ethnicity Data for Pediatricians and Pediatric Trainees.* https://www.abp.org/dashboards/latest-race-and-ethnicity-data-pediatricians-and-pediatric-trainees (accessed May 30, 2023).

American Immigration Council. n.d. *Immigrants in the United States.* https://www.americanimmigrationcouncil.org/sites/default/files/research/immigrants_in_the_united_states_0.pdf (accessed March 18, 2023).

Arce, J. 2021. *The Long History of Forced Sterilization of Latinas.* https://unidosus.org/blog/2021/12/16/the-long-history-of-forced-sterilization-of-latinas/ (accessed May 2, 2023).

Arizona MMRC. 2020. *Maternal mortalities and severe maternal morbidity in Arizona.* Phoenix, AZ: Arizona Department of Health Services.

Arrazola, J., M. M. Masiello, S. Joshi, A. E. Dominguez, A. Poel, C. M. Wilkie, J. M. Bressler, J. McLaughlin, J. Kraszewski, K. K. Komatsu, X. Peterson Pompa, M. Jespersen, G. Richardson, N. Lehnertz, P. LeMaster, B. Rust, A. Keyser Metobo, B. Doman, D. Casey, J. Kumar, A. L. Rowell, T. K. Miller, M. Mannell, O. Naqvi, A. M. Wendelboe, R. Leman, J. L. Clayton, B. Barbeau, S. K. Rice, S. J. Rolland, V. Warren-Mears, A. Echo-Hawk, A. Apostolou, and M. Landen. 2020. COVID-19 mortality among American Indian and Alaska Native persons—14 states, January–June 2020. *Morbidity and Mortality Weekly Report* 69:1853–1856.

Artiga, S., J. Kates, J. Michaud, and L. Hill. 2021. *Racial diversity within COVID-19 vaccine clinical trials: Key questions and answers.* San Francisco, CA: Kaiser Family Foundation.

Artiga, S., L. H. Follow, U. Ranji, and I. Gomez. 2022a. *What are the implications of the overturning of Roe v. Wade for racial disparities?* San Francisco, CA: Kaiser Family Foundation.

Artiga, S., L. Hill, and A. Damico. 2022b. *Health coverage by race and ethnicity, 2010–2021.* San Francisco, CA: Kaiser Family Foundation.

Asad, A. L., and M. Clair. 2018. Racialized legal status as a social determinant of health. *Social Science & Medicine* 199:19–28.

ASPE (Assistant Secretary for Planning and Evaluation). 2021a. *Social Risk Factors and Medicare's Value-Based Purchasing Programs: Background: Request from Congress for a Study of Social Risk Factors and Medicare's Value-Based Purchasing Programs.* https://aspe.hhs.gov/topics/health-health-care/social-drivers-health/social-risk-factors-medicares-value-based-purchasing-programs (accessed May 30, 2023).

ASPE. 2021b. *Social Risk Factors and Medicare's Value-Based Purchasing Programs: Building the Evidence Base for Social Determinants of Health Interventions.* https://aspe.hhs.gov/topics/health-health-care/social-drivers-health/social-risk-factors-medicares-value-based-purchasing-programs/social-risk-factors-medicares-value-based-purchasing-programs-reports (accessed May 30, 2023).

ASPE. 2022a. *How increased funding can advance the mission of the Indian Health Service to improve health outcomes for American Indians and Alaska Natives.* Washington, DC: Office of the Assistant Secretary for Planning and Evaluation.

ASPE. 2022b. *Unwinding the Medicaid continuous enrollment provision: Projected enrollment effects and policy approaches.* Washington, DC: Office of the Assistant Secretary for Planning and Evaluation.

Bahn, K., A. Kugler, M. H. Mahoney, and A. McGrew. 2020. Do U.S. TRAP laws trap women into bad jobs? *Feminist Economics* 26(1):44–97.

Baicker, K., S. L. Taubman, H. L. Allen, M. Bernstein, J. H. Gruber, J. P. Newhouse, E. C. Schneider, B. J. Wright, A. M. Zaslavsky, and A. N. Finkelstein. 2013. The Oregon experiment—effects of Medicaid on clinical outcomes. *New England Journal of Medicine* 368(18):1713–1722.

Baicker, K., H. L. Allen, B. J. Wright, and A. N. Finkelstein. 2017. The effect of Medicaid on medication use among poor adults: Evidence from Oregon. *Health Affairs* 36(12):2110–2114.

Baicker, K., H. L. Allen, B. J. Wright, S. L. Taubman, and A. N. Finkelstein. 2018. The effect of Medicaid on management of depression: Evidence from the Oregon health insurance experiment. *The Milbank Quarterly* 96(1):29–56.

Baicker, K., A. Chandra, and M. Shepard. 2023. Achieving universal health insurance coverage in the United States: Addressing market failures or providing a social floor? *Journal of Economic Perspectives* 37(2):99–122.

Bailey, Z. D., N. Krieger, M. Agénor, J. Graves, N. Linos, and M. T. Bassett. 2017. Structural racism and health inequities in the USA: Evidence and interventions. *The Lancet* 389(10077):1453–1463.

Banerjee, A. 2023. *The economics of abortion bans*. Washington, DC: Economic Policy Institute.

Bergman, A. B., D. C. Grossman, A. M. Erdrich, J. G. Todd, and R. Forquera. 1999. A political history of the Indian Health Service. *The Milbank Quarterly* 77(4):571–604.

Berkman, N. D., S. L. Sheridan, K. E. Donahue, D. J. Halpern, A. Viera, K. Crotty, A. Holland, M. Brasure, K. N. Lohr, E. Harden, E. Tant, I. Wallace, and M. Viswanathan. 2011. *Health literacy interventions and outcomes: An updated systematic review: Evidence report/technology assessment no. 199*. Rockville, MD: Agency for Healthcare Research and Quality.

Bernstein, H., D. Gonzalez, P. Echave, and D. Guelespe. 2022. *Immigrant families faced multiple barriers to safety net programs in 2021*. Washington, DC: Urban Institute.

Black Maternal Health Caucus. n.d. *Momnibus*. https://blackmaternalhealthcaucus-underwood.house.gov/Momnibus (accessed March 18, 2023).

Bohren, M. A., G. J. Hofmeyr, C. Sakala, R. K. Fukuzawa, and A. Cuthbert. 2017. Continuous support for women during childbirth. *Cochrane Database of Systematic Reviews* (7):CD003766.

Boozang, P., C. Brooks-LaSure, and G. Mauser. 2020. *Medicaid's crucial role in combating the maternal mortality and morbidity crisis*. Princeton, NJ: State Health and Value Strategies, Princeton University Woodrow Wilson School of Public and International Affairs.

Brach, C., D. Keller, L. M. Hernandez, C. Baur, R. Parker, B. Dreyer, P. Schyve, A. J. Lemerise, and D. Schillinger. 2012. *Ten attributes of health literate health care organizations*. Washington, DC: National Academy of Medicine.

Brantley, E., and L. Ku. 2021. Continuous eligibility for Medicaid associated with improved child health outcomes. *Medical Care Research and Review* 79(3):404–413.

Broder, T., G. Lessard, and A. Moussavian. 2022. *Overview of immigrant eligibility for federal programs*. Los Angeles, CA: National Immigration Law Center.

Brown, D. W., A. E. Kowalski, and I. Z. Lurie. 2020. Long-term impacts of childhood Medicaid expansions on outcomes in adulthood. *The Review of Economic Studies* 87(2):792–821.

Brown, E. J., D. Polsky, C. M. Barbu, J. W. Seymour, and D. Grande. 2016. Racial disparities in geographic access to primary care in Philadelphia. *Health Affairs* 35(8):1374–1381.

Cabral, J., and A. G. Cuevas. 2020. Health inequities among Latinos/Hispanics: Documentation status as a determinant of health. *Journal of Racial and Ethnic Health Disparities* 7(5):874–879.

Camhi, N., D. Mistak, and V. Wachino. 2020. *Medicaid's evolving role in advancing the health of people involved in the justice system*. New York, NY: The Commonwealth Fund.

Camillo, C. A. 2021. Understanding the mechanisms of administrative burden through a within-case study of Medicaid expansion implementation. *Journal of Behavioral Public Administration* 4(1):1–12.

Campbell, K. M., I. Corral, J. L. Infante Linares, and D. Tumin. 2020. Projected estimates of African American medical graduates of closed historically Black medical schools. *JAMA Network Open* 3(8):e2015220.

Capps, R., M. Fix, and J. Batalova. 2020. *Anticipated "Chilling Effects" of the Public-Charge Rule Are Real: Census Data Reflect Steep Decline in Benefits Use by Immigrant Families*. https://www.migrationpolicy.org/news/anticipated-chilling-effects-public-charge-rule-are-real (accessed March 18, 2023).

Carpenter, D. 2019. The social transformation of American medicine: The rise of a sovereign profession and the making of a vast industry. *Journal of Health Politics, Policy and Law* 44(5):812–817.

Carpio, M. V. 2004. The lost generation: American Indian women and sterilization abuse. *Social Justice* 31(4(98)):40–53.

Castañeda, H., S. M. Holmes, D. S. Madrigal, M.-E. D. Young, N. Beyeler, and J. Quesada. 2015. Immigration as a social determinant of health. *Annual Review of Public Health* 36(1):375–392.

Castro, J. 2022. *Castro, Booker, Jayapal Lead 83 Members Calling on Biden Administration to Remove Barriers to Affordable Health Care for DACA Recipients.* https://castro. house.gov/media-center/press-releases/castro-booker-jayapal-lead-83-members-calling-on-biden-administration-to-remove-barriers-to-affordable-health-care-for-daca-recipients (accessed March 18, 2023).

Caucci, L. n.d. *Hospital presumptive eligibility.* Atlanta, GA: Office for State, Tribal, Local and Territorial Support, Centers for Disease Control and Prevention.

CBPP (Center on Budget and Policy Priorities). 2021. *The Medicaid coverage gap in Georgia.* Washington, DC: Center on Budget and Policy Priorities.

CBPP. 2022. *Policy Basics: Where Do Our Federal Tax Dollars Go?* https://www.cbpp.org/ research/federal-budget/where-do-our-federal-tax-dollars-go (accessed May 18, 2023).

CDC (Centers for Disease Control and Prevention). 2021. *Unintended Pregnancy.* https:// www.cdc.gov/reproductivehealth/contraception/unintendedpregnancy/index.htm (accessed March 18, 2023).

CDC. 2022a. *CDC's Health Literacy Action Plan.* https://www.cdc.gov/healthliteracy/planact/ cdcplan.html (accessed March 15, 2023).

CDC. 2022b. *Four in 5 Pregnancy-Related Deaths in the U.S. Are Preventable.* https://www. cdc.gov/media/releases/2022/p0919-pregnancy-related-deaths.html#:~:text=Most%20 pregnancy%2Drelated%20deaths%20of,to%201%20year%20after%20pregnancy.& text=More%20than%20half%20(53%25),to%20one%20year%20after%20delivery. (accessed March 18, 2023).

CDC. 2022c. *Health Literacy.* https://www.cdc.gov/healthliteracy/index.html (accessed March 15, 2023).

CDC. 2022d. *Numeracy.* https://www.cdc.gov/healthliteracy/researchevaluate/numeracy.html (accessed March 18, 2023).

Census Bureau. 2020. *People That Speak English Less Than "Very Well" in the United States.* https://www.census.gov/library/visualizations/interactive/people-that-speak-english-less-than-very-well.html (accessed June 2, 2023).

Center for Mississippi Health Policy. 2020. *Presumptive Medicaid eligibility for pregnant women.* Jackson, MS: Center for Mississippi Health Policy.

Chapman, E. N., A. Kaatz, and M. Carnes. 2013. Physicians and implicit bias: How doctors may unwittingly perpetuate health care disparities. *Journal of General Internal Medicine* 28(11):1504–1510.

CHCS (Center for Health Care Strategies). 2019. *Fact sheet: Medicaid: A brief history of publicly financed health care in the United States.* Hamilton, NJ: Center for Health Care Strategies.

Chen, A. H., M. K. Youdelman, and J. Brooks. 2007. The legal framework for language access in healthcare settings: Title VI and beyond. *Journal of General Internal Medicine* 22(Suppl 2):362–367.

Choi, J. 2022. Biden administration approves Washington state request to offer health insurance to undocumented immigrants. *The Hill,* December 12.

Chokshi, D. A., M. M. K. Foote, and M. E. Morse. 2022. How to act upon racism—not race—as a risk factor. *JAMA Health Forum* 3(2):e220548.

CIS (U.S. Citizenship and Immigration Services). 2022a. *Count of Active DACA Recipients by Month of Current DACA Expiration as of June 30, 2022.* https://www.uscis.gov/ sites/default/files/document/data/Active_DACA_Recipients_June_30_2022.pdf (accessed March 18, 2023).

CIS. 2022b. *DHS Publishes Fair and Humane Public Charge Rule.* https://www.uscis.gov/ newsroom/news-releases/dhs-publishes-fair-and-humane-public-charge-rule (accessed June 1, 2023).

CIS. n.d. *DACA Litigation Information and Frequently Asked Questions.* https://www.uscis. gov/humanitarian/consideration-of-deferred-action-for-childhood-arrivals-daca/daca-litigation-information-and-frequently-asked-questions (accessed March 18, 2023).

Clark, M. 2023. *Permanent Medicaid Postpartum Coverage Option, Maternal Health Infrastructure Investments in 2022 Year-End Omnibus Bill.* https://ccf.georgetown. edu/2023/01/04/permanent-medicaid-postpartum-coverage-option-maternal-health-infrastructure-investments-in-2022-year-end-omnibus-bill/ (accessed March 18, 2023).

Clark, M., and K. Johnson. 2022. *Maternal Health Policies: Will Congress Act During the Lame Duck Session?* https://ccf.georgetown.edu/2022/12/12/maternal-health-policies-will-congress-act-during-the-lame-duck-session/ (accessed March 18, 2023).

CMMI (Center for Medicare and Medicaid Innovation). n.d. *The Accountable Health Communities Health-Related Social Needs Screening tool.* Baltimore, MD: Center for Medicare and Medicaid Innovation, Centers for Medicare and Medicaid Services.

CMS (Centers for Medicare & Medicaid Services). 2020. *Value-Based Care State Medicaid Directors Letter.* https://www.cms.gov/newsroom/fact-sheets/value-based-care-state-medicaid-directors-letter (accessed March 18, 2023).

CMS. 2021a. *News Alert: CMS Releases Latest Enrollment Figures for Medicare, Medicaid, and Children's Health Insurance Program (CHIP).* https://www.cms.gov/newsroom/news-alert/cms-releases-latest-enrollment-figures-medicare-medicaid-and-childrens-health-insurance-program-chip (accessed March 18, 2023).

CMS. 2021b. *Opportunities in Medicaid and CHIP to Address Social Determinants of Health (SDOH).* Baltimore, MD: Centers for Medicare and Medicaid Services.

CMS. 2022a. *CMS framework for health equity 2022–2032.* Baltimore, MD: Office of Minority Health, Centers for Medicare and Medicaid Services.

CMS. 2022b. *HHS Proposes Rule to Strengthen Beneficiary Protections, Improve Access to Behavioral Health Care, and Promote Equity for Millions of Americans with Medicare Advantage and Medicare Part D.* https://www.cms.gov/newsroom/press-releases/hhs-proposes-rule-strengthen-beneficiary-protections-improve-access-behavioral-health-care-and (accessed March 18, 2023).

CMS. 2022c. *Washington: State Innovation Waiver.* https://www.cms.gov/files/document/1332-wa-fact-sheet.pdf (accessed March 18, 2023).

CMS. 2023a. *Accountable Health Communities Model.* https://innovation.cms.gov/innovation-models/ahcm (accessed May 30, 2023).

CMS. 2023b. *HHS Approves California's Medicaid and Children's Health Insurance Plan (CHIP) Demonstration Authority to Support Care for Justice-Involved People.* https://www.cms.gov/newsroom/press-releases/hhs-approves-californias-medicaid-and-childrens-health-insurance-plan-chip-demonstration-authority (accessed March 18, 2023).

CMS. 2023c. *Hospital Quality Initiative Public Reporting.* https://www.cms.gov/medicare/quality-initiatives-patient-assessment-instruments/hospitalqualityinits/hospitalcompare (accessed March 16, 2023).

CMS. 2023d. *NHE Fact Sheet.* https://www.cms.gov/research-statistics-data-and-systems/statistics-trends-and-reports/nationalhealthexpenddata/nhe-fact-sheet (accessed March 3, 2023).

CMS. n.d. *Section 1332: State Innovation Waivers.* https://www.cms.gov/CCIIO/Programs-and-Initiatives/State-Innovation-Waivers/Section_1332_State_Innovation_Waivers-#:~: text=Section%201332%3A%20State%20Innovation%20Waivers%20Section%201332 %20of,while%20retaining%20the%20basic%20protections%20of%20the%20ACA. (accessed March 18, 2023).

CMS.gov. 2022. *National Health Expenditure Data: Historical.* https://www.cms.gov/research-statistics-data-and-systems/statistics-trends-and-reports/nationalhealthexpenddata/nationalhealthaccountshistorical (accessed March 17, 2023).

CMS.gov. 2023a. *ACO Reach.* https://innovation.cms.gov/innovation-models/aco-reach (accessed May 30, 2023).

CMS.gov. 2023b. *Medicare Advantage Value-Based Insurance Design Model.* https:// innovation.cms.gov/innovation-models/vbid (accessed May 25, 2023).

Cohodes, S. R., D. S. Grossman, S. A. Kleiner, and M. F. Lovenheim. 2016. The effect of child health insurance access on schooling: Evidence from public insurance expansions. *The Journal of Human Resources* 51(3):727–759.

Collins, F. S., A. B. Adams, C. Aklin, T. K. Archer, M. A. Bernard, E. Boone, J. Burklow, M. K. Evans, S. Jackson, A. C. Johnson, J. Lorsch, M. R. Lowden, A. M. Napoles, A. E. Ordonez, R. Rivers, V. Rucker, T. Schwetz, J. A. Segre, L. A. Tabak, M. W. Hooper, C. Wolinetz, and U. Nih. 2021. Affirming NIH's commitment to addressing structural racism in the biomedical research enterprise. *Cell* 184(12):3075–3079.

Corallo, B., R. Garfield, J. Tolbert, and R. Rudowitz. 2021. *Medicaid enrollment churn and implications for continuous coverage policies.* San Francisco, CA: Kaiser Family Foundation.

Cornell Law School. n.d. *National Federation of Independent Business v. Sebelius (2012).* https:// www.law.cornell.edu/wex/national_federation_of_independent_business_v._sebelius_(2012) (accessed March 11, 2023).

Corner, M., R. Carey, and C. Parry. 2023. Moving the needle? Recent CMS efforts to advance health equity. *Health Law Connections*, March 1.

Coyte, P. C., G. A. Hawker, R. Croxford, C. Attard, and J. G. Wright. 1996. Variation in rheumatologists' and family physicians' perceptions of the indications for and outcomes of knee replacement surgery. *The Journal of Rheumatology* 23(4):730–738.

Crocker, A. B., A. Zeymo, J. McDermott, D. Xiao, T. J. Watson, T. DeLeire, N. Shara, K. S. Chan, and W. B. Al-Refaie. 2019. Expansion coverage and preferential utilization of cancer surgery among racial and ethnic minorities and low-income groups. *Surgery* 166(3):386–391.

CRS (Congressional Research Service). 2011. *The tax exclusion for employer-provided health insurance: Issues for Congress.* Washington, DC: Congressional Research Service.

Currie, J., and J. Gruber. 1996a. Health insurance eligibility, utilization of medical care, and child health. *The Quarterly Journal of Economics* 111(2):431–466.

Currie, J., and J. Gruber. 1996b. Saving babies: The efficacy and cost of recent changes in the Medicaid eligibility of pregnant women. *Journal of Political Economy* 104(6):1263–1296.

Daw, J. R., K. B. Backes Kozhimannil, and L. K. Admon. 2019. *High Rates of Perinatal Insurance Churn Persist After the ACA.* https://www.healthaffairs.org/content/forefront/ high-rates-perinatal-insurance-churn-persist-after-aca (accessed June 1, 2023).

Daw, J. R., G. E. Kolenic, V. K. Dalton, K. Zivin, T. Winkelman, K. B. Kozhimannil, and L. K. Admon. 2020. Racial and ethnic disparities in perinatal insurance coverage. *Obstetrics & Gynecology* 135(4):917–924.

Dawes, A. J., R. Louie, D. K. Nguyen, M. Maggard-Gibbons, P. Parikh, S. L. Ettner, C. Y. Ko, and D. S. Zingmond. 2014. The impact of continuous Medicaid enrollment on diagnosis, treatment, and survival in six surgical cancers. *Health Services Research* 49:1787–1811.

Declercq, E., R. Barnard-Mayers, L. Zephyrin, and K. Johnson. 2022. *Issue brief: The U.S. maternal health divide: The limited maternal health services and worse outcomes of states proposing new abortion restrictions.* New York, NY: The Commonwealth Fund.

Dehlendorf, C., M. I. Rodriguez, K. Levy, S. Borrero, and J. Steinauer. 2010. Disparities in family planning. *American Journal of Obstetrics & Gynecology* 202(3):214–220.

DeNavas-Walt, C., B. D. Proctor, and J. C. Smith. 2008. *Income, poverty, and health insurance coverage in the United States: 2007.* Washington, DC: Census Bureau.

Dent, R. B., A. Vichare, and J. Casimir. 2021. Addressing structural racism in the health workforce. *Medical Care* 59(10 Suppl 5):S409.

Department of the Treasury. 2023. *Tax expenditures: FY2024.* Washington, DC: Office of Tax Analysis, Department of the Treasury.

Desisto, C. L., A. Rohan, A. Handler, S. S. Awadalla, T. Johnson, and K. Rankin. 2020. The effect of continuous versus pregnancy-only Medicaid eligibility on routine postpartum care in Wisconsin, 2011–2015. *Maternal and Child Health Journal* 24(9):1138–1150.

DHA (Defense Health Agency). 2022. *Evaluation of the Tricare program: Fiscal year 2022 report to Congress.* Washington, DC: Defense Health Agency.

Diamond, L., K. Izquierdo, D. Canfield, K. Matsoukas, and F. Gany. 2019. A systematic review of the impact of patient–physician non-English language concordance on quality of care and outcomes. *Journal of General Internal Medicine* 34(8):1591–1606.

Domurat, R., I. Menashe, and W. Yin. 2021. The role of behavioral frictions in health insurance marketplace enrollment and risk: Evidence from a field experiment. *American Economic Review* 111(5):1549–1574.

Donohue, J. M., E. S. Cole, C. V. James, M. Jarlenski, J. D. Michener, and E. T. Roberts. 2022. The U.S. Medicaid program: Coverage, financing, reforms, and implications for health equity. *Journal of the American Medical Association* 328(11):1085–1099.

Duff-Brown, B. 2021. Desegregating hospitals: How Medicare's architect forced hospitals to admit Black people. *Stanford Medicine Magazine*, May 10.

Duke University Medical Center Library. 2022. *Black History Month: A Medical Perspective: Hospitals.* https://guides.mclibrary.duke.edu/blackhistorymonth/hospitals (accessed March 10, 2023).

East, C. N., S. Miller, M. Page, and L. R. Wherry. 2023. Multigenerational impacts of childhood access to the safety net: Early life exposure to Medicaid and the next generation's health. *American Economic Review* 113(1):98–135.

Eberth, J. M., P. Hung, G. A. Benavidez, J. C. Probst, W. E. Zahnd, M. K. McNatt, E. Toussaint, M. A. Merrell, E. Crouch, and O. J. Oyesode. 2022. The problem of the color line: Spatial access to hospital services for minoritized racial and ethnic groups. *Health Affairs* 41(2):237–246.

Etchegary, H., A. Pike, A. M. Patey, E. Gionet, B. Johnston, S. Goold, V. Francis, J. Grimshaw, and A. Hall. 2022. Operationalizing a patient engagement plan for health research: Sharing a codesigned planning template from a national clinical trial. *Health Expectations* 25(2):697–711.

Fahrenbach, J., M. H. Chin, E. S. Huang, M. K. Springman, S. G. Weber, and E. L. Tung. 2020. Neighborhood disadvantage and hospital quality ratings in the Medicare hospital compare program. *Medical Care* 58(4):376–383.

FDA (Food and Drug Administration). 2022. *Diversity plans to improve enrollment of participants from underrepresented racial and ethnic populations in clinical trials guidance for industry: Draft guidance.* Rockville, MD: Food and Drug Administration.

Feagin, J., and Z. Bennefield. 2014. Systemic racism and U.S. health care. *Social Science & Medicine* 103:7–14.

Feinglass, J., J. M. Cooper, K. Rydland, L. S. Tom, and M. A. Simon. 2019. Using public claims data for neighborhood level epidemiologic surveillance of breast cancer screening: Findings from evaluating a patient navigation program in Chicago's Chinatown. *Progress in Community Health Partnerships: Research, Education, and Action* 13(5):95–102.

Finer, L. B., and S. K. Henshaw. 2006. Disparities in rates of unintended pregnancy in the United States, 1994 and 2001. *Perspectives on Sexual and Reproductive Health* 38(2):90–96.

Finkelstein, A., S. Taubman, B. Wright, M. Bernstein, J. Gruber, J. P. Newhouse, H. Allen, K. Baicker, and G. Oregon Health Study. 2012. The Oregon health insurance experiment: Evidence from the first year. *The Quarterly Journal of Economics* 127(3):1057–1106.

Finkelstein, A. N., S. L. Taubman, H. L. Allen, B. J. Wright, and K. Baicker. 2016. Effect of Medicaid coverage on ED use—further evidence from Oregon's experiment. *New England Journal of Medicine* 375(16):1505–1507.

Flores, G. 2005. The impact of medical interpreter services on the quality of health care: A systematic review. *Medical Care Research and Review* 62(3):255–299.

Flores, G., and Committee on Pediatric Research. 2010. Racial and ethnic disparities in the health and health care of children. *Pediatrics* 125(4):e979–e1020.

Flores, G., M. B. Laws, S. J. Mayo, B. Zuckerman, M. Abreu, L. Medina, and E. J. Hardt. 2003. Errors in medical interpretation and their potential clinical consequences in pediatric encounters. *Pediatrics* 111(1):6–14.

Flores, G., M. Abreu, V. Brown, and S. C. Tomany-Korman. 2005. How Medicaid and the state children's health insurance program can do a better job of insuring uninsured children: The perspectives of parents of uninsured Latino children. *Ambulatory Pediatrics* 5(6):332–340.

Flores, G., C. Bridon, S. Torres, R. Perez, T. Walter, J. Brotanek, H. Lin, and S. Tomany-Korman. 2009. Improving asthma outcomes in minority children: A randomized, controlled trial of parent mentors. *Pediatrics* 124(6):1522–1532.

Flores, G., M. Abreu, C. P. Barone, R. Bachur, and H. Lin. 2012. Errors of medical interpretation and their potential clinical consequences: A comparison of professional versus ad hoc versus no interpreters. *Annals of Emergency Medicine* 60(5):545–553.

Flores, G., H. Lin, C. Walker, M. Lee, J. M. Currie, R. Allgeyer, M. Fierro, M. Henry, A. Portillo, and K. Massey. 2016. Parent mentors and insuring uninsured children: A randomized controlled trial. *Pediatrics* 137(4).

Flores, G., H. Lin, C. Walker, M. Lee, J. M. Currie, R. Allgeyer, A. Portillo, M. Henry, M. Fierro, and K. Massey. 2017. The health and healthcare impact of providing insurance coverage to uninsured children: A prospective observational study. *BMC Public Health* 17(1):553.

Flores, G., H. Lin, C. Walker, M. Lee, J. Currie, R. Allgeyer, M. Fierro, M. Henry, A. Portillo, and K. Massey. 2018. Parent mentoring program increases coverage rates for uninsured Latino children. *Health Affairs* 37(3):403–412.

Foster, D. G., M. A. Biggs, L. Ralph, C. Gerdts, S. Roberts, and M. M. Glymour. 2022. Socioeconomic outcomes of women who receive and women who are denied wanted abortions in the United States. *American Journal of Public Health* 112(9):1290–1296.

Fox, A. M., E. C. Stazyk, and W. Feng. 2020. Administrative easing: Rule reduction and Medicaid enrollment. *Public Administration Review* 80(1):104–117.

Frayne, S. M., R. B. Burns, E. J. Hardt, A. K. Rosen, and M. A. Moskowitz. 1996. The exclusion of non-English-speaking persons from research. *Journal of General Internal Medicine* 11(1):39–43.

Fraze, T., V. A. Lewis, H. P. Rodriguez, and E. S. Fisher. 2016. Housing, transportation, and food: How ACOS seek to improve population health by addressing nonmedical needs of patients. *Health Affairs* 35(11):2109–2115.

Frost, J. J., L. B. Finer, and A. Tapales. 2008. The impact of publicly funded family planning clinic services on unintended pregnancies and government cost savings. *Journal of Health Care for the Poor and Underserved* 19(3):778–796.

GAO (Government Accountability Office). 2016. *Indian Health Service: Actions needed to improve oversight of patient wait times.* Washington, DC: Government Accountability Office.

GAO. 2018. *Indian Health Service: Spending levels and characteristics of IHS and three other federal health care programs.* Washington, DC: Government Accountability Office.

Gasoyan, H., S. R. Hussain, W. G. Wright, and D. B. Sarwer. 2022. Disparities in diabetes-related lower extremity amputations in the United States: A systematic review. *Health Affairs* 41(7):985–993.

Gates, A., S. Artiga, and R. Rudowitz. 2014. *Health coverage and care for the adult criminal justice-involved population.* Menlo Park, CA: The Kaiser Commission on Medicaid and the Uninsured, The Henry J. Kaiser Family Foundation.

Gee, G. C., and C. L. Ford. 2011. Structural racism and health inequities. *Du Bois Review: Social Science Research on Race* 8(1):115–132.

Georgetown University. 2022. *Comparison of Key Maternal Health Components: Black Maternal Health Momnibus Act, House Build Back Better Language, FY 22 Appropriations and President's FY23 Budget Proposal.* https://ccf.georgetown.edu/wp-content/uploads/2022/05/Maternal-Health-Investments.pdf (accessed March 18, 2023).

Gifford, K., A. Lashbrook, S. Barth, M. Nardone, E. Hinton, M. Guth, L. Stolyar, and R. Rudowitz. 2021. *States respond to COVID-19 challenges but also take advantage of new opportunities to address long-standing issues: Results from a 50-state Medicaid budget survey for state fiscal years 2021 and 2022.* San Francisco, CA: Kaiser Family Foundation.

Gilmore, B., and E. McAuliffe. 2013. Effectiveness of community health workers delivering preventive interventions for maternal and child health in low- and middle-income countries: A systematic review. *BMC Public Health* 13(1):847.

Ginther, D. K., W. T. Schaffer, J. Schnell, B. Masimore, F. Liu, L. L. Haak, and R. Kington. 2011. Race, ethnicity, and NIH research awards. *Science* 333(6045):1015–1019.

Glied, S. A., S. R. Collins, and S. Lin. 2020. Did the ACA lower Americans' financial barriers to health care? *Health Affairs* 39(3):379–386.

Goold, S. D., C. D. Myers, M. Danis, J. Abelson, S. Barnett, K. Calhoun, E. G. Campbell, H. L. La, A. Hammad, R. P. Rosenbaum, H. M. Kim, C. Salman, L. Szymecko, and Z. E. Rowe. 2018. Members of minority and underserved communities set priorities for health research. *The Milbank Quarterly* 96(4):675–705.

Goold, S. D., M. Danis, J. Abelson, M. Gornick, L. Szymecko, C. D. Myers, Z. Rowe, H. M. Kim, and C. Salman. 2019. Evaluating community deliberations about health research priorities. *Health Expectations* 22(4):772–784.

Grady, C. D., C. Dehlendorf, E. D. Cohen, E. B. Schwarz, and S. Borrero. 2015. Racial and ethnic differences in contraceptive use among women who desire no future children, 2006–2010 National Survey of Family Growth. *Contraception* 92(1):62–70.

Green, A. R., D. R. Carney, D. J. Pallin, L. H. Ngo, K. L. Raymond, L. I. Iezzoni, and M. R. Banaji. 2007. Implicit bias among physicians and its prediction of thrombolysis decisions for Black and White patients. *Journal of General Internal Medicine* 22(9):1231–1238.

Gruber, J., and K. Simon. 2008. Crowd-out 10 years later: Have recent public insurance expansions crowded out private health insurance? *Journal of Health Economics* 27(2):201–217.

Gruber, K. J., S. H. Cupito, and C. F. Dobson. 2013. Impact of doulas on healthy birth outcomes. *The Journal of Perinatal Education* 22(1):49–58.

Guarnizo, T. 2022. *Doula Services in Medicaid: State Progress in 2022.* https://ccf.georgetown.edu/2022/06/02/doula-services-in-medicaid-state-progress-in-2022/ (accessed March 17, 2023).

Guglielminotti, J., G. Samari, A. M. Friedman, A. Lee, R. Landau, and G. Li. 2022. Nurse workforce diversity and reduced risk of severe adverse maternal outcomes. *American Journal of Obstetrics and Gynecology MFM* 4(5):100689.

Guth, M. 2022. *Section 1115 waiver watch: Approvals to address health-related social needs.* San Francisco, CA: Kaiser Family Foundation.

Guth, M., and S. Artiga. 2022. *Medicaid and Racial Health Equity.* https://www.kff.org/medicaid/issue-brief/medicaid-and-racial-health-equity/ (accessed March 18, 2023).

Guttmacher Institute. 2017. *Abortion Is a Common Experience for U.S. Women, Despite Dramatic Declines in Rates.* https://www.guttmacher.org/news-release/2017/abortion-common-experience-us-women-despite-dramatic-declines-rates (accessed March 18, 2023).

Guttmacher Institute. 2019. *Unintended Pregnancy in the United States.* https://www.guttmacher.org/fact-sheet/unintended-pregnancy-united-states (accessed March 18, 2023).

Hacker, K., M. Anies, B. L. Folb, and L. Zallman. 2015. Barriers to health care for undocumented immigrants: A literature review. *Risk Management and Healthcare Policy*
8:175–183.

Haldar, S., and M. Guth. 2021. *State Policies Connecting Justice-Involved Populations to
Medicaid Coverage and Care*. https://www.kff.org/medicaid/issue-brief/state-policies-
connecting-justice-involved-populations-to-medicaid-coverage-and-care/ (accessed March
18, 2023).

Haley, J. M., G. M. Kenney, H. Bernstein, and D. Gonzalez. 2020. *One in five adults in immigrant families with children reported chilling effects on public benefit receipt in 2019*.
Washington, DC: Urban Institute.

Haley, J. M., G. M. Kenney, H. Bernstein, and D. Gonzalez. 2021. *Many immigrant families with children continued to avoid public benefits in 2020, despite facing hardships*.
Washington, DC: Urban Institute.

Han, D. 2023. *Biden Administration Will Use Medicaid to Allow Coverage for Incarcerated Substance Use Treatment*. https://subscriber.politicopro.com/article/2023/02/
biden-administration-will-use-medicaid-to-allow-coverage-for-incarcerated-substance-
use-treatment-00083869?source=email (accessed March 18, 2023).

Hardeman, R. R., and K. B. Kozhimannil. 2016. Motivations for entering the doula profession: Perspectives from women of color. *Journal of Midwifery & Women's Health*
61(6):773–780.

Harley, E. 2006. The forgotten history of defunct Black medical schools in the 19th and 20th
centuries and the impact of the Flexner Report. *Journal of the National Medical Association* 98 9:1425–1429.

Hatcher, S. M., C. Agnew-Brune, M. Anderson, L. D. Zambrano, C. E. Rose, M. A. Jim,
A. Baugher, G. S. Liu, S. V. Patel, M. E. Evans, T. Pindyck, C. L. Dubray, J. J. Rainey,
J. Chen, C. Sadowski, K. Winglee, A. Penman-Aguilar, A. Dixit, E. Claw, C. Parshall,
E. Provost, A. Ayala, G. Gonzalez, J. Ritchey, J. Davis, V. Warren-Mears, S. Joshi, T. Weiser,
A. Echo-Hawk, A. Dominguez, A. Poel, C. Duke, I. Ransby, A. Apostolou, and J. McCol-
lum. 2020. COVID-19 among American Indian and Alaska Native persons—23 states,
January 31–July 3, 2020. *Morbidity and Mortality Weekly Report* (69):1166–1169.

Hawker, G. A., J. G. Wright, P. C. Coyte, J. I. Williams, B. Harvey, R. Glazier, and E. M.
Badley. 2000. Differences between men and women in the rate of use of hip and knee
arthroplasty. *New England Journal of Medicine* 342(14):1016–1022.

HCPLAN (Health Care Payment Learning and Action Network). 2021. *Advancing health
equity through APMS*. McLean, VA: MITRE Corporation.

HCPLAN. 2022. *Advancing health equity through APMS: Guidance on social risk adjustment*.
Baltimore, MD: Health Care Payment Learning and Action Network.

HCPLAN. n.d. *Advancing Health Equity Through APMS: Theory of Change*. https://hcp-lan.
org/apms-theory-of-change/ (accessed March 16, 2023).

Heckler, M. 1985. *Report of the Secretary's Task Force on Black & Minority Health*.
Washington, DC: Department of Health and Human Services.

Heisler, E. J., and K. P. McClanahan. 2020. *Advance Appropriations for the Indian Health Service: Issues and Options for Congress*. Washington, DC: Congressional Research Service.

HHS (Department of Health and Human Services). 2013a. *Enforcement Success Stories
Involving Persons with Limited English Proficiency*. https://www.hhs.gov/civil-rights/
for-providers/compliance-enforcement/examples/limited-english-proficiency/index.html
(accessed May 30, 2023).

HHS. 2013b. *Language access plan*. Washington, DC: Department of Health and Human
Services.

HHS. 2020. *Limited English Proficiency (LEP)*. https://www.hhs.gov/civil-rights/for-individuals/
special-topics/limited-english-proficiency/index.html (accessed March 18, 2023).

HHS. 2022a. *Equity action plan summary: U.S. Department of Health and Human Services.* Washington, DC: Department of Health and Human Services.

HHS. 2022b. *HHS Approves Groundbreaking Medicaid Initiatives in Massachusetts and Oregon.* https://www.hhs.gov/about/news/2022/09/28/hhs-approves-groundbreaking-medicaid-initiatives-in-massachusetts-and-oregon.html (accessed March 18, 2023).

HHS. 2022c. *HHS equity action plan.* Washington, DC: Department of Health and Human Services.

HHS. 2023a. *HHS Releases Report to Increase Language Access for Persons with Limited English Proficiency.* https://www.hhs.gov/about/news/2023/05/24/hhs-releases-report-increase-language-access-persons-with-limited-english-proficiency.html (accessed May 30, 2023).

HHS. 2023b. *Section 1557 of the Patient Protection and Affordable Care Act.* https://www.hhs.gov/civil-rights/for-individuals/section-1557/index.html (accessed March 18, 2023).

HHS. n.d.-a. *Education.* https://thinkculturalhealth.hhs.gov/education (accessed March 18, 2023).

HHS. n.d.-b. *Healthy People 2030 Social Determinants of Health.* https://health.gov/healthypeople/priority-areas/social-determinants-health (accessed March 7, 2023).

HHS. n.d.-c. *Healthy People 2030: Access to Primary Care.* https://health.gov/healthypeople/priority-areas/social-determinants-health/literature-summaries/access-primary-care (accessed March 18, 2023).

HHS. n.d.-d. *Healthy People 2030: Increase the Proportion of Adults Who Get Recommended Evidence-Based Preventive Health Care—AHS-08.* https://health.gov/healthypeople/objectives-and-data/browse-objectives/health-care-access-and-quality/increase-proportion-adults-who-get-recommended-evidence-based-preventive-health-care-ahs-08/data?group=Race/Ethnicity&state=United+States&from=2015&to=2 (accessed March 3, 2023).

HHS. n.d.-e. *National Culturally and Linguistically Appropriate Services Standards.* https://thinkculturalhealth.hhs.gov/clas/standards (accessed March 18, 2023).

HHS OCR (Office for Civil Rights). 2023. *Language Access Annual Progress Report.* Washington, DC: Office for Civil Rights, Department of Health and Human Services.

Hill, L., S. Artiga, and U. Ranji. 2022. Racial disparities in maternal and infant health: Current status and efforts to address them. Washington, DC: Kaiser Family Foundation.

Hill, L., N. Ndugga, and S. Artiga. 2023. *Key data on health and health care by race and ethnicity.* San Francisco, CA: Kaiser Family Foundation.

Hiraishi, K. 2022. *Native Hawaiian Health Care Will Receive $22 Million in Federal Funds.* https://www.hawaiipublicradio.org/local-news/2022-07-06/native-hawaiian-health-care-will-receive-22-million-in-federal-funds (accessed May 30, 2023).

Hoppe, T. A., A. Litovitz, K. A. Willis, R. A. Meseroll, M. J. Perkins, B. I. Hutchins, A. F. Davis, M. S. Lauer, H. A. Valantine, J. M. Anderson, and G. M. Santangelo. 2019. Topic choice contributes to the lower rate of NIH awards to African-American/black scientists. *Science Advances* 5(10):eaaw7238.

Howard University Hospital. n.d. *About Howard University Hospital.* https://www.huhealthcare.com/about-us/ (accessed March 10, 2023).

Hoyert, D. L. 2023. *Maternal mortality rates in the United States, 2021.* Atlanta, GA: National Center for Health Statistics, Centers for Disease Control and Prevention.

HRSA (Health Resources and Services Administration). 2023. *Native Hawaiian Health Care Improvement Act.* https://bphc.hrsa.gov/funding/funding-opportunities/native-hawaiian-health-care-improvement-act (accessed May 17, 2023).

HRSA. n.d. *Health Workforce Shortage Areas.* https://data.hrsa.gov/topics/health-workforce/shortage-areas (accessed March 17, 2023).

Hudson, S., and R. V. Rikard. 2018. *The case for health literacy—moving from equality to liberation.* Washington, DC: National Academy of Medicine.

Hui No Ke Ola Pono. n.d. *Get to Know Hui No Ke Ola Pono: Who we are*. https://hnkop.
  org/who-we-are/ (accessed May 17, 2023).
IHS (Indian Health Service). 2014. *Trends in Indian health: 2014 edition*. Washington, DC:
  Indian Health Service.
IHS. 2020. *IHS Profile*. https://www.ihs.gov/sites/newsroom/themes/responsive2017/display_
  objects/documents/factsheets/IHSProfile.pdf (accessed March 17, 2023).
IHS. n.d. *Locations*. https://www.ihs.gov/locations/ (accessed March 18, 2023).
ILRC (Immigrant Legal Resource Center). 2021. *Public Charge Timeline*. https://www.ilrc.
  org/sites/default/files/resources/public_charge_timeline_updated.pdf (accessed March 18,
  2023).
Inouye, D. 1993. *Perspectives on Indian health care. Remarks to forum on American In-
  dian health care reform, March 15, 1993, Washington, DC*. https://www.c-span.org/
  video/?38768-1/native-american-health-care-reform (accessed July 3, 2023).
IOM (Institute of Medicine). 2003. *Unequal treatment: Confronting racial and ethnic dispari-
  ties in health care*. Washington, DC: The National Academies Press.
IOM. 2004. *Health literacy: A prescription to end confusion*. Washington, DC: The National
  Academies Press.
IOM. 2015. *Health literacy: Past, present, and future: Workshop summary*. Washington, DC:
  The National Academies Press.
Jaffery, J. B., and D. Gelb Safran. 2021. *Addressing Social Risk Factors in Value-Based Payment:
  Adjusting Payment Not Performance to Optimize Outcomes and Fairness*. https://www.
  healthaffairs.org/do/10.1377/forefront.20210414.379479/full/ (accessed March 18, 2023).
Jim, M. A., E. Arias, D. S. Seneca, M. J. Hoopes, C. C. Jim, N. J. Johnson, and C. L.
  Wiggins. 2014. Racial misclassification of American Indians and Alaska Natives by
  Indian Health Service contract health service delivery area. *American Journal of Public
  Health* 104(Suppl 3):S295–302.
The Joint Commission. 2016. *Quick Safety 23: Implicit Bias in Health Care*. https://www.
  jointcommission.org/resources/news-and-multimedia/newsletters/newsletters/quick-
  safety/quick-safety-issue-23-implicit-bias-in-health-care/implicit-bias-in-health-care/#.
  ZBSJfRXMI2z (accessed March 17, 2023).
Jones, C. P. 2000. Levels of racism: A theoretic framework and a gardener's tale. *American
  Journal of Public Health* 90(8):1212–1215.
Jones, E., S. R. Lattof, and E. Coast. 2017. Interventions to provide culturally-appropriate
  maternity care services: Factors affecting implementation. *BMC Pregnancy and Child-
  birth* 17(1):267.
Jones, N., R. Marks, R. Ramirez, and M. Rios-Vargas. 2021. *2020 Census Illuminates
  Racial and Ethnic Composition of the Country*. https://www.census.gov/library/
  stories/2021/08/improved-race-ethnicity-measures-reveal-united-states-population-much-
  more-multiracial.html (accessed May 10, 2023).
Jordan, J. 2022. Detroit had 18 Black-owned and operated hospitals: Why they vanished.
  Detroit Free Press, February 27.
Kaiser Commission on Medicaid and the Uninsured. 2012. *A historical review of how states
  have responded to the availability of federal funds for health coverage*. Washington, DC:
  The Henry J. Kaiser Family Foundation.
Karliner, L. S., E. A. Jacobs, A. H. Chen, and S. Mutha. 2007. Do professional interpreters
  improve clinical care for patients with limited English proficiency? A systematic review
  of the literature. *Health Services Research* 42(2):727–754.
Katznelson, I. 2013. *Fear itself: The new deal and the origins of our time*. New York, NY:
  Liveright.
Katznelson, I., and Q. Mulroy. 2012. Was the South pivotal? Situated partisanship and policy
  coalitions during the New Deal and Fair Deal. *The Journal of Politics* 74(2):604–620.

Keisler-Starkey, K., and L. N. Bunch. 2022. *Health insurance coverage in the United States: 2021.* Washington, DC: Census Bureau, Department of Commerce.

Kennell, J., M. Klaus, S. McGrath, S. Robertson, and C. Hinkley. 1991. Continuous emotional support during labor in a U.S. hospital. A randomized controlled trial. *Journal of the American Medical Association* 265(17):2197–2201.

Kenney, G. M., J. M. Haley, C. Pan, V. Lynch, and M. Buettgens. 2017. *Medicaid/CHIP participation rates rose among children and parents in 2015.* Washington, DC: Urban Institute.

KFF (Kaiser Family Foundation). 2009. *New Option for States to Provide Federally Funded Medicaid and CHIP Coverage to Additional Immigrant Children and Pregnant Women.* https://www.kff.org/wp-content/uploads/2013/01/7933.pdf (accessed March 18, 2023).

KFF. 2022a. *Health Coverage and Care of Immigrants.* San Francisco, CA: Kaiser Family Foundation.

KFF. 2022b. *Table 3: State Adoption of Options to Cover Immigrant Populations, January 2022.* https://files.kff.org/attachment/Table-3-Medicaid-and-CHIP-Eligibility-and-Enrollment-Policies-as-of-January-2022.pdf (accessed March 18, 2023).

KFF. 2023a. *Explaining Litigation Challenging the ACA's Preventive Services Requirements: Braidwood Management Inc. V. Becerra.* https://www.kff.org/womens-health-policy/issue-brief/explaining-litigation-challenging-the-acas-preventive-services-requirements-braidwood-management-inc-v-becerra/ (accessed May 16, 2023).

KFF. 2023b. *Medicaid Postpartum Coverage Extension Tracker.* https://www.kff.org/medicaid/issue-brief/medicaid-postpartum-coverage-extension-tracker/ (accessed March 18, 2023).

KFF. 2023c. *Status of State Medicaid Expansion Decisions: Interactive Map.* https://www.kff.org/medicaid/issue-brief/status-of-state-medicaid-expansion-decisions-interactive-map/ (accessed March 3, 2023).

KFF. n.d.-a. *Abortion in the United States Dashboard.* https://www.kff.org/womens-health-policy/dashboard/abortion-in-the-u-s-dashboard/ (accessed March 18, 2023).

KFF. n.d.-b. *Federal Medical Assistance Percentage (FMAP) for Medicaid and Multiplier.* https://www.kff.org/medicaid/state-indicator/federal-matching-rate-and-multiplier/?currentTimeframe=0&sortModel=%7B%22colId%22:%22FMAP%20Percentage%22,%22sort%22:%22desc%22%7D (accessed March 18, 2023).

KFF. n.d.-c. *Medicaid Income Eligibility Limits for Adults as a Percent of the Federal Poverty Level.* https://www.kff.org/health-reform/state-indicator/medicaid-income-eligibility-limits-for-adults-as-a-percent-of-the-federal-poverty-level/?currentTimeframe=0&sortModel=%7B%22colId%22:%22Location%22,%22sort%22:%22asc%22%7D (accessed March 18, 2023).

KFF. n.d.-d. *Presumptive Eligibility in Medicaid and CHIP.* https://www.kff.org/health-reform/state-indicator/presumptive-eligibility-in-medicaid-chip/?currentTimeframe=0&sortModel=%7B%22colId%22:%22Location%22,%22sort%22:%22asc%22%7D# (accessed March 15, 2023).

KFF. n.d.-e. *State Health Facts: Distribution of the Nonelderly with Medicaid by Race/Ethnicity.* https://www.kff.org/medicaid/state-indicator/medicaid-distribution-nonelderly-by-raceethnicity/?currentTimeframe=0&sortModel=%7B%22colId%22:%22Location%22,%22sort%22:%22asc%22%7D (accessed March 18, 2023).

KFF. n.d.-f. *States Reporting Corrections-Related Medicaid Enrollment Policies in Place for Prisons or Jails.* https://www.kff.org/medicaid/state-indicator/states-reporting-corrections-related-medicaid-enrollment-policies-in-place-for-prisons-or-jails/?currentTimeframe=0&sortModel=%7B%22colId%22:%22Location%22,%22sort%22:%22asc%22%7D (accessed March 15, 2023).

Khalil, L., M. Leary, N. Rouphael, I. Ofotokun, P. A. Rebolledo, and Z. Wiley. 2022. Racial and ethnic diversity in SARS-COV-2 vaccine clinical trials conducted in the United States. *Vaccines* 10(2):290.

Khanijou, S. 2005. Rebalancing healthcare inequities: Language service reimbursement may ensure meaningful access to care for LEP patients. *DePaul Journal of Health Care Law* 9(1):855–884.

Khurshid, S. 2020. *"They're Conditioned to Just Ignore or Erase Us": Native Americans in New York Fear Another Census Undercount.* https://www.gothamgazette.com/state/9189-goverment-conditioned-ignore-or-erase-us-native-americans-in-new-york-2020-census-undercount (accessed March 18, 2023).

Kim, H., T. H. A. Meath, A. R. Quiñones, K. J. McConnell, and S. A. Ibrahim. 2021. Association of Medicare mandatory bundled payment program with the receipt of elective hip and knee replacement in White, Black, and Hispanic beneficiaries. *JAMA Network Open* 4(3):e211772.

Kozhimannil, K. B., L. B. Attanasio, R. R. Hardeman, and M. O'Brien. 2013. Doula care supports near-universal breastfeeding initiation among diverse, low-income women. *Journal of Midwifery & Women's Health* 58(4):378–382.

Kozhimannil, K. B., C. A. Vogelsang, and R. R. Hardeman. 2015. *Medicaid coverage of doula services in Minnesota: Preliminary findings from the first year: Interim report to the Minnesota Department of Human Services.* St. Paul, MN: Minnesota Department of Human Services.

Kozhimannil, K. B., A. Hassan, and R. R. Hardeman. 2022. Abortion access as a racial justice issue. *New England Journal of Medicine* 387(17):1537–1539.

Kozlov, M. 2023. *FDA to Require Diversity Plan for Clinical Trials.* https://www.nature.com/articles/d41586-023-00469-4?utm_source=Daily+Clips+5%2F10%2F18&utm_campaign=8c5ffce383-EMAIL_CAMPAIGN_2023_02_17_01_58&utm_medium=email&utm_term=0_-8c5ffce383-%5BLIST_EMAIL_ID%5D (accessed May 3, 2023).

Krase, K. 1996. *Sterilization Abuse: The Policies Behind the Practice.* https://nwhn.org/sterilization-abuse-the-policies-behind-the-practice/ (accessed May 2, 2023).

Ku, L., and A. Vichare. 2023. The association of racial and ethnic concordance in primary care with patient satisfaction and experience of care. *Journal of General Internal Medicine* 38(3):727–732.

Lawrence, J. 2000. The Indian health service and the sterilization of Native American women. *American Indian Quarterly* 24(3):400–419.

Lee, H., D. Hodgkin, M. P. Johnson, and F. W. Porell. 2021. Medicaid expansion and racial and ethnic disparities in access to health care: Applying the National Academy of Medicine definition of health care disparities. *INQUIRY: The Journal of Health Care Organization, Provision, and Financing* 58:004695802199129.

Lee, J. 2015. The impact of health information technology on disparity of process of care. *International Journal for Equity in Health* 14:34.

Lee, J. T., D. Polsky, R. Fitzsimmons, and R. M. Werner. 2020. Proportion of racial minority patients and patients with low socioeconomic status cared for by physician groups after joining accountable care organizations. *JAMA Network Open* 3(5):e204439.

Levine, P. B., and D. Schanzenbach. 2009. The impact of children's public health insurance expansions on educational outcomes. *Forum for Health Economics & Policy* 12(1).

Liao, J. M., A. S. Navathe, and R. M. Werner. 2020. The impact of Medicare's alternative payment models on the value of care. *Annual Review of Public Health* 41(1):551–565.

Liao, J. M., Q. Huang, S. A. Ibrahim, J. Connolly, D. S. Cousins, J. Zhu, and A. S. Navathe. 2021. Between-community low-income status and inclusion in mandatory bundled payments in Medicare's comprehensive care for joint replacement model. *JAMA Network Open* 4(3):e211016.

Lieberman, R. C. 2001. *Shifting the color line: Race and the American welfare state.* Cambridge, MA: Harvard University Press.

Lo, L. 2011. The right to understand your doctor: Protecting language access rights in health-care. *Boston College Third World Law Journal* 31:377–403.

Lofthouse, J. 2022. *Increasing funding for the Indian Health Service to improve Native American health outcomes*. Arlington, VA: Mercatus Center, George Mason University.

Logan, R. A., W. F. Wong, M. Villaire, G. Daus, T. A. Parnell, E. WIllis, and M. K. Paasche-Orlow. 2015. *Health literacy: A necessary element for achieving health equity*. Washington, DC: National Academy of Medicine.

Lundie, K., B. D'Avanzo, I. Mohyeddin, I. Rodriguez Kmec, T. Broder, G. Lessard, and T. K. Wong. 2022. *Tracking DACA recipients' access to health care*. Los Angeles, CA: National Immigration Law Center.

Lykens, K. A., and P. A. Jargowsky. 2002. Medicaid matters: Children's health and Medicaid eligibility expansions. *Journal of Policy Analysis and Management* 21(2):219–238.

Ma, M. A., D. E. Gutiérrez, J. M. Frausto, and W. K. Al-Delaimy. 2021. Minority representation in clinical trials in the United States. *Mayo Clinic Proceedings* 96(1):264–266.

MACPAC (Medicaid and CHIP Payment and Access Commission). 2018. *State children's health insurance program (CHIP)*. Washington, DC: Medicaid and CHIP Payment and Access Commission.

MACPAC. 2021a. *Chapter 3: Medicaid estate recovery: Improving policy and promoting equity*. Washington, DC: Medicaid and CHIP Payment and Access Commission.

MACPAC. 2021b. *Fact sheet: Medicaid and CHIP in the territories*. Washington, DC: Medicaid and CHIP Payment and Access Commission.

MACPAC. 2023a. *Pregnant Women*. https://www.macpac.gov/subtopic/pregnant-women/ (accessed March 15, 2023).

MACPAC. 2023b. *Section 1115 Waivers for Substance Use Disorder Treatment*. https://www.macpac.gov/subtopic/section-1115-waivers-for-substance-use-disorder-treatment/ (accessed March 15, 2023).

Manafò, E., L. Petermann, V. Vandall-Walker, and P. Mason-Lai. 2018. Patient and public engagement in priority setting: A systematic rapid review of the literature. *PLOS ONE* 13(3):e0193579.

March of Dimes. 2020. *Nowhere to go: Maternity care deserts across the U.S.: 2020 report*. Arlington, VA: March of Dimes.

Marchi, K. S., P. A. Braveman, K. Martin, M. Curtis, T. Stancil, and L. Harrison. 2013. Eligibility and enrollment in the Special Supplemental Nutrition Program for Women, Infants, and Children (WIC)—27 states and New York City, 2007–2008. *Morbidity and Mortality Weekly Report* 62(10):189–193.

Martinez, O., E. Wu, T. Sandfort, B. Dodge, A. Carballo-Dieguez, R. Pinto, S. D. Rhodes, E. Moya, and S. Chavez-Baray. 2015. Evaluating the impact of immigration policies on health status among undocumented immigrants: A systematic review. *Journal of Immigrant and Minority Health* 17(3):947–970.

Martínez Rosas, G. 2022. *Congress Has Once Again Failed Immigrant Youths*. https://www.nytimes.com/2022/12/22/opinion/daca-immigration-republicans-democrats.html (accessed March 18, 2023).

MassHealth. 2022. *Fact Sheet: Masshealth's Newly Approved 1115 Demonstration Extension Supports Accountable Care and Advances Health Equity*. https://www.mass.gov/doc/1115-waiver-extensionfact-sheet/download (accessed March 18, 2023).

Maternal Health Learning & Innovation Center. 2022. *New Black Maternal Health Momnibus Bill Tracker Provides Latest Details on Federal Legislative Activity, Visually Stunning Resources for Education and Advocacy*. https://maternalhealthlearning.org/2022/momnibus-bill-tracker-provides-latest-details-visually-stunning-resources/?utm_source=rss&utm_medium=rss&utm_campaign=momnibus-bill-tracker-provides-latest-details-visually-stunning-resources (accessed March 18, 2023).

McBride, E. 2022. Life and death of Mississippi's four Black-owned hospitals. *Jackson Advocate*, February 25.

McCoy, C., and A. Wheatley. 2023. *Bringing the U.S. Territories Closer to Medicaid Equity.* https://www.astho.org/communications/blog/bringing-us-territories-closer-to-medicaid-equity/ (accessed March 18, 2023).

McIntyre, A., M. Shepard, and M. Wagner. 2021. Can automatic retention improve health insurance market outcomes? *AEA Papers and Proceedings* 111:560–566.

McMorrow, S., and G. Kenney. 2018. *Despite Progress Under the ACA, Many New Mothers Lack Insurance Coverage.* https://www.healthaffairs.org/content/forefront/despite-progress-under-aca-many-new-mothers-lack-insurance-coverage (accessed June 1, 2023).

McMorrow, S., L. Dubay, G. M. Kenney, E. M. Johnston, and C. A. Caraveo. 2020. *Uninsured new mothers' health and health care challenges highlight the benefits of increasing postpartum Medicaid coverage.* Washington, DC: Urban Institute.

Medicaid.gov. 2021. *Medicaid and CHIP Coverage of Lawfully Residing Children & Pregnant Women.* https://www.medicaid.gov/medicaid/enrollment-strategies/medicaid-and-chip-coverage-lawfully-residing-children-pregnant-women (accessed March 18, 2023).

Medicaid.gov. 2022. *December 2021 and January 2022 Medicaid and CHIP Enrollment Trends Snapshot.* https://www.medicaid.gov/medicaid/national-medicaid-chip-program-information/downloads/dec-2021-jan-2022-medicaid-chip-enrollment-trend-snapshot.pdf (accessed March 18, 2023).

Medicaid.gov. n.d.-a. *CHIP Eligibility.* https://www.medicaid.gov/chip/eligibility/index.html (accessed May 2, 2023).

Medicaid.gov. n.d.-b. *Medicaid Eligibility.* https://www.medicaid.gov/medicaid/eligibility/index.html (accessed March 18, 2023).

Menand, L. 2001. Morton, Agassiz, and the origins of scientific racism in the United States. *The Journal of Blacks in Higher Education* (34):110–113.

Miller, S., N. Johnson, and L. R. Wherry. 2021. Medicaid and mortality: New evidence from linked survey and administrative data. *The Quarterly Journal of Economics* 136(3):1783–1829.

Miller, T. A. 2016. Health literacy and adherence to medical treatment in chronic and acute illness: A meta-analysis. *Patient Education and Counseling* 99(7):1079–1086.

Mirin, A. A. 2021. Gender disparity in the funding of diseases by the U.S. National Institutes of Health. *Journal of Women's Health* 30(7):956–963.

Misra, S., S. C. Kwon, A. F. Abraído-Lanza, P. Chebli, C. Trinh-Shevrin, and S. S. Yi. 2021. Structural racism and immigrant health in the United States. *Health Education & Behavior* 48(3):332–341.

Mohottige, D., T. S. Purnell, and L. E. Boulware. 2023. Redressing the harms of race-based kidney function estimation. *Journal of the American Medical Association* 329(11):881–882.

Montgomery Rice, V. 2021. Diversity in medical schools: A much-needed new beginning. *Journal of the American Medical Association* 325(1):23–24.

Morey, B. N. 2018. Mechanisms by which anti-immigrant stigma exacerbates racial/ethnic health disparities. *American Journal of Public Health* 108(4):460–463.

Moriya, A. S., and S. Chakravarty. 2023. Racial and ethnic disparities in preventable hospitalizations and ED visits five years after ACA Medicaid expansions. *Health Affairs* 42(1):26–34.

Morris, D. B., P. A. Gruppuso, H. A. McGee, A. L. Murillo, A. Grover, and E. Y. Adashi. 2021. Diversity of the national medical student body—four decades of inequities. *New England Journal of Medicine* 384(17):1661–1668.

Musa, A., and J. Bonifield. 2023. *Maternity Units Are Closing Across America, Forcing Expectant Mothers to Hit the Road.* https://www.cnn.com/2023/04/07/health/maternity-units-closing/index.html (accessed May 19, 2023).

Muthukumar, A. V., W. Morrell, and B. E. Bierer. 2021. Evaluating the frequency of English language requirements in clinical trial eligibility criteria: A systematic analysis using clinicaltrials.gov. *PLOS Medicine* 18(9):e1003758.

Myers, C. D., E. C. Kieffer, A. M. Fendrick, H. M. Kim, K. Calhoun, L. Szymecko, L. LaHahnn, C. Ledón, M. Danis, Z. Rowe, and S. D. Goold. 2020. How would low-income communities prioritize Medicaid spending? *Journal of Health Politics, Policy and Law* 45(3):373–418.

Mykyta, L., K. Keisler-Starkey, and L. Bunch. 2022. *Uninsured Rate of U.S. Children Fell to 5.0% in 2021.* https://www.census.gov/library/stories/2022/09/uninsured-rate-of-children-declines.html (accessed March 18, 2023).

NAM (National Academy of Medicine). 2022. *Assessing meaningful community engagement: A conceptual model to advance health equity through transformed systems for health.* Washington, DC: National Academy of Medicine.

NASEM (National Academies of Sciences, Engineering, and Medicine). 2016. *Accounting for social risk factors in Medicare payment: Identifying social risk factors.* Washington, DC: The National Academies Press.

NASEM. 2017a. *Accounting for social risk factors in Medicare payment.* Washington, DC: The National Academies Press.

NASEM. 2017b. *Communities in action: Pathways to health equity.* Washington, DC: The National Academies Press.

NASEM. 2017c. *Facilitating health communication with immigrant, refugee, and migrant populations through the use of health literacy and community engagement strategies: Proceedings of a workshop.* Washington, DC: The National Academies Press.

NASEM. 2018a. *An American crisis: The growing absence of Black men in medicine and science: Proceedings of a joint workshop.* Washington, DC: The National Academies Press.

NASEM. 2018b. *Immigration as a social determinant of health: Proceedings of a workshop.* Washington, DC: The National Academies Press.

NASEM. 2018c. *The safety and quality of abortion care in the United States.* Washington, DC: The National Academies Press.

NASEM. 2019a. *Integrating social care into the delivery of health care: Moving upstream to improve the nation's health.* Washington, DC: The National Academies Press.

NASEM. 2019b. *Vibrant and healthy kids: Aligning science, practice, and policy to advance health equity.* Washington, DC: The National Academies Press.

NASEM. 2020. *Health literacy in clinical research: Practice and impact: Proceedings of a workshop.* Washington, DC: The National Academies Press.

NASEM. 2021a. *Exploring the role of critical health literacy in addressing the social determinants of health: Proceedings of a workshop—in brief.* Washington, DC: The National Academies Press.

NASEM. 2021b. *The future of nursing 2020–2030: Charting a path to achieve health equity.* Washington, DC: The National Academies Press.

NASEM. 2021c. *Implementing high-quality primary care: Rebuilding the foundation of health care.* Washington, DC: The National Academies Press.

NASEM. 2022. *Improving representation in clinical trials and research: Building research equity for women and underrepresented groups.* Washington, DC: The National Academies Press.

NASEM. 2023a. *The roles of trust and health literacy in achieving health equity: Clinical settings: Proceedings of a workshop—in brief.* Washington, DC: The National Academies Press.

NASEM. 2023b. *The roles of trust and health literacy in achieving health equity: Community settings: Proceedings of a workshop—in brief.* Washington, DC: The National Academies Press.

NASEM. 2023c. *The roles of trust and health literacy in achieving health equity: Public health institutions: Proceedings of a workshop—in brief.* Washington, DC: The National Academies Press.

NASEM. n.d. *Roundtable on Health Literacy.* https://www.nationalacademies.org/our-work/roundtable-on-health-literacy (accessed March 18, 2023).

National Indian Health Board. 2021. *Testimony of the National Indian Health Board for the U.S. Department of Health and Human Services 23rd annual tribal budget and policy consultation.* Washington, DC: National Indian Health Board.

NBER (National Bureau of Economic Research). n.d.-a. *Oregon Health Insurance Experiment—Background.* https://www.nber.org/programs-projects/projects-and-centers/oregon-health-insurance-experiment/oregon-health-insurance-experiment-background (accessed March 17, 2023).

NBER. n.d.-b. *Oregon Health Insurance Experiment—Results.* https://www.nber.org/programs-projects/projects-and-centers/oregon-health-insurance-experiment?page=1&perPage=50 (accessed March 17, 2023).

NCUIH (National Council of Urban Indian Health). 2023a. *Final FY2023 Omnibus Bill Includes Advance Appropriations for the Indian Health Service and Several Other Priorities.* https://ncuih.org/2023/01/09/final-fy2023-omnibus-bill-includes-advance-appropriations-for-the-indian-health-service-and-several-other-priorities/ (accessed June 1, 2023).

NCUIH. 2023b. *Tribal Leaders Highlight Need for Increased Urban Indian Health Funding in Fiscal Year 2025 IHS Budget Requests.* https://ncuih.org/2023/02/02/tribal-leaders-highlight-need-for-increased-urban-indian-health-funding-in-fiscal-year-2025-ihs-budget-requests/ (accessed March 18, 2023).

Nguyen, K. H., N. C. Giron, and A. N. Trivedi. 2023. Parental immigration status, Medicaid expansion, and Supplemental Nutrition Assistance Program participation. *Health Affairs* 42(1):53–62.

NICHD (National Institute of Child Health and Human Development). 2017. *What Is Prenatal Care and Why Is It Important?* https://www.nichd.nih.gov/health/topics/pregnancy/conditioninfo/prenatal-care (accessed March 15, 2023).

NIH (National Institutes of Health). n.d. *Impact of NIH Research.* https://www.nih.gov/about-nih/what-we-do/impact-nih-research (accessed June 2, 2023).

NILC (National Immigration Law Center). 2013. *Frequently Asked Questions: Exclusion of Youth Granted "Deferred Action for Childhood Arrivals" from Affordable Care Act.* https://www.nilc.org/wp-content/uploads/2015/10/DACA-and-health-care-2013-09-25.pdf (accessed March 18, 2023).

Nirappil, F., and F. Stead Sellers. 2023. Abortion ban states see steep drop in OB/GYN residency applications. *The Washington Post*, April 21.

Nolen, L. T., A. L. Beckman, and E. Sandoe. 2020. *How Foundational Moments in Medicaid's History Reinforced Rather Than Eliminated Racial Health Disparities.* https://www.healthaffairs.org/do/10.1377/forefront.20200828.661111/ (accessed March 18, 2023).

NQF (National Quality Forum). 2014. *Risk adjustment for socioeconomic status or other sociodemographic factors.* Washington, DC: National Quality Forum.

NQF. n.d. *Risk Adjustment Guidance.* https://www.qualityforum.org/Risk_Adjustment_Guidance.aspx (accessed May 25, 2023).

O'Rourke, L. 2019. *Congress Is Holding Health, Wellbeing of U.S. Territory Residents in the Balance.* https://www.clasp.org/blog/congress-holding-health-wellbeing-us-territory-residents-balance/ (accessed March 18, 2023).

OASH (Office of the Assistant Secretary for Health). 2010. *National action plan to improve health literacy.* Washington, DC: Office of Disease Prevention and Health Promotion, Department of Health and Human Services.

OASH. 2020. *Policy of Inclusion of Women in Clinical Trials.* https://www.womenshealth.gov/30-achievements/04 (accessed March 16, 2023).

Office for Civil Rights. 2013. *Compliance review initiative: Advancing effective communication in critical access hospitals*. Washington, DC: Office for Civil Rights, Department of Health and Human Services.

Office of Inspector General. 2010a. *Guidance and standards on language access services: Medicare plans*. Washington, DC: Department of Health and Human Services.

Office of Inspector General. 2010b. *Guidance and standards on language access services: Medicare providers*. Washington, DC: Department of Health and Human Services.

Office of Senator Schatz. 2022. *Schatz: Federal Funding for Hawai'i Increases in New Appropriations Deal*. https://www.schatz.senate.gov/news/press-releases/schatz-federal-funding-for-hawaii-increases-in-new-appropriations-deal (accessed May 30, 2023).

OMB (Office of Management and Budget). 2021. *Study to identify methods to assess equity: Report to the president*. Washington, DC: Office of Management and Budget.

OMH (Office of Minority Health). 2016. *National standards for culturally and linguistically appropriate services in health and health care: Compendium of state-sponsored national CLAS standards implementation activities*. Washington, DC: Department of Health and Human Services.

OMH. 2019. *About the Office of Minority Health*. https://www.minorityhealth.hhs.gov/omh/browse.aspx?lvl=1&lvlid=1 (accessed March 18, 2023).

OMH. 2023. *Culturally and Linguistically Appropriate Standards (CLAS)*. https://minorityhealth.hhs.gov/omh/browse.aspx?lvl=1&lvlid=6 (accessed March 18, 2023).

Orgera, K., R. Rudowitz, and A. Damico. 2021. *A Closer Look at the Remaining Uninsured Population Eligible for Medicaid and CHIP*. https://www.kff.org/uninsured/issue-brief/a-closer-look-at-the-remaining-uninsured-population-eligible-for-medicaid-and-chip/ (accessed March 18, 2023).

Ornelas, I. J., T. J. Yamanis, and R. A. Ruiz. 2020. The health of undocumented Latinx immigrants: What we know and future directions. *Annual Review of Public Health* 41:289–308.

Osterman, M. J. K., B. E. Hamilton, J. A. Martin, A. K. Driscoll, and C. P. Valenzuela. 2023. *National vital statistics reports: Births: Final data for 2021*. Hyattsville, MD: National Center for Health Statistics.

Paradise, J. 2014. *The impact of the children's health insurance program (CHIP): What does the research tell us?* Menlo Park, CA: The Kaiser Commission on Medicaid and the Uninsured, The Henry J. Kaiser Family Foundation.

Paradise, J., B. Lyons, and D. Rowland. 2015. *Medicaid at 50*. Menlo Park, CA: The Kaiser Commission on Medicaid and the Uninsured, The Henry J. Kaiser Family Foundation.

Park, E., J. Alker, and A. Corcoran. 2020. *Jeopardizing a sound investment: Why short-term cuts to Medicaid coverage during pregnancy and childhood could result in long-term harm*. New York, NY: The Commonwealth Fund.

Partridge, S., J. Balayla, C. A. Holcroft, and H. A. Abenhaim. 2012. Inadequate prenatal care utilization and risks of infant mortality and poor birth outcome: A retrospective analysis of 28,729,765 U.S. deliveries over 8 years. *American Journal of Perinatology* 29(10):787–794.

Pearson, C. 2019. *Protecting and Expanding Medicaid Means Confronting Racism Baked into the Program*. https://nwhn.org/protecting-and-expanding-medicaid-means-confronting-racism-baked-into-the-program/ (accessed March 6, 2023).

Petersen, E. E., N. L. Davis, D. Goodman, S. Cox, C. Syverson, K. Seed, C. Shapiro-Mendoza, W. M. Callaghan, and W. Barfield. 2019. Racial/ethnic disparities in pregnancy-related deaths—United States, 2007–2016. *Morbidity and Mortality Weekly Report* 68(35):762.

Philbin, M. M., M. Flake, M. L. Hatzenbuehler, and J. S. Hirsch. 2018. State-level immigration and immigrant-focused policies as drivers of Latino health disparities in the United States. *Social Science & Medicine* 199:29–38.

Pierson, L. 2021. *The NIH Has the Opportunity to Address Research Funding Disparities*. https://blog.petrieflom.law.harvard.edu/2021/10/14/nih-research-funding-disparities/ (accessed June 2, 2023).

Platt, T., and N. Kaye. 2020. *Four state strategies to employ doulas to improve maternal health and birth outcomes in Medicaid*. Portland, ME: National Academy for State Health Policy.

Poll-Hunter, N. I., Z. Brown, A. Smith, S. M. Starks, R. Gregory-Bass, D. Robinson, M. D. Cullins, Q. I. Capers, A. Landry, A. Bush, K. Bellamy, N. Lubin-Johnson, C. J. Fluker, D. A. Acosta, G. H. Young, G. C. Butts, and C. M. Bright. 2023. Increasing the representation of Black men in medicine by addressing systems factors. *Academic Medicine* 98(3):304–312.

Potter, J. E., K. Coleman-Minahan, K. White, D. A. Powers, C. Dillaway, A. J. Stevenson, K. Hopkins, and D. Grossman. 2017. Contraception after delivery among publicly insured women in Texas: Use compared with preference. *Obstetrics & Gynecology* 130(2):393–402.

Provost Peters, C. 2008. *Issue brief no. 828: Medicaid financing: How the FMAP formula works and why it falls short*. Washington, DC: National Health Policy Forum, George Washington University.

Race Forward, and PolicyLink. 2023. *Assessment of federal equity action plans*. Oakland, CA: PolicyLink.

Radley, D. C., J. C. Baumgartner, S. R. Collins, L. Zephyrin, and E. C. Schneider. 2021. *Achieving racial and ethnic equity in U.S. health care: A scorecard of state performance*. New York, NY: The Commonwealth Fund.

Ramamoorthy, A., M. Pacanowski, J. Bull, and L. Zhang. 2015. Racial/ethnic differences in drug disposition and response: Review of recently approved drugs. *Clinical Pharmacology & Therapeutics* 97(3):263–273.

Redd, S. K., W. S. Rice, M. S. Aswani, S. Blake, Z. Julian, B. Sen, M. Wingate, and K. S. Hall. 2021. Racial/ethnic and educational inequities in restrictive abortion policy variation and adverse birth outcomes in the United States. *BMC Health Services Research* 21(1):1139.

Reyes, R. A. 2016. *"No Mas Bebes" Looks Back at L.A. Mexican Moms' Involuntary Sterilizations*. https://www.nbcnews.com/news/latino/no-m-s-beb-s-looks-back-l-mexican-moms-n505256 (accessed May 2, 2023).

Robles-Fradet, A. 2021. *Medicaid Coverage for Doula Care: State Implementation Efforts*. https://healthlaw.org/medicaid-coverage-for-doula-care-state-implementation-efforts/ (accessed June 1, 2023).

Rosenbaum, S. 2022. *A Public Health Paradox: States with Strictest Abortion Laws Have Weakest Maternal and Child Health Outcomes*. https://www.commonwealthfund.org/blog/2022/public-health-paradox-states-abortion-laws-maternal-child-health-outcomes (accessed March 18, 2023).

Rudich, J., D. K. Branham, C. Peters, and B. D. Sommers. 2022. *Estimates of uninsured adults newly eligible for Medicaid if remaining non-expansion states expand*. Washington, DC: Office of the Assistant Secretary for Planning and Evaluation, Department of Health and Human Services.

Rudowitz, R., R. Garfield, and E. Hinton. 2019. *10 things to know about Medicaid: Setting the facts straight*. San Francisco, CA: Kaiser Family Foundation.

Saadi, A., U. Sanchez Molina, A. Franco-Vasquez, M. Inkelas, and G. W. Ryan. 2020. Assessment of perspectives on health care system efforts to mitigate perceived risks among immigrants in the United States: A qualitative study. *JAMA Network Open* 3(4):e203028.

Sabin, J. A. 2022. Tackling implicit bias in health care. *New England Journal of Medicine* 387(2):105–107.

Saenz, R., and D. L. Poston, Jr. 2020. *Children of Color Projected to Be Majority of U.S. Youth This Year*. https://www.pbs.org/newshour/nation/children-of-color-projected-to-be-majority-of-u-s-youth-this-year (accessed May 10, 2023).

Schaettle, R. P., R. S. Kapaln, V. S. Lee, M. D. Parkinsin, G. H. Gorman, and M. Browne. 2021. Mobilizing the U.S. military's Tricare program for value-based care: A report from the Defense Health Board. *Military Medicine* 187(1-2):12–16.

Schwartz, M. B., H. O. N. Chambliss, K. D. Brownell, S. N. Blair, and C. Billington. 2003. Weight bias among health professionals specializing in obesity. *Obesity Research* 11(9):1033–1039.

Sequist, T. D., T. Cullen, K. Bernard, S. Shaykevich, E. J. Orav, and J. Z. Ayanian. 2011. Trends in quality of care and barriers to improvement in the Indian Health Service. *Journal of General Internal Medicine* 26(5):480–486.

Shane, L. 2022. *VA to Get $300b, Its Biggest Budget Ever, Under Federal Spending Deal.* https://www.militarytimes.com/veterans/2022/12/20/va-to-get-300b-its-biggest-budget-ever-under-federal-spending-deal/ (accessed March 18, 2023).

Shepard, M., and M. Wagner. 2022. *NBER working paper 30781: Reducing ordeals through automatic enrollment: Evidence from a health insurance exchange.* Cambridge, MA: National Bureau of Economic Research.

Sheridan, S. L., D. J. Halpern, A. J. Viera, N. D. Berkman, K. E. Donahue, and K. Crotty. 2011. Interventions for individuals with low health literacy: A systematic review. *Journal of Health Communication* 16(Sup3):30–54.

Simon, M. A., L. S. Tom, N. J. Nonzee, K. R. Murphy, R. Endress, X. Dong, and J. Feinglass. 2015. Evaluating a bilingual patient navigation program for uninsured women with abnormal screening tests for breast and cervical cancer: Implications for future navigator research. *American Journal of Public Health* 105(5):e87–e94.

Simon, M. A., L. S. Tom, I. Leung, E. Wong, E. E. Knightly, D. P. Vicencio, A. Yau, K. Ortigara, and X. Dong. 2019. The Chinatown Patient Navigation Program: Adaptation and implementation of breast and cervical cancer patient navigation in Chicago's Chinatown. *Health Services Insights* 12:1178632919841376.

Simon, M., C. Baur, S. Guastello, K. Ramiah, J. Tufte, K. Wisdom, M. Johnston-Fleece, A. Cupito, and A. Anise. 2020. *NAM perspectives: Patient and family engaged care: An essential element of health equity.* Washington, DC: National Academy of Medicine.

Skocpol, T. 1995. *Protecting soldiers and mothers: The political origins of social policy in the United States.* Cambridge, MA: The Belknap Press of Harvard University Press.

Smedley, A., and B. D. Smedley. 2005. Race as biology is fiction, racism as a social problem is real: Anthropological and historical perspectives on the social construction of race. *American Psychologist* 60(1):16–26.

Smedley, B. D. 2012. The lived experience of race and its health consequences. *American Journal of Public Health* 102(5):933–935.

Snowden, L. R., and E. Michaels. 2023. Racial bias correlates with states having fewer health professional shortage areas and fewer federally qualified community health center sites. *Journal of Racial and Ethnic Health Disparities* 10(1):325–333.

Snyder, L., and R. Rudowitz. 2015. *Issue brief: Medicaid financing: How does it work and what are the implications?* Menlo Park, CA: The Kaiser Commission on Medicaid and the Uninsured, The Henry J. Kaiser Family Foundation.

Solomon, J. 2021. *Closing the coverage gap would improve Black maternal health.* Washington, DC: Center on Budget and Policy Priorities.

Sonenberg, A., and D. J. Mason. 2023. Maternity care deserts in the U.S. *JAMA Health Forum* 4(1):e225541.

Steenland, M. W., and L. R. Wherry. 2023. Medicaid expansion led to reductions in postpartum hospitalizations: Study examines the impact of Medicaid expansion on postpartum hospitalizations of low-income enrollees. *Health Affairs* 42(1):18–25.

Stevenson, A. J. 2021. The pregnancy-related mortality impact of a total abortion ban in the United States: A research note on increased deaths due to remaining pregnant. *Demography* 58(6):2019–2028.

Stolyar, L., J. Tolbert, B. Corallo, R. Rudowitz, J. Sharac, P. Shin, and S. Rosenbaum. 2021. *Community health centers in the U.S. territories and the freely associated states*. San Francisco, CA: Kaiser Family Foundation.

Sudhinaraset, M., I. Ling, T. M. To, J. Melo, and T. Quach. 2017. Dreams deferred: Contextualizing the health and psychosocial needs of undocumented Asian and Pacific Islander young adults in northern California. *Social Science & Medicine* 184:144–152.

Taffe, M. A., and N. W. Gilpin. 2021. Racial inequity in grant funding from the U.S. National Institutes of Health. *eLife* 10:e65697.

Tax Policy Center. 2020. *The Tax Policy Center's briefing book: A citizen's guide to the tax system and tax policy*. Washington, DC: Urban-Brookings Tax Policy Center.

Taylor, C. R., G. R. Alexander, and J. T. Hepworth. 2005. Clustering of U.S. women receiving no prenatal care: Differences in pregnancy outcomes and implications for targeting interventions. *Maternal and Child Health Journal* 9(2):125–133.

Tikkanen, R., M. Z. Gunja, M. FitzGerald, and L. Zephyrin. 2020. *Maternal mortality and maternity care in the United States compared to 10 other developed countries*. New York, NY: The Commonwealth Fund.

Tolbert, J., and M. Ammula. 2023. *10 Things to Know About the Unwinding of the Medicaid Continuous Enrollment Provision*. https://www.kff.org/medicaid/issue-brief/10-things-to-know-about-the-unwinding-of-the-medicaid-continuous-enrollment-provision/ (accessed March 18, 2023).

Tolbert, J., K. Orgera, N. Singer, and A. Damico. 2022. *Key facts about the uninsured population*. San Francisco, CA: Kaiser Family Foundation.

Tollestrup, J. 2021. *Overview of funding mechanisms in the federal budget process, and selected examples*. Washington, DC: Congressional Research Service.

Tollestrup, J., and K. P. McClanahan. 2019. *Advance appropriations, forward funding, and advance funding: Concepts, practice, and budget process considerations*. Washington, DC: Congressional Research Service.

Tong, M., and S. Artiga. 2021. *Use of race in clinical diagnosis and decision making: Overview and implications*. San Francisco, CA: Kaiser Family Foundation.

Torpy, S. J. 2000. Native American women and coerced sterilization: On the Trail of Tears in the 1970s. *American Indian Culture and Research Journal* 24(2):1–22.

Tribal Budget Formulation Workgroup. 2022. *Advancing health equity through the federal trust responsibility: Full mandatory funding for the Indian Health Service and strengthening nation-to-nation relationships*. Washington, DC: National Indian Health Board.

Trost, S., J. Beauregard, G. Chandra, F. Njie, J. Berry, A. Harvey, and D. A. Goodman. 2022. *Pregnancy-related deaths: Data from maternal mortality review committees in 36 U.S. states, 2017–2019*. Atlanta, GA: Centers for Disease Control and Prevention.

Troutman, M., S. Rafique, and T. C. Plowden. 2020. Are higher unintended pregnancy rates among minorities a result of disparate access to contraception? *Contraception and Reproductive Medicine* 5(1):16.

University of Wisconsin Population Health Institute. 2023. *County Health Rankings Model*. https://www.countyhealthrankings.org/explore-health-rankings/county-health-rankings-model (accessed June, 2023).

USAFacts. 2022. *Our Changing Population: New York*. https://usafacts.org/data/topics/people-society/population-and-demographics/our-changing-population/state/new-york?utm_source=google&utm_medium=cpc&utm_campaign=ND-DemPop&gclid=Cj0KCQjwwt WgBhDhARIsAEMcxeB_txs_li1ejD1ToTjm00Uz3m6_0Y1NWUOk6fHHczoojqzf2fWF kzQaAr8jEALw_wcB (accessed March 17, 2023).

U.S. Commission on Civil Rights. 2004. *Broken promises: Evaluating the Native American health care system.* Washington, DC: U.S. Commission on Civil Rights.

U.S. Commission on Civil Rights. 2019. *Are rights a reality? Evaluating federal civil rights enforcement.* Washington, DC: U.S. Commission on Civil Rights.

VA (Department of Veterans Affairs). 2022. *Veterans Health Administration.* https://www.va.gov/health/ (accessed May 9, 2023).

Van Eijk, M. S., G. A. Guenther, A. D. Jopson, S. M. Skillman, and B. K. Frogner. 2022a. Health workforce challenges impact the development of robust doula services for underserved and marginalized populations in the United States. *The Journal of Perinatal Education* 31(3):133–141.

Van Eijk, M. S., G. A. Guenther, P. M. Kett, A. D. Jopson, B. K. Frogner, and S. M. Skillman. 2022b. Addressing systemic racism in birth doula services to reduce health inequities in the United States. *Health Equity* 6(1):98–105.

Van Ryn, M., D. J. Burgess, J. F. Dovidio, S. M. Phelan, S. Saha, J. Malat, J. M. Griffin, S. S. Fu, and S. Perry. 2011. The impact of racism on clinician cognition, behavior, and clinical decision making. *Du Bois Review: Social Science Research on Race* 8(1):199–218.

Varney, S., and M. Lenei Buhre. 2023. *Idaho's Strict Abortion Laws Create Uncertainty for OB-Gyns in the State.* https://www.pbs.org/newshour/show/idahos-strict-abortion-laws-create-uncertainty-for-ob-gyns-in-the-state (accessed May 19, 2023).

Vespa, J., L. Medina, and D. M. Armstrong. 2020. *Demographic turning points for the United States: Population projections for 2020 to 2060.* Washington, DC: United States Census Bureau.

Vyas, D. A., D. S. Jones, A. R. Meadows, K. Diouf, N. M. Nour, and J. Schantz-Dunn. 2019. Challenging the use of race in the Vaginal Birth After Cesarean Section Calculator. *Women's Health Issues* 29(3):201–204.

Vyas, D. A., L. G. Eisenstein, and D. S. Jones. 2020. Hidden in plain sight—reconsidering the use of race correction in clinical algorithms. *New England Journal of Medicine* 383(9):874–882.

Wallace, D., and X. Wang. 2020. Does in-prison physical and mental health impact recidivism? *SSM—Population Health* 11:100569.

Wallace, J., A. Lollo, K. A. Duchowny, M. Lavallee, and C. D. Ndumele. 2022. Disparities in health care spending and utilization among Black and White Medicaid enrollees. *JAMA Health Forum* 3(6):e221398.

Wallis, B. 1995. Black bodies, White science: Louis Agassiz's slave daguerreotypes. *American Art* 9(2):39–61.

Washington, V., K. DeSalvo, F. Mostashari, and D. Blumenthal. 2017. The HITECH era and the path forward. *New England Journal of Medicine* 377(10):904–906.

Watson, M. M. 2018. Documentation and coding practices for risk adjustment and hierarchical condition categories. *Journal of AHIMA* 89(6).

Werner, R. M. 2005. The unintended consequences of publicly reporting quality information. *Journal of the American Medical Association* 293(10):1239–1244.

Werner, R. M., D. A. Asch, and D. Polsky. 2005. Racial profiling: The unintended consequences of coronary artery bypass graft report cards. *Circulation* 111(10):1257–1263.

Wherry, L. R., and B. D. Meyer. 2016. Saving teens: Using a policy discontinuity to estimate the effects of Medicaid eligibility. *Journal of Human Resources* 51(3):556–588.

The White House. 2022. *White House blueprint for addressing the maternal health crisis.* Washington, DC: White House.

The White House. 2023. *Budget of the U.S. government: Fiscal year 2024.* Washington, DC: Office of Management and Budget.

Whitener, K., and J. Alker. 2020. *Covering all children.* Washington, DC: Georgetown University Center for Children and Families.

Whitner, K. 2022. *Research Shows More Can Be Done to Ensure Eligible Immigrant Children and Families Get Access to Health Coverage.* https://ccf.georgetown.edu/2022/09/07/research-shows-more-can-be-done-to-ensure-eligible-immigrant-children-and-families-get-access-to-health-coverage/ (accessed March 18, 2023).

Wikle, S., J. Wagner, F. Erzouki, and J. Sullivan. 2022. *States can reduce Medicaid's administrative burdens to advance health and racial equity.* Washington, DC: Center on Budget and Policy Priorities.

Williams, D. R., J. A. Lawrence, B. A. Davis, and C. Vu. 2019. Understanding how discrimination can affect health. *Health Services Research* 54:1374–1388.

Williams, E., B. Corallo, J. Tolbert, A. Burns, and R. Rudowitz. 2022. *Implications of continuous eligibility policies for children's Medicaid enrollment churn.* San Francisco, CA: Kaiser Family Foundation.

Williams, M. V., L. T. Martin, L. M. Davis, L. Warren May, and A. Y. Kim. 2018. *Evaluation of the national CLAS standards: Tips and resources.* Washington, DC: Office of Minority Health, Department of Health and Human Services.

Wilson, F. A., Y. Wang, L. N. Borrell, S. Bae, and J. P. Stimpson. 2018. Disparities in oral health by immigration status in the United States. *Journal of the American Dental Association* 149(6):414–421.e413.

Wint, K., T. I. Elias, G. Mendez, D. D. Mendez, and T. L. Gary-Webb. 2019. Experiences of community doulas working with low-income, African American mothers. *Health Equity* 3(1):109–116.

Wright, B. J., G. Garcia-Alexander, M. A. Weller, and K. Baicker. 2017. Low-cost behavioral nudges increase Medicaid take-up among eligible residents of Oregon. *Health Affairs* 36(5):838–845.

Wright, J. G., P. Coyte, G. Hawker, C. Bombardier, D. Cooke, D. Heck, R. Dittus, and D. Freund. 1995. Variation in orthopedic surgeons' perceptions of the indications for and outcomes of knee replacement. *Canadian Medical Association Journal* 152(5):687–697.

Yasaitis, L. C., W. Pajerowski, D. Polsky, and R. M. Werner. 2016. Physicians' participation in ACOS is lower in places with vulnerable populations than in more affluent communities. *Health Affairs* 35(8):1382–1390.

Yearby, R., B. Clark, and J. F. Figueroa. 2022. Structural racism in historical and modern U.S. health care policy. *Health Affairs* 41(2):187–194.

6

Neighborhood and Built Environment

The places where people live, work, learn, play, age, and pray can have significant effects on individual and community health outcomes. This includes, for example, homes, schools, workplaces, places of worship, grocery stores, transportation infrastructure, green spaces, and playgrounds. Each of these environments affects the availability, accessibility, affordability, placement, and condition of the goods and services that enable communities to live and thrive. This chapter reviews the ways that federal policies related to the built environment contribute to or help alleviate racial, ethnic, and tribal health inequities. The chapter examines underlying issues around four key themes within the neighborhood and built environment domain:

1. Housing insecurity and segregation (redlining, housing on American Indian and Alaska Native [AIAN] reservations and Native Hawaiian homelands, and federal rental assistance);
2. Disinvestment in infrastructure and the built environment (policies related to water, transportation, and aging and green infrastructure);
3. Environmental exposures that threaten health and well-being, particularly in the workplace (the Worker Protection Standard [WPS] and exposure to pesticides); and
4. Food access and production (the Farm Bill and Food Distribution Program on Indian Reservations).

Examples throughout the chapter illustrate the role that federal policies play in creating or mitigating inequities within neighborhoods and built environments; such inequities require solutions that account for different needs in rural, tribal, and urban areas. A comprehensive approach is necessary because many of these problems are pervasive and overlapping. For instance, historical housing discrimination and redlining (and, conversely, "greenlining") caused inequities that continue today, including reduced homeownership and reduced access to affordable housing for many racially and ethnically minoritized populations (see the section later in this chapter and Chapter 3 for more information on redlining). Discrimination leads to segregation, which is made worse by disinvestment in low-income communities (Banaji et al., 2021; NASEM, 2017; Ray et al., 2021; Solomon et al., 2019; Turner and Greene, n.d.; Williams and Collins, 2001). Social and economic segregation can have negative effects on housing quality, location, surrounding resources, including food and green spaces, and ability to build wealth (NASEM, 2017; Ray et al., 2021; Williams and Collins, 2001). Exposure to toxic pollutants in the air, soil, and water are more common in areas with a heavier concentration of racially and ethnically minoritized populations and made worse by inadequate and degrading infrastructure in segregated and disinvested neighborhoods. As discussed in Chapter 1, this and other report chapters could not cover all relevant topics and federal policies (see Chapter 1 for the committee's policy selection process). Rather, the committee reviewed a range of topics to illustrate how federal policies—historical and current—have impacted racial, ethnic, and tribal inequities.

STRUCTURED INSECURITY:
HOUSING SEGREGATION AND DISPLACEMENT

Having a safe, high-quality, and affordable place to live is an important component of a healthy life. This section reviews how housing conditions, locations, and federal underinvestment have increased racial, ethnic, and tribal health inequities and describes an effective federal-level intervention to help more people and families afford homes and improve well-being of adults and children alike. Housing location and neighborhood conditions also affect health, from factors such as multiresidence housing and housing density, to neighborhood violence and crime, to walkability and accessibility of green spaces, and proximity to supermarkets, public transportation options, and other integral community resources (NASEM, 2017).

On average, Americans spend more than 90 percent of their time indoors, in environments from schools to offices to homes (EPA, 2021). Physical conditions of housing, including home structure and design, can affect health through inadequate ventilation, lack of air conditioning or heating, and the infiltration of air pollution and noise. Biological and chemical factors, such as mold, allergens (e.g., dust mites), pests, lead, radon, and carbon monoxide, also affect health (NASEM, 2017, 2019b; Taylor, 2018). For example, mold and allergens can exacerbate asthma and other respiratory symptoms (CDC, 2022a; CDC and HUD, 2006; IOM, 2004). Insect and rodent pests can aggravate respiratory conditions and introduce other health risks (CDC and HUD, 2006). Radon exposure causes lung cancer. In homes with a lack of adequate ventilation, carbon monoxide can accumulate and cause fatalities. Particulate matter exacerbates respiratory and cardiovascular conditions (EPA, 2022b). Conditions of homes and surrounding areas were also associated with COVID-19 incidence and mortality, including factors such as lack of access to adequate plumbing, crowding, inadequate air circulation, air pollution, and lack of access to parks and health care services (Ahmad et al., 2020; Frumkin, 2021; Rollston and Galea, 2020). For each of these harmful living conditions, research has shown that low-income and racialized groups are disproportionately exposed (Hanna-Attisha et al., 2016; Jacobs, 2011; Tessum et al., 2021). Consideration of structure durability, efficiency, long-term maintenance, and reinvestment in home design and construction are also important factors (Department of Energy, n.d.; Gibson, 2017; Newport Partners and ARES Consulting, 2015).

Household lead is a particular issue for children. Exposure to this neurotoxin from old paint and water infrastructure slows child growth and development and damages the brain and central nervous system, influencing learning and academic achievement, behavior and attention span, hearing, and speech (CDC, 2022c). Lead poisoning prevention policies, such as the bans on lead in paint (in 1978), gasoline, and canned food and the federal Residential Lead-Based Paint Hazard Reduction Act of 1992,[1] are public health successes and have drastically reduced childhood lead exposure (NASEM, 2019b; Weitzman et al., 2013). However, lead poisoning continues to disproportionately affect racially and ethnically minoritized children, children from low-income families, and those living in older housing (CDC, 2021; Hanna-Attisha et al., 2016; Jacobs, 2011; Weitzman et al., 2013). The Department of Housing and Urban Development (HUD) is responsible for identifying lead paint hazards in HUD-assisted housing but has not completed a comprehensive evaluation of the Project-Based Rental Assistance Program to distinguish properties presenting the greatest risk to children under age 6 (GAO, 2020). According to the Government Accountability Office, about one in five such properties have at least one building from 1978 or earlier and are home to more than 138,000 children under age 6 (GAO, 2020); similarly, approximately 229,000 children under age 6 in HUD's voucher program live in units built before 1978 (GAO, 2021). Remediating lead paint is part of the Biden-Harris Lead Pipe and Paint Action Plan (The White House, 2021). Additionally, in 2023, HUD announced $165 million in grant opportunities for public housing agencies to evaluate

---

[1] 42 U.S.C. § 4851 *et seq.*

and mitigate lead-based paint, among other threats to residents' health; additional grant money is available for state and local governments to reduce lead-based paint hazards in privately owned housing (HUD, 2023).

Segregation and Health

Redlining

The disparity in access to and quality of U.S. homes has been exacerbated by federal policies—past and present—that segregate neighborhoods, exposing specific communities to precarious health outcomes. For example, although redlining, an explicitly racist mortgage lending policy of the federal government from the 1930s to the 1960s, is now unlawful,[2] its legacy of structural racism is still observable today in patterns of neighborhood disinvestment and residential segregation by race and consequent effects on other social determinants of health (SDOH), such as intergenerational wealth accumulation (Bailey et al., 2017; Barber et al., 2022; Braveman et al., 2022; Williams et al., 2019). Differences in home values and ownership and credit scores by race and ethnicity endure in formerly redlined areas (Braveman et al., 2022). Furthermore, residential segregation is associated with increased rates of homicides and other crimes in disinvested Black and Latino/a neighborhoods, which then reinforce racialized punitive policing and community depletion (Bailey et al., 2017). Redlining and the norms, policies, and structures that sustained it also continue to adversely affect the natural environment and human health in the selective placement of mobile and stationary pollution sources, such as roads and traffic, rail lines, ports, and industrial facilities (Bailey et al., 2017). For example, studies have found historically redlined neighborhoods are consistently associated with modern air pollution levels (NO_2 and $PM_{2.5}$) (Lane et al., 2022) and with higher flood risk (Conzelmann et al., 2023; Katz, 2021). Additionally, a 2020 study of 108 U.S. cities found that a lack of tree canopy and extensive infrastructure amplified temperatures in historically redlined areas, such as parts of Denver, Colorado; Minneapolis, Minnesota; and Portland, Oregon (Hoffman et al., 2020). Redlining is associated with other negative health outcomes as well (Jadow et al., 2023; Lee et al., 2022). A meta-analysis and systematic review found the odds of a preterm birth were 41 percent higher in a historically redlined neighborhood than in a nonredlined neighborhood (95 percent CI: 1.05–1.88, p = 0.02) (Lee et al., 2022). Researchers found other health outcomes, such as gunshot injuries, heat-related illness, and multiple chronic conditions, including

---

[2] Discriminatory lending practices by private lenders resulting in redlining still occur (see, for example, DOJ, 2023; Glantz and Martinez, 2018; Zaru, 2023).

asthma and some cancers, were also associated with living in a historically redlined neighborhood (Lee et al., 2022). More recent research has shown that historic redlining practices continue to produce unhealthy food access options for low-income and racialized neighborhoods (Shaker et al., 2022).

Homeownership plays a significant role in wealth generation. As a system, redlining produced disinvested Black neighborhoods by denying access to credit while valuing and directing investment to White neighborhoods, which increased in appraisal value and concentrated wealth ("greenlining") (Aaronson et al., 2021; Domonoske, 2016; Faber, 2020; Howell, 2006; Perry and Harshbarger, 2019; Rothstein, 2017; Szto, 2013). The systematic advantaging of high-income, predominately White communities continues in policies and practices by public and private actors, including through gentrification patterns that see an influx of residents with higher socioeconomic status in neighborhoods after reinvestment and development, usually accompanied by higher home values and rents. Although gentrification can provide economic benefits and improved neighborhood conditions, it can also displace the incumbent neighborhood residents and businesses; there is a role for government to reduce these risks (Dorazio, 2022; Hwang and Ding, 2020; Levy et al., 2006; NASEM, 2017; O'Regan, 2016; Rothstein, 2017; Smith et al., 2020; Zuk et al., 2015; Zuliaga, 2019). For example, gentrification is associated with more economic change in formerly redlined neighborhoods and also greater city-level economic inequality (Mitchell and Franco, 2018). See Chapter 3 for more information on wealth and homeownership and the connection to health.

Displacement and Health: Housing for American Indian and Alaska Native and Native Hawaiian People

Federally mandated and supported segregation and displacement have been uniquely harmful to AIAN individuals. Federal government actions encouraging settler colonialism through, in part, forcible removal of AIAN people from their traditional, ancestral lands caused intergenerational physical, spiritual, mental, emotional, economic, and environmental harms, including death and population loss (Hoss, 2019; NASEM, 2017). The United States has had five major federal Indian policy periods spanning from the early 1800s to the present day (see Chapter 2 for more information). The first of these was Removal and Reservation (1830–1886). The goal was to remove American Indians from their lands, starting on the east coast as more Europeans arrived. President Andrew Jackson used the Removal Act[3] to buy lands in the west to remain under federal trust to move American Indians away from the European settlers. These became known

---

[3] Act of May 28, 1830.

as "reserved lands" or "reservations." Today, 326 areas are held in reserve and 574 tribes are federally recognized (BIA, 2017; Schwartz, 2023). Some tribes have no reserved lands, and multiple tribes are sometimes assigned to the same land (Fitzpatrick, 2021). A study estimated the effects of this dispossession and found present-day land density and spread has been reduced almost 99 percent (Farrell et al., 2021). These predominantly rural reservations frequently have fewer resources and are far from the tribes' native lands, often undesirable and unfarmable, and in environments now more at risk for climate change hazards (Farrell et al., 2021; Maillacheruvu, 2022; Nikolaus et al., 2022). The built environment is often still lacking or subpar. These past federal policies affect contemporary SDOH for these populations, including the neighborhood and built environment (Miletić et al., 2022; NASEM, 2017; U.S. Commission on Civil Rights, 2018).

For example, housing is often inadequate and substandard, leaving portions of the trust obligation unfulfilled (NCAI, 2021; Pindus et al., 2017; U.S. Commission on Civil Rights, 2018). Reservations have both a lack of affordable housing and pervasive poor conditions within the existing housing stock (U.S. Commission on Civil Rights, 2018). As a report from the U.S. Commission on Civil Rights concluded, this is tied to inadequate federal funding for programs meant for AIAN people across the government (U.S. Commission on Civil Rights, 2018). This is echoed by the National Congress of American Indians, which finds that 40 percent of reservation housing is inadequate (NCAI, n.d.). Housing conditions vary regionally, but overcrowding is more common than among the nation as a whole, as are severe deficiencies in necessities, such as plumbing, water and sanitation, heating, electricity, and other utilities (NCAI, n.d.; Pindus et al., 2017; U.S. Commission on Civil Rights, 2018), putting AIAN people living in these conditions at risk of the health effects described early in this chapter.

The Native American Housing Assistance and Self-Determination Act of 1996[4] is the main source of federal assistance for affordable, safe, accessible housing for AIAN and Native Hawaiian people. A bipartisan group of senators introduced the Native American Housing Assistance and Self-Determination Reauthorization Act of 2021[5] to reauthorize the bill's programs through FY2032 (National Low Income Housing Coalition, 2021); the act was favorably passed out of the Senate Committee on Indian Affairs in February 2022 but has not yet been voted on by the full senate (Senate Committee on Indian Affairs, 2022). The act includes the Indian Housing Block Grant, a formula-based program that directly funds tribes (or tribally designated housing entities) to build, acquire, or rehabilitate affordable housing. It furthers tribal self-determination by providing direct funds to tribes and supporting them in developing housing programs based on

---

[4] 25 U.S.C. § 4101 *et seq.*
[5] S. 2264, 117th Congress (2021).

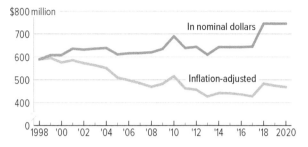

FIGURE 6-1 Funding for the tribal housing program has less buying power now than when created: Amount of Indian Housing Block Grant funds appropriated, 1998–2020.
NOTE: The increases in funding starting in fiscal year 2018 are largely from a pot of funding allocated to some tribes through a competition instead of to all tribes through the established formula.
SOURCE: Acosta, 2021. This material was created by the Center on Budget and Policy Priorities (www.cbpp.org).

community needs and priorities (U.S. Commission on Civil Rights, 2018). The grant provides funds that tribal governments can use to finance rental assistance for AIAN people living on tribal lands (CBPP, 2022b). However, grant funding has remained relatively flat since its inception and not kept pace with inflation or demand for housing, eroding tribes' buying power and limiting their ability to increase total housing available and maintain aging housing (Acosta, 2021; Pindus et al., 2017; U.S. Commission on Civil Rights, 2018) (see Figure 6-1).

The American Rescue Plan included $555 million for the Indian Housing Block Grant, half allocated through its traditional formula and half through a competitive grant process. The plan also included funds for the Indian Community Development Block Grant, which could be used for housing (Acosta, 2021). This is needed progress and in line with the U.S. Commission on Civil Rights recommendation that the federal government provide steady, direct funding to support housing, reauthorize the Native American Housing Assistance and Self-Determination Act of 1996, and increase appropriations to the Indian Housing Block Grant (U.S. Commission on Civil Rights, 2018).

Native Hawaiians were also dispossessed of their traditional land in the illegal annexation and colonization of Hawaii (Harvard Law Review, 2020; Perez, 2021a). The Hawaiian Homes Commission Act was signed in 1921 "to enable native Hawaiians to return to their lands in order to fully support self-sufficiency for native Hawaiians and the self-determination of native Hawaiians in the administration of this Act, and the preservation of the values, traditions, and culture of native Hawaiians."[6] The Hawaiian Homes

---

[6] Act of July 9, 1921, ch. 42, 42 Stat 108.

Commission administers 200,000 acres of public land for homesteads for Native Hawaiians (defined as people having at least 50 percent Hawaiian blood); beneficiaries receive 99-year residential, agricultural, pastoral, or aquaculture leases for $1 per year (leases can be extended to 199 years) to help build generational wealth (Department of Hawaiian Home Lands, n.d.; Hiraishi, 2021). Despite the size of the land trust, less than a quarter of the acreage is being used for homesteads, with only approximately 10,000 lessees and more than 28,000 people on the waitlist (Andrade, 2022). Funding levels and land inventory have been deemed inadequate; the commission must provide new sites to waitlist applicants (including the cost of infrastructure development) and continue serving existing sites with utility maintenance (Andrade, 2022; Department of Hawaiian Home Lands, n.d.; Hiraishi, 2021). The Department of Hawaiian Home Lands estimated it would cost $6 billion and take more than 180 years to clear the wait list at the current level of funding (Burnett, 2021). Many people on the waitlist are homeless, and people can wait decades to receive a lease (Consillio, 2022; Perez, 2021b). Additionally, federal government actions involving excess property have sometimes undermined the land debt repayment (Andrade, 2022; Perez, 2021b).

Federal Rental Assistance

Affordability is an important component of housing. Access to housing that families can afford is associated with positive health outcomes; without it, low-income people may live in substandard, unsafe housing with fewer community assets and have fewer resources available for other needs, like health care, food, and transportation (Braveman et al., 2011; Los Angeles County Department of Public Health, 2015; Maqbool et al., 2015; NASEM, 2019b). However, housing policy decisions are mainly made at the state and local levels, rather than the federal level (Cho, 2022). For example, zoning is largely set at the local level (this determines land use and density at which residential properties can be built), and housing development is done in large part by the private sector; these factors directly impact residents' ability to access homes and homeownership. Renters are more likely to be racially and ethnically minoritized and have lower income than homeowners; housing costs are more likely to burden[7] racially and ethnically minoritized renters, especially Black and Latino/a households, than White renters and those with lower income than those with higher household incomes (CBPP, 2022a; JCHS, 2022). The federal government's role in housing policy is in four primary areas: (1) provides rental assistance that helps low-income people afford modest housing, (2) provides funding sources to build below-market rental housing, (3) insures mortgages for homeownership, and (4)

---

[7] A cost-burdened household pays more than 30 percent of income on housing.

acts as the largest source of funding for homeless assistance and services (Cho, 2022).

A robust and growing evidence base exists on the health effects of federal policies related to rental assistance, neighborhoods, and housing (see for example, Sard et al., 2018). An important body of knowledge draws on the HUD Moving to Opportunity (MTO) research demonstration, which began 1994–1998 and has continued to follow low-income families moving from extremely poor neighborhoods to "neighborhoods of opportunity" (HUD, n.d.-b). The 4,600 families in the study were randomly assigned to one of three arms: one group offered "a housing voucher that could only be used to move to a low-poverty neighborhood, a group offered a traditional Section 8 housing voucher, and a control group" (NBER, n.d.). Families were followed 2004–2007 and 2008–2010. Longer-term findings included better physical and mental health status for adults who moved to lower-poverty neighborhoods and better mental health for female youth. These findings echoed the earlier results, which had also included a large decrease in violent-crime arrests (NBER, n.d.). In a follow-up of the MTO participants, Chetty and colleagues found the most noteworthy effects in children who were moved to lower-poverty neighborhoods in early childhood. They found

> that moving a child out of public housing to a low-poverty area when young (at age eight on average) using an MTO-type experimental voucher will increase the child's total lifetime earnings by about $302,000. This is equivalent to a gain of $99,000 per child moved in present value at age eight, discounting future earnings at a 3 percent interest rate. . . The additional tax revenue obtained from these children will itself offset the incremental cost of the experimental voucher treatment relative to providing public housing. (Chetty et al., 2016, p. 859–860)

The work of Chetty and colleagues (2018) also shows that the level of poverty in a close-by neighborhood (less than 0.6 mile radius) has causal effects on a child's outcomes, so the design of housing vouchers is extremely important for housing stability and getting to and remaining in a neighborhood that will improve a child's economic outcomes in later life.

Two federal agencies are involved with federal rental assistance. The Department of Agriculture (USDA) administers the USDA Section 521 Rural Rental Assistance program. HUD administers three major programs, including housing choice vouchers,[8] public housing,[9] and Section 8 project-based

---

[8] This a federally funded program in which low-income households use tenant-based vouchers to obtain rental housing in the private market; it is administered by state and local housing agencies (Mazzara, 2017).

[9] Public housing units are for eligible low-income families; they are owned and managed by local housing agencies (Mazzara, 2017).

rental assistance[10] (Mazzara, 2017); these three programs aid approximately 84 percent of those receiving federal rental assistance (CBPP, 2022b). Other HUD programs serve specific populations, such as those with disabilities, living with HIV/AIDS, or experiencing homelessness (Mazzara, 2017).

Approximately 10 million people receive federal rental assistance (CBPP, 2022c). About 5 million people use housing choice vouchers, the majority of whom are Black or Latino (CBPP, 2021). Federal rental assistance programs provided almost $49 billion in 2020 (CBPP, 2022c), and the fiscal year (FY) 2023 budget proposed funding to expand to 200,000 more families, prioritizing those who are homeless or escaping domestic violence (HUD, 2022). However, room for improvement remains in the federal government's role in rental assistance; funding is discretionary and historically has been severely underfunded relative to how many people are eligible (Cho, 2022; HUD, 2022). For example, because of limited funding, only one in four low-income renter households who qualify receive assistance (CBPP, 2022b; Cho, 2022). More than half of households in need are headed by racially and ethnically minoritized people (Fischer et al., 2021). Furthermore, due to limited program funding creating long waitlists, households awarded a housing choice voucher often wait close to 2.5 years to receive it, placing them at risk for housing instability during that time (Acosta and Gartland, 2021). Black households make up a disproportionate share of voucher waitlists, as Black people are among the minoritized communities disproportionately likely to experience housing insecurity and negative economic outcomes because of discriminatory housing and economic policies that have limited opportunities across generations (Acosta and Gartland, 2021). Tenant-based voucher programs also differ in eligibility criteria, such as income level (determined by the administering public housing agency and based on median income of the county or metropolitan area in which a recipient chooses to live); rental processes, including time allowed to find a unit; assistance, such as counseling in finding rental housing; and availability of short-term payments to cover moving expenses like rental deposits (CPSTF, 2021; HUD, n.d.-a).

The federal government offers other programs to build or rehabilitate rental housing with tax credits,[11] grants, and reduced-interest loans, but without rental assistance, these units are often unaffordable to families with the lowest incomes (CBPP, 2022b; NASEM, 2022b; National Housing Law Project, 2021; National Low Income Housing Coalition, 2022).

---

[10] The Project-Based Rental Assistance program contracts with private owners to rent at least some units in housing developments to low-income households (Mazzara, 2017).

[11] For example, the Low-Income Housing Tax Credit creates new affordable rental housing by encouraging private developers to build or rehabilitate housing for low-income individuals. Once compliance periods conclude, however, affordability requirements end, and owners can raise rents (National Low Income Housing Coalition, 2022; Tax Policy Center, 2020).

Additional, sustained federal investment in rental assistance could help reduce waiting times for vouchers, ease housing insecurity and crowded conditions, and alleviate rates of homelessness (Acosta and Gartland, 2021; Fischer et al., 2019; Schapiro et al., 2022). Rental assistance has also been shown to improve mental and physical well-being, reduce health care costs and food insecurity, and improve outcomes for children, including improvements in educational outcomes and behavioral development (Acosta and Gartland, 2021; CPSTF, 2021; Denary et al., 2021; Fischer et al., 2019). Expanding housing choice through vouchers increases access to neighborhoods with more resources and lower poverty (Acosta and Gartland, 2021). For example, Black and Latino children in families with housing vouchers are less likely to live in a high-poverty neighborhood (Fenelon et al., 2022). Additionally, expanding the housing choice voucher program could reduce poverty and racial and ethnic disparities. Using 2019 data, one study estimated that 9.3 million people could be lifted above the poverty line by providing vouchers to all eligible households; this would also reduce gaps in poverty rates between White and racially and ethnically minoritized households (Acosta and Gartland, 2021) (see Figure 6-2). Based on a

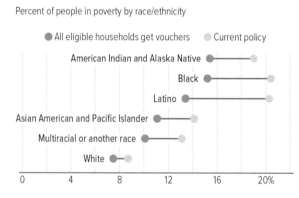

FIGURE 6-2 Expanding housing vouchers to all eligible households would cut poverty and reduce racial disparities.
NOTE: Currently about one in four households eligible for a voucher receives any type of federal rental assistance. Latino category may contain individuals of any race who identify as Latino or Hispanic; other categories exclude individuals that identify as Latino or Hispanic. Results for American Indian and Alaska Native and multiracial individuals calculated using data from the 2017–2019 Current Population Survey. Results for these groups need to be interpreted with caution due to sample size constraints. Results for Pacific Islanders when combined with Asian need to be interpreted with caution due to sample size constraints and masking of inequities of the Native Hawaiian and Pacific Islander population as a distinct racial Office of Management and Budget minimum category (see Chapter 2 for more details). SOURCE: CBPP, 2022a. This material was created by the Center on Budget and Policy Priorities (www.cbpp.org).

systemic review, the Community Preventive Services Task Force recommends vouchers as an effective intervention to advance equity and improve health and health-related outcomes, such as health care use, housing security and quality, and neighborhood opportunities (CPSTF, 2021). In addition to overall funding issues, the program could also be improved by giving participants more time to find HUD-certified housing with a landlord who accepts vouchers, providing assistance with housing searches, and recruiting more landlords (CPSTF, 2021).

> *Conclusion 6-1: Redlining and associated policies and structures resulted in residential segregation and neighborhood disinvestment, which have led to measurable health inequities present today. Safe, quality housing is necessary for maintaining an adequate standard of living, and there is a compelling link between housing and health equity. Increased federal investment in housing interventions for low-income people, such as the housing voucher program, could improve housing security and health outcomes for children and adults, especially among Black, Latino/a, American Indian and Alaska Native, and Native Hawaiian and Pacific Islander populations, and advance racial and ethnic health equity. Federal investment in housing would benefit from evidence-based guidelines to ensure that such investments do not contribute to future health inequities.*

INFRASTRUCTURE:
INVESTMENT, DISINVESTMENT, AND COMMUNITY HEALTH

Introduction

As illustrated with the example of redlining, historical federal policies heavily influence the neighborhood and built environment domain. The historical, deliberate siting and continued presence of freeways and other large, land-intensive infrastructure, such as manufacturing, industrial land uses, or landfills, for example, are well-established physical forms at neighborhood scales that have direct, long-standing negative effects on individual and community health (Ash and Boyce, 2018; Mikati et al., 2018; Mohai et al., 2009; Mohai and Saha, 2015; NASEM, 2021; Rothstein, 2017). Historical disinvestment in select neighborhoods reduces land rent prices, which enables land-intensive developments to locate to these areas, thereby establishing a long-lasting source of air pollution, extreme heat, or other hazards to human health; segregation is explicitly connected to disinvestment in infrastructure that supports community health. Racially and ethnically minoritized communities and low-income communities are consistently and disproportionately exposed to environmental hazards, such as air and water pollution and ambient noise, such as through water contamination events and the siting of waste facilities and petrochemical plants and refineries (Baurick et al., 2019; Brulle and Pellow, 2006; Bullard et al., 2007; Campbell et al., 2016; Deep South Center for Environmental Justice, 2020; Mohai et al., 2009; Paul, 2016). Race and ethnicity are significantly correlated with hazardous exposure after controlling for income; research has found new facilities are often sited where racially and ethnically minoritized communities already existed (Ash and Boyce, 2018; Bullard, 1983; Liu et al., 2021; Mikati et al., 2018; Mohai and Saha, 2015). Executive Order 14096[12] *Revitalizing our Nation's Commitment to Environmental Justice for All* aims to confront environmental injustice through a variety of mechanisms, including meaningful public participation and investment in mitigation efforts.

Additionally, as described in Chapter 2, racially and ethnically minoritized populations have disproportionately higher rates of disability, which shapes one's experience with SDOH, including the built environment (Krahn et al., 2015; NASEM, 2018a). Although the Americans with Disabilities Act[13] (ADA) prohibits discrimination on the basis of disability in employment, state and local government services, public transit, businesses that are open to the public, and telecommunications, it relies on complaints from members of the public who encounter violations. However, people may be unaware of their rights under the ADA or lack the resources to file a complaint (ADA.gov, n.d.; IOM, 2007). This is evident, for example, in transportation infrastructure.

Transportation services vary in ADA compliance, which can result in limited options and/or routes, high fares, and long wait and commute times, affecting access to employment, health care, and community participation (AAPD, n.d.; Blick et al., 2015; Martin-Proctor, 2022; Senate HELP Committee, 2014). The literature shows that people from racially and ethnically minoritized groups experience these and other factors that constitute transportation inequities, underscoring the important intersections of disability status and race and ethnicity (Karner et al., 2020). Built environment design for people with disabilities is important for realizing equity and the full participation of people of all ages and abilities in public spaces. Improving accessibility, mobility, safety, and inclusivity in public spaces can encompass audible, visual, and tactile design elements in street environments and public transit options (NACTO, 2016; National Endowment for the Arts, 2021). The federal government has a role to play in encouraging disability-inclusive design in urban planning and development.

---

[12] Exec. Order No. 14096, 88 FR 25251 (April 2023).
[13] 42 U.S.C. § 12101 *et seq.*

For example, the Infrastructure Investment and Jobs Act[14] included funding to modernize and improve accessibility of transit for people with disabilities and older people (FTA, 2022). It also established the All Stations Accessibility Program to improve accessibility of rail system stations built before the ADA (DOT, 2022a). In July 2022, the Department of Transportation (DOT) announced the Disability Policy Priorities, which include enabling "safe and accessible air travel; multimodal accessibility of public transportation facilities, vehicles, and rights-of-way; access to good-paying jobs and business opportunities for people with disabilities; and accessibility of electric vehicles and automated vehicles" (DOT, n.d.).

This section provides additional detail and examples of how federal investment and disinvestment in infrastructure can help or harm community health and contribute to racial, ethnic, and tribal health inequities. In an overview of the scholarly research on Hurricane Katrina's impact on New Orleans, Jampel (2018) points out that "those most likely to be subject to and bear the greatest burdens of environmental injustice often occupy multiple marginalized social locations" and describes how an array of infrastructure failures presented an issue of disability justice in addition to issues of racial, climate, and environmental justice. Disability status played a role in people's ability to evacuate and compounded the plight of many who sought refuge in the Superdome (Jampel, 2018).

The federal government has long recognized that the country's infrastructure strengthens economic growth and national security while bolstering global competitiveness, and the 2021 Infrastructure Investment and Jobs Act provided $1 trillion for transportation and other infrastructure investment (Goubert and Austin, 2022). However, the federal responsibility is shared with state and local governments, which provide the majority of the funding for transportation and infrastructure (CBO, 2018; Shirley, 2017; Sprunt, 2021; Zhao et al., 2019). Infrastructure consists of the physical materials used to support, for example, transportation (e.g., mass transit, bridges, highways, railroads, aviation, waterway infrastructure, as well as the transportation of hazardous materials and of resources via pipeline). In terms of public health, it plays a direct role in ensuring clean water, wastewater management, and flood damage reduction and other disaster preparedness and response. It also includes the management of federally owned buildings and the development of economically depressed areas. Several federal agencies and standing congressional committees are directly responsible for assessing infrastructure, including DOT, Environmental Protection Agency (EPA), Federal Emergency Management Agency, as well as Amtrak, U.S. Army Corps of Engineers, U.S. Coast Guard, Economic Development Administration, and others.

---

[14]Pub. L. 117–58, 135 Stat. 429 (Nov. 15, 2021).

Despite the federal responsibility for infrastructure, the United States lacks a national comprehensive infrastructure planning system that integrates federal decision making with state and local land-use policies. The legal power to regulate infrastructure largely rests with the states and local governments, not federal agencies, which can assist in building and maintaining infrastructure and evaluating related projects. The limited role of the federal government in local land-use is related to the United States' background of settlement and development. The historical idea that, given the country's size and relatively low population density, abundant space was available for development (Kayden, 2001) led in part to the rapid expansion of Europeans across the western United States in the 1800s on land belonging to AIAN tribes. The U.S. government supported and legally enforced settlers' claims; this dispossession of land, along with decades of other federal Indian policies, is at the core of inequity, especially for AIAN and NHPI people (see Chapter 7 for a more in-depth discussion of dispossession from land, historical and ongoing trauma, and the landback movement). This homesteading ethos contributes to the inequities in land and the built environment and assigns high reverence for private property that manifests in legal debates. In addition to the lack of federal emphasis on infrastructure, most states minimize their degree of intervention with infrastructure policies of the local governments (Cullingworth and Caves, 2009; Kayden, 2001).

Despite the emphasis on local land-use decisions in infrastructure planning and the importance of private property, the federal government has used land-use controls to achieve public health objectives such as establishing mitigation regulations and emission and waste treatment standards as well as procedural tools like environmental impact assessments. Four federal laws, in particular, have driven debate over the federal role in infrastructure planning and public health: (1) the Clean Air Act,[15] which establishes standards for criteria of air pollutants; (2) Safe Drinking Water Act,[16] which ensures that communities have access to potable water; (3) the Clean Water Act,[17] which establishes the necessary guidelines for ensuring clean and swimmable waters; and (4) the National Environmental Policy Act,[18] which is triggered any time federal money funds an infrastructure project and requires an environmental impact statement. These and other policies regulate the quality of infrastructure and its potential implications, but only the Clean Air and Water Acts directly reduce harms to public health by establishing thresholds for compounds found in air and water known

---

[15] 42 U.S.C. § 7401 *et seq.*
[16] Pub. L. 93–523, 88 Stat. 1660 (Dec. 16, 1974).
[17] Pub. L. 92–500, 86 Stat. 816 (Oct. 18, 1972).
[18] 42 U.S.C. § 4321 *et seq.*

to adversely affect human health. The National Environmental Policy Act does not reference community public health in the administration of the environmental impact statement.

Water

Water infrastructure is a concern that disproportionately impacts racially and ethnically minoritized communities across the country, affecting both sanitation and potable water. Evidence indicates that nearly 500,000 U.S. households lacked complete plumbing (meaning access to a bath or shower, a sink with a faucet, and hot and cold water); these were clustered mainly in Alaska, Puerto Rico, the Four Corners area, and parts of Texas and Appalachia (Mueller and Gasteyer, 2021). Water infrastructure issues are acute on AIAN reservations, where 58 out of every 1,000 households do not have complete plumbing; AIAN households are also 19 times more likely to lack indoor plumbing than White households. Many people on reservations also lack access to clean water because of old or deficient pipes or because pipes or water systems do not exist at all, forcing use of bottled or boiled water (Tebor, 2021; U.S. Water Alliance and DigDeep, 2019).

The Safe Drinking Water Act regulates the public drinking water supply and authorized EPA to set national minimum standards to protect against contamination from naturally occurring and anthropogenic health risks. It applies to all public water systems (which can be publicly or privately owned); responsibility is shared among EPA, states, and water systems, but state drinking water programs have the most direct oversight of water systems. States and EPA can take legal action, fine utilities, or take other enforcement actions against systems not meeting standards (EPA, 2004). The Clean Water Act governs pollution control; it regulates quality standards of surface waters and pollutant discharge into waterways. In 2021, across the United States, 1,165 community water systems were serious violators of the Safe Drinking Water Act and 9,457 permittees of the Clean Water Act were in significant noncompliance, indicating poor water quality in these communities for millions of residents. Violators of the Safe Drinking Water Act were clustered in Alaska, Puerto Rico, Appalachia, New Mexico, and parts of the Northwest. Noncompliance with the Clean Water Act was clustered in parts of the Northwest, including much of Washington; Appalachia; the upper Midwest; and lower Mississippi; this pattern illustrates variable state monitoring (Mueller and Gasteyer, 2021). Lack of adequate water infrastructure is especially important in Black, Latino, and AIAN communities, where data indicate that violations of the Safe Drinking Water Act are significantly higher (Switzer and Teodoro, 2017). On tribal land, researchers have found that regulatory agencies less vigorously enforce both acts (Teodoro et al., 2018). EPA data reveal that communities with a higher proportion of Hispanic residents were more likely to have community water systems contaminated by high nitrate levels (Schaider et al., 2019), which have been associated with increased risk of birth defects, thyroid disease, and cancers (Ward et al., 2018). Water infrastructure issues related to sanitation, clean and potable water, and unpolluted waterways are likely to become more widespread as climate change intensifies.

Transportation

Transportation is an essential resource for health through multiple pathways. Accessible and safe transportation and mobility options help people of all abilities access schools, employment, social networks, grocery stores, and health care and social services. The variety of transportation options available to a household corresponds to the extent to which communities have access to basic necessities. For example, research has found that more than 3.6 million people have delayed or missed medical care because of transportation barriers (NASEM, 2016a); people with chronic conditions that require regular care are especially vulnerable. Rural counties are particularly challenged because they have a higher concentration of federally designated primary care health professional shortage areas (NASEM, 2016a). This means that individuals who are mobility challenged or lack their own transportation must often travel farther to receive care. Furthermore, unsafe transportation systems and infrastructure can lead to injuries or death for motorists, cyclists, and pedestrians (GHSA, 2021; Hamann et al., 2020; Raifman and Choma, 2022). Infrastructure contributes to inequitable outcomes here as well, with racial disparities in traffic fatalities and pedestrian injury hospitalizations. Neighborhoods with lower-income, racially and ethnically minoritized communities are less likely to have features such as well-marked crosswalks and sidewalks or other types of infrastructure that lower speeds and improve pedestrian safety (Montgomery, 2021). Complete Streets may be a way to improve equity; they support safe, efficient, and inclusive mobility and multimodal transportation for all users. Complete Streets design approaches depend on community context but can address components such as sidewalks and accessible pedestrian signals and crossing opportunities, bicycle lanes, bus lanes and public transportation stops, and streetscape and landscape (City of Saint Paul, 2016; DOT, 2015a; Smart Growth America, n.d.). When appropriately designed and implemented, they can reduce motor vehicle crashes and reduce risk to pedestrians and bicyclists; more walkable and bikeable communities can also encourage physical activity and help reduce transportation's contribution to greenhouse gas emissions (Aytur et al., 2007; DOT, 2015a,b; FHWA, 2022; Frank et al., 2006; Pineda et al., 2017; Reynolds et al., 2009). Implementing Complete Streets plans and other infrastructure investments could also help prioritize and address outdated, inappropriate, and aging infrastructure in underserved communities (Huang and Taylor, 2019; Smart Growth America, 2023).

It is not coincidental that some of the major battles of the Civil Rights Movement occurred around bus transportation—an essential conduit to work, school, and other essential destinations (Brenman, 2007). Planning and transportation have also harmed many communities in the name of "urban renewal" in the 1950s and 1960s, displacing families, tearing apart social fabric, and uprooting entire neighborhoods (NASEM, 2016b, 2022a). Like housing and education, transportation can serve as a path to expanded opportunity, improved health and well-being, and thriving communities but can also represent an array of strategies that create and deepen social, environmental, and economic inequities that shape health outcomes.

DOT is the federal agency responsible for building and upkeep of the interstate highway system, and its agencies oversee public transit, airports, railroads, gas pipelines, bridges, and tunnels. Approximately 80 percent of the federal DOT budget is passed through to state DOTs. The federal department also sets standards, provides resources for innovations, collaborates with and provides technical assistance to state DOTs and local and regional planning organizations, and operates a research program with multiple academic partners, among other functions. State DOTs "are the primary state agency responsible for planning and programming mobility needs, as well as constructing, managing, and operating the statewide transportation system" (Flanigan and Howard, 2008). Federal coordination is needed to link health outcomes to transportation funding.

Given the range of linkages between transportation and health and the legacy of structural racism in land-use and planning decisions (e.g., devaluing the Black communities displaced by a new highway project), transportation agencies at all levels of government can play robust roles in furthering health equity. DOT has recognized its potential contribution and taken steps to focus considerable resources and effort on improving transportation equity and mitigating past harms. One important dimension of this work has been to center community voices (see Box 6-1).

Aging Infrastructure

These issues are exacerbated by aging infrastructure. Figure 6-3 shows that the average age of major components of infrastructure (e.g., roads, dams, water treatment plants) are beyond the average life expectancy. Road wear and tear and lack of maintenance, for example, have left just under half of public roadways in mediocre or poor condition (ASCE, 2021). The American Society of Civil Engineers produces a report card for U.S. infrastructure every 4 years; in 2021, it scored a C- (ASCE, 2021). The United

BOX 6-1
Reconnecting Communities Pilot Program

The Federal-Aid Highway Act of 1956 (also known as the "National Interstate and Defense Highways Act")[1] funded the national highway system. In addition to shifting jobs and homes to suburban areas and contributing to sprawl and diminished public transit, the interstate highway system "disproportionately cut through communities of color, contributing to the racial and economic segregation of cities and concentrated poverty that persist today" (Heaps et al., 2021, p. 2). Highway siting has a long and well-documented history of purposeful displacement, division, and isolation of neighborhoods, exacerbating existing socioeconomic and racial and ethnic inequities (Archer, 2020; NASEM, 2021; National Archives, 2022; Reft, 2023; Walker, 2023). It also displaced communities and contributed to air pollution and blight. Using highways to usher in the "era of mobility" highlights the ramifications of exercising eminent domain and subsequent displacement of communities for local infrastructure projects. Black households and business districts were disproportionately displaced or destroyed in original siting decisions (Archer, 2020; NASEM, 2021; Walker, 2023), and present-day freeway expansion in places such as Houston, Texas, Tampa, Florida, and Los Angeles County continues to reproduce inequities by affecting predominantly Black and Latino neighborhoods (Dillon and Poston, 2021; NASEM, 2022a). Research indicates that widening these roadways often only reduces traffic temporarily and can increase congestion overall by encouraging more driving (Dillon and Poston, 2021; Duranton and Turner, 2011; Hymel, 2019; Mogridge, 1997; Volker et al., 2020; Weingart, 2023); estimates of this effect could be included in studies of where to site and widen highways. Siting highways in these communities results in environmental injustice, exposing them to more toxic vehicle emissions and noise pollution, and affecting community structure and the accumulation of intergenerational wealth (NASEM, 2021, 2022a).

Transportation agencies at all levels of government are required by Title VI of the 1964 Civil Rights Act[2] and Executive Order 12898[3] *Federal Actions to Address Environmental Justice in Minority Populations and Low-Income Populations* to assess whether infrastructure projects will affect low-income and racially and ethnically minoritized communities. Although such statutory and regulatory frameworks around environmental justice and related issues in transportation are helpful, transformative action involves engaging the affected communities and centering their needs, such as by linking residents and planners, using local data, and working with community-based organizers (Velasco, 2020).

In June 2022, the Department of Transportation announced Reconnecting Communities, a $1 billion pilot program in the Bipartisan Infrastructure Plan designed to help undo some of the harms created decades ago by the interstate highway system and reconnect communities by removing, replacing, or mitigating infrastructure. The program notice stated that preference would "be given to applications from economically disadvantaged communities, especially those with projects that are focused on equity and environmental justice, have strong community engagement and stewardship, and a commitment to shared prosperity and equitable development" (DOT, 2022b). A discretionary grant program under the Reconnecting Communities pilot was intended specifically for rural and tribal

---

BOX 6-1 Continued

communities (Rural Health Information Hub, n.d.). DOT awarded 45 community-led projects $185 million in 2023, including for projects that improve access and connectivity around existing infrastructure and capping interstates with parks (DOT, 2023; Walker, 2023).

---

[1] Pub. L. 84–627, 70 Stat. 374 (June 29, 1956).
[2] 42 U.S.C. § 2000d *et seq.*
[3] Exec. Order No. 12898, 59 FR 7629 (February 1994).

States falls short on funding maintenance of vital infrastructure, such as transit, stormwater systems, bridges, and dams (ASCE, 2021), with needed repairs totaling an estimated $1 trillion (Zhao et al., 2019). The American Society of Civil Engineers forecasts $10.3 trillion in gross domestic product (GDP) loss by 2039 if the investment gap is not addressed (ASCE, 2021; EBP and ASCE, 2021).

The effects of aging or substandard infrastructure are felt by all but particularly by racially and ethnically minoritized communities. For example, Illinois has the most lead pipes of any state, and Black and Latino households are two times more likely than White households to live in a neighborhood

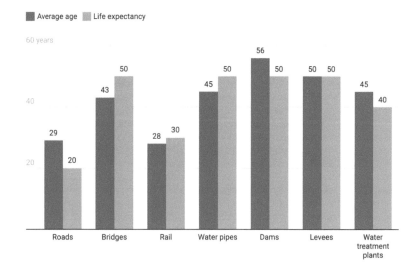

FIGURE 6-3 Average age and life expectancy of U.S. infrastructure.
NOTE: U.S. = United States.
SOURCE: Chinowsky, 2022.

with the most lead pipes. Puerto Rico, which has a majority Latino population, has among the worst energy infrastructure, leading to blackouts and
high electricity prices (ASCE, 2019; Goubert and Austin, 2022). Similarly, the
U.S. Commission on Civil Rights (2018) states that infrastructure projects on
reservations have been underfunded for decades, which compounds the back-
log of needed maintenance, let alone new projects to improve the physical
infrastructure and built environment (NCAI, 2021). Indian Country has over
160,000 miles of roads eligible for federal funding, yet transportation systems
are underdeveloped. Additionally, thousands of miles of roads owned by Bureau of Indian Affairs on reservations are among the most unsafe and poorly
maintained (NCAI, 2021; U.S. Commission on Civil Rights, 2018). The lack
of public transportation on many reservations, combined with roads in need
of repair and often rural locations, complicates access to quality health care,
food, education, and employment for many AIAN people.

Natural Environment

The natural world and environmental conditions are directly affected by
infrastructure decisions, which are direct determinants of health outcomes
(NASEM, 2017; Shilling et al., 2007; Thacker et al., 2021). Large developments, such as highways, industrial and manufacturing facilities, hazardous
waste sites, and rail lines (and depots), are often sited in disinvested areas
of cities and generate atmospheric pollutants that are harmful to human
health (Ash and Boyce, 2018; Kay and Katz, 2012; Mikati et al., 2018;
Mohai and Saha, 2015; Spencer-Hwang et al., 2014). They also reduce the
available land for green spaces, such as tree canopies in neighborhoods and
safe and accessible parks and playgrounds that provide opportunities for
physical activity and social connectedness (Arnold and Resilience Justice
Project Researchers, 2021). Such green spaces also help mitigate the effects
of extreme heat and noise pollution. Moreover, the increase in temperatures
correspond to poor air and water quality (and lack of water), contaminated
soil, pollution, and proximity to toxic sites, which negatively affect human
health (Arnold and Resilience Justice Project Researchers, 2021). Green
spaces also benefit mental health (NASEM, 2017).

Although climate change is a global phenomenon, communities experience the effects differentially. Health risk is shaped by adjacent infrastructure, which drives potential exposure, sensitivity, and ability to adapt to
climate change–related extreme weather events (e.g., heatwaves, wildfires,
drought, floods, storms) and rising temperatures. Changes in precipitation,
increasing hurricane and tornado intensity, and rising sea levels will have
more acute impacts on those already living precariously, who are consistently in areas where policies have "locked in" infrastructure that exacerbates extreme events. These climate change processes lead to temperature

and precipitation extremes, air pollution, altered food and water supply and quality, environmental degradation, increased allergens, and changes in disease vector ecology (Romanello et al., 2022). Outcomes include heat-related illnesses; respiratory and cardiovascular conditions; injuries; adverse pregnancy outcomes; increased prevalence and altered distribution of water-, food-, and vector-borne diseases; malnutrition; harmful algal blooms; mental health effects; forced migration; civil conflict; and death (CDC, 2022b,d; Frumkin and Haines, 2019). At every income level, racially and ethnically minoritized people are exposed to higher levels of air pollution than White people in the United States (Clark et al., 2014, 2017; Lane et al., 2022; Liu et al., 2021; Tessum et al., 2021) and, on average, face higher heat island intensity in all but 6 of the 175 largest urbanized areas (Hsu et al., 2021). In a study of wildfire potential and vulnerability, Davies and colleagues (2018) found that majority Black, Hispanic, and American Indian census tracts were more vulnerable and less likely to be able to adapt and respond to wildfires than majority White tracts.

Furthermore, climate change is likely to intensify challenges presented by aging infrastructure, especially among racially and ethnically minoritized communities (Arnold and Resilience Justice Project Researchers, 2021; USGCRP, 2018). Extreme heat and storms, for instance, will put pressure on old infrastructure and worsen racial and ethnic health inequities. For example, Black neighborhoods have been disproportionately harmed by flooding, as seen in the damage caused by Hurricane Katrina in New Orleans and Hurricane Harvey in Houston; these neighborhoods also have lower capacity to recover from flooding (Frank, 2020; Goubert and Austin, 2022; NASEM, 2019a). As mentioned, a study found that AIAN reservations experience more climate change–related days of extreme heat and long-term drought and less precipitation than their historical lands (Farrell et al., 2021).

Despite a few direct mechanisms for engaging local communities through federal support, programs that offer promising directions need greater visibility in infrastructure planning. This could include, for example, using community scientists to understand how past planning policies affect human health through measurement of air temperatures. For example, Heat Watch, administered through the National Integrated Heat Health Information System, is a public–private partnership that brings together almost a dozen federal agencies in addressing the disproportionate exposure to extreme heat events (National Integrated Heat Health Information System, n.d.). Through engaging directly with local organizations, investing in local communities, the participants are able to directly describe the differences in air temperatures across the built environment and work toward locally equitable solutions (Hoffman et al., 2022). If more federal agencies developed similar programs that engage local communities and public health partners in addressing known causes of health risk, pernicious effects on racially and ethnically minoritized communities could be more effectively averted.

Green Infrastructure

Essential in the built environment is the need for gray infrastructure— traditional infrastructure that allows the seamless movement of goods, removal of wastewater, housing of residents, businesses, and other buildings, and myriad other services. Yet, establishing these assets has led to removing green infrastructure (GI),[19] which can play a critical role in improving population health. GI is becoming an important component of the built environment, especially as cities respond to both climate change and environmental quality degradation. Discussion of GI in urban planning highlights benefits such as air quality improvements (Nowak et al., 2006), stormwater management (Copeland, 2016; Eaton, 2018), flood and heat control (Webber et al., 2020; Zölch et al., 2016), and carbon capture and climate change mitigation (Foster et al., 2011; Romanello et al., 2022; USGCRP, 2018). Yet, an emerging area of research points to the disparate access to GI across the built environment. Past federal policies, such as redlining, are associated with racial inequities in GI, including green spaces and tree canopy (Locke et al., 2021; Nardone et al., 2021).

Studies are catalyzing actions in U.S. cities in establishing large tracts of GI, even within highly populated neighborhoods (Grabowski et al., 2023). GI can be traditional systems, such as parks and greenways, but recently is expanding into green roofs and walls, bioswales, street trees, and other forms of greening that sometimes create networks across metropolitan regions. However, GI can be more than a physical barrier to environmental hazards; "it is a gateway through which urban planners and policy makers might respond to underlying disparities that create socioecological vulnerability and inhibit resilience" (Bowen and Lynch, 2017; Jennings et al., 2012; Shandas and Hellman, 2022, p. 290; Zhu et al., 2019). Although several factors, such as home value, perceptions of crime, and polluting infrastructure, can preclude access to high-quality green spaces in neighborhoods, it is crucial that cities' GI plans acknowledge causes of racial and ethnic health inequity and displacement and use inclusive processes to design and evaluate GI so that the systems do not perpetuate harms (Arnold and Resilience Justice Project Researchers, 2021; Barber et al., 2022; Grabowski et al., 2023). For example, a study of 122 GI plans from 20 cities found that

---

[19] Defined in 33 U.S.C. § 1362 as "the range of measures that use plant or soil systems, permeable pavement or other permeable surfaces or substrates, stormwater harvest and reuse, or landscaping to store, infiltrate, or evapotranspirate stormwater and reduce flows to sewer systems or to surface waters."

fewer than 15 percent defined equity or justice, and few plans recognized houselessness and gentrification as related issues (Grabowski et al., 2023). Communities without effective and appropriately scaled GI are more vulnerable and less resilient to pollution, disasters, and climate change (Arnold and Resilience Justice Project Researchers, 2021). If properly planned and integrated with a focus on inclusion and community voice, "GI could be an essential tool enabling environmental justice and equity in the urban environment, alongside climate change mitigation, cost-effective risk reduction, and ecological protection" (Shandas and Hellman, 2022, p. 290).

Two essential and practical applications are necessary for sustaining GI in the long term. The first is developing maintenance and operations systems that align new GI to specific public agencies and/or related partner organizations. With concerns about increasing costs for municipal parks and recreation agencies and a general lack of resources for maintaining existing GI, municipal leaders will need to prioritize long-term care and support for expanding GI facilities. Federal agencies can be instrumental in providing additional incentives, such as through expanding revolving block grants, cost-share programs, and other capacity-building approaches; the Inflation Reduction Act of 2022[20] focus on greening urban communities is a positive example of federal investment in this area (Copeland, 2016; EPA, 2023c; NCSL, 2022; The White House, 2022). At the local level, municipal leaders can champion equity-centered applications of GI. Second, data are essential for integrating tools, yet sufficient quality data for improving the overall assessment of new building in relation to future environmental and climate threats and systematic investments are still lacking. Consideration of a set of guidelines for improving the resolution of environmental and climate data at subneighborhood scales can serve as an important first step. This means establishing GI standards in federally sponsored programs that also account for racial and ethnic health inequities.

> *Conclusion 6-2: The federal infrastructure policies governed by the Department of Housing and Urban Development, the Environmental Protection Agency, the Department of Transportation, and other agencies play critical roles to ensure health equity. Essential in these policies is the protection for those most vulnerable to the health effects of infrastructure investments, since, in many cases, federal funding propels infrastructure spending from state and local governments. While the role of federal funding may be limited in terms of the types of state and local infrastructure projects, there are missed opportunities for the federal government to monitor and address the health inequities tied to infrastructure. Coordination, monitoring, and guidance on infrastructure spending are lacking across federal agencies.*

---

[20] Pub. L. 117–169, 136 Stat. 1818 (Aug. 16, 2022).

ENVIRONMENTAL EXPOSURES: WORKPLACE VULNERABILITIES

Occupational health inequities have been recognized by the Centers for Disease Control and Prevention as increased rates of work-related illness and injury for vulnerable populations (NIOSH, 2019). Some workplace hazards pose direct risks to employee health and safety. For instance, in 2021, 2.6 million people suffered workplace-related injuries or illness in the private sector; one worker died from a work-related injury every 111 minutes during 2020 (BLS, 2021, 2022). As a report from the National Institute for Occupational Safety and Health found, "not all workers have the same risk of being injured at work, even when they are in the same industry or have the same job" (NIOSH and ASSE, 2015, p. 6). This was especially true for Latino/a workers, who represented 18 percent of the labor force in 2020 but almost 23 percent of all work-related deaths; most fatalities were in the construction, agriculture, and transportation industries (Frederick, 2022). According to the Department of Labor, Latino/a workers have the highest fatal injury rate in the country (Frederick, 2022).

The workplace can present a variety of psychosocial health risks that are compounded by other SDOH. Where someone works can also be an SDOH (Healthy People 2030 includes work as one of the environments that affects health outcomes) (HHS, n.d.). For example, financial stability can determine vulnerability to illness and life expectancy. The gender pay gap contributes to financial stability, and it is larger for AIAN, Hispanic or Latina, Black, and Native Hawaiian and Pacific Islander (NHPI) women than for White and Asian women. According to Census Bureau data, for every dollar White men earned in 2021, White and Asian women earned $0.79 and $0.97, respectively. AIAN and Hispanic or Latina women each earned $0.58, Black women $0.63, and NHPI women $0.66 (GAO, 2022). See Chapter 3 for more information on income, employment, and health. Additionally, workplace discrimination and harassment have been shown to affect physical and psychological health, such as elevated blood pressure levels for Black and Latina women and general poor mental health (Okechukwu et al., 2014). This is particularly true when it comes to workplace-based racial discrimination, which contributes to occupational health disparities (Okechukwu et al., 2014).

Congress passed the Occupational Safety and Health Act of 1970[21] because it found that "personal injuries and illnesses arising out of work situations impose a substantial burden upon, and are a hindrance to, interstate commerce in terms of lost production, wage loss, medical expenses, and disability compensation payments" (OSHA, n.d.-b). Even with these protections, hazardous work conditions contribute to racial health

---

[21] 29 U.S.C. § 651 et seq.

inequities (Baron et al., 2013; Bui et al., 2020; NASEM, 2017; Rho et al., 2020; Seabury et al., 2017). The National Institute for Occupational Safety and Health has recognized occupational health inequities as "differences in work-related disease incidence, mental illness, or morbidity and mortality that are closely linked with social, economic, and/or environmental disadvantage such as work arrangements (e.g. contingent work), sociodemographic characteristics (e.g. age, sex, race, and class), and organizational factors (e.g. business size)" (NIOSH, 2019); food production is one of the industries where such inequities manifest (Newman et al., 2015).

Agricultural food production provides an example of how work-related health risks exacerbate social and economic inequities. Such work is among the most hazardous occupations; direct hazards include exposure to heat, extreme conditions, toxic pesticides, and chemicals; musculoskeletal injuries and use of nonergonomic tools; and unsanitary conditions, among other threats to health and safety (Newman et al., 2015; OSHA, n.d.-a). For example, a study of agricultural workers in California found heat strain was associated with increased odds of acute kidney injury (Moyce et al., 2017). Farmworkers can be exposed to pesticides during mixing and application, or because of direct spray, drift, or residue on crops or in soil (Damalas and Koutroubas, 2016; OSHA, n.d.-a). Pesticides can drift to schools, residences, and other facilities nearby. Farmworkers can also carry residue home on skin, clothes, or hair, exposing children and family members. Exposure causes acute health effects, such as rash, headaches, nausea, and difficulty breathing; long-term health effects can include cancers, neurological disorders like Parkinson's disease, and reproductive health issues (Kim et al., 2017).

Federal policy can contribute to inequities in workplace toxic exposure. This happens in the agricultural sector, where about 80 percent of all workers identify as Latino/a (Donley et al., 2022; Ornelas et al., 2021); occupational risks will disproportionately affect one ethnically minoritized group. Furthermore, according to the Department of Labor's 2017–2018 National Agricultural Workers Survey, approximately 44 percent of farmworkers reported they did not have health insurance (Ornelas et al., 2021). Regulators have taken steps to protect consumers from harmful pesticides, including the Federal Insecticide, Fungicide, and Rodenticide Act[22] and Federal Food, Drug, and Cosmetic Act,[23] which together form the basis of pesticide regulation in the United States. However, the combination of disproportionate exposure at the workplace and lack of health insurance can produce more negative outcomes for agricultural workers (APHA, 2011; Donley et al., 2022; Liebman et al., 2013; Ornelas et al., 2021).

---

[22] 7 U.S.C. § 136 et seq.
[23] 21 U.S.C. § 301 et seq.

The production and extensive use of industrial agriculture also exposes non-workers to health dangers. Pesticide production tends to expose surrounding low-income Black and Latino/a communities. In Kentucky, a major DDT producer was designated a Superfund site after it contaminated a community in which 84 percent of the residents were Black (Donley et al., 2022). California EPA has found that pesticide exposure during the use phase also exposes low-income and Latino/a communities to health risks (Donley et al., 2022); pesticide use in California is greatest in majority Latino/a counties (Cushing et al., 2015). Consequently, farmworkers and people who live in areas where pesticides are produced and/or used have higher concentrations of toxins in their bodies. For example, strawberry fieldworkers in Monterey County, California, had median urinary pesticide metabolite levels that were about 61 to 395 times higher than national levels (Salvatore et al., 2008). In Washington state, researchers discovered that 85 percent of farmworker homes contained pesticide-laden dust and 88 percent of children who lived with farmworkers had pesticides in their urine (Curl et al., 2002). In sum, pesticide exposure is responsible for thousands (estimated 10,000–20,000) of medical visits for acute health needs (Donley et al., 2022). EPA has acknowledged these inequities and proposed to resolve them by drafting the "Revised Risk Assessment Methods for Workers, Children of Workers in Agricultural Fields, and Pesticides with No Food Uses," but it faced opposition and has been stalled since 2009 (Donley et al., 2022).

The Occupational Health and Safety Administration (OSHA) oversees most occupational sector safety standards, but EPA exerts authority over agricultural worker safety through the federal WPS, which is largely administered by states and meant to reduce risk of pesticide poisoning and injuries among agricultural workers (EPA, 2023a). Lack of compliance monitoring and enforcement of the WPS disincentivizes inspections for violations; federal data show that more than half of violations have no enforcement action, and many that do only result in a warning (Guarna et al., 2022). When penalties are assessed, they are often low. For example, fines in California for pesticide-related violations from 2019 to 2021 were $50–12,000, but the majority were $500 or less (Guarna et al., 2022). Despite improvements to the standard in 2015, worker protection from pesticides could be improved further (APHA, 2011; Bohme, 2015; Donley et al., 2022; Guarna et al., 2022; Liebman et al., 2013). Future efforts need to address exposure in the workplace, residential communities, and the production site, such as requiring no-spray buffer zones to protect workers and communities from pesticide drift. This idea is supported by a new rule[24] proposed by EPA in 2023 aimed at reducing exposure for farmworkers and

---

[24]Pesticides; Agricultural Worker Protection Standard; Reconsideration of the Application Exclusion Zone Amendments, 88 FR 15346 (March 2023).

their communities by updating the pesticide application exclusion zone (EPA, 2023b). Other ideas for change include extending worker protection to agricultural workers that enables access to safety training and information in Spanish and other languages; it could be a requirement that pesticide labels be printed in Spanish, as well. Federal policies that explicitly protect essential workers or workers who are most vulnerable (such as making sure that farmworkers are covered by policies that have excluded them or adding a federal heat safety standard) could be implemented, or OSHA's jurisdiction over regulation of pesticide-related occupational hazards could be restored. EPA could also be granted effective, meaningful tools to respond to states that fail to enforce the WPS, and penalties for violations could be increased (Guarna et al., 2022).

Conclusion 6-3: There is a lack of coordination among relevant federal agencies to address workplace protection from pesticides, such as among the Occupational Safety and Health Administration, the Environmental Protection Agency, and the Centers for Disease Control and Prevention. Inadequate workplace protections from pesticides for agricultural workers disproportionately impact Latino/a workers, their children, and surrounding communities.

FOOD ACCESS AND PRODUCTION

Healthy neighborhoods require access to healthy food systems. Access to nutritious, affordable food and to supermarkets and grocery stores, corner stores, convenience stores, and other food venues is an important factor in health outcomes across the life span. USDA defines food insecurity as a "household-level economic and social condition of limited or uncertain access to adequate food" (USDA, 2022b). Poor nutrition and food insecurity (or access to only nonnutritious foods) are associated with increased risk of chronic diseases, from obesity, cardiovascular disease, and hypertension to type 2 diabetes and certain cancers, and, among children, frequent infections (e.g., ear or upper respiratory infections), iron-deficiency anemia, poor oral health, and overall poor health (Pflipsen and Zenchenko, 2017; Seligman and Berkowitz, 2019; Thorndike et al., 2022). According to data from the Current Population Survey Food Security Supplement, approximately 10 percent of U.S. households were food insecure in 2021, as were 12.5 percent of households with children. The prevalence of food insecurity in 2021 was higher among lower-income (26.5 percent), Black (19.8 percent), and Hispanic (16.2 percent) households than among non-Hispanic White (7.0 percent) households and those with incomes higher than 185 percent of the poverty threshold (5.0 percent) (USDA, 2022c). About 20–25 percent of AIAN people are food insecure (Feeding America, n.d.; Jernigan et al., 2017).

Additionally, distribution of supermarkets, which can provide more nutritious food options at lower prices, is inequitable in the United States. USDA estimates that, in 2019, 11–27 percent of the U.S. population lived in census tracts that have both low income[25] and low access[26] to large food stores, such as grocery stores and supermarkets (Rhone et al., 2022). Areas of low income and low access are sometimes referred to as "food deserts" in popular culture. People who are Black, Asian, Hispanic, and NHPI generally live closer to food stores than do people who are White or AIAN (Rhone et al., 2019). Much of this variation across racial, ethnic, and tribal groups is correlated with differences in living in urban versus rural areas. Within urban and rural areas, in general, White people lived further away from food stores (Rhone et al., 2019). However, Bower and colleagues (2014) found that majority Black census tracts had the fewest supermarkets and White census tracts had the most at equal levels of poverty. Higher census tract poverty was associated with lower supermarket availability and higher grocery[27] and convenience store availability (Bower et al., 2014). In rural areas, 12 percent of AIAN people lived more than 20 miles away from the nearest food store, compared with less than 1 percent of rural residents overall (Rhone et al., 2019), and the largest proportion of AIAN people in tribal areas live 1–10 miles from a grocery store (driving distance) (Kaufman et al., 2014). Access to healthy food is also more difficult for those who do not own a car or must rely on often inadequate public transportation infrastructure.

Climate change will continue to affect food systems through an array of mechanisms, such as more frequent heavy precipitation, which can erode soil and deplete nutrients; stronger storms and sea level rise, which can affect agricultural land and water supplies; and increased threat of wildfire, which poses risk to farmlands and rangelands; it may also affect pollinator ecology. Climate change is also likely to negatively affect livestock health and productivity (e.g., heat stress) (EPA, 2022a; USGCRP, 2018).

The Agriculture Improvement Act (commonly referred to as the "Farm Bill") is a major piece of federal legislation that influences what and how food is produced in the United States. It affects the composition of the food supply, nutrition and public health, food prices, agricultural producers

---

[25]Defined as "a tract with either a poverty rate of 20 percent or more, or a median family income less than 80 percent of the state-wide median family income; or a tract in a metropolitan area with a median family income less than 80 percent of the surrounding metropolitan area median family income" (USDA, 2022a).

[26]Defined as "at least 500 people, or 33 percent of the population, living more than one-half mile (urban areas) or more than 10 miles (rural areas) from the nearest supermarket, supercenter, or large grocery store" (USDA, 2022a). USDA also produces estimates using the distance threshold as 1 mile for urban areas and 20 miles for rural areas.

[27]In this study, the authors differentiated supermarkets from grocery stores if the store had more than 50 employees or was classified as a franchise.

and practices, the use and conservation of natural resources, and trade (Shannon et al., 2015). The omnibus law is typically reauthorized every 5 years (Johnson and Monke, 2023); the 2018 act expires at the end of FY2023 and included 12 titles.[28] The nutrition title comprised the majority of funding in the 2018 bill (the largest part of which was for the Supplemental Nutrition Assistance Program [SNAP], followed by crop insurance, commodities, and conservation) (Johnson and Monke, 2023). Given the bill's size, scope, and impact, it could benefit from an equity audit to review its effects on racial, ethnic, and tribal health equity; the USDA Equity Commission's interim report recommends equity audits across USDA's services (USDA Equity Commission, 2023).

As described, reservations are often in rural areas and frequently underresourced. The reservation system destroyed traditional food systems; sources of nutritious food may be sparse and/or difficult to reach (Maillacheruvu, 2022; Nikolaus et al., 2022). Part of the nutrition title in the Farm Bill includes the Food Distribution Program on Indian Reservations. This program provides USDA food commodities, in lieu of SNAP benefits, to eligible low-income households on reservations and American Indians living in Oklahoma or near reservations in designated areas; eligible households cannot participate in both SNAP and the Food Distribution Program on Indian Reservations during the same month (Aussenberg and Billings, 2019; Croft, 2022; Maillacheruvu, 2022). The 2018 Farm Bill increased the federal administrative funding, requiring the government to pay a minimum of 80 percent of administrative costs, and authorized a demonstration project for tribes to enter self-determination contracts to purchase their own commodities, giving them more flexibility in selecting foods (Croft, 2022; Johnson and Monke, 2023). This is in accordance with the USDA Equity Action Plan (and its commission's interim report) and its Indigenous Food Sovereignty Initiative, both of which acknowledge and support enabling tribal self-determination and self-governance, strengthening tribes' efforts to protect and build traditional food systems, and responding to dietary needs as they see fit with traditional and culturally appropriate food, including tribally grown food (Johnson, 2022; Maillacheruvu, 2022; USDA Equity Commission, 2023). These changes (among 63 new tribal-specific provisions in 11 of the 12 titles to support food, farm and agriculture, infrastructure, and research programs for tribal governments, communities, and food producers) came about in part

---

[28] Pub. L. 115–334, 132 Stat. 4490 (Dec. 20, 2018). Title I: Commodity Programs, Title II: Conservation, Title III: Trade, Title IV: Nutrition, Title V: Credit, Title VI: Rural Development, Title VII: Research, Extension, and Related Matters, Title VIII: Forestry, Title IX: Energy, Title X: Horticulture, Title XI: Crop Insurance, Title XII: Miscellaneous (Johnson and Monke, 2023).

because of the sustained efforts of the Native Farm Bill Coalition, an initiative made up of 170 tribal governments (Duren, 2020).

Racial inequities extend beyond access to food and federal nutrition support to the production portion of the food system. From the late 1990s to the 2010s, USDA settled multiple class action suits from Black, Latino/a, and AIAN farmers who claimed the agency engaged in systemic discrimination when deciding on farm loans and access to land. In *Pigford v. Glickman*,[29] the federal government was ordered to pay more than $2 billion in monetary relief to a group of Black farmers for damages caused by discriminatory loan and land access practices (NSAC, 2017). Similarly, *Keepseagle v. Vilsack*[30] found USDA had systematically discriminated against American Indian farmers and ranchers since the 1980s by denying them access to low interest rate loans in the Farm Loan Program; the settlement was $760 million (CohenMilstein, n.d.; NSAC, 2017). Discrimination and restricted access to opportunities and resources (e.g., land, infrastructure, credit, capital, information) results in generational wealth loss for racially and ethnically minoritized farmers and reduces their numbers (Ackoff et al., 2022; Aminetzah et al., 2021; Casey, 2021; Union of Concerned Scientists, 2020). In response to advocacy by organizations such as Rural Coalition and 1890 land-grant colleges (historically Black universities established under the Second Morrill Act of 1890[31]) (USDA, n.d.), the 1990 Farm Bill created a formal designation of socially disadvantaged farmer and rancher: "a group whose members have been subjected to racial or ethnic prejudice because of their identity as members of a group without regard to their individual qualities"[32]; this includes Black, Latino/a, Asian, NHPI, and AIAN farmers and ranchers (NSAC, 2017). Some, but not all, USDA programs also include women (USDA, 2022d). The 2018 Farm Bill included expanded support for this group in crop insurance, farm credit, and conservation programs. Additionally, USDA leadership signaled intention to address possible discrimination involving this group across USDA programs and offices (Johnson, 2021).

Adding provisions to the 2018 Farm Bill aimed specifically at tribal governments and communities is a positive example of incorporating community voice in federal policy making; building strong community leadership and capacity is an important way to improve public health (NASEM, 2017; NCAI, 2021). However, room for improvement remains in the next iteration of the Farm Bill, and the federal government can do more to promote racial, ethnic, and tribal equity in the food and agricultural system.

---

[29] *Pigford v. Glickman*, 185 F.R.D. 82 (D.D.C. 1999).
[30] *Keepseagle v. Vilsack*, Case No. 99-CV-3119 (D.D.C. 2011) (EGS).
[31] 7 U.S.C. § 321 *et seq.*
[32] 7 U.S.C. § 2279.

See, for example, the priorities of the Native Farm Bill Coalition (Parker et al., 2022), the National Young Farmers Coalition (Ackoff et al., 2022), and the National Sustainable Agriculture Coalition (NSAC, 2023) for the 2023 Farm Bill, which include additional ways to address racial, ethnic, and tribal equity. For more information on racial, ethnic, and tribal food and land issues in this report, see Chapter 3 (SNAP and the Special Supplemental Nutrition Program for Women, Infants, and Children), Chapter 4 (National School Lunch Program), and Chapter 7 (land dispossession and restoration).

> *Conclusion 6-4: Community voice through advocacy has played a positive role in shaping iterations of the Agriculture Improvement Act. However, given the bill's size and scope, an audit of the equity implications of the bill could identify additional areas of improvement, such as areas to expand further tribal self-determination and self-governance in relevant programs and other mechanisms to advance racial and ethnic health equity.*

CONCLUDING OBSERVATIONS

This chapter has outlined some of the key ways that the built environment functions as an SDOH and how federal policies in this area positively and negatively impact racial, ethnic, and tribal equity. Although this report provides crosscutting recommendations for federal action (see Chapter 8), many National Academies reports have evidence-based and promising recommendations for federal action on specific policies to advance racial, ethnic, and tribal health equity in the area of neighborhood and built environment (including and beyond the federal policies reviewed in this chapter) that are still relevant (see Box 6-2 for examples of such recommendations from two reports also focused on health equity).

Given the broad scope of this SDOH domain, the committee could not review all relevant federal policies. However, the policies in this chapter highlight several crosscutting themes—access barriers for existing programs, program implementation issues, and the need to include community voice. Where people work, live, play, and age can have major repercussions on health outcomes, and the current system of federal laws and policies can play a supporting role in furthering inequities. Because of the relatively fixed nature of the built environment, past federal policies that were key to shaping it still have major implications for processes that affect racial, ethnic, and tribal health outcomes and inequities. For example, redlining continues to harm some communities and benefit others today.

BOX 6-2
Example Recommendations from
National Academies Reports

Vibrant and Healthy Kids: Aligning Science, Practice, and Policy to Advance Health Equity (NASEM, 2019b)
Recommendation 6-3: The U.S. Department of Housing and Urban Development, states, and local, territorial, and tribal public housing authorities should increase the supply of high-quality affordable housing that is available to families, especially those with young children.

Recommendation 6-4: The Secretary of the U.S. Department of Health and Human Services, in collaboration with the U.S. Department of Housing and Urban Development and other relevant agencies, should lead the development of a comprehensive plan to ensure access to stable, affordable, and safe housing in the prenatal through early childhood period. This strategy should particularly focus on priority populations who are disproportionately impacted by housing challenges and experience poor health outcomes.

Communities in Action: Pathways to Health Equity (NASEM, 2017)
Recommendation 6-1: All government agencies that support or conduct planning related to land use, housing, transportation, and other areas that affect populations at high risk of health inequity should:

- Add specific requirements to outreach processes to ensure robust and authentic community participation in policy development.
- Collaborate with public health agencies and others to ensure a broad consideration of unintended consequences for health and well-being, including whether the benefits and burdens will be equitably distributed.
- Highlight the co-benefits of—or shared "wins" that could be achieved by—considering health equity in the development of comprehensive plans (e.g., improving public transit in transit-poor areas supports physical activity, promotes health equity, and creates more sustainable communities).
- Prioritize affordable housing, implement strategies to mitigate and avoid displacement (and its serious health effects), and document outcomes.

Permanent Supportive Housing: Evaluating the Evidence for Improving Health Outcomes Among People Experiencing Chronic Homelessness (NASEM, 2018b)
Recommendation 7-1: The Department of Housing and Urban Development and the Department of Health and Human Services should undertake a review of their programs and policies for funding permanent supportive housing with the goal of maximizing flexibility and the coordinated use of funding streams for supportive services, health-related care, housing-related services, the capital costs of housing, and operating funds such as Housing Choice Vouchers.

The evidence in this chapter illustrates several examples of how policies have resulted in intergenerational health outcomes disproportionately burdening communities who have faced segregation, disinvestment, and exposure to environmental hazards—a foundational context that needs to be accounted for when implementing or creating federal policy.

The committee identified federal actions, supported by evidence, that can address racial and ethnic health inequities in this domain. First, expanding access to effective programs such as federal rental assistance can improve housing security and health outcomes among racially and ethnically minoritized communities. Second, federal support for infrastructure projects provides opportunities to prevent health inequities from being built into racially and ethnically minoritized communities; integrating several existing tools into infrastructure investment decisions will need to be a priority. Third, government agencies that work on housing, transportation, food, and other areas related to the built environment need to review their policies and practices to verify that they collaborate with community stakeholders and public health partners to avoid or minimize health risks; a positive example is the inclusion of AIAN community voice in parts of the Farm Bill. The chapter also highlights future challenges. Federal actions will need to face the reality that, gone unchecked, climate change will further amplify harms in the built environment.

REFERENCES

AAPD (American Association of People with Disabilities). n.d. *Equity in transportation for people with disabilities*. Washington, DC: American Association of People with Disabilities.

Aaronson, D., D. Hartley, and B. Mazumder. 2021. The effects of the 1930s HOLC "redlining" maps. *American Economic Journal: Economic Policy* 13(4):355–392.

Ackoff, S., E. Flom, V. G. Polanco, D. Howard, J. Manly, C. Mueller, H. Rippon-Butler, and L. Wyatt. 2022. *Building a future with farmers 2022: Results and recommendations from the National Young Farmer Survey*. Hudson, NY: National Young Farmers Coalition.

Acosta, S. 2021. *Tribal Housing Funding a Critical Component of Build Back Better*. https://www.cbpp.org/blog/tribal-housing-funding-a-critical-component-of-build-back-better (accessed March 2, 2023).

Acosta, S., and E. Gartland. 2021. *Families wait years for housing vouchers due to inadequate funding: Expanding program would reduce hardship, improve equity*. Washington, DC: Center on Budget and Policy Priorities.

ADA.gov. n.d. *Introduction to the Americans with Disabilities Act*. https://www.ada.gov/topics/intro-to-ada/ (accessed May 28, 2023).

Ahmad, K., S. Erqou, N. Shah, U. Nazir, A. R. Morrison, G. Choudhary, and W. C. Wu. 2020. Association of poor housing conditions with COVID-19 incidence and mortality across U.S. counties. *PLOS ONE* 15(11):e0241327.

Aminetzah, D., J. Brennan, W. Davis, B. Idoniboye, N. Noel, J. Palowski, and S. Stewart. 2021. *Black Farmers in the U.S.: The Opportunity for Addressing Racial Disparities in Farming*. https://www.mckinsey.com/industries/agriculture/our-insights/black-farmers-in-the-us-the-opportunity-for-addressing-racial-disparities-in-farming (accessed March 2, 2023).

Andrade, T. J. H. 2022. Belated justice: The failures and promise of the Hawaiian Homes Commission Act. *American Indian Law Review* 46(1):1–56.

APHA (American Public Health Association). 2011. *Ending Agricultural Exceptionalism: Strengthening Worker Protection in Agriculture Through Regulation, Enforcement, Training, and Improved Worksite Health Safety: Policy Number 201110.* https://www.apha.org/policies-and-advocacy/public-health-policy-statements/policy-database/2014/07/09/10/ending-agricultural-exceptionalism-strengthening-worker-protection-in-agriculture (accessed May 31, 2023).

Archer, D. N. 2020. "White men's roads through Black men's homes": Advancing racial equity through highway reconstruction. *Vanderbilt Law Review* 73(5):1259–1330.

Arnold, C. A., and Resilience Justice Project Researchers. 2021. Resilience justice and community-based green and blue infrastructure. *William & Mary Environmental Law and Policy Review* 45(3):665–737.

ASCE (American Society of Civil Engineers). 2019. *2019 report card for Puerto Rico's infrastructure.* Reston, VA: American Society of Civil Engineers.

ASCE. 2021. *2021 report card for America's infrastructure.* Reston, VA: American Society of Civil Engineers.

Ash, M., and J. K. Boyce. 2018. Racial disparities in pollution exposure and employment at U.S. industrial facilities. *Proceedings of the National Academy of Sciences* 115(42):10636–10641.

Aussenberg, R. A., and K. C. Billings. 2019. *2018 Farm Bill primer: SNAP and nutrition title programs.* Washington, DC: Congressional Research Service.

Aytur, S. A., D. A. Rodriguez, K. R. Evenson, D. J. Catellier, and W. D. Rosamond. 2007. Promoting active community environments through land use and transportation planning. *American Journal of Health Promotion* 21(4 Suppl):397–407.

Bailey, Z. D., N. Krieger, M. Agénor, J. Graves, N. Linos, and M. T. Bassett. 2017. Structural racism and health inequities in the USA: Evidence and interventions. *The Lancet* 389(10077):1453–1463.

Banaji, M. R., S. T. Fiske, and D. S. Massey. 2021. Systemic racism: Individuals and interactions, institutions and society. *Cognitive Research: Principles and Implications* 6(1):82.

Barber, S., A. Ferreira, A. B. Gripper, and J. L. Jahn. 2022. Healthy and thriving: Advancing anti-racism evidence and solutions to transform the health of Black communities. *The Lancet* 400(10368):2016–2018.

Baron, S. L., A. L. Steege, S. M. Marsh, C. C. Menendez, J. R. Myers, and CDC (Centers for Disease Control and Prevention). 2013. Nonfatal work-related injuries and illnesses—United States, 2010. *Morbidity and Mortality Weekly Report Supplements* 62(3):35–40.

Baurick, T., L. Younes, and J. Meiners. 2019. *Welcome to "Cancer Alley," Where Toxic Air Is About to Get Worse.* https://www.propublica.org/article/welcome-to-cancer-alley-where-toxic-air-is-about-to-get-worse (accessed May 28, 2023).

BIA (Bureau of Indian Affairs). 2017. *What Is a Federal Indian Reservation?* https://www.bia.gov/faqs/what-federal-indian-reservation (accessed March 17, 2023).

Blick, R. N., M. D. Franklin, D. W. Ellsworth, S. M. Havercamp, and B. L. Kornblau. 2015. *The double burden: Health disparities among people of color living with disabilities.* Columbus, OH: Ohio Disability and Health Program.

BLS (Bureau of Labor Statistics). 2021. *The Economics Daily: Number of Fatal Work Injuries in 2020 the Lowest Since 2013.* https://www.bls.gov/opub/ted/2021/number-of-fatal-work-injuries-in-2020-the-lowest-since-2013.htm (accessed March 17, 2023).

BLS. 2022. *Employer-Reported Workplace Injuries and Illnesses, 2021.* https://www.bls.gov/news.release/osh.nr0.htm (accessed March 17, 2023).

Bohme, S. R. 2015. EPA's proposed worker protection standard and the burdens of the past. *International Journal of Occupational and Environmental Health* 21(2):161–165.

Bowen, K. J., and Y. Lynch. 2017. The public health benefits of green infrastructure: The potential of economic framing for enhanced decision-making. *Current Opinion in Environmental Sustainability* 25:90–95.

Bower, K. M., R. J. Thorpe, Jr., C. Rohde, and D. J. Gaskin. 2014. The intersection of neighborhood racial segregation, poverty, and urbanicity and its impact on food store availability in the United States. *Preventive Medicine* 58:33–39.

Braveman, P., M. Dekker, S. Egerter, T. Sadegh-Nobari, and C. Pollack. 2011. *Issue brief #7 exploring the social determinants of health: Housing and health*. Princeton, NJ: Robert Wood Johnson Foundation.

Braveman, P. A., E. Arkin, D. Proctor, T. Kauh, and N. Holm. 2022. Systemic and structural racism: Definitions, examples, health damages, and approaches to dismantling. *Health Affairs* 41(2):171–178.

Brenman, M. 2007. *Transportation inequity in the United States: A historical overview*. https://www.americanbar.org/groups/crsj/publications/human_rights_magazine_home/human_rights_vol34_2007/summer2007/hr_summer07_brenma/ (accessed March 23, 2023).

Brulle, R. J., and D. N. Pellow. 2006. Environmental justice: Human health and environmental inequalities. *Annual Review of Public Health* 27(1):103–124.

Bui, D. P., K. McCaffrey, M. Friedrichs, N. LaCross, N. M. Lewis, K. Sage, B. Barbeau, D. Vilven, C. Rose, S. Braby, S. Willardson, A. Carter, C. Smoot, A. Winquist, and A. Dunn. 2020. Racial and ethnic disparities among COVID-19 cases in workplace outbreaks by industry sector—Utah, March 6–June 5, 2020. *Morbidity and Mortality Weekly Report* 69(33):1133–1138.

Bullard, R. D. 1983. Solid waste sites and the Black Houston community. *Sociological Inquiry* 53(2–3):273–288.

Bullard, R. D., P. Mohai, R. Saha, and B. Wright. 2007. *Toxic wastes and race at twenty: 1987–2007*. Cleveland, OH: United Church of Christ.

Burnett, J. 2021. Officials mark 100th anniversary of signing of Hawaiian Homes Commission Act. *Hawaii Tribune-Herald*, July 10.

Campbell, C., R. Greenberg, D. Mankikar, and R. D. Ross. 2016. A case study of environmental injustice: The failure in Flint. *International Journal of Environmental Research and Public Health* 13(10):951.

Casey, A. R. 2021. *Racial equity in U.S. farming: Background in brief*. Washington, DC: Congressional Research Service.

CBO (Congressional Budget Office). 2018. *Federal Support for Financing State and Local Transportation and Water Infrastructure*. Washington, DC: Congressional Budget Office.

CBPP (Center on Budget and Policy Priorities). 2021. *Policy Basics: The Housing Choice Voucher Program*. https://www.cbpp.org/research/housing/the-housing-choice-voucher-program (accessed March 2, 2023).

CBPP. 2022a. *Chart book: Housing and health problems are intertwined. So are their solutions*. Washington, DC: Center on Budget and Policy Priorities.

CBPP. 2022b. *Policy Basics: Federal Rental Assistance*. https://www.cbpp.org/research/housing/federal-rental-assistance (accessed March 2, 2023).

CBPP. 2022c. *United States Federal Rental Assistance Fact Sheet*. https://www.cbpp.org/research/housing/federal-rental-assistance-fact-sheets#US (accessed March 2, 2023).

CDC (Centers for Disease Control and Prevention). 2021. *Childhood Lead Poisoning Prevention: Populations at Higher Risk*. https://www.cdc.gov/nceh/lead/prevention/populations.htm (accessed May 23, 2023).

CDC. 2022a. *Basic Facts About Mold and Dampness*. https://www.cdc.gov/mold/faqs.htm (accessed March 2, 2023).

CDC. 2022b. *Climate Effects on Health*. https://www.cdc.gov/climateandhealth/effects/default.htm (accessed March 2, 2023).

CDC. 2022c. *Health Effects of Lead Exposure.* https://www.cdc.gov/nceh/lead/prevention/health-effects.htm (accessed March 2, 2023).

CDC. 2022d. *Justice, Equity, Diversity, and Inclusion in Climate Adaptation Planning.* https://www.cdc.gov/climateandhealth/JEDI.htm (accessed March 2, 2023).

CDC and HUD (Department of Housing and Urban Development). 2006. *Healthy housing reference manual.* Atlanta, GA: Department of Health and Human Services.

Chetty, R., N. Hendren, and L. F. Katz. 2016. The effects of exposure to better neighborhoods on children: New evidence from the Moving to Opportunity experiment. *American Economic Review* 106(4):855-902.

Chetty, R., J. N. Friedman, N. Hendren, M. R. Jones, and S. R. Porter. 2018. *The opportunity atlas: Mapping the childhood roots of social mobility: Working paper 25147.* Cambridge, MA: National Bureau of Economic Research.

Chinowsky, P. 2022. *Intense Heat and Flooding Are Wreaking Havoc on Power and Water Systems as Climate Change Batters America's Aging Infrastructure.* https://theconversation.com/intense-heat-and-flooding-are-wreaking-havoc-on-power-and-water-systems-as-climate-change-batters-americas-aging-infrastructure-189761 (accessed March 2, 2023).

Cho, R. 2022. *Presentation to the Committee on the Review of Federal Policies That Contribute to Racial and Ethnic Health Inequities.* July 26. Paper presented at Meeting 3, Part 1: Committee on the Review of Federal Policies That Contribute to Racial and Ethnic Health Inequities, Washington, DC.

City of Saint Paul. 2016. *Saint Paul street design manual.* Saint Paul, MN: City of Saint Paul.

Clark, L. P., D. B. Millet, and J. D. Marshall. 2014. National patterns in environmental injustice and inequality: Outdoor NO2 air pollution in the United States. *PLOS ONE* 9(4):e94431.

Clark, L. P., D. B. Millet, and J. D. Marshall. 2017. Changes in transportation-related air pollution exposures by race-ethnicity and socioeconomic status: Outdoor nitrogen dioxide in the United States in 2000 and 2010. *Environmental Health Perspectives* 125(9):097012.

CohenMilstein. n.d. *Keepseagle.* https://www.cohenmilstein.com/case-study/keepseagle (accessed March 2, 2023).

Consillio, K. 2022. *More Than 3,000 Lots Proposed for Native Hawaiians on Housing Waitlist; Advocates Say More Needed.* https://www.kitv.com/news/local/more-than-3-000-lots-proposed-for-native-hawaiians-on-housing-waitlist-advocates-say-more/article_66d3fff6-33de-11ed-b542-87d7cb86a334.html (accessed May 21, 2023).

Conzelmann, C., A. Salazar-Miranda, T. Phan, and J. Hoffman. 2023. *Working paper series: Long-term causal effects of redlining on environmental risk exposure.* Richmond, VA: Federal Reserve Bank of Richmond.

Copeland, C. 2016. *Green infrastructure and issues in managing urban stormwater.* Washington, DC: Congressional Research Service.

CPSTF (Community Preventive Services Task Force). 2021. *Social determinants of health: Tenant-based housing voucher programs: Finding and rationale statement.* Atlanta, GA: Office of the Associate Director for Policy and Strategy, Centers for Disease Control and Prevention.

Croft, G. K. 2022. *Preparing for the next Farm Bill.* Washington, DC: Congressional Research Service.

Cullingworth, J. B., and R. W. Caves. 2009. *Planning in the USA: Policies, issues, and processes,* 3rd ed. London, UK: Routledge.

Curl, C. L., R. A. Fenske, J. C. Kissel, J. H. Shirai, T. F. Moate, W. Griffith, G. Coronado, and B. Thompson. 2002. Evaluation of take-home organophosphorus pesticide exposure among agricultural workers and their children. *Environmental Health Perspectives* 110(12):A787–A792.

Cushing, L., J. Faust, L. M. August, R. Cendak, W. Wieland, and G. Alexeeff. 2015. Racial/ethnic disparities in cumulative environmental health impacts in California: Evidence from a statewide environmental justice screening tool (CalEnviroScreen 1.1). *American Journal of Public Health* 105(11):2341–2348.

Damalas, C. A., and S. D. Koutroubas. 2016. Farmers' exposure to pesticides: Toxicity types and ways of prevention. *Toxics* 4(1).

Davies, I. P., R. D. Haugo, J. C. Robertson, and P. S. Levin. 2018. The unequal vulnerability of communities of color to wildfire. *PLOS ONE* 13(11):e0205825.

Deep South Center for Environmental Justice. 2020. *Surviving cancer alley: The stories of five communities.* New Orleans, LA: Deep South Center for Environmental Justice.

Denary, W., A. Fenelon, P. Schlesinger, J. Purtle, K. M. Blankenship, and D. E. Keene. 2021. Does rental assistance improve mental health? Insights from a longitudinal cohort study. *Social Science & Medicine* 282:114100.

Department of Energy. n.d. *Energy Saver: Efficient Home Design.* https://www.energy.gov/energysaver/efficient-home-design (accessed May 20, 2023).

Department of Hawaiian Home Lands. n.d. *About the Department of Hawaiian Home Lands.* https://dhhl.hawaii.gov/dhhl/ (accessed May 21, 2023).

Dillon, L., and B. Poston. 2021. Freeways force out residents in communities of color—again. *Los Angeles Times*, November 11.

DOJ (Department of Justice). 2023. *Justice Department Announces New Initiative to Combat Redlining.* https://www.justice.gov/opa/pr/justice-department-announces-new-initiative-combat-redlining (accessed May 22, 2023).

Domonoske, C. 2016. *Interactive Redlining Map Zooms in on America's History of Discrimination.* https://www.npr.org/sections/thetwo-way/2016/10/19/498536077/interactive-redlining-map-zooms-in-on-americas-history-of-discrimination (accessed May 23, 2023).

Donley, N., R. D. Bullard, J. Economos, I. Figueroa, J. Lee, A. K. Liebman, D. N. Martinez, and F. Shafiei. 2022. Pesticides and environmental injustice in the USA: Root causes, current regulatory reinforcement and a path forward. *BMC Public Health* 22(1).

Dorazio, J. 2022. *Localized anti-displacement policies: Ways to combat the effects of gentrification and lack of affordable housing.* Washington, DC: Center for American Progress.

DOT (Department of Transportation). 2015a. *Complete Streets.* https://www.transportation.gov/mission/health/complete-streets (accessed May 23, 2023).

DOT. 2015b. *Complete Streets Policies.* https://www.transportation.gov/mission/health/complete-streets-policies (accessed May 28, 2023).

DOT. 2022a. *Biden-Harris Administration Announces $686 Million in Grants to Modernize Older Transit Stations and Improve Accessibility Across the Country.* https://www.transportation.gov/briefing-room/biden-harris-administration-announces-686-million-grants-modernize-older-transit (accessed May 23, 2023).

DOT. 2022b. *Biden Administration Announces First-Ever Funding Program Dedicated to Reconnecting American Communities.* https://www.transportation.gov/briefing-room/biden-administration-announces-first-ever-funding-program-dedicated-reconnecting (accessed May 31, 2023).

DOT. 2023. *Reconnecting Communities Pilot Program.* https://www.transportation.gov/grants/reconnecting-communities (accessed May 31, 2023).

DOT. n.d. *U.S. Department of Transportation's Disability Policy Priorities.* https://www.transportation.gov/mission/accessibility/priorities (accessed May 23, 2023).

Duranton, G., and M. A. Turner. 2011. The fundamental law of road congestion: Evidence from U.S. cities. *American Economic Review* 101(6):2616–2652.

Duren, C. D. 2020. The native Farm Bill coalition and the 2018 Farm Bill: Building a strong, sustained voice on food and agriculture issues in Indian country. *Renewable Agriculture and Food Systems* 35(4):463–464.

Eaton, T. T. 2018. Approach and case-study of green infrastructure screening analysis for urban stormwater control. *Journal of Environmental Management* 209:495–504.

EBP and ASCE. 2021. *Failure to act: Economic impacts of status quo investment across infrastructure systems.* Reston, VA: American Society of Civil Engineers.

EPA (Environmental Protection Agency). 2004. *Understanding the Safe Drinking Water Act.* https://www.epa.gov/sites/default/files/2015-04/documents/epa816f04030.pdf (accessed March 14, 2023).

EPA. 2021. *Indoor Air Quality.* https://www.epa.gov/report-environment/indoor-air-quality (accessed March 2, 2023).

EPA. 2022a. *Climate Change Impacts on Agriculture and Food Supply.* https://www.epa.gov/climateimpacts/climate-change-impacts-agriculture-and-food-supply (accessed March 2, 2023).

EPA. 2022b. *Health and Environmental Effects of Particulate Matter (PM).* https://www.epa.gov/pm-pollution/health-and-environmental-effects-particulate-matter-pm (accessed March 2, 2023).

EPA. 2023a. *Agricultural Worker Protection Standard (WPS).* https://www.epa.gov/pesticide-worker-safety/agricultural-worker-protection-standard-wps (accessed March 15, 2023).

EPA. 2023b. *EPA Proposes Rule to Protect Farmworkers and Pesticide Handlers from Exposure.* https://www.epa.gov/newsreleases/epa-proposes-rule-protect-farmworkers-and-pesticide-handlers-exposures (accessed March 15, 2023).

EPA. 2023c. *Overcoming Barriers to Green Infrastructure.* https://www.epa.gov/green-infrastructure/overcoming-barriers-green-infrastructure (accessed May 22, 2023).

Faber, J. W. 2020. We built this: Consequences of New Deal Era intervention in America's racial geography. *American Sociological Review* 85(5):739–775.

Farrell, J., P. B. Burow, K. McConnell, J. Bayham, K. Whyte, and G. Koss. 2021. Effects of land dispossession and forced migration on Indigenous peoples in North America. *Science* 374(6567):eabe4943.

Feeding America. n.d. *Hunger Impacts Native American Families and Communities.* https://www.feedingamerica.org/hunger-in-america/native-american (accessed March 2, 2023).

Fenelon, A., N. Slopen, and S. J. Newman. 2022. The effects of rental assistance programs on neighborhood outcomes for U.S. children: Nationwide evidence by program and race/ethnicity. *Urban Affairs Review* 59(3):832–865.

FHWA (Federal Highway Administration). 2022. *Complete Streets in FHWA.* https://highways.dot.gov/complete-streets/complete-streets-fhwa (accessed May 28, 2023).

Fischer, W., D. Rice, and A. Mazzara. 2019. *Research shows rental assistance reduces hardship and provides platform to expand opportunity for low-income families.* Washington, DC: Center on Budget and Policy Priorities.

Fischer, W., S. Acosta, and E. Gartland. 2021. *More housing vouchers: Most important step to help more people afford stable homes.* Washington, DC: Center on Budget and Policy Priorities.

Fitzpatrick, T. 2021. *Tribal land and ownership statuses: Overview and selected issues for Congress.* Washington, DC: Congressional Research Service.

Flanigan, E., and M. Howard. 2008. *An interim guidebook on the congestion management process in metropolitan transportation planning.* Washington, DC: Federal Highway Administration.

Foster, J., A. Lowe, and S. Winkelman. 2011. *The value of green infrastructure for urban climate adaptation.* Washington, DC: The Center for Clean Air Policy.

Frank, L. D., J. F. Sallis, T. L. Conway, J. E. Chapman, B. E. Saelens, and W. Bachman. 2006. Many pathways from land use to health: Associations between neighborhood walkability and active transportation, body mass index, and air quality. *Journal of the American Planning Association* 72(1):75–87.

Frank, T. 2020. Flooding disproportionately harms black neighborhoods. *Scientific American,* June 2.

Frederick, J. 2022. *Expanding Efforts to Ensure the Health and Safety of Hispanic Workers.* https://blog.dol.gov/2021/09/27/expanding-efforts-to-ensure-the-health-and-safety-of-hispanic-workers (accessed March 3, 2023).

Frumkin, H. 2021. COVID-19, the built environment, and health. *Environmental Health Perspectives* 129(7):075001.

Frumkin, H., and A. Haines. 2019. Global environmental change and noncommunicable disease risks. *Annual Review of Public Health* 40:261–282.

FTA (Federal Transit Administration). 2022. *Fact Sheet: Enhanced Mobility of Seniors and Individuals with Disabilities.* https://www.transit.dot.gov/funding/grants/fact-sheet-enhanced-mobility-seniors-and-individuals-disabilities (accessed May 23, 2023).

GAO (Government Accountability Office). 2020. *Lead paint in housing: HUD has not identified high-risk project-based rental assistance properties.* Washington, DC: Government Accountability Office.

GAO. 2021. *Lead paint in housing: Key considerations for adopting stricter lead evaluation methods in HUD's voucher program.* Washington, DC: Government Accountability Office.

GAO. 2022. *Women in the workforce: The gender pay gap is greater for certain racial and ethnic groups and varies by education level.* Washington, DC: Government Accountability Office.

GHSA (Governors Highway Safety Administration). 2021. *An analysis of traffic fatalities by race and ethnicity.* Washington, DC: Governors Highway Safety Association.

Gibson, S. 2017. *A House to Last for 500 Years.* https://www.greenbuildingadvisor.com/article/a-house-to-last-for-500-years (accessed May 20, 2023).

Glantz, A., and E. Martinez. 2018. *For People of Color, Banks Are Shutting the Door to Homeownership.* https://revealnews.org/article/for-people-of-color-banks-are-shutting-the-door-to-homeownership/ (accessed May 22, 2023).

Goubert, A., and A. Austin. 2022. *The Historic Opportunities for Racial Equity in the Infrastructure Investment and Jobs Act.* https://cepr.net/the-historic-opportunities-for-racial-equity-in-the-infrastructure-investment-and-jobs-act/ (accessed March 2, 2023).

Grabowski, Z. J., T. McPhearson, and S. T. A. Pickett. 2023. Transforming U.S. urban green infrastructure planning to address equity. *Landscape and Urban Planning* 229:104591.

Guarna, O. N., L. J. Beyranevand, L. S. Nelson, and T. Pulaski. 2022. *Exposed and at risk: Opportunities to strengthen enforcement of pesticide regulations for farmworker safety.* South Royalton, VT: Center for Agriculture and Food Systems, Vermont Law and Graduate School.

Hamann, C., C. Peek-Asa, and B. Butcher. 2020. Racial disparities in pedestrian-related injury hospitalizations in the United States. *BMC Public Health* 20(1):1459.

Hanna-Attisha, M., J. LaChance, R. C. Sadler, and A. C. Schnepp. 2016. Elevated blood lead levels in children associated with the Flint drinking water crisis: A spatial analysis of risk and public health response. *American Journal of Public Health* 106(2):283–290.

Harvard Law Review. 2020. Chapter 4: Aloha 'āina: Native Hawaiian land restitution. *Harvard Law Review* 133(6):2148–2171.

Heaps, W., E. Abramsohn, and E. Skillen. 2021. *Health Affairs Policy Brief: Public Transportation in the U.S.: A Driver of Health and Equity.* https://www.healthaffairs.org/do/10.1377/hpb20210630.810356/full/health-affairs-brief-public-transportation-health-equity-heaps-1632491696172.pdf (accessed March 2, 2023).

HHS (Department of Health and Human Services). n.d. *Healthy People 2030: Promote the Health and Safety of People at Work.* https://health.gov/healthypeople/objectives-and-data/browse-objectives/workplace (accessed May 30, 2023).

Hiraishi, K. 2021. *100 Years of Hawaiian Home Lands Creates Generational Wealth for Some, Lost Opportunity for Many.* https://www.hawaiipublicradio.org/local-news/2021-07-09/100th-anniversary-of-the-hawaiian-homes-commission-act (accessed May 21, 2023).

Hoffman, J. S., V. Shandas, and N. Pendleton. 2020. The effects of historical housing policies on resident exposure to intra-urban heat: A study of 108 U.S. urban areas. *Climate* 8(1):12.

Hoffman, J. S., V. Shandas, and L. Johnson. 2022. Community science for the climate win: An equity-based framework for understanding and acting on extreme urban heat. In *Collaborating for climate equity: Researcher–practitioner partnerships in the Americas*, edited by V. Shandas and D. Hellman. New York, NY: Routledge.

Hoss, A. 2019. Federal Indian law as a structural determinant of health. *Journal of Law, Medicine & Ethics* 47(S4):34–42.

Howell, B. 2006. Exploiting race and space: Concentrated subprime lending as housing discrimination. *California Law Review* 94(1):101–147.

Hsu, A., G. Sheriff, T. Chakraborty, and D. Manya. 2021. Disproportionate exposure to urban heat island intensity across major U.S. cities. *Nature Communications* 12(1):2721.

Huang, C.-C., and R. Taylor. 2019. *Any federal infrastructure package should boost investment in low-income communities*. Washington, DC: Center on Budget and Policy Priorities.

HUD (Department of Housing and Urban Development). 2022. *2023 budget in brief*. Washington, DC: Department of Housing and Urban Development.

HUD. 2023. *HUD Announces $568 Million Available to Address Lead-Based Paint and Additional Housing-Related Hazards*. https://www.hud.gov/press/press_releases_media_advisories/ hud_no_23_012 (accessed May 23, 2023).

HUD. n.d.-a. *Housing Choice Vouchers Fact Sheet*. https://www.hud.gov/topics/housing_ choice_voucher_program_section_8#hcv02 (accessed March 14, 2023).

HUD. n.d.-b. *Moving to Opportunity for Fair Housing*. https://www.hud.gov/ programdescription/mto (accessed March 17, 2023).

Hwang, J., and L. Ding. 2020. Unequal displacement: Gentrification, racial stratification, and residential destinations in Philadelphia. *American Journal of Sociology* 126(2):354–406.

Hymel, K. 2019. If you build it, they will drive: Measuring induced demand for vehicle travel in urban areas. *Transport Policy* 76:57–66.

IOM (Institute of Medicine). 2004. *Damp indoor spaces and health*. Washington, DC: The National Academies Press.

IOM. 2007. *The future of disability in America*. Washington, DC: The National Academies Press.

Jacobs, D. E. 2011. Environmental health disparities in housing. *American Journal of Public Health* 101(S1):S115–S122.

Jadow, B. M., L. Hu, J. Zou, D. Labovitz, C. Ibeh, B. Ovbiagele, and C. Esenwa. 2023. Historical redlining, social determinants of health, and stroke prevalence in communities in New York City. *JAMA Network Open* 6(4):e235875.

Jampel, C. 2018. Intersections of disability justice, racial justice and environmental justice. *Environmental Sociology* 4(1):122–135.

JCHS (Joint Center for Housing Studies). 2022. *American's rental housing 2022*. Cambridge, MA: Joint Center for Housing Studies of Harvard University.

Jennings, V., C. Johnson Gaither, and R. Schulterbrandt Gragg. 2012. Promoting environmental justice through urban green space access: A synopsis. *Environmental Justice* 5(1):1–7.

Jernigan, V. B. B., K. R. Huyser, J. Valdes, and V. W. Simonds. 2017. Food insecurity among American Indians and Alaska Natives: A national profile using the Current Population Survey—Food Security Supplement. *Journal of Hunger & Environmental Nutrition* 12(1):1–10.

Johnson, R. 2021. *Defining a socially disadvantaged farmer or rancher (SDFR): In brief*. Washington, DC: Congressional Research Service.

Johnson, R. 2022. *Farm bill primer: Support for native agricultural producers*. Washington, DC: Congressional Research Service.

Johnson, R., and J. Monke. 2023. *What is the Farm Bill?* Washington, DC: Congressional Research Service.

Karner, A., J. London, D. Rowangould, and K. Manaugh. 2020. From transportation equity to transportation justice: Within, through, and beyond the state. *Journal of Planning Literature* 35(4):440–459.

Katz, L. 2021. *A racist past, a flooded future: Formerly redlined areas have $107 billion worth of homes facing high flood risk—25% more than non-redlined areas.* Seattle, WA: Redfin Corporation.

Kaufman, P., C. Dicken, and R. Williams. 2014. *Measuring access to healthful, affordable food in American Indian and Alaska Native tribal areas.* Washington, DC: Economic Research Service, Department of Agriculture.

Kay, J., and C. Katz. 2012. Pollution, poverty and people of color: Living with industry. *Scientific American*, June 4.

Kayden, J. S. 2001. National land-use planning and regulation in the United States: Understanding its fundamental importance. In *National-level planning in democratic countries: An international comparison of city and regional policy-making*, edited by R. Alterman. Liverpool, UK, Liverpool University Press. Pp. 43–64.

Kim, K.-H., E. Kabir, and S. A. Jahan. 2017. Exposure to pesticides and the associated human health effects. *Science of the Total Environment* 575:525–535.

Krahn, G. L., D. K. Walker, and R. Correa-De-Araujo. 2015. Persons with disabilities as an unrecognized health disparity population. *American Journal of Public Health* 105(S2):S198–S206.

Lane, H. M., R. Morello-Frosch, J. D. Marshall, and J. S. Apte. 2022. Historical redlining is associated with present-day air pollution disparities in U.S. cities. *Environmental Science & Technology Letters* 9(4):345–350.

Lee, E. K., G. Donley, T. H. Ciesielski, I. Gill, O. Yamoah, A. Roche, R. Martinez, and D. A. Freedman. 2022. Health outcomes in redlined versus non-redlined neighborhoods: A systematic review and meta-analysis. *Social Science & Medicine* 294:114696.

Levy, D. K., J. Comey, and S. Padilla. 2006. *In the face of gentrification: Case studies of local efforts to mitigate displacement.* Washington, DC: The Urban Institute.

Liebman, A. K., M. F. Wiggins, C. Fraser, J. Levin, J. Sidebottom, and T. A. Arcury. 2013. Occupational health policy and immigrant workers in the agriculture, forestry, and fishing sector. *American Journal of Industrial Medicine* 56(8):975–984.

Liu, J., L. P. Clark, M. J. Bechle, A. Hajat, S. Y. Kim, A. L. Robinson, L. Sheppard, A. A. Szpiro, and J. D. Marshall. 2021. Disparities in air pollution exposure in the United States by race/ethnicity and income, 1990–2010. *Environmental Health Perspectives* 129(12):127005.

Locke, D. H., B. Hall, J. M. Grove, S. T. A. Pickett, L. A. Ogden, C. Aoki, C. G. Boone, and J. P. M. O'Neil-Dunne. 2021. Residential housing segregation and urban tree canopy in 37 U.S. cities. *NPJ Urban Sustainability* 1(1):15.

Los Angeles County Department of Public Health. 2015. *Social determinants of health: Housing and health in Los Angeles County.* Los Angeles County, CA: Los Angeles County Department of Public Health.

Maillacheruvu, S. U. 2022. *The historical determinants of food insecurity in native communities.* Washington, DC: Center on Budget and Policy Priorities.

Maqbool, N., J. Viveiros, and M. Ault. 2015. *The impacts of affordable housing on health: A research summary.* Washington, DC: Center for Housing Policy, National Housing Conference.

Martin-Proctor, K. 2022 August 1. *Presentation to the Committee on the Review of Federal Policies That Contribute to Racial and Ethnic Health Inequities.* Paper presented at Meeting 3, Part 2: Committee on the Review of Federal Policies That Contribute to Racial and Ethnic Health Inequities.

Mazzara, A. 2017. *Federal rental assistance provides affordable homes for vulnerable people in all types of communities.* Washington, DC: Center on Budget and Policy Priorities.

Mikati, I., A. F. Benson, T. J. Luben, J. D. Sacks, and J. Richmond-Bryant. 2018. Disparities in distribution of particulate matter emission sources by race and poverty status. *American Journal of Public Health* 108(4):480–485.

Miletić, M., F. Shahine, M. Sarkar, and A. Quandt. 2022. A Native American perspective on sustainable and resilient infrastructure in southern California. *Sustainability* 14(19):12811.

Mitchell, B., and J. Franco. 2018. *HOLC "redlining" maps: The persistent structure of segregation and economic inequality.* Washington, DC: National Community Reinvestment Coalition.

Mogridge, M. J. H. 1997. The self-defeating nature of urban road capacity policy: A review of theories, disputes and available evidence. *Transport Policy* 4(1):5–23.

Mohai, P., and R. Saha. 2015. Which came first, people or pollution? Assessing the disparate siting and post-siting demographic change hypotheses of environmental injustice. *Environmental Research Letters* 10(11):115008.

Mohai, P., D. Pellow, and J. T. Roberts. 2009. Environmental justice. *Annual Review of Environment and Resources* 34(1):405–430.

Montgomery, D. 2021. *Low-Income People of Color Bear Brunt of Rising Pedestrian Deaths.* https://www.pewtrusts.org/en/research-and-analysis/blogs/stateline/2021/07/02/low-income-people-of-color-bear-brunt-of-rising-pedestrian-deaths (accessed March 2, 2023).

Moyce, S., D. Mitchell, T. Armitage, D. Tancredi, J. Joseph, and M. Schenker. 2017. Heat strain, volume depletion and kidney function in California agricultural workers. *Occupational and Environmental Medicine* 74(6):402-409.

Mueller, J. T., and S. Gasteyer. 2021. The widespread and unjust drinking water and clean water crisis in the United States. *Nature Communications* 12(1):3544.

NACTO (National Association of City Transportation Officials). 2016. *Transit street design guide: Universal design elements.* New York, NY: National Association of City Transportation Officials.

Nardone, A., K. E. Rudolph, R. Morello-Frosch, and J. A. Casey. 2021. Redlines and greenspace: The relationship between historical redlining and 2010 greenspace across the United States. *Environmental Health Perspectives* 129(1):017006.

NASEM (National Academies of Sciences, Engineering, and Medicine). 2016a. *Exploring data and metrics of value at the intersection of health care and transportation: Proceedings of a workshop.* Washington, DC: The National Academies Press.

NASEM. 2016b. *Framing the dialogue on race and ethnicity to advance health equity: Proceedings of a workshop.* Washington, DC: The National Academies Press.

NASEM. 2017. *Communities in action: Pathways to health equity.* Washington, DC: The National Academies Press.

NASEM. 2018a. *People living with disabilities: Health equity, health disparities, and health literacy: Proceedings of a workshop.* Washington, DC: The National Academies Press.

NASEM. 2018b. *Permanent supportive housing: Evaluating the evidence for improving health outcomes among people experiencing chronic homelessness.* Washington, DC: The National Academies Press.

NASEM. 2019a. *Framing the challenge of urban flooding in the United States.* Washington, DC: The National Academies Press.

NASEM. 2019b. *Vibrant and healthy kids: Aligning science, practice, and policy to advance health equity.* Washington, DC: The National Academies Press.

NASEM. 2021. *Racial equity addendum to critical issues in transportation.* Washington, DC: The National Academies Press.

NASEM. 2022a. *Racial equity, Black America, and public transportation, volume 1: A review of economic, health, and social impacts.* Washington, DC: The National Academies Press.

NASEM. 2022b. *Rental eviction and the COVID-19 pandemic: Averting a looming crisis.* Washington, DC: The National Academies Press.

National Archives. 2022. *National Interstate and Defense Highways Act (1956).* https://www.archives.gov/milestone-documents/national-interstate-and-defense-highways-act (accessed March 2, 2023).

National Endowment for the Arts. 2021. *Disability design: Summary report from a field scan.* Washington, DC: National Endowment for the Arts.

National Housing Law Project. 2021. *An advocate's guide to tenants' rights in the Low-Income Housing Tax Credit Program.* San Francisco, CA: National Housing Law Project.

National Integrated Heat Health Information System. n.d. *Mapping Campaigns.* https://www.heat.gov/pages/mapping-campaigns (accessed March 13, 2023).

National Low Income Housing Coalition. 2021. *NAHASDA Reauthorization Reintroduced in Senate.* https://nlihc.org/resource/nahasda-reauthorization-reintroduced-senate (accessed March 2, 2023).

National Low Income Housing Coalition. 2022. *Reforms to the low-income housing tax credit.* Washington, DC: National Low Income Housing Coalition.

NBER (National Bureau of Economic Research). n.d. *Moving to Opportunity (MTO) for Fair Housing Demonstration Project.* http://www2.nber.org/mtopublic/ (accessed March 17, 2023).

NCAI (National Congress of American Indians). 2021. *Fiscal year 2022 Indian country budget request: Restoring promises.* Washington, DC: National Congress of American Indians.

NCAI. n.d. *Housing & Infrastructure.* https://www.ncai.org/policy-issues/economic-development-commerce/housing-infrastructure (accessed March 2, 2023).

NCSL (National Conference of State Legislatures). 2022. *State policy options for green infrastructure.* Denver, CO: National Conference of State Legislatures.

Newman, K. L., J. S. Leon, and L. S. Newman. 2015. Estimating occupational illness, injury, and mortality in food production in the United States: A farm-to-table analysis. *Journal of Occupational and Environmental Medicine* 57(7):718–725.

Newport Partners and ARES Consulting. 2015. *Durability by design: A professional's guide to durable home design.* Washington, DC: Office of Policy Development and Research, Department of Housing and Urban Development.

Nikolaus, C. J., S. Johnson, T. Benally, T. Maudrie, A. Henderson, K. Nelson, T. Lane, V. Segrest, G. L. Ferguson, D. Buchwald, V. Blue Bird Jernigan, and K. Sinclair. 2022. Food insecurity among American Indian and Alaska Native people: A scoping review to inform future research and policy needs. *Advances in Nutrition* 13(5):1566–1583.

NIOSH (National Institute for Occupational Safety and Health). 2019. *Occupational Health Equity.* https://www.cdc.gov/niosh/programs/ohe/default.html (accessed March 3, 2023).

NIOSH and ASSE (American Society for Safety Engineers). 2015. *Overlapping vulnerabilities: The occupational safety and health of young workers in small construction firms.* Cincinnati, OH: National Institute for Occupational Safety and Health, Centers for Disease Control and Prevention.

Nowak, D. J., D. E. Crane, and J. C. Stevens. 2006. Air pollution removal by urban trees and shrubs in the United States. *Urban Forestry & Urban Greening* 4(3):115–123.

NSAC (National Sustainable Agriculture Coalition). 2017. *Racial Equity in the Farm Bill: Context and Foundations.* https://sustainableagriculture.net/blog/racial-equity-in-the-farm-bill/ (accessed March 2, 2023).

NSAC. 2023. *2023 Farm Bill platform.* Washington, DC: National Sustainable Agriculture Coalition.

O'Regan, K. M. 2016. Commentary: A federal perspective on gentrification. *Cityscape* 18(3):151–162.

Okechukwu, C. A., K. Souza, K. D. Davis, and A. B. de Castro. 2014. Discrimination, harassment, abuse, and bullying in the workplace: Contribution of workplace injustice to occupational health disparities. *American Journal of Industrial Medicine* 57(5):573–586.

Ornelas, I., W. Fung, S. Gabbard, and D. Carroll. 2021. *Findings from the National Agricultural Workers Survey (NAWS) 2017–2018: A demographic and employment profile of United States farmworkers.* Rockville, MD: JBS International.

OSHA (Occupational Safety and Health Administration). n.d.-a. *Agricultural Operations: Hazards & Controls.* https://www.osha.gov/agricultural-operations/hazards (accessed March 3, 2023).

OSHA. n.d.-b. *OSH Act of 1970: Sec. 2: Congressional Findings and Purpose.* https://www.osha.gov/laws-regs/oshact/section_2 (accessed March 15, 2023).

Parker, E., C. Griffith Hotvedt, J. VanPool, K. Case, M. B. Zook, S. Wilkie, J. Damaso, and K. Coutu. 2022. *Gaining ground: A report on the 2018 Farm Bill successes for Indian country and opportunities for 2023.* Prior Lake, MN: Shakopee Mdewakanton Sioux Community.

Paul, J. 2016. Navajo president says farmers continue to struggle after Gold King spill. *The Denver Post,* April 22.

Perez, R. 2021a. The U.S. broke its promise to return land to Hawaiians. My family knows something about land loss. *ProPublica,* May 26.

Perez, R. 2021b. The U.S. owes Hawaiians millions of dollars worth of land. Congress helped make sure the debt wasn't paid. *ProPublica,* May 7.

Perry, A. M., and D. Harshbarger. 2019. *America's formerly redlined neighborhoods have changed, and so must solutions to rectify them.* Washington, DC: The Brookings Institution.

Pflipsen, M., and Y. Zenchenko. 2017. Nutrition for oral health and oral manifestations of poor nutrition and unhealthy habits. *General Dentistry* 65(6):36–43.

Pindus, N., G. T. Kingsley, J. Biess, D. Levy, J. Simington, C. Hayes, and Urban Institute. 2017. *Housing needs of American Indians and Alaska Natives in tribal areas: A report from the assessment of American Indian, Alaska Native, and Native Hawaiian housing needs.* Washington, DC: Office of Policy Development and Research, Department of Housing and Urban Development.

Pineda, V. S., S. Meyer, and J. P. Cruz. 2017. The inclusion imperative. Forging an inclusive new urban agenda. *The Journal of Public Space* 2(4):1–20.

Raifman, M. A., and E. F. Choma. 2022. Disparities in activity and traffic fatalities by race/ethnicity. *American Journal of Preventive Medicine* 63(2):160–167.

Ray, R., A. M. Perry, D. Harshbarger, S. Elizondo, and A. Gibbons. 2021. *Homeownership, racial segregation, and policy solutions to racial wealth.* Washington, DC: The Brookings Institution.

Reft, R. 2023. We mythologize highways, but they've damaged communities of color. *The Washington Post,* January 19.

Reynolds, C. C. O., M. A. Harris, K. Teschke, P. A. Cripton, and M. Winters. 2009. The impact of transportation infrastructure on bicycling injuries and crashes: A review of the literature. *Environmental Health* 8(1):47.

Rho, H. J., H. Brown, and S. Fremstad. 2020. *A basic demographic profile of workers in frontline industries.* Washington, DC: Center for Economic and Policy Research.

Rhone, A., M. Ver Ploeg, R. Williams, and V. Breneman. 2019. *Understanding low-income and low-access census tracts across the nation: Subnational and subpopulation estimates of access to healthy food.* Washington, DC: Economic Reserch Service, Department of Agriculture.

Rhone, A., R. Williams, and C. Dicken. 2022. *Low-income and low-foodstore-access census tracts, 2015-19.* Washington, DC: Economic Research Service, Department of Agriculture.

Rollston, R., and S. Galea. 2020. COVID-19 and the social determinants of health. *American Journal of Health Promotion* 34(6):687–689.

Romanello, M., C. Di Napoli, P. Drummond, C. Green, H. Kennard, P. Lampard, D. Scamman, N. Arnell, S. Ayeb-Karlsson, L. B. Ford, K. Belesova, K. Bowen, W. Cai, M. Callaghan, D. Campbell-Lendrum, J. Chambers, K. R. van Daalen, C. Dalin, N. Dasandi, S. Dasgupta, M. Davies, P. Dominguez-Salas, R. Dubrow, K. L. Ebi, M. Eckelman, P. Ekins, L. E. Escobar, L. Georgeson, H. Graham, S. H. Gunther, I. Hamilton, Y. Hang, R. Hänninen, S. Hartinger, K. He, J. J. Hess, S.-C. Hsu, S. Jankin, L. Jamart, O. Jay, I. Kelman, G. Kiesewetter, P. Kinney, T. Kjellstrom, D. Kniveton, J. K. W. Lee, B. Lemke, Y. Liu, Z. Liu, M. Lott, M. L. Batista, R. Lowe, F. MacGuire, M. O. Sewe, J. Martinez-Urtaza, M. Maslin, L. McAllister, A. McGushin, C. McMichael, Z. Mi, J. Milner, K. Minor, J. C. Minx, N. Mohajeri, M. Moradi-Lakeh, K. Morrissey, S. Munzert, K. A. Murray, T. Neville, M. Nilsson, N. Obradovich, M. B. O'Hare, T. Oreszczyn, M. Otto, F. Owfi, O. Pearman, M. Rabbaniha, E. J. Z. Robinson, J. Rocklöv, R. N. Salas, J. C. Semenza, J. D. Sherman, L. Shi, J. Shumake-Guillemot, G. Silbert, M. Sofiev, M. Springmann, J. Stowell, M. Tabatabaei, J. Taylor, J. Triñanes, F. Wagner, P. Wilkinson, M. Winning, M. Yglesias-González, S. Zhang, P. Gong, H. Montgomery, and A. Costello. 2022. The 2022 report of the Lancet countdown on health and climate change: Health at the mercy of fossil fuels. *The Lancet* 400(10363):1619–1654.

Rothstein, R. 2017. *The color of law: A forgotten history of how our government segregated America*. New York, NY: Liveright Publishing Corporation.

Rural Health Information Hub. n.d. *Reconnecting Communities Pilot Discretionary Grant Program*. https://www.ruralhealthinfo.org/funding/5593 (accessed March 2, 2023).

Salvatore, A., A. Bradman, R. Castorina, J. Camacho, J. Lopez, D. Barr, J. Snyder, N. Jewell, and B. Eskenazi. 2008. Occupational behaviors and farmworkers' pesticide exposure: Findings from a study in Monterey County, California. *American Journal of Industrial Medicine* 51:782–794.

Sard, B., M. Cunningham, and R. Greenstein. 2018. *Helping young children move out of poverty by creating a new type of rental voucher*. Washington, DC: U.S. Partnership on Mobility from Poverty.

Schaider, L. A., L. Swetschinski, C. Campbell, and R. A. Rudel. 2019. Environmental justice and drinking water quality: Are there socioeconomic disparities in nitrate levels in U.S. drinking water? *Environmental Health* 18(1):3.

Schapiro, R., K. Blankenship, A. Rosenberg, and D. Keene. 2022. The effects of rental assistance on housing stability, quality, autonomy, and affordability. *Housing Policy Debate* 32(3):456–472.

Schwartz, M. A. 2023. *The 574 federally recognized Indian tribes in the United States*. Washington, DC: Congressional Research Service.

Seabury, S. A., S. Terp, and L. I. Bioden. 2017. Racial and ethnic differences in the frequency of workplace injuries and prevalence of work-related disability. *Health Affairs* 36(2):266–273.

Seligman, H. K., and S. A. Berkowitz. 2019. Aligning programs and policies to support food security and public health goals in the United States. *Annual Review of Public Health* 40:319–337.

Senate Committee on Indian Affairs. 2022. *Schatz, Murkowski Lead Committee Passage of Bipartisan Bill to Advance Native American Housing Programs*. https://www.indian. senate.gov/news/press-release/schatz-murkowski-lead-committee-passage-bipartisan-bill-advance-native-american (accessed March 2, 2023).

Senate HELP Committee. 2014. *Fulfilling the promise: Overcoming persistent barriers to economic self-sufficiency for people with disabilities: Majority committee staff report*. Washington, DC: U.S. Senate Committe on Health, Education, Labor and Pensions.

Shaker, Y., S. E. Grineski, T. W. Collins, and A. B. Flores. 2022. Redlining, racism and food access in U.S. urban cores. *Agriculture and Human Values* 40:101–112.

Shandas, V., and D. Hellman. 2022. Toward an equitable distribution of urban green spaces for people and landscapes: An opportunity for Portland's green grid. In *Green infrastructure and climate change adaptation: Function, implementation and governance*, edited by F. Nakamura. Singapore: Springer Nature. Pp. 289–301.

Shannon, K. L., B. F. Kim, S. E. McKenzie, and R. S. Lawrence. 2015. Food system policy, public health, and human rights in the United States. *Annual Review of Public Health* 36(1):151–173.

Shilling, J. D., K. Chomitz, and A. E. Flanagan. 2007. *The nexus between infrastructure and environment*. Washington, DC: The World Bank.

Shirley, C. 2017. *Spending on Infrastructure and Investment*. https://www.cbo.gov/publication/52463 (accessed March 2, 2023).

Smart Growth America. 2023. *The Complete Streets policy framework*. Washington, DC: Smart Growth America.

Smart Growth America. n.d. *Complete Streets*. https://smartgrowthamerica.org/what-are-complete-streets/ (accessed May 28, 2023).

Smith, G. S., H. Breakstone, L. T. Dean, and R. J. Thorpe, Jr. 2020. Impacts of gentrification on health in the U.S.: A systematic review of the literature. *Journal of Urban Health* 97(6):845–856.

Solomon, D., C. Maxwell, and A. Castro. 2019. *Systemic inequality: Displacement, exclusion, and segregation:How America's housing system undermines wealth building in communities of color*. Washington, DC: Center for American Progress.

Spencer-Hwang, R., S. Montgomery, M. Dougherty, J. Valladares, S. Rangel, P. Gleason, and S. Soret. 2014. Experiences of a rail yard community: Life is hard. *Journal of Environmental Health* 77(2):8–17.

Sprunt, B. 2021. *Here's What's Included in the Bipartisan Infrastructure Law*. https://www.npr.org/2021/06/24/1009923468/heres-whats-included-in-the-infrastructure-deal-that-biden-struck-with-senators (accessed March 23, 2023).

Switzer, D., and M. P. Teodoro. 2017. The color of drinking water: Class, race, ethnicity, and Safe Drinking Water Act compliance. *Journal AWWA* 109(9):40–45.

Szto, M. 2013. Real estate agents as agents of social change: Redlining, reverse redlining, and greenlining. *Seattle Journal for Social Justice* 12(1):1–59.

Tax Policy Center. 2020. *The Tax Policy Center's briefing book: A citizen's guide to the tax system and tax policy*. Washington, DC: Urban-Brookings Tax Policy Center.

Taylor, L. T. 2018. *Health Affairs Policy Brief: Housing and Health: An Overview of the Literature*. https://www.healthaffairs.org/do/10.1377/hpb20180313.396577/full/ (accessed February 28, 2023).

Tebor, C. 2021. On Native American reservations, the push for more clean water and sanitation. *Los Angeles Times*, June 26.

Teodoro, M. P., M. Haider, and D. Switzer. 2018. U.S. environmental policy implementation on tribal lands: Trust, neglect, and justice. *Policy Studies Journal* 46(1):37–59.

Tessum, C. W., D. A. Paolella, S. E. Chambliss, J. S. Apte, J. D. Hill, and J. D. Marshall. 2021. PM2.5 polluters disproportionately and systemically affect people of color in the United States. *Science Advances* 7(18):eabf4491.

Thacker, S., D. Adshead, C. Fantini, R. Palmer, R. Ghosal, T. Adeoti, G. Morgan, and S. Stratton-Short. 2021. *Infrastructure for climate action*. Copenhagen, Denmark: United Nations Office for Project Services.

Thorndike, A. N., C. D. Gardner, K. B. Kendrick, H. K. Seligman, A. L. Yaroch, A. V. Gomes, K. N. Ivy, S. Scarmo, C. J. Cotwright, and M. B. Schwartz. 2022. Strengthening U.S. food policies and programs to promote equity in nutrition security: A policy statement from the American Heart Association. *Circulation* 145(24):e1077–e1093.

Turner, M. A., and S. Greene. n.d. *Causes and consequences of separate and unequal neighborhoods*. Washington, DC: Urban Institute.

Union of Concerned Scientists. 2020. *Leveling the fields: Creating farming opportunities for Black people, Indigenous people, and other people of color*. Cambridge, MA: Union of Concerned Scientists.

U.S. Commission on Civil Rights. 2018. *Broken promises: Continuing federal funding shortfall for Native Americans*. Washington, DC: U.S. Commission on Civil Rights.

USDA (United States Department of Agriculture). 2022a. *Food Access Research Atlas: Documentation*. https://www.ers.usda.gov/data-products/food-access-research-atlas/documentation/ (accessed March 2, 2023).

USDA. 2022b. *Food Security in the U.S.: Definitions of Food Security*. https://www.ers.usda.gov/topics/food-nutrition-assistance/food-security-in-the-u-s/definitions-of-food-security/ (accessed March 2, 2023).

USDA. 2022c. *Food Security in the U.S.: Key Statistics and Graphics*. https://www.ers.usda.gov/topics/food-nutrition-assistance/food-security-in-the-u-s/key-statistics-graphics/ (accessed March 2, 2023).

USDA. 2022d. *Socially Disadvantaged, Beginning, Limited Resource, and Female Farmers and Ranchers*. https://www.ers.usda.gov/topics/farm-economy/socially-disadvantaged-beginning-limited-resource-and-female-farmers-and-ranchers/ (accessed March 2, 2023).

USDA. n.d. *1890 Land-Grant Institutions Programs*. https://www.nifa.usda.gov/grants/about-programs/program-operational-areas/1890-land-grant-institutions-programs (accessed March 2, 2023).

USDA Equity Commission. 2023. *Interim report 2023: Recommendations made to the U.S. Department of Agriculture to advance equity for all*. Washington, DC: USDA Equity Commission.

USGCRP (United States Global Change Research Program). 2018. *Impacts, risks, and adaptation in the United States: Fourth national climate assessment, volume II*. Washington, DC: U.S. Global Change Research Program.

U.S. Water Alliance and DigDeep. 2019. *Closing the water access gap in the United States: A national action plan*. Washington, DC: U.S. Water Alliance.

Velasco, G. 2020. *How Transportation Planners Can Advance Racial Equity and Environmental Justice*. https://www.urban.org/urban-wire/how-transportation-planners-can-advance-racial-equity-and-environmental-justice (accessed March 2, 2023).

Volker, J. M. B., A. E. Lee, and S. Handy. 2020. Induced vehicle travel in the environmental review process. *Transportation Research Record* 2674(7):468–479.

Walker, M. 2023. Highways have sliced through city after city. Can the U.S. undo the damage? *The New York Times*, May 25.

Ward, M. H., R. R. Jones, J. D. Brender, T. M. de Kok, P. J. Weyer, B. T. Nolan, C. M. Villanueva, and S. G. van Breda. 2018. Drinking water nitrate and human health: An updated review. *International Journal of Environmental Research and Public Health* 15(7):1557.

Webber, J. L., T. D. Fletcher, L. Cunningham, G. Fu, D. Butler, and M. J. Burns. 2020. Is green infrastructure a viable strategy for managing urban surface water flooding? *Urban Water Journal* 17(7):598–608.

Weingart, E. 2023. Widening highways doesn't fix traffic. So why do we keep doing it? *The New York Times*, January 6.

Weitzman, M., A. Baten, D. G. Rosenthal, R. Hoshino, E. Tohn, and D. E. Jacobs. 2013. Housing and child health. *Current Problems in Pediatric and Adolescent Health Care* 43(8):187–224.

The White House. 2021. *Fact Sheet: The Biden-Harris Lead Pipe and Paint Action Plan*. https://www.whitehouse.gov/briefing-room/statements-releases/2021/12/16/fact-sheet-the-biden-harris-lead-pipe-and-paint-action-plan/ (accessed May 23, 2023).

The White House. 2022. *Fact Sheet: Inflation Reduction Act Advances Environmental Justice.* https://www.whitehouse.gov/briefing-room/statements-releases/2022/08/17/fact-sheet-inflation-reduction-act-advances-environmental-justice/ (accessed May 28, 2023).

Williams, D. R., and C. Collins. 2001. Racial residential segregation: A fundamental cause of racial disparities in health. *Public Health Reports* 116(5):404–416.

Williams, D. R., J. A. Lawrence, and B. A. Davis. 2019. Racism and health: Evidence and needed research. *Annual Review of Public Health* 40:105-125.

Zaru, D. 2023. *City National Bank to Pay $31M in Redlining Settlement with DOJ.* https://abcnews.go.com/US/city-national-bank-pay-31m-redlining-settlement-doj/story?id=96400698 (accessed May 22, 2023).

Zhao, J. Z., C. Fonseca-Sarmiento, and J. Tan. 2019. *America's trillion-dollar repair bill: Capital budgeting and the disclosure of state infrastructure needs.* New York, NY: The Volcker Alliance.

Zhu, Z., J. Ren, and X. Liu. 2019. Green infrastructure provision for environmental justice: Application of the equity index in Guangzhou, China. *Urban Forestry & Urban Greening* 46:126443.

Zölch, T., J. Maderspacher, C. Wamsler, and S. Pauleit. 2016. Using green infrastructure for urban climate-proofing: An evaluation of heat mitigation measures at the micro-scale. *Urban Forestry & Urban Greening* 20:305–316.

Zuk, M., A. H. Bierbaum, K. Chapple, K. Gorska, A. Loukaitou-Sideris, P. Ong, and T. Thomas. 2015. *Working paper 2015-05: Gentrification, displacement and the role of public investment: A literature review.* San Francisco, CA: Federal Reserve Bank of San Francisco.

Zuliaga, D. 2019. *How a 40-Year-Old Federal Law Is Speeding Gentrification.* https://www.politico.com/agenda/story/2019/07/24/gentrification-credit-discrimination-000937/ (accessed May 23, 2023).

7

Social and Community Context

INTRODUCTION

Health outcomes reflect the social and community context in which people live. Accordingly, efforts to address health inequities must consider the social and community factors that impact health and well-being. Social relationships, which provide people with critical support and can act as a buffer against negative conditions, such as unsafe neighborhoods, discrimination, and financial instability, are needed for thriving. The Healthy People 2030 initiative emphasizes that "relationships and interactions with family, friends, coworkers, and community members" and "the social support [one needs] where they live, work, learn, and play" are important factors in determining health outcomes (HHS, 2020). Likewise, the National Academies *Communities in Action* report notes that "individuals, families, businesses, and organizations within a community; the interactions among them; and norms and culture . . . social networks, capital,[1] cohesion,[2] trust, participation, and willingness to act for the common good" all function as

---

[1] Social capital refers to "features of social structures—such as levels of interpersonal trust and norms of reciprocity and mutual aid—which act as resources for individuals and facilitate collective action. Social capital thus forms a subset of the notion of social cohesion" (Coleman, 1990; Kawachi and Berkman, 2000, p. 175; Putnam, 1993).

[2] Social cohesion refers to "(1) the absence of latent social conflict . . . and (2) the presence of strong social bonds," measuring "the extent of connectedness and solidarity among groups in society." A cohesive society is characterized by abundant social capital, and social cohesion and social capital are "collective, or ecological, dimensions of society, to be distinguished from the concepts of social networks and social support, which are characteristically measured at the level of the individual" (Kawachi and Berkman, 2000, p. 175).

important social determinants of health (SDOH) (NASEM, 2017a, p.152). The social and community context is itself shaped by the structural context, namely, structural inequities, including the societal-level norms, policies, laws, regulations, institutions, and practices that underlie, maintain, and reinforce structural racism (see also Health Affairs, 2022; Hicken et al., 2018; NASEM, 2017a). These structural inequities stem from historical processes, such as slavery and settler colonialism, that have ongoing effects. Social and community context—from families, neighborhoods, and the institutions where people learn, work, and play to norms and culture—is also shaped by the SDOH outlined in previous chapters (e.g., economic instability, housing quality, climate change) (see Figure 1-2).

Despite recognizing this interplay with other SDOH, this chapter focuses on the relational, cultural, and normative elements of context. The following considerations within the social and community context domain offer significant opportunities to address racial, ethnic, and tribal health inequities and are explored in the chapter: violence, public safety, and the criminal legal system; historical trauma and healing; civic infrastructure and engagement; and one's sense of community and belonging, which is impacted by experience, such as criminal legal system contact and various aspects of identity, including race, ethnicity, immigration status, disability status, sexual orientation, and gender identity. Although this report is unable to comprehensively cover all racial, ethnic, and tribal equity issues under this umbrella (see Chapter 1 for more information on how policies were selected), it provides policy examples that highlight how federal intervention in the social and community context can address health inequities. Specifically, the chapter explores the following policies: waiting periods for gun purchases; policies that increase accountability in policing and data collection, such as the George Floyd Justice in Policing Act; mass incarceration policies, such as long and mandatory minimum sentences; policies that acknowledge and provide redress for historical actions, practices, laws, and policies that caused enduring harm; and policies that build civic engagement and a sense of community and belonging. These examples include both policies that perpetuate inequities (i.e., mass incarceration) and policies that are successful and can be expanded or better funded for further improvement (i.e., the Special Diabetes Program for Indians and efforts to increase costewardship of federal lands, such as Joint Secretarial Order 3403).

VIOLENCE, PUBLIC SAFETY,
AND THE CRIMINAL LEGAL SYSTEM

Structural racism, other structural inequities, and the legacy of federal laws and policies have contributed to racially and ethnically minoritized populations experiencing disproportionate violence, public safety issues, and contact with the criminal legal system. For example, redlining and residential segregation have been linked to violent crime and racial disparities in police violence (Siegel et al., 2019; Townsley et al., 2021). These structural factors have also contributed to a disproportionate impact of gun homicide, fatal police shootings, and incarceration on Black, Latino/a, and American Indian and Alaska Native (AIAN) people (Davis et al., 2022; Edwards et al., 2019; Giffords, n.d.; Gramlich, 2020; NAACP, n.d.). Research has linked these inequities to health and well-being. Data demonstrate that incarcerated individuals have poorer mental and physical health, including higher rates of mental health disorders, chronic illness, and infectious disease, compared to the general population (HHS, n.d.-c). The impacts extend to incarcerated individuals' children, families, friends, and communities; research documents mental health, economic, and other effects on communities and families and increased risk for poverty, homelessness, learning and developmental disabilities and delays, attention disorders, aggressive behavior, and involvement with the criminal legal system among children with an incarcerated parent (HHS, n.d.-c; Lee and Wildeman, 2021; NASEM, 2017a). Police brutality has been linked to mental and physical health outcomes through physical injury and death, psychological distress, racist public reactions, financial strain, and systematic disempowerment of communities (Alang et al., 2017).

This section discusses three interrelated dimensions of social and community context: violence, public safety, and the criminal legal system. It reviews examples of federal policies that have impacted or, if enacted, could impact racial and ethnic health inequities and summarizes the relevant evidence. The criminal legal system is also relevant to other SDOH, including economic stability and health care quality and access, which are discussed in Chapters 3 and 5, respectively.

For the purposes of this report, the committee used the World Health Organization (WHO) definition of violence: "the intentional use of physical and psychological force or power, threatened or actual, against oneself, another person, or against a group or community, that either results in or has a high likelihood of resulting in injury, death, psychological harm, maldevelopment, or deprivation" (WHO, 2002, p. 5). This definition encompasses more than just criminal acts; it also considers the impact of "feelings of insecurity and differential perceptions of threat and harm . . . deprivation, psychological abuse, and neglect" (Aisenberg et al., 2010, p. 17). Public safety concerns are central to public policy decisions and laws. Like the definition of violence, the definition of public safety used in this report moves beyond the absence of crime and the notion that the criminal legal system apparatus is the only way to deliver safety to communities. It also considers the role of that system in promoting safety but also enacting violence (e.g., police use of lethal force against racially and ethnically minoritized individuals). Drawing from work attempting to link population health and public safety, public safety is conceptualized as "a sense of physical, emotional, social, and material security that fosters stability and is accompanied by support from community and society when needed" (Gourevitch et al., 2022, p. 716). More expansive notions conceptualize it as "a core human need that comprises not only physical safety but also security in health, housing, education, and living-wage jobs" (Gourevitch et al., 2022, p. 716). These definitions overlap with areas covered in other chapters of this report (i.e., housing, education, and economic stability).[3] With these definitions in mind, this section reviews some examples of federal policies related to violence, public safety, and the criminal legal system.

Gun Violence

The lack of federal regulation of firearm access is one example of a policy directly related to violence and public safety impacting racial and ethnic health inequities. A history of disinvestment, structural inequities, and the legacy of past policies have had lasting effects on minoritized communities and contributed to Black, Latino/a, and AIAN people being disproportionately impacted by gun homicide compared to their White counterparts. Together, Black and Latino/a communities make up less than one-third of the population but three-quarters of gun homicide deaths (Giffords, n.d.). Centers for Disease Control and Prevention (CDC) firearm fatality data demonstrate that firearm-related deaths reached a peak in 2020 at over 45,000 people. An analysis of these data by the Johns Hopkins Center for Gun Violence Solutions reveals that, compared to their White counterparts, AIAN and Hispanic/Latino people were 3.7 times and twice as likely to be a victim of firearm homicide, respectively (Davis et al., 2022). Black people faced the highest risks—they were over 12 times more likely—and the risk for young Black men was especially high; Black men aged 15–34 were more than 20 times more likely to die by gun homicide. Although they make up only 2 percent of the total population, they made up about 38 percent of gun homicide deaths in 2020 (Davis et al., 2022).

For racially and ethnically minoritized women, who are disproportionately impacted by domestic violence, including intimate partner violence (IPV) (Breiding et al., 2014; Wertheimer and Hill, 2022), a recent decision by the Fifth Circuit Court of Appeals (*United States v. Rahimi*) has serious ramifications: the federal prohibition on firearm possession by those subject to domestic violence protection orders was ruled unconstitutional under

---

[3] The committee acknowledges that multiple definitions of public safety exist and continue to be debated, adapted, and reimagined.

the Second Amendment.[4] According to data reported from 18 states to the National Violent Death Reporting System, from 2003 to 2014, most female homicides were IPV related (55.3 percent) and involved firearms (53.9 percent) (Petrosky et al., 2017). Data demonstrate that transgender men and women are also disproportionately impacted by IPV (Peitzmeier et al., 2020). The ruling in *United States v. Rahimi* cited the Supreme Court's 2022 decision in *New York State Rifle & Pistol Association, Inc. v. Bruen*, which deemed unconstitutional a New York State law that required individuals to provide "proper cause" to receive a concealed carry license.[5] Additional lawsuits challenging gun regulations (and directly citing *Bruen*) have been mounted, suggesting that the decision is likely to complicate ongoing firearm regulation efforts (Finerty, 2022).

Gun violence is also a children's health problem, disproportionately so for racially and ethnically minoritized children. In the United States, firearm-related injuries are now the leading cause of death for children 1–19. Before being surpassed by firearm-related injuries in 2020, motor vehicle crashes were the leading cause of death from 1999 to 2019 (Goldstick et al., 2022). Data suggest that this increase, which coincided with the onset of the COVID-19 pandemic, is driven by increases in firearm-related injuries among minoritized children. One analysis found that child shootings among non-Hispanic White children did not increase during the pandemic, whereas rates for non-Hispanic Black, Hispanic, and Asian children did (Jay et al., 2023). The authors hypothesize that this may be explained by the pandemic's exacerbation of inequities in health, employment, and education. Other research has found that rates of violence from March to July 2020 were higher in low-income, racially and ethnically minoritized neighborhoods (Schleimer et al., 2022).

Evidence also demonstrates significant increases in firearm suicides among young Black adults: between 2013 and 2019, it increased by 84.5 percent and 76.9 percent, respectively, for young Black men and women (Kaplan et al., 2022). Gun violence also has implications for the health and well-being of the broader community (Collins and Swoveland, n.d.; NASEM, 2017b). Research demonstrates that exposure to violence by direct victimization is a predictor of gun-related delinquency (McGee et al., 2017) and links witnessing a severe injury or murder to depression and antisocial behavior (Schilling et al., 2007). Gun violence is a clear health equity issue and provides an opportunity for federal legislation to improve outcomes for racially and ethnically minoritized populations.

Although *Bruen* is likely to complicate efforts to regulate firearms, enacting a federal waiting period for gun purchases is one potential avenue

---

[4] *United States v. Rahimi*, 59 F.4th 163 (5th Cir. 2023).
[5] *New York State Rifle & Pistol Association, Inc. v. Bruen*, 597 U.S. __ (2022).

to address this issue. Waiting periods serve several purposes. First, they interrupt the impulsivity that characterizes many acts of gun violence. Additionally, they provide time for law enforcement to uncover purchases being made on behalf of a prohibited person and complete background checks, which can take longer than the 3-day window provided by federal law. In 2021, 5,203 firearms were sold from federally licensed dealers to prohibited persons due to delays from the National Instant Criminal Background Check System that surpassed 3 business days (RAND, 2023c). Although four states and DC have passed waiting period laws that apply to any firearm purchase (the length varies by state, and five additional states have passed waiting period laws for certain firearms), most states have not passed such legislation, and there is no waiting period at the federal level (RAND, 2023c).

Recent causal evidence suggests that waiting period laws at the state level that delay a purchase by a few days may reduce gun homicides and suicides (Luca et al., 2017). In a 2017 study, researchers compared firearm deaths in states with and without waiting period laws over the same time and found that the laws were associated with a 17 percent reduction in gun homicides, these laws prevent about 750 gun homicides per year, and expansion to all states would prevent 910 additional gun homicides per year. The study also found these laws reduced gun suicide by 7–11 percent (Luca et al., 2017). A study similarly found that handgun purchase delays reduced gun suicides by about 3 percent (Edwards et al., 2018). Data about effects of such laws on racial and ethnic inequities in gun violence and on the implications of a federal waiting period law are still needed. In addition to limited evidence on effectiveness, it has been argued that a waiting period creates unnecessary additional burdens on first-time gun owners who have no intent to harm themselves or others and may need a firearm for protection. However, Luca et al. (2017) note that their findings point to waiting period laws as a method to reduce gun violence without restricting gun ownership. Although research is needed, given the disproportionate impact of gun homicide on Black, Latino/a, and AIAN populations and recent increases in firearm suicide among young Black adults, a federal waiting period is one potential policy lever that may counteract the impact of gun violence in these communities. Other firearm regulation policies that have received attention in recent years and may be worth exploring as avenues to address racial and ethnic inequities in gun homicides include policies for safe storage, background checks (for private sales/gun shows), firearm safety training requirements, mental health restrictions, a national gun registry, and banning high-capacity or assault-style weapons (APA, 2013; IOM and NRC, 2013; Johns Hopkins Center for Gun Violence Prevention and Policy, n.d.-a,b; Monmouth University, 2019; RAND, 2023a,b).

Policing and the Criminal Legal System

Generations of discrimination and disinvestment and systemic inequalities within the criminal legal system have had a lasting impact on racially and ethnically minoritized communities, contributing to disproportionate crime and violence (NASEM, 2017a). Many policies intended to combat these issues and improve public safety have also caused harm. For example, data on policing policies, such as stop-and-frisk, and extremely punitive criminal legal policies, such as long sentences and mandatory minimums, show that such policies disproportionately impact Black, Latino/a, and AIAN people yet do little or nothing to address crime and violence (Dunn and Shames, 2019; The Educational Fund to Stop Gun Violence et al., 2022; Keating and Stevens, 2020; MacDonald, n.d.; Siegler, 2021). Combating these issues in minoritized communities will require not only considering potential new policies from a racial equity lens but also reexamining existing policies from this same perspective. The George Floyd Justice in Policing Act of 2021 (JIPA), which passed the House but not the Senate, is one example of proposed reforms to address racial inequities in policing.[6] JIPA aims to address not only the disproportionate impact of policing on Black, Latino/a, and AIAN communities but also the need for improved collection of data on racial and ethnic inequities in policing. The bill would end qualified immunity and the use of chokeholds and no-knock warrants in drug cases by federal law enforcement (Collins, 2021).

Administrative data are limited, and improved collection on inequities in law enforcement is needed, including on racial and ethnic inequities for chokeholds and no-knock warrants, cases dismissed due to qualified immunity by race and ethnicity of the plaintiff, and other outcomes. However, existing data reveal clear inequities in policing and police violence. Of 92,383 recorded stop-and-frisk stops in New York City between 2014 and 2017, 53 and 28 percent were of Black and Latino/a people, respectively, and only 11 percent were of White people (Dunn and Shames, 2019). Figure 7-1 illustrates inequities in lifetime risk of being killed by police use of force by sex and race and ethnicity at 2013 to 2018 risk levels (Edwards et al., 2019). The red bars indicate mortality rate ratios (relative to White people) for African American, Latinx, Asian and Pacific Islander, and AIAN women. The blue bars indicate mortality rate ratios (relative to White people) for men. African American, Latinx, and AIAN men are about 2.5, 1.3–1.4, and 1.2–1.7 times more likely, respectively, to be killed by police than White men. African American and AIAN women are about 1.4 and 1.1–2.1 times more likely, respectively, to be killed by police than White women. Latina women are 12–23 percent less likely to be killed

---

[6]H.R. 1280, 117th Congress (2021).

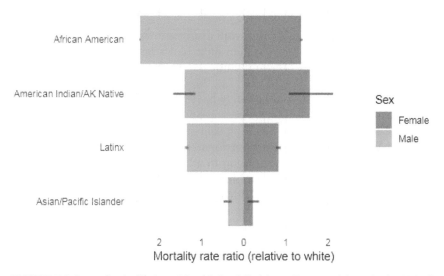

FIGURE 7-1 Inequality in lifetime risk of being killed by police use of force in the United States by sex and race/ethnicity at 2013–2018 risk levels.
NOTE: Dashes indicate 90 percent uncertainty intervals. Life tables were calculated using model simulations from 2013–2018 Fatal Encounters data and 2017 National Vital Statistics System data. Data for the Native Hawaiian and Pacific Islander (NHPI) population were combined with the Asian population—this provides an inaccurate representation of the NHPI population as a distinct racial Office of Management and Budget minimum category and masks inequities for NHPI people and within-group differences for Asian people.
SOURCE: Edwards et al., 2019.

by police than White women, and both Asian and Pacific Islander men and women are over 50 percent less likely to be killed by police than White men and women (Edwards et al., 2019). As noted above, police brutality has been linked to mental and physical health outcomes (Alang et al., 2017). Data suggest that officer-involved killings of individuals from racially and ethnically minoritized communities may negatively influence the educational performance of Black and Hispanic students who live nearby, and research is underway investigating how fatal police shootings might affect pregnancy-related and infant health in impacted communities (Ang, 2021; Noguchi, 2020). Improved data collection efforts are needed, but federal interventions that increase accountability in policing, such as JIPA, may help reduce inequities given that Black, Latino/a, and AIAN communities are disproportionately impacted.

Although the federal government has limited power over policing at the state and local level, JIPA attempts to address the issue at these levels by "[requiring] federal, state, tribal, and local law enforcement agencies to report data to DOJ on traffic violation stops, pedestrian stops, frisks and body searches, and the use of deadly force by their law enforcement officers. Reporting agencies would be required to include in these data the race, ethnicity, age, and gender of the officers and members of the public involved" (James and Finklea, 2021, p. 2). The bill attaches conditions to the Edward Byrne Memorial Justice Assistance Grant and Community Oriented Policing Services programs that are meant to incentivize compliance, but it is uncertain whether these programs provide enough funding to state and local governments to allow the loss of or reduced funding to actually do so (James and Finklea, 2021). Data compiled by the Urban Institute indicate that federal grants account for only a small fraction of spending on police and corrections (Urban Institute, 2023). Prior and related data collection mandates, such as the Death in Custody Reporting Act,[7] have also been stymied by lack of enforcement (Bryant, 2022). JIPA could be improved by developing other incentives for state and local governments, such as grants to help them afford the staff and technology needed to comply with data reporting requirements (James and Finklea, 2021). With such improvements, full passage of this bill has the potential to address both the disproportionate impact of police misconduct on Black, Latino/a, and AIAN communities and the need to collect data on racial and ethnic inequities in law enforcement.

Federal policy changes related to incarceration also provide an opportunity to address the disparate impact of the criminal legal system on racially and ethnically minoritized communities. The United States has the highest rate of incarceration in the world; it accounts for almost 25 percent of the global prison population despite making up only 5 percent of the global population overall (NAACP, n.d.). Moreover, this mass incarceration, which research has tied to poorer mental and physical health, disproportionately impacts minoritized communities (HHS, n.d.-c). In 2010, the incarceration rates for Latinx, Native Hawaiian or Pacific Islander (NHPI), AIAN, and Black people were about 1.85, 2.26, 2.87, and 5.12 times the incarceration rate for White non-Latinx people, respectively (Prison Policy Initiative, n.d.). Black and Hispanic people account for 33 and 23 percent of the prison population despite representing only 12 and 16 percent of the U.S. adult population, respectively. Conversely, White people represent 63 percent of the adult population but only 30 percent of the prison population (Gramlich, 2020). Upon release, incarcerated individuals face significant barriers to accessing SDOH, as they must navigate "stigma, limited employment and housing opportunities, and the lack of a cohesive social network" (NASEM, 2017a, p. 160).

---

[7]Pub. L. 106–297, 114 Stat. 1045 (Oct. 13, 2000) and Pub. L. 113–242, 128 Stat. 2860 (Dec. 18, 2014).

Incarceration also adversely affects children, families, and communities, as discussed previously. Mass incarceration has been tied to the "breakdown of educational opportunities, family structures, economic mobility, housing options, and neighborhood cohesion, especially in low-income communities of color" (NASEM, 2017a, p. 160). Heavily impacted communities also have higher rates of mental health disorders, such as major depressive disorder and generalized anxiety disorder (Hatzenbuehler et al., 2015). Children with an incarcerated parent are at higher risk for negative outcomes, such as poverty, homelessness, abuse, learning and developmental disabilities and delays, attention disorders, aggressive behavior, and criminal legal system involvement (HHS, n.d.-c). Adult family members (e.g., romantic partners and mothers) are also impacted via a variety of pathways, including loss of income, increased child care burden, stigma, and loss of social support, which increase the risk of poor physical and mental health (Lee and Wildeman, 2021; Wildeman and Lee, 2021).

Re-examination of federal policies regarding mandatory minimum sentences and long sentences could address the disproportionate impact of mass incarceration on minoritized communities (NRC, 2014). Data suggest that mass incarceration has had minimal effect on reducing crime and may actually result in more crime, as incarcerated individuals miss career opportunities and become part of shrunken social networks that consist primarily of other individuals engaged in criminal behavior and/or whose access to resources and opportunities have also been stymied due to incarceration (Roodman, 2017; Stemen, 2017), limiting their access to SDOH. A Brennan Center state-level analysis estimates that increased incarceration was only responsible for 0–7 percent of the decline in property crime from 1990 to 2013 and had no net effect on the decline in violent crime during this time (Roeder et al., 2015). A 2017 review estimated the impact of additional incarceration on crime at 0, noting that the deterrent effect of incarceration is mild or 0, while its incapacitation effect appears to be cancelled out by its crime-increasing "aftereffects" (Roodman, 2017). No consistent evidence indicates that punishment severity has a deterrent effect, contrary to arguments made to justify longer sentences and mandatory minimums. Furthermore, that both crime and recidivism rates decrease with age indicates that long sentences are an ineffective strategy for preventing crime via incapacitation and that, over long sentences, benefits to public safety are increasingly outweighed by the costs of incarceration (NRC, 2014; Roeder et al., 2015; Roodman, 2017). For the majority of crimes, criminal activity peaks from the mid-teens to early or mid-twenties, declining by more than half by the late twenties, across race and class. The median age range of people in federal prison is past this peak, at 36–40 years old (Mauer, 2018; NRC, 2014). Although addressing sentence length alone will not eliminate inequities in the mass incarceration of Black, Latino/a, NHPI, and AIAN people, it is a meaningful step, with important implications for health inequities.

As noted, the committee was unable to comprehensively examine all policies under the violence, public safety, and criminal legal system umbrella; other areas merit examination to assess impacts on health equity—for example, violence against women and juvenile incarceration (see Box 7-1).

Conclusion 7-1: Community safety is critical for health and well-being. Racial and ethnic inequities in gun homicides and recent increases in firearm suicide among young Black adults suggest the need for more evidence-based policies that can prevent harm.

BOX 7-1
One Million Experiments

One Million Experiments showcases community-based projects that expand ideas about what keeps communities safe, moving beyond the paradigm that centers policing, incarceration, and other forms of punishment (One Million Experiments, n.d.-a)

Youth incarceration is decreasing overall, but significant racial and ethnic inequities persist (NASEM, 2019a). According to data from 2019, Black, tribal, and Latinx youth are 4.4, 3.3, and 1.3 times, respectively, more likely detained or committed than their White peers (Rovner, 2021a,b,c).

The community projects that One Million Experiments showcases cover a broad range of categories, including economic justice, food and environmental justice, education and recreation, and children and families. Youth-centered projects include Detroit Heals Detroit, a group designed to connect Detroit youth to peers also working to heal from trauma, and the Radical Monarchs, an organization similar to Girl Scouts but focused on girls from racially and ethnically minoritized communities (One Million Experiments, n.d.-b,c).

Federal support for community programs like these, along with broader efforts toward improving the criminal legal system, could have important implications for youth and for racial and ethnic inequities in violence, public safety, and public health. Research demonstrates that youth programming may reduce violence and criminal legal system involvement. Summer youth employment programs, for example, may reduce involvement in violent crime by up to 43 percent, and the effects are seen not only during but also after the employment period, even 2–3 years later (Davis and Heller, 2017; Heller, 2014; Modestino, 2019). Becoming a Man, a school-based program designed to help male youth develop cognitive and decision-making skills, and a similar program based at a juvenile temporary detention center, have been found to reduce total arrests, violent crime arrests, and juvenile detention readmission rates and increase graduation rates, based on randomized controlled trials in Chicago (Heller et al., 2017; Sebastian et al., 2022; University of Chicago Crime Lab, 2018, n.d.).

Conclusion 7-2: There are clear racial and ethnic inequities in policing. Improved data collection is needed to increase accountability, better understand the extent of these inequities, and determine which policy changes may help reduce them.

Conclusion 7-3: The criminal legal system is an important driver of health across the life course, as well as the health of communities and families. Racially and ethnically minoritized communities have experienced and continue to experience disproportionate contact with the criminal legal system. Evidence suggests that policies regarding mandatory minimum sentences, long sentences, and mass incarceration merit re-examination.

TRAUMA AND HEALING

In addition to issues related to violence, public safety, and the criminal legal system, historical traumas continue to affect the health and well-being of racially and ethnically minoritized populations and tribal communities. A deep literature illustrates how past trauma influences health—for example, on toxic stress (from adversity and intergenerational poverty) and allostatic load (McEwen and McEwen, 2017; NASEM, 2019a,b); posttraumatic stress disorder and racial trauma (Williams et al., 2021); the impact of discrimination on allostatic load in adults (Geronimus et al., 2006; Miller et al., 2021); how the evidence about intergenerational trauma could inform social policy (Njaka and Peacock, 2021); and race-related stress and trauma and emotional dysregulation in minoritized youth (Roach et al., 2023). This section explores how federal policy interventions that address the ongoing impact of historical traumas could advance health equity.

The repercussions of past actions, practices, policies, and laws continue to heavily affect health outcomes for minoritized racial, ethnic, and tribal communities today. Historical processes, such as colonialism, imperialism, genocide, slavery, and broken treaties, have inflicted lasting harm and undermined access to social, economic, and political resources and opportunities for Black, AIAN, NHPI, Latino/a, Asian, and Compact of Free Association (COFA) communities in both the past and present. These harms, resultant trauma, and lack of access to resources and opportunities have impeded the ability of these communities to reach their full potential for health, happiness, and overall well-being. For Black communities, significant trauma stems from a history of slavery, segregation, discrimination (NASEM, 2017a; Rothstein, 2017), racial terror and violence (e.g., lynching) (Equal Justice Initiative, 2020), systematic disinvestment in and destruction of Black communities (Lee et al., 2022; NASEM, 2017a; Rothstein, 2017), denial of voting and civil rights (National Archives, 2022a), forced sterilization

(Stern, 2020), and past and present policies such as voting literacy tests (National Archives, 2022a), redlining (Lee et al., 2022; NASEM, 2017a; Rothstein, 2017), aggressive policing (NASEM, 2017a), and criminal legal system policies, such as the convict leasing system (Equal Justice Initiative, 2013) and mandatory minimum sentences (NRC, 2014).

For AIAN communities, a history of forced assimilation, removal, extermination, forced sterilization, broken treaties, and intrusion on sovereignty has led to cultural loss, wealth depletion, and poor physical and mental health outcomes (Newland, 2022; Stern, 2020). The U.S. nuclear testing program on the Marshall Islands from 1946 to 1958 is another example. Today, the Marshallese people grapple with displacement, increased rates of cancer, and residual radiation in their land and water (Palafox, 2010; Rapaport and Nikolić Hughes, 2022). The U.S. government's role in the overthrow of Hawaii's monarchy in 1893, and eventual annexation of Hawaii as a territory and later state, is yet another example (Sai, 2018). These actions have had a lasting impact on mental and physical health and well-being and economic and cultural preservation for Native Hawaiians (Blaisdell, 2019). For Latino/a people, significant trauma stems from racial terror and violence (e.g., lynching) (Carrigan and Webb, 2003), forced sterilization (Novak et al., 2018), immigration detention, and immigration policies such as family separation (Hampton et al., 2021) and delousing at the U.S.–Mexico border (Stern, 1999) (see Box 7-2). The legacy of

---

BOX 7-2
Trauma and Healing for Latino/a Communities

For Latino/a communities, U.S. immigration policies, both historical and modern, represent a significant source of trauma. In 1917, the United States passed an immigration act imposing (among other restrictions) new barriers to entry at the Mexico border, including a passport requirement for Mexican nationals, a literacy test, a head tax, and a ban on contract labor. That same year, Customs also instituted a policy of mandatory delousing of individuals crossing the Mexican border at the bridge between El Paso and Juarez, to control the spread of typhus (Romo, n.d.). As part of this policy, those crossing were made to strip, have their clothes sterilized, and be examined for lice. Anyone found to have lice had their hair clipped or covered in kerosene and vinegar (Stern, 1999). Then individuals were "directed into sex-segregated showers where they were sprayed with a mixture of soap, kerosene, and water" (Stern, 1999, p. 46). When first instituted, the new measures sparked protests known as the "Bath Riots" among individuals from Juarez. After a few days, however, these protests subsided and anyone looking to enter the United States at El Paso had to submit to this "decontamination" process. Afterward, individuals were provided a certificate from the U.S. Public Health Service verifying what they had undergone and then had to complete a general medical and

BOX 7-2 Continued

psychological examination and interrogation about themselves and their citizenship. Individuals could be denied entry due to "physical or mental defects" identified during this additional examination (Stern, 1999, p. 46).

The family separations that occurred at the U.S.–Mexico border between 2017 and 2021 as part of the federal government's "Zero Tolerance" immigration policy are another example (Hampton et al., 2021). The Interagency Task Force on the Reunification of Families, established in February 2021 through Executive Order 14011,[1] has identified 3,925 children that were separated from their families as a result (DHS, 2023). These children were as young as 4 months old (Dickerson, 2019). Family separations were carried out despite warnings of their potential for harm from the Department of Health and Human Services (Fram, 2018) and overwhelming evidence from the scientific literature on the impact this practice could have—childhood trauma and Adverse Childhood Experiences are linked to developmental disruption, learning and behavioral challenges, and increased risk of depression, post-traumatic stress disorder (PTSD), stroke, and diabetes (Hampton et al., 2021; NASEM, 2019b).

Although limited, data on those impacted by the policy support predictions that it would cause harm. For example, an analysis of 31 medico-legal affidavits from families impacted by family separation showed "nearly uniform negative mental health outcomes" (Hampton et al., 2021, p. 7). Based on clinician evaluation, nearly all individuals met the diagnostic criteria for PTSD, major depressive disorder, or generalized anxiety disorder. Moreover, the data suggest that these impacts could be long term. For example, in two of these cases, the children were evaluated long after reunification but continued to meet the diagnostic criteria for PTSD and both PTSD and separation anxiety disorder 1 year and 2 years later, respectively (Hampton et al., 2021). Another study of children and mothers who had been detained revealed that forcibly separated children had more emotional symptoms (i.e., being unhappy or excessively fearful) and total difficulties than those who had not been forcibly separated (MacLean et al., 2019).

Of the 3,925 separated children identified by the reunification task force, 2,317 had been reunified prior to its formation. As of March 2023, the task force was responsible for 652 reunifications, with an additional 164 in progress.

---

[1] Exec. Order No. 14011, 86 FR 8273 (February 2021).

colonialism in Puerto Rico and its status as a territory, which constrains its self-governance, congressional representation, and the federal support it can receive (Cheatham and Roy, 2022); Japanese American internment during World War II (National Archives, 2022b); and immigration policies, such as the Chinese Exclusion Act are additional examples (Department of State, n.d.; National Archives, 2023) (see Box 7-3).

How the United States might begin to rectify these harms and therefore advance health equity is a topic of ongoing discussion. Proposed solutions typically include a combination of official acknowledgement of harms,

BOX 7-3
Trauma and Healing for Asian Communities

After the emergence of SARS-CoV-2 in Wuhan, China, its worldwide spread, and the World Health Organization's declaration of a global pandemic, the United States saw an increase in anti-Asian racism, including violent attacks. FBI data document a 77 percent increase in hate crimes against Asian people from 2019 to 2020 (DOJ, 2023). In an April 2021 poll from the AP-NORC Center for Public Affairs Research at the University of Chicago, 57 percent of Asian respondents reported feeling often or sometimes unsafe in public due to their race or ethnicity, compared to 16 percent of White and 63 percent of Black respondents (AP-NORC Center for Public Affairs Research, 2021).

Based on surveys administered at various points in the pandemic, Huang et al. (2023) found that 17–27 percent of respondents blamed Asian people as most responsible for bringing COVID-19 into the United States. The other answer options included Black, Latino, and White people and "don't know," and "no racial or ethnic group is responsible." In the fourth wave of their survey (administered in April 2021), half of the sample was shown the same question with a different set of answers; 38 percent of respondents blamed Chinese people as most responsible. The other answer options included Japanese, Italian, French, Mexican, Greek, Indian, and Thai people and "other," "don't know," and "no racial or ethnic group is responsible." Their data also suggest that this rhetoric impacted consumer behavior, documenting an 18.4 percent decrease in traffic at Asian restaurants relative to comparable non-Asian restaurants (Huang et al., 2023), on top of the challenges that all businesses faced during the pandemic. Huang et al. (2023) estimate that this decrease translates to about $7.42 billion USD in lost revenue in 2020.

These patterns echo examples of anti-Asian racism and xenophobia throughout U.S. history (Chen, 2000), which have often been perpetuated by federal actions, practices, policies, and laws. For example, in 1882, the Chinese Exclusion Act banned Chinese laborers from immigrating to the United States for 10 years. Its requirements also made it difficult for Chinese non-laborers to enter the country and existing Chinese immigrants to re-enter if they left (National Archives, 2023). The act followed growing anti-Chinese sentiment that stemmed from resentment from other workers, cultural tension, and racism (Department of State, n.d.). When it expired in 1892, the act was extended for 10 years as the Geary Act[1] and then made permanent in 1902. Following World War I, the United States expanded its policies to limit immigration from all of Asia using census-based quotas. The exclusion acts were repealed when China joined the Allied Nations during War II, but quotas continued to limit immigration based on the "national origin system" until the Immigration Act of 1965.[2] In 2011 and 2012, the Senate and House of Representatives unanimously passed resolutions condemning the Chinese Exclusion Act and committing to protect the civil and constitutional rights of all people (National Archives, 2023).[3]

The treatment of Japanese American citizens following the attack on Pearl Harbor during World War II is another example. Two months after the attack, President Roosevelt issued Executive Order 9066, which authorized

BOX 7-3 Continued

the military to forcibly remove anyone believed to be threat to national security from the West Coast. Although a specific group was not named, the order resulted in curfews, the encouragement of voluntary evacuation, and later forced removal and internment of Japanese Americans in "relocation centers." Almost 70,000 of these 112,000 people were U.S. citizens, and none had charges of disloyalty brought against them. Many lost the homes, farms, businesses, and belongings they were forced to leave behind, with no avenue for them to appeal the loss of their freedom and property. In 1988, the federal government formally apologized for Japanese internment and the Civil Liberties Act[4] provided monetary redress for those who had been interned (National Archives, 2022b).

---

[1] May 5, 1892, ch. 60, 27 Stat. 25.
[2] Pub. L. 89–236, 79 Stat 911 (Oct. 3, 1965).
[3] S. Res. 201, 112th Congress (2011) and H. Res. 683, 112th Congress (2012).
[4] 50 U.S.C. § 4211 et seq.

---

financial redress, and structural redress (for example, policies that advance asset building to address intergenerational poverty). The Civil Liberties Act of 1988, which formally acknowledged the injustice of internment of Japanese American citizens and residents during World War II and provided monetary reparations to survivors and their heirs (National Archives, 2022b), and Public Law 103–150, wherein the federal government apologized for its role in overthrowing the Hawaiian monarchy, provide precedent for such federal action (Kana'iaupuni and Malone, 2006). Redress provided by the federal government to Vietnam War veterans exposed to Agent Orange and survivors of the Tuskegee Syphilis Study and their families provide additional precedent (CDC, 2022b; VA, 2022). Although acknowledgement of past injustice is a meaningful step, further action is needed to address the long-lasting harm of past actions and ultimately advance health equity.

Experts on racial and ethnic equity issues assert that inequities cannot be eliminated without changes that address historical wrongs and their ongoing impact on the structural and social determinants of health, and evidence increasingly supports this view, as this section discusses (Christopher, 2022; Galea, 2022; Welburn et al., 2022). Given the scope of this area of study, the committee was unable to comprehensively lay out the repercussions of past actions, practices, policies, and laws for all racially and ethnically minoritized populations. However, the following section details how some policies have led to lasting trauma and harm for minoritized communities and potential avenues for redress that scholars have proposed.

Trauma and Healing for Black Communities

Chapters 3–7 describe significant racial inequities in income, wealth, homeownership, educational quality and attainment, health care quality and access, health outcomes, neighborhood quality, policing, incarceration, and more. These inequities are part of the legacy of slavery, failed Reconstruction, segregation, redlining, the destruction of Black communities, and structural racism, which persists today (Du Bois, 1998; Equal Justice Initiative, 2020; Foner, 2014; Lee et al., 2022; NASEM, 2017a; Rothstein, 2017). Following the Civil War, the opportunity that the Reconstruction era provided to address structural racism and inequities, offer redress to formerly enslaved individuals, and chart a path toward racial equity went unfulfilled (Equal Justice Initiative, 2020). Although the 13th,[8] 14th,[9] and 15th[10] amendments abolished slavery, granted citizenship to formerly enslaved people, and granted Black men voting rights, respectively, the realization of fully equal citizenship, status, and opportunity for Black people was stymied by political opposition (Equal Justice Initiative, 2020). Other factors crucial for Black advancement and equality, such as economic growth, were obstructed by practices such as sharecropping and debt peonage (Du Bois, 1998; Equal Justice Initiative, 2020). Following the Compromise of 1877, Reconstruction efforts were abandoned by the federal government (Equal Justice Initiative, 2020). Black Codes, discriminatory laws passed at the state level, and Jim Crow laws restricted freedoms and reversed gains, such as Black voting rights (Equal Justice Initiative, 2020; National Geographic, 2022).

The persistence of racial inequity can be traced to the failure of Reconstruction (Du Bois, 1998; Equal Justice Initiative, 2020; Foner, 2014). For example, Darity and Mullen argue that these failures, starting with the reversal of Special Field Order No.15, which promised to provide formerly enslaved Black people with 40 acres of farmland and a mule after the end of the Civil War, helped create the Black-White wealth gap that persists today (Darity and Mullen, 2020). Beyond economic inequities, structural racism, slavery, the failure of Reconstruction, and policies that harmed Black communities have also paved the way for persistent inequities in health outcomes and other structural and social determinants of health (NASEM, 2017a). The influence of redlining is evident in not only present levels of wealth and rates of homeownership for Black families and individuals but also the built environment in Black communities, including lack of access to public transit and exposure to air pollution (Lane et al., 2022; Lee et al., 2022; Townsley et al., 2021). Ongoing discrimination in the

---

[8] U.S. Constitution, amend. 13, sec. 1.
[9] U.S. Constitution, amend. 14, sec. 1.
[10] U.S. Constitution, amend. 15, sec. 1.

health care system, which echoes past harms, such as the sterilization of Black women (Stern, 2020), the Tuskegee Syphilis Study (CDC, 2022b), and J. Marion Sims' medical experimentation and abuse of Lucy, Anarcha, Betsey, and other enslaved Black women (Wailoo, 2018; Wall, 2006), has resulted in lingering mistrust of medicine, including early pandemic COVID-19 vaccine hesitancy (Martin et al., 2022; Ober, 2022). The legacies of the Fugitive Slave Act, Black Codes, and Jim Crow laws are evident in today's inequitable policing and criminal legal policies that have disproportionately removed Black individuals from their families and communities, which has economic and physical and mental health implications for them and their children, partners, and other family and has been tied to community disempowerment (Dyer et al., 2019; Mason, 2021; Maxwell and Solomon, 2018; National Geographic, 2022; Paul, 2016). In these varied ways, harmful policies and their legacy of structural racism have inflicted lasting trauma and discrimination on Black communities, impacting access to resources and opportunities critical for health and well-being.

For Black communities that have been destroyed by past actions, practices, policies, and laws and their legacy of structural racism, healing has been a challenging process. The aftermath of the 1921 Race Massacre in Tulsa, Oklahoma, is one example. This racial violence, which followed the arrest of a young Black man accused of attempting to rape a young White woman, is estimated to have killed 100–300 people in Tulsa's Greenwood District, an affluent Black community then known as "Black Wall Street" (Monroe, 2021; Ross et al., 2001). Before the massacre, the district was a "symbol of Black prosperity" and entrepreneurship against the backdrop of Jim Crow America (Monroe, 2021). According to records analyzed by the Oklahoma Commission to Study the Tulsa Race Riot of 1921, 1,256 homes were burned and an additional 215 looted. Businesses, churches, schools, a hospital, and a library—"virtually every other structure" in the neighborhood—were also destroyed (Ross et al., 2001, p. 12). The Tulsa Real Estate Exchange Commission reported that $1.5 million worth of property damage resulted from the massacre, one-third of this in the business district (Ross et al., 2001). Denial of insurance claims and lack of restitution from local, state, and federal government left Greenwood residents to rebuild on their own. These rebuilding efforts were successful, but during the 1960s–1980s, eminent domain, rezoning, highway construction, and redlining devastated the community once again (Perry et al., 2021).

Today, Tulsa's Black community still struggles to heal from the violence and harmful policies it endured. A Brookings Institution analysis reveals that Tulsa's predominately Black neighborhoods are no longer hubs for finance, insurance, and real estate jobs, and only 1.25 percent of Tulsa's 20,000 businesses are Black owned (Perry et al., 2021). Displaced by the "urban renewal" policies of the 1960s to 1980s, many Black residents now live in North Tulsa, where over one-third of people live in poverty, and where there are "fewer businesses (including grocers) and more abandoned or dilapidated buildings, as well as fewer banks and more payday lenders" (Perry et al., 2021). The 1921 race massacre and urban renewal policies also decreased Black homeownership in Tulsa and today, homes in Tulsa's Black neighborhoods are valued at 40 percent less than similar homes in non-Black neighborhoods (Perry et al., 2021). Building off a 2018 study that estimated the total losses from the race massacre would be worth $200 million today (Messer et al., 2018), Brookings Institution found that a restitution package to recoup these losses could fully fund the education of 2,173–4,545 Black residents, purchase 4,187 median-priced homes in Black neighborhoods, or help start 6,421 Black-owned businesses (Perry et al., 2021). This type of event is not unique to Tulsa; the urban renewal policies of the 1960s–1980s affected Black communities all across U.S. cities (Fullilove, 2001), and incidents similar to the massacre in Tulsa also devastated Black communities in Wilmington, North Carolina, Rosewood, Florida, and other cities (González-Tennant, 2023; Wilmington Race Riot Commission, 2006).

Although past actions, practices, policies, and laws have inflicted lasting trauma on Black communities and undermined access to social, economic, and political resources and opportunity, this history is also characterized by Black perseverance and resistance to injustice, from slavery, to Reconstruction, to the Civil Rights Movement, to the present (American Social History Project, n.d.-a). Uprisings by enslaved people and historical documents, such as accounts from formerly enslaved individuals and advertisements offering rewards for the return of those who escaped enslavement, chronicle such resistance (American Social History Project, n.d.-b). During Reconstruction, Black activists founded Equal Rights Leagues, fought for equal citizenship, opportunity, and suffrage, and against Black Codes (NMAAHC, n.d.; Villanova University, n.d.). The Civil Rights Movement of the 1950s–1960s, and the racial justice protests that followed the killing of George Floyd in 2020, offer additional examples of how Black organizing and resistance has played a role in the movement toward healing and racial equity for Black communities (Library of Congress, n.d.; McLaughlin, 2020).

Evidence demonstrates that redress for harms inflicted on Black communities would improve health and other aspects of well-being. As discussed in Chapter 3, significant racial inequities in economic stability, particularly wealth, stem from past policies. Given the systemic nature of inequities in income and wealth, and their persistence over the last 30 years, they will not resolve without intervention. A recent analysis from RAND explores several strategies and amounts (e.g., equal allocations to all Black households, equal allocations to all households, targeted allocations to all households, and targeted allocations to Black households) for wealth allocation policies to address inequities and their projected impact on the racial wealth gap. The analysis considers wealth allocations funded through the sale of sovereign bonds rather than wealth reallocation to some households funded by taxing others. Using data from the Survey of Consumer Finances, the analysis finds that $500 billion, $1.5 trillion, or $3 trillion equally allocated to all Black households could reduce median wealth disparity by 17, 50, or 100 percent, respectively (Welburn et al., 2022). It also finds that policies targeting $760 billion or $1.6 trillion to Black households at the lower end of the wealth distribution could halve or eliminate the median wealth disparity, respectively (Welburn et al., 2022).

A 2021 study showed that a restitutive wealth redistribution program for Black individuals would have decreased COVID-19 risk for recipients, and the resultant decrease in transmission would benefit the broader population (Richardson et al., 2021). The authors hypothesized that several mechanisms might be responsible for this effect: a narrowed racial wealth gap, differences in built environment that increase the ability to social distance, a more equitable racial distribution of frontline workers, and decreased race-based allostatic load (Richardson et al., 2021). Additionally, a recent study by Himmelstein et al. (2022) aimed to determine what share of the Black–White gap in longevity could be explained by differences in wealth and how much reparations payments that aimed to close this wealth gap might reduce differences in that longevity gap. In models adjusting for income or educational attainment alone, racial gaps in longevity persisted. However, adjusting for differences in wealth eliminated differences in survival by race, and simulations indicated that payments that aimed to decrease the mean racial wealth gap were associated with longevity gap reductions of 65.0–102.5 percent (Himmelstein et al., 2022). As discussed in prior chapters, decades of research have established how social and structural factors, such as wealth, impact health outcomes and have created racial and ethnic inequities (Chapter 1 and 2). Critically, wealth enables access to other SDOH and enables individuals to engage in health-promoting behaviors (Chapter 3). Welburn et al. (2022), Richardson et al. (2021), and Himmelstein et al. (2022) provide evidence that targeting wealth could be an effective strategy to address inequities and redress for past actions, practices, policies, and laws that continue to harm Black communities. Such policies may also apply to other racially and ethnically minoritized populations, who also experience inequities in wealth due to structural racism.

Similar policies to redress harm caused to Black communities are being explored and implemented at the state and local levels. In Evanston, Illinois, for example, the Reparations Restorative Housing Program was designed to address the city's history of discriminatory housing policies and practices. With an initial budget of $400,000, it has provided payments of up to $25,000 for 16 Black residents to put toward homeownership, home improvement, or mortgage assistance. It is the first initiative of the reparations fund that Evanston established in 2019 and was implemented after the city's Equity and Empowerment Commission concluded that in Evanston, the strongest case (that is, the most politically feasible and justifiable) for reparations was around housing (City of Evanston, n.d.; Richardson, 2021; Robinson and Thompson, 2021).

In California, Assembly Bill 3121 established the Task Force to Study and Develop Reparation Proposals for African Americans, with a Special Consideration for African Americans Who Are Descendants of Persons Enslaved in the United States.[11] The task force is meant to recommend appropriate redress based on its findings. Through its deliberations thus far, the task force has identified housing, the dispossession and destruction of Black-owned property and businesses, education, mass incarceration and policing, and health, among others, as areas of harm. It continues to deliberate on this and other aspects of the proposals for reparations it will develop and policy changes it may recommend (Austin and Har, 2022; California Task Force, 2022).

In 2010, North Carolina established the Office of Justice for Sterilization Victims to address the injustices carried out by the North Carolina Eugenics Board program (NCDOA, n.d.). North Carolina was not the only state to forcibly sterilize people deemed "unfit" for reproduction. In 1935, 27 states had laws that allowed for forced sterilization of people who were deemed mentally unfit, were on welfare, or had genetic defects. Black, Latino/a, and AIAN women were overrepresented among victims of state programs and federally funded "family planning" efforts (Novak et al., 2018; Stern, 2020; Washington, 2006). The North Carolina Eugenics Board program sterilized almost 7,600 people between 1929 and 1974. Many of them were low income or had a disability, and 40 percent were racially or ethnically minoritized (Mennel, 2014; NCDOA, 2014). Although North Carolina's Office of Justice for Sterilization Victims provided compensation in 2014, the process was not without flaws. Residents whose forced sterilizations were approved by judges and social workers but not signed off on by the Eugenics Board found themselves ineligible for compensation based on this technicality (Mennel, 2014).

Efforts such as those by North Carolina, California, and Evanston are also underway in Asheville, North Carolina (The City of Asheville, 2023); Providence, Rhode Island (Providence Municipal Reparations Comission, 2022); Boston, Massachusetts (City of Boston, 2023); Cambridge, Massachusetts (Kingdollar, 2021); and other cities. Although it may be difficult to gain broad support for similar efforts at the federal level, this is one avenue through which the federal government could begin to address

---

[11] A.B. 3121 (CA 2020).

the trauma it has caused Black individuals and communities. H.R.40, which would establish the Commission to Study and Develop Reparation Proposals for African Americans, was introduced in the House of Representatives in 2021 but has yet to advance through Congress.[12] It could serve a similar role as Evanston's equity commission and California's task force in exploring possibilities for redress, to lift impacted communities out of poverty and harmful living conditions, provide access to quality education, and address other social needs to mitigate or eliminate health inequities.

Challenges to the use of affirmative action in college admissions mounted in *Students for Fair Admissions, Inc. v. President & Fellows of Harvard College*[13] and *Students for Fair Admissions, Inc. v. University of North Carolina*[14] (see Chapter 4) suggest that it may be difficult to gain broad support for race-based reparations-like policies compared to those that are targeted more specifically. North Carolina's Office of Justice for Sterilization Victims, for example, targets individuals who were directly affected, and California's task force, though not excluding others, has a special consideration for Black descendants of people who were enslaved in the United States. Reparations-like policies may gain broader support if they are structured to target particular communities based on ancestry or poverty, rather than being race-based. However, structural racism affects all Black people in the United States today, regardless of ancestry.

Trauma and Healing for American Indian and Alaska Native Communities

AIAN tribes have a unique legal relationship with the United States, which includes hundreds of treaties that mandate support for economic well-being, public safety, education, and health care (U.S. Commission on Civil Rights, 2018) (see Chapter 2 for more information). Despite numerous challenges, courts have consistently upheld these rights. For example, in *Rosebud Sioux Tribe v. United States*, the Eighth Circuit Court of Appeals upheld the right of Tribal Nations to physician-directed health care.[15] However, despite this legal acknowledgment, the Indian Health Service (IHS) remains chronically underfunded (see Chapter 5) (Tribal Budget Formulation Workgroup, 2022). Additionally, an insufficient federal response to the crisis of missing and murdered AIAN women and girls and inadequate collection of and access to related data perpetuate this crisis (Urban Indian

---

[12] H.R. 40, 117th Congress (2021).
[13] 600 U.S. ___ (2023).
[14] 600 U.S. ___ (2023).
[15] *Rosebud Sioux Tribe v. United States*, 9 F.4th 1018 (8th Circ. 2021).

Health Institute, 2018a), economic deprivation of urban and rural tribal communities has built a system of pervasive poverty (Davis et al., 2016), and a lack of quality educational opportunities has resulted in low high school graduation and college enrollment rates (Keith et al., 2016). A lack of data related to inequities and resiliencies for AIAN people, discussed more extensively in Chapter 2, also directly impacts the allocation of resources legally owed through treaty and trust responsibility.

In addition to this failure to honor treaty obligations, past and present federal actions, practices, policies, and laws, such as forced assimilation, territorial dispossession, extermination, and intrusion on sovereignty, have also resulted in ongoing trauma and negatively affected health and well-being for AIAN people. The legacy of Indian boarding schools is one example. From 1819 to 1869, schools established and supported by federal policies removed AIAN and Native Hawaiian children from their families and incarcerated them in "educational" institutions as a method of forced cultural assimilation. Sexual, physical, and emotional abuse were common, as were school cemeteries for an estimated hundreds of children who died while in attendance (Newland, 2022). In addition to this cultural loss, abuse, and death, these experiences have contributed to ongoing trauma and effects on the health and well-being of AIAN and Native Hawaiian communities. A study by Running Bear found that various aspects of the Indian boarding school experience, including limited family contact, punishment for use of American Indian language, and prohibition on practicing American Indian culture and traditions, were independently linked to poorer physical health in adulthood (Running Bear et al., 2018). Running Bear et al. (2019) found that now-adult attendees of Indian boarding schools were more likely to have cancer, tuberculosis, high cholesterol, diabetes, anemia, arthritis, and gallbladder disease compared to adult nonattendees. Indian boarding schools have also been linked with increased risk for mental health outcomes, such as substance use disorders, suicidal ideation, and attempted suicide in now-adult attendees and anxiety, PTSD, and suicidal ideation in people raised by attendees (Evans-Campbell et al., 2012). In June 2021, Secretary of the Interior Deb Haaland issued a memorandum to the Department of the Interior that launched the Federal Indian Boarding School Initiative. In consultation with impacted communities, the initiative collected data and reviewed records to document the scope of the system and its effects. This initiative provides a positive example of federal action to address past harms and improve equity that can be built upon. In May 2022, the department released the Federal Indian Boarding School Initiative Investigative Report, outlining its activities and recommending, among other actions, continued investigation, the advancement of Native language revitalization, and research into the health effects of the boarding school system on AIAN and Native Hawaiian individuals and communities (Newland, 2022).

The removal of AIAN and Native Hawaiian children from their communities occurred in parallel with territorial dispossession (Newland, 2022). The forced removal and relocation of AIAN from their traditional lands was embedded into federal policy as a means to handle the "Indian problem" and ensure land was available for encroaching European settlers (Kiel, 2017; Moss, 2019). Although precise estimates as to the scope of territorial dispossession and forced migration have been largely lacking, a recent analysis demonstrates a "near total" reduction in aggregate land, with 42.1 percent of tribes with historical lands having no federally or state-recognized land base (Farrell et al., 2021). For tribes that do, their lands average 2.6 percent of the estimated size of their historical lands. Estimates of migration distances averaged 148 miles, with a maximum of 1,724 miles (Farrell et al., 2021). Although data on the mental and physical health impacts of territorial dispossession and forced migration have been limited, studies suggest that AIAN people think regularly about broken treaties and historical loss of land, language, culture, traditional spiritual ways, and family ties from relocation or boarding schools and experience associated sadness, anger, anxiety, and shame (Urban Indian Health Institute, 2018b; Whitbeck et al., 2004).

Decades of tribal advocacy have focused on restoring land that was taken. In 2020, protest by AIAN activists at the Lakota sacred site known as Mount Rushmore birthed NDN Collective's LANDBACK campaign, continuing the legacy of tribal advocacy and demanding restoration of land and land management (NDN Collective, 2020a,b). Landback efforts have seen success (Thompson, 2020); however, much remains to be done to fully undo historical harm and restore land to its original owners.[16] Ample opportunities exist for federal agencies and Congress to restore ancestral homelands to AIAN tribes and address the harmful impacts of territorial dispossession and forced migration. Although laws that reduced the size of reservations took this land for the purpose of private ownership and settlement by non-AIAN people, 140 years later, one-third of the land that had been part of reservations is managed by six federal agencies. One-quarter of land within 10 miles of present-day reservations is managed by one of six federal agencies. These lands are strong candidates for federal landback efforts (Taylor and Jorgensen, 2022). Another option for addressing the impacts of territorial dispossession is establishing "first right of refusal" for Tribal Nations on sales of federal lands in their ancestral territories. This potential solution was proposed in H.R. 8108, the Advancing Tribal Parity

---

[16] In federal Indian policy, it is understood that the original owners of land are the original peoples inhabiting and stewarding the lands under the auspices of inherent sovereignty for 10 to 20,000 years pre-European contact.

on Public Land Act, which was introduced in the House in 2022.[17] The California Public Utilities Commission implemented a similar policy of first right of refusal that applies to the disposition of land by investor-owned utilities (California Public Utilities Commission, n.d.).

In addition to restoration of land, ensuring access for AIAN communities to federal lands and waters for traditional hunting, fishing, and gathering activities and costewardship is another avenue to address ongoing historical trauma and emotional distress related to loss of land and traditional ways (Gordon, 2022; Whitbeck et al., 2004). Alaska Natives, for example, depend on hunting, fishing, and gathering for subsistence (Gordon, 2022). Territorial dispossession and the ecological impacts of climate change on Alaskan flora and fauna are threatening their traditional ways of life and life-sustaining foods (Green et al., 2021). Mandating access to federal lands and waters for Alaska Natives to maintain subsistence lifestyles could thus help address not only historical trauma but also the impact of climate change on health (Green et al., 2021). Expanding CLEAR30[18] to federal, state, and tribal lands to increase their accessibility for hunting and gathering rights is one strategy that could help achieve this.

An association between 27 tribes and Yellowstone National Park provides one example of how costewardship can address the trauma of loss of land and traditional ways. Formed with just a few tribes in 1996, this association creates the opportunity for tribes to participate in resource management and decision making, conduct ceremonies and other events in the park, collect plants and minerals for traditional uses, and hunt bison outside of the park in coordination with park officials (NPS, 2022). Holding agencies accountable to Joint Secretarial Order 3403 between the Departments of the Interior and Agriculture could help to increase such opportunities. Joint Secretarial Order 3403 directs the departments' bureaus and offices to do the following:

a. Ensure that all decisions by the departments related to federal stewardship of federal lands, waters, and wildlife under their jurisdiction include consideration of how to safeguard the interests of any Indian tribes such decisions may affect;
b. Make agreements with Indian tribes to collaborate in the costewardship of federal lands and waters under the departments' jurisdiction, including for wildlife and its habitat;

---

[17]H.R. 8108, 117th Congress (2022).
[18]CLEAR30 (the Clean Lakes, Estuaries, And Rivers initiative) is an opportunity for landowners and agricultural producers implementing water quality practices through the Conservation Reserve Program to receive incentives by enrolling in 30-year contracts, strengthening and extending the implementation of these existing water quality practices (USDA, 2021).

   c. Identify and support tribal opportunities to consolidate tribal homelands and empower tribal stewardship of those resources;

   d. Complete a preliminary legal review of current land, water, and wildlife treaty responsibilities and authorities that can support costewardship and tribal stewardship within 180 days and finalize the legal review within one year of the date of this order; and

   e. Issue a report within one year of this order, and each year thereafter, on actions taken to fulfill the purpose of this order (Haaland and Vilsack, 2021, p. 2).

Thirteen costewardship agreements have followed the order's signing, per the first annual report released in November 2022, and the Bureau of Land Management, National Park Service, and U.S. Fish and Wildlife Service have also released guidance to improve costewardship (DOI, 2022).

Incorporating Indigenous knowledge into policies, programs, and decision making is another avenue to address the health inequity that past and present federal actions, practices, policies, and laws have wrought and uphold trust responsibility at the federal, state, and local levels. Scholars have defined Indigenous knowledge as "diverse knowledge preferences and practices of Indigenous peoples, whether modern or traditional, but even modern Indigenous knowledges typically trace some continuity with the Indigenous past" (Gone, forthcoming, p. 20). However, efforts to recognize and incorporate Indigenous knowledge need to consider the unique cultural differences of each Tribal Nation and urban AIAN community and not take a one-size-fits-all approach. Despite overwhelming odds, tribal communities have survived and, in many instances, thrived when given the opportunity and resources to apply Indigenous knowledge systems to address inequities. For example, diabetes has long been an issue within AIAN communities; however, despite a disproportionately high diabetes prevalence, that rate has not increased since 2011. This is attributed to the Special Diabetes Program for Indians, a national program funding urban and rural tribal communities whose programing incorporated local and regional cultural traditions and teachings into Western evidenced-based diabetes prevention programing (ASPE, 2019). A study found that after the implementation of this program among AIAN adults, age-adjusted diabetes-related end-stage renal disease rates per 100,000 population decreased 54 percent, and overall cost savings for this program was up to $520 million (ASPE, 2019; Bullock et al., 2017). However, despite overwhelming data supporting its impact, tribal leaders are consistently forced to fight and advocate to Congress for minimal funding appropriations to keep the program operational, illustrating the lack of investment in AIAN knowledge systems and failure by the federal government to uphold treaty rights. In late 2022, the Biden Administration released the first-of-its-kind Indigenous Knowledge Guidance for federal agencies.

This document provides guidance on the incorporation of Indigenous traditional ecological knowledge in federal scientific and policy processes, highlighting an opportunity to advance equity for AIAN communities, with an accompanying memorandum on implementation (The White House OSTP and Council on Environmental Quality, 2022a,b). Drawing upon decades of feedback from tribes, tribal leaders, tribal and urban Indian organizations, and community members, this guidance offers a plan to ensure the appropriate application of Indigenous knowledge across federal agencies (The White House, 2022b). Although these efforts are commendable and necessary to repair the harm inflicted on AIAN communities, to address long-standing inequities, they must be embedded in policy and not depend on who is in office.

Health inequities and historical trauma in AIAN communities are directly tied to the political status of Tribal Nations and past and present federal actions, practices, policies, and laws, such as forced assimilation, territorial dispossession, extermination, intrusion on sovereignty, and the failure to uphold treaty and trust responsibilities. Given its scope, this report is unable to expansively review all strategies to address these wrongs. In addition to the policies covered above, other avenues to address historical trauma and improve health equity for AIAN communities include permanently providing advanced appropriations to IHS (National Indian Health Board, n.d.) (see Chapters 5 and 8), improving data collection for AIAN communities (Erickson et al., 2021; Friedman et al., 2023) (see Chapters 2 and 8), properly implementing Savanna's Act[19] and Not Invisible Act,[20] and other strategies to address the maze of injustice related to missing and murdered AIAN women, girls, and people (GAO, 2021). By addressing historical trauma through strategies such as restoring land, expanding costewardship opportunities, and grappling with the legacy of the Federal Indian boarding school system, and by upholding treaty and trust responsibilities to provide for tribes' well-being, the federal government can begin to address the legacy of harm to AIAN communities, improving access to health care and life-sustaining food, supporting restoration of traditional ways of life, improving mental health outcomes related to past losses, and addressing other community needs to mitigate or eliminate health inequities.

Trauma and Healing for Native Hawaiian and Pacific Islander Communities

Federal actions, practices, policies, and laws in Hawaii that have led to lasting harm include the illegal overthrow of the Hawaiian monarchy and annexation of the Hawaiian Islands, driven by business and

---

[19] 25 U.S.C. § 5701 *et seq.*
[20] Pub. L. 116–166, 134 Stat. 766 (Oct. 10, 2020).

agricultural interests, and U.S. military deployment of personnel and weapons (Blaisdell, 2019; Sai, 2018). In 1921, Congress passed the Hawaiian Homes Commission Act,[21] which created the term "native Hawaiian" to refer to "any descendant of not less than one-half part of the blood of the races inhabiting the Hawaiian Islands previous to 1778" (referring to the arrival of Captain Cook) and defined "the United States as trustee and 'native Hawaiians' as wards" (Blaisdell, 2019, p. 256). Since that time, the U.S. military has established an extensive network of bases as part of its Pacific strategic defense framework.

Western colonialism in Hawaii introduced diseases and violence; displaced people and dispossessed them of their land; ended self-government; degraded the quality of land, water, and air (Kanaʻiaupuni and Malone, 2006; Levy, 1975; MacKenzie et al., 2007; Martin et al., 1996); and created cultural conflict, physiological stress, and trauma (Kaholokula et al., 2012; Liu and Alameda, 2011; Pokhrel and Herzog, 2014). Although, in 1993, Public Law 103–150 acknowledged that "the indigenous Hawaiian people never directly relinquished their claims to their inherent sovereignty," no action has been taken to reinstate this sovereignty (Kanaʻiaupuni and Malone, 2006; The Learning Network, 2012; Sai, 2018; University of Hawaiʻi at Mānoa, n.d.).[22] As discussed in Chapter 2, lack of sufficient data collection has also impacted NHPI communities. Until 1997, Native Hawaiians and Other Pacific Islanders were aggregated in the Asian or Pacific Islander category, which masked a high level of heterogeneity in outcomes and made it difficult to characterize the needs of NHPI communities, let alone analyze data for Native Hawaiians specifically (OMB, 1997). More accurate and complete data allowed a clearer picture of the health inequities experienced by Native Hawaiians, ranging from chronic conditions to mental illness (Liu and Alameda, 2011). However, data for the NHPI population are still often not separately reported or sometimes combined with the Asian population, rendering these populations invisible or masking inequities (AAPI Data and National Council of Asian Pacific Americans, 2022; OMB, 1997; Panapasa et al., 2011).

Chapter 2 provides an overview of the COFA that governs U.S. relations to the Republic of the Marshall Islands (RMI). In March 2023, the United States and RMI "signed a memorandum of understanding on a new Compact of Free Association agreement that will govern relations between the two nations for the next 20 years," once the final compact is approved by Congress (Kimball, 2023). The health inequities of the Marshallese people have been shaped by layers of U.S. federal

---

[21] July 9, 1921, ch. 42, 42 Stat. 108.
[22] Pub. L. 103–150, 107 Stat. 1510 (Nov. 23, 1993).

policies that have displaced them, appropriated their lands, and exposed them to health-harming environmental hazards (including nuclear tests). The health effects of nuclear testing radiation and in-utero effects have led to higher levels of certain cancers (Pineda et al., 2023). Moreover, "increased levels of background radiation may continue to pose future problems to the ecosystem and people living in adjacent areas" and "[y] ears of trauma associated with radiation testing has led to generations of perceived radiation-related birth defects, cancers, and other chronic disease, which may explain in part why Pacific Islanders are particularly at risk of refusing potentially curative radiation therapy in the U.S." (Pineda et al., 2023).

For Marshallese who have moved to the United States seeking safety from radiation and the effects of climate change, relocation has created new challenges. For example, they face issues ranging from racism to administrative hurdles to obtaining essential benefits, such as health care and unemployment. Climate change will likely exacerbate the movement of Marshallese and other Pacific Islands people to the United States, and it will be important to examine and address structural and systemic factors likely to continue to play a role in worsening health inequities (Jetñil-Kijiner and Heine, 2020).

Conclusion 7-4: Generations of Black, American Indian, Alaska Native, Native Hawaiian, Pacific Islander, Latino/a, and Asian communities have been negatively affected by past actions, practices, policies, and laws that inflicted lasting harm and undermined access to social, economic, and political resources and opportunities, contributing to current racial and ethnic health inequities. There is a need to continue to study and address the impacts of historical and contemporaneous laws and policies that sustain racial inequity.

CIVIC ENGAGEMENT AND BELONGING

Systems of civic engagement and belonging are critical to the well-being of individuals, families, and entire communities. The path to racial, ethnic, and tribal health equity requires enlarging the contours of civic life. Specifically, it is important to expand the circle of who feels they belong—leaving no one behind—and strengthen the civic muscle necessary to establish systems that are built for everyone to thrive together in a multiracial, multicultural society. Cultivating belonging is distinct from assimilation; such efforts value each individual's and community's unique culture and knowledge system and recognize that valuing these differences is an essential part of achieving equity.

Systems of civic engagement and belonging involve critical components of *civic infrastructure* (including the presence and strength of civil society institutions, such as faith-based groups, community-serving news media, and well-resourced educational institutions, cultural organizations, governing institutions, and electoral infrastructure). These systems also involve *processes* of belonging and engagement (such as civic association, freedom from stigma and discrimination, access to information and opportunities to participate in voting, volunteering, and public work, and access to—and making contributions to—arts, culture, and spiritual life).

In 2022, the federal government, through various agencies, published a whole-of-government plan to enhance well-being and equity: the Federal Plan for Equitable Long-Term Recovery and Resilience (ELTRR). It placed "belonging and civic muscle" as the core of seven vital conditions for health and well-being (see Figure 7-2), building on a broad coalition effort during the pandemic called the "Thriving Together Springboard" (Milstein et al., 2023; Thriving Together, n.d.). That component crystallizes a rich history of eclectic efforts to strengthen connections and build shared power with a focus on civic agency, civic capacity, deliberative democracy, public participation, public work, constructive nonviolence, and collaborative problem solving (Thriving Together, n.d.). It also builds on a large body of work that connects civic engagement, feelings of efficacy and belonging, and various aspects of health and well-being (HHS, n.d.-b; NASEM, 2023; University of Wisconsin Population Health Institute, 2023).

It is a universal human need to feel loved and valued by others and to feel a sense of belonging to one's community, organization, nation, and culture (Milstein et al., 2020). Belonging instills a feeling of connection to others and to the world. A lack of belonging is tied a multitude of negative outcomes, including loneliness, isolation, anxiety, depression, substance use disorder, and suicide, and greater risk of chronic illness, infectious disease, environmental hazards, and violence (Murthy, 2020; NASEM, 2020). True belonging does not entail only passive membership in a group, but action, "typically marked by the ability to do productive work and be accountable for both contributions and consequences" (Milstein et al., 2020, p. 49). Belonging bestows both the privilege of receiving resources from society and also the responsibility to add value to society (this value can take many forms, including economic, civic, and spiritual value). The literature on human development indicates that humans develop a strong "need to contribute" by adolescence in part because of the benefit that contribution confers to the contributor (Fuligni, 2019). This balance of autonomy and interdependence is critical for human agency and human dignity (Arendt, 1958; Milstein et al., 2020).

Similarly, civic capacity and civic muscle relate to health equity and community well-being through individual, social, and institutional capacities,

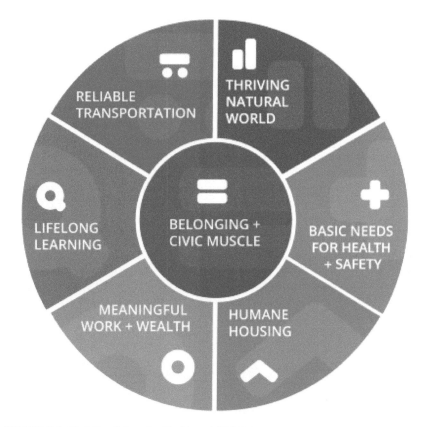

FIGURE 7-2 Vital Conditions for Health and Well-Being.
SOURCE: Federal Plan for Equitable Long-Term Recovery and Resilience ELTRR Interagency Workgroup, 2022.

activities, and processes. Civic capacity is "a stock that may expand or erode, depending on how people relate to each other, both directly and through institutions. Civic muscle explains how diverse people can work together around common values" (Milstein et al., 2020, p. 49). It is a way of weaving vested interests, "multiplying energy, and doing work that no one person or organization could do alone" (Milstein et al., 2020, p. 49). Norris (2019) describes the importance of belonging and civic muscle by explaining that "people are healthier when they are connected to others"— social networks confer resilience, support mental and emotional well-being, and encourage positive health behaviors (Norris, 2019, p. 80). Additionally, cohesive communities work together to create and ensure conditions that support health and well-being (Norris, 2019).

Civic Engagement and Belonging Are Important for Health Equity

Civic Engagement has Powerful Effects on Population Health and Well-being, Including Health Equity

An extensive analysis conducted by RAND concluded that increases in civic engagement are associated with increases in physical and mental health and well-being (Nelson et al., 2019). Likewise, communities facing fewer barriers to civic engagement are more likely to have their needs met than those with limited access or greater barriers (Ballard, 2019; Center for Social Innovation and University of Wisconsin Population Health Institute, 2021). Civic engagement among youth in particular is important for democracy and youth development; this has key implications for equity, given that racially and ethnically minoritized youth and those from immigrant and lower socioeconomic backgrounds have less access to these opportunities (Ballard, 2019).

Furthermore, a sweeping examination on the psychology of citizenship and civic engagement concluded that civic engagement in community organizations makes them "more representative, inclusive, accountable, and effective" and leads to the provision of "more appropriate, accessible, and better utilized" services (Pancer, 2015). It also found that greater neighborhood-level civic engagement is associated with a stronger sense of community, better leadership, lower crime rates, and happier, healthier citizens. States and countries with high civic participation have better physical and mental health and lower rates of disease, suicide, and crime. Research also indicates that they are more economically successful, have better-educated children, and are better governed (Pancer, 2015).

Better-connected Networks and Inclusionary Processes Tend to Produce Better Outcomes

Raj Chetty and colleagues showed how cross-class friendship networks open up opportunities for economic mobility (Chetty et al., 2022); similarly, Glen Mays and colleagues demonstrated that preventable death rates fell in communities that conduct population health activities through well-connected multisector networks (Mays et al., 2016). In addition, insights from research and the practice of planning indicates that community inclusion in program design, program implementation, and regional planning leads to better outcomes, by benefiting from a diversity of expertise, including among those affected by policies and programs, as well as anticipating and avoiding stalemates and costly mistakes in design and implementation (Innes and Booher, 2004; Klosterman, 2013; Ramakrishnan and Tamayose, 2022). Past practice also suggests that decision making, planning, and policy/program implementation need to be explicit about the type of inclusionary processes used, from a process of community informing to one of consultation, collaboration, and empowerment (Nabatchi, 2012).

Racism, Stigma, Discrimination, and Misinformation are Lethal

The Centers for Disease Control and Prevention (CDC), along with scores of municipalities nationwide, has stated unequivocally that racism is a public health threat (CDC, 2021; City of Chicago, 2021; Martin, 2020; New York State Department of Health, 2022). Similarly, the World Health Organization (WHO) confirms that stigma and discrimination contribute to global health inequities (Commission on Social Determinants of Health, 2008). The Surgeon General issued a formal Advisory on Health Misinformation emphasizing that everyone needs access to trustworthy sources of information (Office of the Surgeon General, 2021).

Sustained Investments to Strengthen Shared Power and Build a Unifying Movement for Equitable Health and Well-being Can Generate Significant Results

After investing more than $1 billion into one of the most extensive initiatives for health equity, leaders at The California Endowment concluded that improving democracy, especially by building community power and funding power-building organizations, is essential for achieving health equity (Iton et al., 2022; UCLA Center for Health Policy Research, n.d.). Evaluators concluded that movement-building approaches, such as organizing, base-building, investing in organizational capacity, and forming alliances, could advance progress toward health equity, be inclusive of and responsive to communities, and build collective power and capacity for advocacy in those communities (Sims et al., 2023).

Likewise, after more than a decade leading the County Rankings and Roadmaps project, leaders at the University of Wisconsin are asking whether power imbalance may be the most fundamental cause of health inequity. They argue that addressing socioeconomic status and social networks alone will not lead to equity, but that a transdisciplinary effort to understand, measure, and address power imbalance is necessary. They reason that sustained power imbalance becomes "reinforced in the systems and structures that affect decision making and resource allocation," resulting in persistent inequities in opportunity, including the opportunity to accrue money, knowledge, or influence, thereby producing inequities in health. They conclude that addressing power imbalance as a determinant of health is critical and that building community power through organizing and advocacy is a promising strategy to do so (Givens et al., 2018).

Crafting Federal Action on Civic Engagement
and Belonging for Health Equity

Existing Authorities

When developing new policies specifically aimed at addressing and reversing the harms that have created today's health inequities, it is important to recognize and leverage the power agencies already hold and implement existing policies. How career officials interpret, implement, and enforce the policies under their authority has as much to do with the outcome as drafting and passing a given policy. Often, this is overlooked when well-intentioned problem solving begins to craft a better way forward. The act of drafting and passing new policies is a long-term endeavor and not always guaranteed to succeed with the intended effect.

Leveraging authorities and interpretation of existing policies is a both pragmatic and effective solution in terms of expedience and durability; policies, once passed, tend to have staying power. Furthermore, recently established policies and actions need time to have an effect, and carefully monitoring implementation for effectiveness is just as important as perpetually drafting new policies that need new infrastructure and political will to pass and carry out.

Scouring the landscape of the vast federal government is a daunting task. However, this has already been accomplished to a large extent. Potential levers to enhance health and well-being—specifically opportunities to improve belonging and civic muscle—are outlined in the recently released federal interagency plan for ELTRR (ELTRR Interagency Workgroup, 2022).

The ELTRR plan was specifically developed with a stated goal to "eliminate disparities and achieve equity for all people and communities." Its recommendations aim to address inequity while improving conditions so that everyone can thrive. Ten crosscutting recommendations speak to the agency coordination and infrastructure needed to support transforming how agencies better align and collaborate in service of eliminating disparities, and eight recommendations speak specifically to agency actions that would improve belonging and civic muscle. These recommendations (see Box 7-4) were initially proposed, vetted, and approved by an interagency body consisting of over 35 agencies (HHS, n.d.-a).

The Justice 40 Initiative is one example of an existing policy that can be sustained and evaluated in order to realize the full intended benefit, rather than starting over with a new approach (The White House, 2022a). Justice 40 requires that 40 percent of federal investments go to communities that are disadvantaged, underserved, and overburdened by pollution. Qualifying investments include "climate change, clean energy and energy efficiency, clean

BOX 7-4
Example Recommendations from the Federal Plan for Equitable Long-Term Recovery and Resilience

Crosscutting

- Demonstrate Continuous Community-Led Planning and Design. Integrate requirements for inclusive constituent-and/or community-owned planning (e.g., master plans, capital improvement, needs assessment), codesign, and performance monitoring that prioritize locally defined needs and goals in all federal resource provision.
- Allow Federal Funds to Facilitate Multisector Collaboration. Expand the allowed use and flexibility of federal funds to support locally determined activities and infrastructure to manage multisector collaboration and planning processes, prioritizing coleadership by communities that have been marginalized.
- Establish Infrastructure to Enable Meaningful Interagency Collaboration. Create and formalize, through adequate resources and authority, federal infrastructures including interagency action labs, training and capacity at all staff levels, consistent collaboration tools, and leadership review that prioritizes continual strategic collective and coordinated action across federal agencies on programs, policies, and initiatives impacting the vital conditions.
- Strengthen Measurement Practices to Increase Collection of Data Measuring Equity and Well-Being. Advance new and existing efforts to assess collection of demographic data across federal agencies to accurately understand disparities and measure progress toward equity.

Civic Agency

- Enhance cross-agency collaboration to increase inclusion of civics topics in Pre-K and K–12 education, higher education, community education, museums, libraries, and arts programs.

Civic Association

- Expand federal agency partnerships with federal civic engagement programs, including Citizens Corps and AmeriCorps, to support locally driven community development and resilience programs.

Collective Efficacy

- Establish a Center of Excellence in Cultivating Community Well-Being to provide technical assistance and training focused on increasing connections between federal agencies and communities working to improve the vital conditions for health and well-being, prioritizing supports for groups that have been economically and socially marginalized and underresourced communities.
- Expand cross-agency collaboration in the development of social cohesion, personal growth, and career exploration among youth by supporting strategic partnerships with community, career development, and educational institutions using positive youth development approaches that align with community workforce needs and engagement goals.

BOX 7-4 Continued

- Expand the use of cross-agency federal funds to build and sustain effective local networks that include organizations vital to community development (e.g., nonprofit organizations, associations, volunteer organizations, foundations) in proactive planning and collaboration on community-based actions for recovery and resilience.

Opportunities for Civic Engagement
- Increase federal program approaches to meaningfully engage youth who have been marginalized to identify local issues, prioritize needs, and design, implement, and monitor strategies to strengthen the vital conditions.
- Allow states to leverage federal funds to support initiatives that meaningfully engage individuals, families, and communities in the design and oversight of service delivery systems.

SOURCE: ELTRR Interagency Workgroup, 2022.

---

transit, affordable and sustainable housing, training and workforce development, remediation and reduction of legacy pollution, and the development of clean water and wastewater infrastructure" (The White House, 2022a).

Policy Design

The nature of policy change as an evergreen tool for all levels of government presents an opportunity to articulate the qualities and attributes of efforts that result in more equitable systems. Articulating requirements to address all phases of the policy life cycle that meet criteria for promoting or detracting from equity would facilitate enduring change and likely foster belonging and civic muscle. Guides for policy development and community inclusion in policy and program implementation already exist within agencies. Examples include the following:

- CDC Policy Process (CDC, 2022a);
- Community engagement associated with the decennial census (in 2020, Census Complete Count Committees composed of government and community leaders developed campaigns to increase awareness of the census and encourage their communities to respond) (Census Bureau, 2022);
- The White House Initiative on Asian Americans and Pacific Islanders Regional Interagency Working Group (which helps coordinate policy making, program development, and outreach efforts across federal agencies to address issues that impact Asian American and NHPI communities) (HHS, 2021);

- Tribal Consultation (a formal dialogue between official tribal and federal agency representatives that precedes decisions on federal proposals) (IHS, n.d.); and
- Mandated processes on community input involving transportation projects (DOT, 2022).

Adding elements that build belonging, community inclusion, and civic muscle into those frameworks would ensure that policy development beyond this study remains consistent with equity aims.

Conclusion 7-5: Research demonstrates that civic engagement and belonging have powerful effects on population health, well-being, and health equity. Civic infrastructure and civic engagement are important factors in building social cohesion and inclusionary decision making that lead to better design and implementation of policies that affect health equity.

Conclusion 7-6: Important considerations when crafting federal action on health equity include leveraging existing policies and authority, considering the limitations of executive orders, and articulating elements that build belonging, community inclusion, and civic muscle into federal agency policy development processes.

CONCLUDING OBSERVATIONS

This report primarily offers crosscutting recommendations, rather than changes to the specific federal policies and programs discussed. However, many past National Academies reports have evidence-based and promising recommendations for federal action to advance health equity in the area of social and community context (including and beyond the federal policies reviewed in this chapter) that have not been implemented and are still relevant today (see Box 7-5 for examples) (NASEM, 2017a, 2019a,b).

In this chapter, the committee was not able to delineate the entire historical landscape of federal interventions (i.e., laws, policies, practices) or lack thereof that have negatively impacted the community and social contexts of racially and ethnically minoritized populations. However, the research suggests that past actions and inaction have had long-lasting effects on communities. It is important to not only recognize this but also identify strategies for intervention and redress. A significant body of research has also shown that social and community context matter for health and well-being and can also serve as important resources for communities to draw upon when faced with adversities/shocks (e.g., pandemics, climate change). Although communities are unique in their histories and require strategies

BOX 7-5
Example Recommendations from National Academies Reports

The Promise of Adolescence: Realizing Opportunity for All Youth (NASEM, 2019a)
Recommendation 9-3: Implement policies that aim to reduce harm to justice-involved youth in accordance with knowledge from developmental science.

- Congress and state legislatures should enact legislation to eliminate the use of sex offender registries for non-violent juveniles.
- Given the robust evidence of the harmful effects of solitary confinement, the federal government or philanthropic organizations should fund research on effective alternatives to solitary confinement so that detention facilities will be able to scale back or eliminate the use of this practice as soon as practicable.

Vibrant and Healthy Kids: Aligning Science, Practice, and Policy to Advance Health Equity (NASEM, 2019b)
Recommendation 4-4: Policy makers at the federal, state, local, territorial, and tribal levels and philanthropic organizations should support the creation and implementation of programs that ensure families have access to high-quality, cost-effective, local community-based programs that support the psychosocial well-being of the primary adult caregivers and contribute to building resilience and reducing family stress.

Recommendation 8-1: Policy makers and leaders in the health care, public health, social service, criminal justice, early care and education/education, and other sectors should support and invest in cross-sector initiatives that align strategies and operate community programs and interventions that work across sectors to address the root causes of poor health outcomes. This includes addressing structural and policy barriers to data integration and cross-sector financing and other challenges to cross-sector collaboration.

Recommendation 8-5: Policy makers and leaders in the health care, public health, social service, criminal justice, early care and education/education, and other sectors should improve access to programs or policies that explicitly provide parental or caregiver supports and help build or promote family attachments and functioning by engaging with the families as a cohesive unit. For families with intensive support needs, develop programs or initiatives designed to provide comprehensive wraparound supports along a number of dimensions, such as health care, education, and social services, designed to address needs related to the social determinants of health that are integrated and community based.

Communities in Action: Pathways to Health Equity (NASEM, 2017a)
Recommendation 7-1: Foundations and other funders should support community interventions to promote health equity by:

- Supporting community organizing around important social determinants of health;
- Supporting community capacity building;

BOX 7-5 Continued

- Supporting education, compliance, and enforcement related to civil rights laws; and
- Prioritizing health equity and equity in the social determinants of health through investments in low-income and racially/ethnically minoritized communities.

tailored to their specific needs, the committee identified some themes shared by promising strategies to address inequity. Several of these themes are relevant to federal policies within the social and community context, including the need for data (and accountability in collection of that data), the importance of community voice, and implementation of federal policy at the state and local levels. For example, there is a need for data on racial and ethnic inequities in law enforcement to better understand the extent of these inequities and which policy changes may help reduce them. Data collection mandates in this area, such as the Death in Custody Reporting Act, have been stymied by lack of enforcement, and incentives for state and local governments, such as grants to help these jurisdictions pay for the staff and technology needed to comply, could improve implementation. Evidence also suggests that federal efforts to integrate community voice by articulating elements that build belonging, community inclusion, and civic engagement into agency policy development processes can also improve health equity.

It is also important to recognize and consider the work being done at the community level to promote safety and well-being, promote healing from historical trauma, and build civic muscle and a sense of belonging. The examples provided in this chapter can be drawn upon to inform federal policy to strengthen communities and promote health for a more equitable future.

REFERENCES

AAPI Data and National Council of Asian Pacific Americans. 2022. *2022 Asian American, Native Hawaiian, and Pacific Islander (AA and NHPI) roadmap for data equity in federal agencies*. Riverside, CA: AAPI Data.

Aisenberg, E., A. Gavin, G. Mehrotra, and J. Bowman. 2010. Defining violence. In *Violence in context: Current evidence on risk, protection, and prevention*, edited by T. I. Herrenkohl, E. Aisenberg, J. H. Williams, and J. M. Jenson. New York, NY: Oxford University Press. Pp. 13–24.

Alang, S., D. McAlpine, E. McCreedy, and R. Hardeman. 2017. Police brutality and Black health: Setting the agenda for public health scholars. *American Journal of Public Health* 107(5):662–665.

American Social History Project. n.d.-a. *Historicizing Black Resistance in the U.S.* https://ashp.cuny.edu/historicizing-black-resistance-us (accessed March 18, 2023).

American Social History Project. n.d.-b. *Slave Communities & Resistance*. https://shec.ashp.cuny.edu/exhibits/show/slavecommunities (accessed March 14, 2023).

Ang, D. 2021. The effects of police violence on inner-city students. *Quarterly Journal of Economics* 136(1):115–168.

AP-NORC Center for Public Affairs Research. 2021. *The April 2021 AP-NORC center poll.* Chicago, IL: Associated Press—NORC Center for Public Affairs Research.

APA (American Psychological Association). 2013. *Gun violence: Prediction, prevention, and policy.* Washington, DC: American Psychological Association.

Arendt, H. 1958. *The human condition,* 2nd ed. Chicago, IL: University of Chicago Press.

ASPE (Assistant Secretary for Planning and Evaluation). 2019. *ASPE issue brief: Special Diabetes Program for Indians: Estimates of Medicare savings.* Washington, DC: Office of the Assistant Secretary for Planning and Evaluation.

Austin, S., and J. Har. 2022. *California Reparations Task Force Dives into What Is Owed.* https://apnews.com/article/california-sacramento-oakland-8941e77405b87c91b9d235f42038380e (accessed March 28, 2023).

Ballard, P. A. 2019. *Youth civic engagement and health, wellbeing, and safety: A review of research.* Washington, DC: Philanthropy for Active Citizen Engagement.

Blaisdell, K. 2019. I hea nā Kānaka Maoli? Whither the Hawaiians? *Hūlili: Multidisciplinary Research on Hawaiian Well-Being* 11(2):253–262.

Breiding, M. J., J. Chen, and M. C. Black. 2014. *Intimate partner violence in the United States—2010.* Atlanta, GA: National Center for Injury Prevention and Control, Centers for Disease Control and Prevention.

Bryant, E. 2022. *Government Can't Say How Many People Die in U.S. Jails and Prisons.* https://www.vera.org/news/government-cant-say-how-many-people-die-in-u-s-jails-and-prisons (accessed March 14, 2023).

Bullock, A., N. R. Burrows, A. S. Narva, K. Sheff, I. Hora, A. Lekiachvili, H. Cain, and D. Espey. 2017. Vital signs: Decrease in incidence of diabetes-related end-stage renal disease among American Indians/Alaska Natives—United States, 1996–2013. *Morbidity and Mortality Weekly Report* 66(1):26–32.

California Public Utilities Commission. n.d. *Investor-Owned Utility Real Property—Land Disposition—First Right of Refusal for Disposition of Real Property Within the Ancestral Territories of California Native American Tribes.* https://www.cpuc.ca.gov/-/media/cpuc-website/divisions/news-and-outreach/documents/bco/tribal/final-land-transfer-policy-116.pdf#:~:text=As%20we%20use%20it%20here%2C%20the%20term%20first,by%20the%20IOU%20is%20provided%20to%20the%20Tribe (accessed March 15, 2023).

California Task Force. 2022. *California Task Force to Study and Develop Reparation Proposals for African Americans: Interim report.* Sacramento, CA: Office of the Attorney General, State of California Department of Justice.

Carrigan, W. D., and C. Webb. 2003. The lynching of persons of Mexican origin or descent in the United States, 1848 to 1928. *Journal of Social History* 37(2):411–438.

CDC (Centers for Disease Control and Prevention). 2021. *Racism and Health.* https://www.cdc.gov/minorityhealth/racism-disparities/index.html (accessed February 24, 2023).

CDC. 2022a. *CDC Policy Process.* https://www.cdc.gov/policy/opaph/process/index.html (accessed March 18, 2023).

CDC. 2022b. *The Syphilis Study at Tuskegee Timeline.* https://www.cdc.gov/tuskegee/timeline.htm (accessed March 14, 2023).

Census Bureau. 2022. *2020 Census: Conducting and Motivating the Count: Complete Count Committees.* https://www.census.gov/programs-surveys/decennial-census/decade/2020/planning-management/count/complete_count.html#:~:text=WHAT%3F,community%20to%20encourage%20a%20respons (accessed March 18, 2023).

Center for Social Innovation and University of Wisconsin Population Health Institute. 2021. *Compendium on civic engagement and population health.* Riverside, CA: University of California, Riverside and University of Wisconsin.

Cheatham, A., and D. Roy. 2022. *Backgrounder: Puerto Rico: A U.S. Territory in Crisis.* https://www.cfr.org/backgrounder/puerto-rico-us-territory-crisis (accessed March 28, 2023).

Chen, T. Y.-L. 2000. Hate violence as border patrol: An Asian American theory of hate violence. *Asian Law Journal* 7(1):69–101.

Chetty, R., M. O. Jackson, T. Kuchler, J. Stroebel, N. Hendren, R. B. Fluegge, S. Gong, F. Gonzalez, A. Grondin, M. Jacob, D. Johnston, M. Koenen, E. Laguna-Muggenburg, F. Mudekereza, T. Rutter, N. Thor, W. Townsend, R. Zhang, M. Bailey, P. Barbera, M. Bhole, and N. Wernerfelt. 2022. Social Capital II: Determinants of economic connectedness. *Nature* 608(7921):122–134.

Christopher, G. C. 2022. *Rx racial healing: A guide to embracing our humanity*. Washington, DC: American Association of Colleges and Universities.

The City of Asheville. 2023. *Community Reparations Commission*. https://www.ashevillenc. gov/department/city-clerk/boards-and-commissions/reparations-commission/ (accessed June 2, 2023).

City of Boston. 2023. *Task Force on Reparations*. https://www.boston.gov/equity-and-inclusion/task-force-reparations (accessed June 2, 2023).

City of Chicago. 2021. *Mayor Lightfoot and Chicago Department of Public Health Jointly Declare Racism a Public Health Crisis in Chicago*. https://www.chicago.gov/city/en/depts/mayor/press_room/press_releases/2021/june/RacismPublicHealthCrisis.html (accessed June 7, 2023).

City of Evanston. n.d. *Evanston Local Reparations*. https://www.cityofevanston.org/government/city-council/reparations (accessed March 14, 2023).

Coleman, J. S. 1990. *Foundations of social theory*. Cambridge, MA: Harvard University Press.

Collins, J., and E. Swoveland. n.d. *The Impact of Gun Violence on Children, Families, & Communities*. https://www.cwla.org/the-impact-of-gun-violence-on-children-families-communities/ (accessed March 28, 2023).

Collins, S. 2021. *The House Has Passed the George Floyd Justice in Policing Act*. https://www.vox.com/2021/3/3/22295856/george-floyd-justice-in-policing-act-2021-passed-house (accessed March 28, 2023).

Commission on Social Determinants of Health. 2008. *Closing the gap in a generation: Health equity through action on the social determinants of health. Final report of the Commission on Social Determinants of Health*. Geneva, Switzerland: World Health Organization.

Darity, W. A., and A. K. Mullen. 2020. *From here to equality: Reparations for Black Americans in the twenty-first century*, 2nd ed. Chapel Hill, NC: The University of North Carolina Press.

Davis, A., L. Geller, R. Kim, S. Villarreal, A. McCourt, J. Cubbage, and C. Crifasi. 2022. *A year in review: 2020 gun deaths in the U.S.* Baltimore, MD: Johns Hopkins Bloomberg School of Public Health.

Davis, J. J., V. J. Roscigno, and G. Wilson. 2016. American Indian poverty in the contemporary United States. *Sociological Forum* 31(1):5–28.

Davis, J. M. V., and S. B. Heller. 2017. *NBER working paper series: Rethinking the benefits of youth employment programs: The heterogeneous effects of summer jobs*. Cambridge, MA: National Bureau of Economic Research.

Department of State. n.d. *Chinese Immigration and the Chinese Exclusion Acts*. https://history.state.gov/milestones/1866-1898/chinese-immigration (accessed March 14, 2023).

DHS (Department of Homeland Security). 2023. *Interim progress report: Interagency Task Force on the Reunification of Families*. Washington, DC: Department of Homeland Security.

Dickerson, C. 2019. The youngest child separated from his family at the border was 4 months old. *The New York Times*, June 16, 2019.

DOI (Department of the Interior). 2022. *First annual report on tribal co-stewardship*. Washington, DC: Department of the Interior.

DOJ (Department of Justice). 2023. *2020 FBI Hate Crimes Statistics*. https://www.justice.gov/crs/highlights/2020-hate-crimes-statistics (accessed May 22, 2023).

DOT (Department of Transportation). 2022. *Promising practices for meaningful public involvement in transportation decision-making*. Washington, DC: Department of Transportation.

Du Bois, W. E. B. 1998. *Black Reconstruction in America 1860–1880*. New York, NY: The Free Press.

Dunn, C., and M. Shames. 2019. *Stop and frisk in the De Blasio era*. New York, NY: New York Civil Liberties Union.

Dyer, L., R. Hardeman, D. Vilda, K. Theall, and M. Wallace. 2019. Mass incarceration and public health: The association between Black jail incarceration and adverse birth outcomes among Black women in Louisiana. *BMC Pregnancy and Childbirth* 19.

The Educational Fund to Stop Gun Violence, DC Justice Lab, Cities United, March for Our Lives, Community Justice Action Fund, Consortium for Risk-Based Firearm Policy, and Johns Hopkins Center for Gun Violence Prevention and Policy. 2022. *Racial equity framework for gun violence prevention*. Washington, DC: The Educational Fund to Stop Gun Violence.

Edwards, F., H. Lee, and M. Esposito. 2019. Risk of being killed by police use of force in the United States by age, race–ethnicity, and sex. *Proceedings of the National Academy of Sciences* 116(34):16793–16798.

Edwards, G., E. Nesson, J. J. Robinson, and F. Vars. 2018. Looking down the barrel of a loaded gun: The effect of mandatory handgun purchase delays on homicide and suicide. *The Economic Journal* 128(616):3117–3140.

ELTRR Interagency Workgroup. 2022. *Federal plan for equitable long-term recovery and resilience for social, behavioral, and community health*. Washington, DC: Department of Health and Human Services.

Equal Justice Initiative. 2013. *Convict Leasing*. https://eji.org/news/history-racial-injustice-convict-leasing/ (accessed March 17, 2023).

Equal Justice Initiative. 2020. *Reconstruction in America: Racial violence after the Civil War, 1865–1876*. Montgomery, AL: Equal Justice Initiative.

Erickson, S., K. Flannery, G. Leipertz, D. Wang, A. Small, N. Ly, A. Dominguez, and A. Echo-Hawk. 2021. *Data genocide of American Indians and Alaska Natives in COVID-19 data*. Seattle, WA: Urban Indian Health Institute.

Evans-Campbell, T., K. L. Walters, C. R. Pearson, and C. D. Campbell. 2012. Indian boarding school experience, substance use, and mental health among urban two-spirit American Indian/Alaska Natives. *The American Journal of Drug and Alcohol Abuse* 38(5):421–427.

Farrell, J., P. B. Burow, K. McConnell, J. Bayham, K. Whyte, and G. Koss. 2021. Effects of land dispossession and forced migration on Indigenous peoples in North America. *Science* 374(6567):eabe4943.

Finerty, M. J. 2022. *The Supreme Court's Bruen Decision and Its Impact: What Comes Next?* https://nysba.org/the-supreme-courts-bruen-decision-and-its-impact-what-comes-next/#_edn36 (accessed May 11, 2023).

Foner, E. 2014. *Reconstruction: America's unfinished revolution, 1863–1877*. New York, NY: Harper Perennial Modern Classics.

Fram, A. 2018. *Official Says Agency Warned Family Separation Bad for Kids*. https://apnews.com/article/health-north-america-ap-top-news-judiciary-az-state-wire-ee8e81ca0c9542df b997f4bef444d0e1 (accessed June 5, 2023).

Friedman, J., H. Hansen, and J. P. Gone. 2023. Deaths of despair and Indigenous data genocide. *The Lancet* 401(10379):874–876.

Fuligni, A. J. 2019. The need to contribute during adolescence. *Perspectives on Psychological Science* 14(3):331–343.

Fullilove, M. T. 2001. Root shock: The consequences of African American dispossession. *Journal of Urban Health* 78(1):72–80.

Galea, S. 2022. Principles to guide the U.S. toward better health for all. *JAMA Health Forum* 3(12):e225359.

GAO (Government Accountability Office). 2021. *Missing or murdered Indigenous women: New efforts are underway but opportunities exist to improve the federal response*. GAO publication no. 22-104045. Washington, DC: Government Accountability Office.

Geronimus, A. T., M. Hicken, D. Keene, and J. Bound. 2006. "Weathering" and age patterns of allostatic load scores among Blacks and Whites in the United States. *American Journal of Public Health* 96(5):826–833.

Giffords. n.d. *Community Violence.* https://giffords.org/issues/community-violence/ (accessed March 14, 2023).

Givens, M., D. Kindig, P. T. Inzeo, and V. Faust. 2018. *Power: The Most Fundamental Cause of Health Inequity?* https://www.healthaffairs.org/content/forefront/power-most-fundamental-cause-health-inequity (accessed March 16, 2023).

Goldstick, J. E., R. M. Cunningham, and P. M. Carter. 2022. Current causes of death in children and adolescents in the United States. *New England Journal of Medicine* 386(20):1955–1956.

Gone, J. P. Forthcoming. Chapter 14: Researching with American Indian and Alaska Native communities: Pursuing partnerships for psychological inquiry in service to Indigenous futurity. In *APA handbook of research methods in psychology, volume 2: Research designs: Quantitative, qualitative, neuropsychological, and biological,* 2nd ed, edited by H. Cooper, M. N. Coutanche, L. M. McMullen, and A. T. Panter. Washington, DC: American Psychological Association.

González-Tennant, E. 2023. *Remembering the Rosewood Massacre.* https://daily.jstor.org/remembering-rosewood-massacre/ (accessed March 14, 2023).

Gordon, H. S. J. 2022. Alaska Native subsistence rights: Taking an anti-racist decolonizing approach to land management and ownership for our children and generations to come. *Societies* 12(3).

Gourevitch, M. N., N. Kleiman, and K. B. Falco. 2022. Public health and public safety: Converging upstream. *American Journal of Public Health* 112(5):716–718.

Gramlich, J. 2020. *Black Imprisonment Rate in the U.S. Has Fallen by a Third Since 2006.* https://www.pewresearch.org/fact-tank/2020/05/06/share-of-black-white-hispanic-americans-in-prison-2018-vs-2006/ (accessed March 18, 2023).

Green, K. M., A. H. Beaudreau, M. H. Lukin, and L. B. Crowder. 2021. Climate change stressors and social-ecological factors mediating access to subsistence resources in Arctic Alaska. *Ecology and Society* 26(4):15.

Haaland, D., and T. J. Vilsack. 2021. *Joint Secretarial Order on Fulfilling the Trust Responsibility to Indian Tribes in the Stewardship of Federal Lands and Waters.* https://www.doi.gov/sites/doi.gov/files/elips/documents/so-3403-joint-secretarial-order-on-fulfilling-the-trust-responsibility-to-indian-tribes-in-the-stewardship-of-federal-lands-and-waters.pdf (accessed March 15, 2023).

Hampton, K., E. Raker, H. Habbach, L. Camaj Deda, M. Heisler, and R. Mishori. 2021. The psychological effects of forced family separation on asylum-seeking children and parents at the U.S.–Mexico border: A qualitative analysis of medico-legal documents. *PLOS ONE* 16(11):e0259576.

Hatzenbuehler, M. L., K. Keyes, A. Hamilton, M. Uddin, and S. Galea. 2015. The collateral damage of mass incarceration: Risk of psychiatric morbidity among nonincarcerated residents of high-incarceration neighborhoods. *American Journal of Public Health* 105(1):138–143.

Health Affairs. 2022. *Health Affairs Vol. 41, No. 2: Racism and Health.* https://www.healthaffairs.org/racism-and-health (accessed April 5, 2023).

Heller, S. B. 2014. Summer jobs reduce violence among disadvantaged youth. *Science* 346(6214):1219–1223.

Heller, S. B., A. K. Shah, J. Guryan, J. Ludwig, S. Mullainathan, and H. A. Pollack. 2017. Thinking, fast and slow? Some field experiments to reduce crime and dropout in Chicago. *The Quarterly Journal of Economics* 132(1):1–54.

HHS (Department of Health and Human Services). 2020. *Healthy People 2030: Social and Community Context.* https://health.gov/healthypeople/objectives-and-data/browse-objectives/social-and-community-context (accessed March 14, 2023).

HHS. 2021. *White House Initiative on Asian Americans, Native Hawaiians, and Pacific Islanders Interagency Working Group.* https://www.hhs.gov/about/whiaanhpi/interagency-working-group/index.html (accessed March 18, 2023).

HHS. n.d.-a. *Equitable Long-Term Recovery and Resilience: Interagency Workgroup.* https://health.gov/our-work/national-health-initiatives/equitable-long-term-recovery-and-resilience/interagency-workgroup (accessed June 8, 2023).

HHS. n.d.-b. *Healthy People 2030: Civic Participation.* https://health.gov/healthypeople/priority-areas/social-determinants-health/literature-summaries/civic-participation (accessed June 8, 2023).

HHS. n.d.-c. *Healthy People 2030: Incarceration.* https://health.gov/healthypeople/priority-areas/social-determinants-health/literature-summaries/incarceration (accessed March 18, 2023).

Hicken, M. T., M. Durkee, N. Kravitz-Wurtz, and J. S. Jackson. 2018. The role of racism in health inequalities: Integrating approaches from across disciplines. *Social Science & Medicine* 199:11–240.

Himmelstein, K. E. W., J. A. Lawrence, J. L. Jahn, J. N. Ceasar, M. Morse, M. T. Bassett, B. P. Wispelwey, W. A. Darity, and A. S. Venkataramani. 2022. Association between racial wealth inequities and racial disparities in longevity among U.S. adults and role of reparations payments, 1992 to 2018. *JAMA Network Open* 5(11):e2240519.

Huang, J. T., M. Krupenkin, D. Rothschild, and J. Lee Cunningham. 2023. The cost of anti-Asian racism during the COVID-19 pandemic. *Nature Human Behaviour* 7:682–695.

IHS (Indian Health Service). n.d. *Tribal Consultation and Urban Confer.* https://www.ihs.gov/dbh/consultationandconfer/ (accessed March 11, 2023).

Innes, J. E., and D. E. Booher. 2004. Reframing public participation: Strategies for the 21st century. *Planning Theory & Practice* 5(4):419–436.

IOM (Institute of Medicine) and NRC (National Research Council). 2013. *Priorities for research to reduce the threat of firearm-related violence.* Washington, DC: The National Academies Press.

Iton, A., R. K. Ross, and P. S. Tamber. 2022. Building community power to dismantle policy-based structural inequity in population health. *Health Affairs* 41(12):1763–1771.

James, N., and K. Finklea. 2021. *Programs to collect data on law enforcement activities: Overview and issues.* Washington, DC: Congressional Research Service.

Jay, J., R. Martin, M. Patel, K. Xie, F. Shareef, and J. T. Simes. 2023. Analyzing child firearm assault injuries by race and ethnicity during the COVID-19 pandemic in 4 major U.S. cities. *JAMA Network Open* 6(3):e233125.

Jetñil-Kijiner, K., and H. Heine. 2020. *Displacement and Out-Migration: The Marshall Islands Experience.* https://www.wilsoncenter.org/article/displacement-and-out-migration-marshall-islands-experience (accessed March 18, 2023).

Johns Hopkins Center for Gun Violence Prevention and Policy. n.d.-a. *Background Checks.* https://www.jhsph.edu/research/centers-and-institutes/johns-hopkins-center-for-gun-violence-prevention-and-policy/research/background-checks/ (accessed March 17, 2023).

Johns Hopkins Center for Gun Violence Prevention and Policy. n.d.-b. *Safe Gun Storage.* https://www.jhsph.edu/research/centers-and-institutes/johns-hopkins-center-for-gun-violence-prevention-and-policy/research/safe-gun-storage/ (accessed March 18, 2023).

Kaholokula, J. K., A. Grandinetti, S. Keller, A. H. Nacapoy, T. K. Kingi, and M. K. Mau. 2012. Association between perceived racism and physiological stress indices in Native Hawaiians. *Journal of Behavioral Medicine* 35(1):27–37.

Kanaʻiaupuni, S. M., and N. Malone. 2006. This land is my land: The role of place in Native Hawaiian identity. *Hūlili: Multidisciplinary Research on Hawaiian Well-Being* 3(1):281–307.

Kaplan, M. S., A. C. Mueller-Williams, S. Goldman-Mellor, and R. Sakai-Bizmark. 2022. Changing trends in suicide mortality and firearm involvement among Black young adults in the United States, 1999–2019. *Archives of Suicide Research* 1–6.

Kawachi, I., and L. Berkman. 2000. Social cohesion, social capital, and health. In *Social epidemiology*, 2nd ed., edited by L. F. Berkman, I. Kawachi, and M. M. Glymour. New York, NY: Oxford University Press. Pp. 174–190.

Keating, D., and H. Stevens. 2020. Bloomberg said "stop and frisk" decreased crime. Data suggests it wasn't a major factor in cutting felonies. *The Washington Post*, February 27.

Keith, F. J., N. S. Stastny, and A. Brunt. 2016. Barriers and strategies for success for American Indian college students: A review. *Journal of College Student Development* 57(6):698–714.

Kiel, D. 2017. *American Expansion Turns to Official Indian Removal*. https://www.nps.gov/articles/american-expansion-turns-to-indian-removal.htm (accessed June 6, 2023).

Kimball, D. G. 2023. *U.S., Marshall Islands Sign Deal on Nuclear Testing Impacts*. https://www.armscontrol.org/act/2023-03/news/us-marshall-islands-sign-deal-nuclear-testing-impacts (accessed March 18, 2023).

Kingdollar, B. L. 2021. *Cambridge City Council to Explore Reparations for Slavery, Restitution for War on Drugs*. https://www.thecrimson.com/article/2021/9/14/city-council-sept-14/ (accessed June 5, 2023).

Klosterman, R. E. 2013. Lessons learned about planning. *Journal of the American Planning Association* 79(2):161–169.

Lane, H. M., R. Morello-Frosch, J. D. Marshall, and J. S. Apte. 2022. Historical redlining is associated with present-day air pollution disparities in U.S. cities. *Environmental Science & Technology Letters* 9(4):345–350.

The Learning Network. 2012. *Jan. 17, 1893 | Hawaiian monarchy Overthrown by America-Backed Businessmen*. https://archive.nytimes.com/learning.blogs.nytimes.com/2012/01/17/jan-17-1893-hawaiian-monarchy-overthrown-by-america-backed-businessmen/ (accessed March 18, 2023).

Lee, E. K., G. Donley, T. H. Ciesielski, I. Gill, O. Yamoah, A. Roche, R. Martinez, and D. A. Freedman. 2022. Health outcomes in redlined versus non-redlined neighborhoods: A systematic review and meta-analysis. *Social Science & Medicine* 294:114696.

Lee, H., and C. Wildeman. 2021. Assessing mass incarceration's effects on families. *Science* 374(6565):277–281.

Levy, N. M. 1975. Native Hawaiian land rights. *California Law Review* 63(4):848–885.

Library of Congress. n.d. *The African American Odyssey: A Quest for Full Citizenship*. https://www.loc.gov/exhibits/african-american-odyssey/civil-rights-era.html (accessed March 17, 2023).

Liu, D. M. K. I., and C. K. Alameda. 2011. Social determinants of health for Native Hawaiian children and adolescents. *Hawai'i Medical Journal* 70(11):9–14.

Luca, M., D. Malhotra, and C. Poliquin. 2017. Handgun waiting periods reduce gun deaths. *Proceedings of the National Academy of Sciences* 114(46):12162–12165.

MacDonald, J. n.d. *Does Stop-and-Frisk Reduce Crime?* https://crim.sas.upenn.edu/fact-check/does-stop-and-frisk-reduce-crime (accessed March 18, 2023).

MacKenzie, M. K., S. K. Serrano, and K. L. Kaulukukui. 2007. Environmental justice for Indigenous Hawaiians: Reclaiming land and resources. *Natural Resources & Environment* 21(3):37–42, 79.

MacLean, S. A., P. O. Agyeman, J. Walther, E. K. Singer, K. A. Baranowski, and C. L. Katz. 2019. Mental health of children held at a United States immigration detention center. *Social Science & Medicine* 230:303–308.

Martin, E. 2020. *L.A. City Council Declares Racism a Public Health Crisis*. https://ktla.com/news/local-news/l-a-city-council-declares-racism-a-public-health-crisis/ (accessed June 7, 2023).

Martin, E. A. H. K. P., D. L. Martin, D. C. Penn, and J. E. McCarty. 1996. Cultures in conflict of Hawai'i: The law and politics of Native Hawaiian water rights. *University of Hawai'i Law Review* 18(1):71–200.

Martin, K. J., A. L. Stanton, and K. L. Johnson. 2022. Current health care experiences, medical trust, and COVID-19 vaccination intention and uptake in Black and White Americans. *Health Psychology* (Advance online publication) *https://doi.org/10.1037/hea0001240*.

Mason, T. 2021. *Extreme Sentences Disproportionately Impact and Harm Black Women*. https://www.nbwji.org/post/extreme-sentences-disproportionately-impact-and-harm-black-women (accessed March 18, 2023).

Mauer, M. 2018. Long-term sentences: Time to reconsider the scale of punishment. *UMKC Law Review* 87(1):113–131.

Maxwell, C., and D. Solomon. 2018. *Mass incarceration, stress, and Black infant mortality: A case study in structural racism*. Washington, DC: Center for American Progress.

Mays, G. P., C. B. Mamaril, and L. R. Timsina. 2016. Preventable death rates fell where communities expanded population health activities through multisector networks. *Health Affairs* 35(11):2005–2013.

McEwen, C. A., and B. S. McEwen. 2017. Social structure, adversity, toxic stress, and intergenerational poverty: An early childhood model. *Annual Review of Sociology* 43:445–472.

McGee, Z. T., K. Logan, J. Samuel, and T. Nunn. 2017. A multivariate analysis of gun violence among urban youth: The impact of direct victimization, indirect victimization, and victimization among peers. *Cogent Social Sciences* 3(1).

McLaughlin, E. C. 2020. *How George Floyd's Death Ignited a Racial Reckoning That Shows No Signs of Slowing Down*. https://www.cnn.com/2020/08/09/us/george-floyd-protests-different-why/index.html (accessed June 5, 2023).

Mennel, E. 2014. *Payments Start for N.C. Eugenics Victims, But Many Won't Qualify*. https://www.npr.org/sections/health-shots/2014/10/31/360355784/payments-start-for-n-c-eugenics-victims-but-many-wont-qualify (accessed April 5, 2023).

Messer, C. M., T. E. Shriver, and A. E. Adams. 2018. The destruction of Black Wall Street: Tulsa's 1921 riot and the eradication of accumulated wealth. *The American Journal of Economics and Sociology* 77(3–4):789–819.

Miller, H. N., S. LaFave, L. Marineau, J. Stephens, and R. J. Thorpe. 2021. The impact of discrimination on allostatic load in adults: An integrative review of literature. *Journal of Psychosomatic Research* 146.

Milstein, B., B. Payne, C. Kelleher, J. Homer, T. Norris, M. Roulier, and S. Saha. 2023. *Organizing Around Vital Conditions Moves the Social Determinants Agenda into Wider Action*. https://www.healthaffairs.org/content/forefront/organizing-around-vital-conditions-moves-social-determinants-agenda-into-wider-action (accessed March 18, 2023).

Milstein, B., P. Stojicic, E. Auchincloss, and C. Kelleher. 2020. Civic life and system stewardship on the job: How can workers in every industry strengthen the belonging and civic muscle we all need to thrive? *The Good Society* 29(1–2):42–73.

Modestino, A. S. 2019. How do summer youth employment programs improve criminal justice outcomes, and for whom? *Journal of Policy Analysis and Management* 38(3):600–628.

Monmouth University. 2019. *National: Public divided on assault weapons policy: Broad support for background checks and "red flag" laws*. West Long Branch, NJ: Monmouth University.

Monroe, I. 2021. *Reparations for the Tulsa Race Massacre Would Begin the Healing*. https://www.wgbh.org/news/commentary/2021/06/01/reparations-for-the-tulsa-race-massacre-would-begin-the-healing (accessed March 18, 2023).

Moss, M. 2019. *Trauma Lives on in Native Americans by Making Us Sick—While the U.S. Looks Away*. https://www.theguardian.com/commentisfree/2019/may/09/trauma-lives-on-in-native-americans-while-the-us-looks-away (accessed March 6, 2023).

Murthy, V. H. 2020. *Together: The healing power of human connection in a sometimes lonely world*. New York: Harper Wave.

NAACP (National Association for the Advancement of Colored People). n.d. *Criminal Justice Fact Sheet*. https://naacp.org/resources/criminal-justice-fact-sheet (accessed March 18, 2023).

Nabatchi, T. 2012. Putting the "public" back in public values research: Designing participation to identify and respond to values. *Public Administration Review* 72(5):699–708.

NASEM (National Academies of Sciences, Engineering, and Medicine). 2017a. *Communities in action: Pathways to health equity*. Washington, DC: The National Academies Press.

NASEM. 2017b. *Community violence as a population health issue: Proceedings of a workshop*. Washington, DC: The National Academies Press.

NASEM. 2019a. *The promise of adolescence: Realizing opportunity for all youth*. Washington, DC: The National Academies Press.

NASEM. 2019b. *Vibrant and healthy kids: Aligning science, practice, and policy to advance health equity*. Washington, DC: The National Academies Press.

NASEM. 2020. *Social isolation and loneliness in older adults: Opportunities for the health care system*. Washington, DC: The National Academies Press.

NASEM. 2023. *Civic engagement and civic infrastructure to advance health equity*. Washington, DC: The National Academies Press.

National Archives. 2022a. *15th Amendment to the U.S. Constitution: Voting Rights (1870)*. https://www.archives.gov/milestone-documents/15th-amendment (accessed March 18, 2023).

National Archives. 2022b. *Japanese-American Incarceration During World War II*. https://www.archives.gov/education/lessons/japanese-relocation (accessed March 18, 2023).

National Archives. 2023. *Chinese Exclusion Act (1882)*. https://www.archives.gov/milestone-documents/chinese-exclusion-act (accessed March 18, 2023).

National Geographic. 2022. *The Black Codes and Jim Crow Laws*. https://education.nationalgeographic.org/resource/black-codes-and-jim-crow-laws/ (accessed March 14, 2023).

National Indian Health Board. n.d. *Advance Appropriations*. https://www.nihb.org/legislative/advance_appropriations.php (accessed March 11, 2023).

NCDOA (North Carolina Department of Administration). 2014. *N.C. Justice for Sterilization Victims Foundation*. https://ncadmin.nc.gov/media/3165/download (accessed March 18, 2023).

NCDOA. n.d. *Welcome to the Office of Justice for Sterilization Victims*. https://ncadmin.nc.gov/about-doa/special-programs/welcome-office-justice-sterilization-victims (accessed March 18, 2023).

NDN Collective. 2020a. *NDN Collective Calls for Closure of Mount Rushmore and for the Black Hills to Be Returned to the Lakota*. https://ndncollective.org/ndn-collective-calls-for-closure-of-mount-rushmore-and-for-the-black-hills-to-be-returned-to-the-lakota/ (accessed June 6, 2023).

NDN Collective. 2020b. *NDN Collective Landback Campaign Launching on Indigenous Peoples' Day 2020*. https://ndncollective.org/ndn-collective-landback-campaign-launching-on-indigenous-peoples-day-2020/ (accessed June 6, 2023).

Nelson, C., J. Sloan, and A. Chandra. 2019. *Examining civic engagement links to health: Findings from the literature and implications for a culture of health*. Santa Monica, CA: RAND Corporation.

Newland, B. 2022. *Federal Indian Boarding School Initiative investigative report*. Washington, DC: The Office of the Assistant Secretary—Indian Affairs.

New York State Department of Health. 2022. *Statement from New York State Health Commissioner Dr. Mary T. Bassett as National Public Health Week Begins with a Spotlight on Racism: A Public Health Crisis*. https://www.health.ny.gov/press/releases/2022/2022-04-04_commissioner_national_health_week.htm (accessed June 7, 2023).

Njaka, I., and D. Peacock. 2021. *Addressing Trauma as a Pathway to Social Change*. https://ssir.org/articles/entry/addressing_trauma_as_a_pathway_to_social_change (accessed March 8, 2023).

NMAAHC (National Museum of African American History and Culture). n.d. *Make Good the Promises: Reconstructing Citizenship*. https://nmaahc.si.edu/explore/exhibitions/reconstruction/citizenship (accessed March 18, 2023).

Noguchi, Y. 2020. *How Police Violence Could Impact the Health of Black Infants*. https://www.npr.org/2020/11/13/933084699/how-police-violence-could-impact-the-health-of-black-infants (accessed April 5, 2023).

Norris, T. 2019. Reclaiming well-being in America: The vital conditions that make people and places healthier and more resilient. *National Civic Review* 108(3):77–81.

Novak, N. L., N. Lira, K. E. O'Connor, S. D. Harlow, S. L. R. Kardia, and A. M. Stern. 2018. Disproportionate sterilization of Latinos under California's eugenic sterilization program, 1920–1945. *American Journal of Public Health* 108(5):611–613.

NPS (National Park Service). 2022. *Yellowstone National Park: Native American Affairs.* https://www.nps.gov/yell/learn/historyculture/native-american-affairs.htm (accessed March 18, 2023).

NRC (National Research Council). 2014. *The growth of incarceration in the United States: Exploring causes and consequences.* Washington, DC: The National Academies Press.

Ober, H. 2022. *Black Americans' COVID Vaccine Hesitancy Stems More from Today's Inequities Than Historical Ones: UCLA Study Urges Medical Community to Pursue Changes That Build Better Trust.* https://newsroom.ucla.edu/releases/causes-of-covid-vaccine-hesitancy-among-black-americans (accessed March 18, 2023).

Office of the Surgeon General. 2021. *Confronting health misinformation: The U.S. Surgeon General's advisory on building a healthy information environment.* Washington, DC: Office of the Surgeon General, Department of Health and Human Services.

OMB (Office of Management and Budget). 1997. Revisions to the standards for the classification of federal data on race and ethnicity. *Federal Register* 62(210):58782–58790.

One Million Experiments. n.d.-a. *About One Million Experiments.* https://millionexperiments.com/about (accessed March 23, 2023).

One Million Experiments. n.d.-b. *Detroit Heals Detroit.* https://millionexperiments.com/projects/detroit-heals-detroit (accessed March 18, 2023).

One Million Experiments. n.d.-c. *The Radical Monarchs.* https://millionexperiments.com/projects/the-radical-monarchs/ (accessed March 18, 2023).

Palafox, N. A. 2010. Health consequences of the Pacific U.S. nuclear weapons testing program in the Marshall Islands: Inequity in protection, health care access, policy, regulation. *Reviews on Environmental Health* 25(1):81–85.

Panapasa, S. V., K. M. Crabbe, and J. K. Kaholokula. 2011. Efficacy of federal data: Revised Office of Management and Budget standard for Native Hawaiian and other Pacific Islanders examined. *AAPI Nexus* 9(1–2):212–220.

Pancer, S. M. 2015. Chapter 8: Impacts of civic engagement on programs, organizations, neighborhoods, and society. In *The psychology of citizenship and civic engagement.* New York: Oxford University Press. Pp. 127–145.

Paul, C. A. 2016. *Social Welfare History Project: Fugitive Slave Act of 1850.* https://socialwelfare.library.vcu.edu/federal/fugitive-slave-act-of-1850/ (accessed March 18, 2023).

Peitzmeier, S. M., M. Malik, S. K. Kattari, E. Marrow, R. Stephenson, M. Agénor, and S. L. Reisner. 2020. Intimate partner violence in transgender populations: Systematic review and meta-analysis of prevalence and correlates. *American Journal of Public Health* 110(9):e1–e14.

Perry, A. M., A. Barr, and C. Romer. 2021. *The true costs of the Tulsa Race Massacre, 100 years later.* Washington, DC: The Brookings Institution.

Petrosky, E., J. M. Blair, C. J. Betz, K. A. Fowler, S. P. D. Jack, and B. H. Lyons. 2017. Racial and ethnic differences in homicides of adult women and the role of intimate partner violence—United States, 2003–2014. *MMWR* 66(28):741–746.

Pineda, E., R. Benavente, M. Y. Gimmen, N. V. DeVille, and K. Taparra. 2023. Cancer disparities among Pacific Islanders: A review of sociocultural determinants of health in the Micronesian region. *Cancers* 15(5).

Pokhrel, P., and T. A. Herzog. 2014. Historical trauma and substance use among Native Hawaiian college students. *American Journal of Health Behavior* 38(3):420–429.

Prison Policy Initiative. n.d. *U.S. Incarceration Rates by Race and Ethnicity, 2010.* https://www.prisonpolicy.org/graphs/raceinc.html (accessed March 10, 2023).

Providence Municipal Reparations Comission. 2022. *Report of the Providence Municipal Reparations Commission*. Providence, RI: Providence Municipal Reparations Comission.

Putnam, R. D. 1993. *Making democracy work: Civic traditions in modern Italy*. Princeton, NJ: Princeton University Press.

Ramakrishnan, S. K., and B. Tamayose. 2022. *UCR SPP working paper series: Ready to rise: A pragmatic framework to improve planning, investment, and community development*. Riverside, CA: University of California, Riverside.

RAND. 2023a. *Research Review: Effects of Assault Weapon and High-Capacity Magazine Bans on Mass Shootings*. https://www.rand.org/research/gun-policy/analysis/ban-assault-weapons/mass-shootings.html (accessed March 18, 2023).

RAND. 2023b. *Research Review: The Effects of Firearm Safety Training Requirements*. https://www.rand.org/research/gun-policy/analysis/firearm-safety-training-requirements. html (accessed June 1, 2023).

RAND. 2023c. *Research Review: The Effects of Waiting Periods*. https://www.rand.org/research/gun-policy/analysis/waiting-periods.html (accessed March 18, 2023).

Rapaport, H., and I. Nikolić Hughes. 2022. The U.S. must take responsibility for nuclear fallout in the Marshall Islands. *Scientific American*, April 4, 2022.

Richardson, E. T., M. M. Malik, W. A. Darity Jr, A. K. Mullen, M. E. Morse, M. Malik, A. Maybank, M. T. Bassett, P. E. Farmer, and L. Worden. 2021. Reparations for Black American descendants of persons enslaved in the U.S. and their potential impact on SARS-CoV-2 transmission. *Social Science & Medicine* 276:113741.

Richardson, K. 2021. *Memorandum: Adoption of Resolution 37-R-27, Authorizing the Implementation of the Evanston Local Reparations Restorative Housing Program and Program Budget*. https://cityofevanston.civicweb.net/document/50624/Adoption%20of%20Resolution%2037-R-27,%20Authorizing%20the.pdf?handle=E11C7B73E1B6470DA42362AB80A50C46 (accessed March 18, 2023).

Roach, E. L., S. L. Haft, J. Huang, and Q. Zhou. 2023. Systematic review: The association between race-related stress and trauma and emotion dysregulation in youth of color. *Journal of the American Academy of Child & Adolescent Psychiatry* 62(2):190–207.

Robinson, M., and J. Thompson. 2021. *Evanston policies and practices directly affecting the African American community, 1900–1960 (and present)*. Evanston, IL: Shorefront Legacy Center and Evanston History Center.

Roeder, O., L. B. Eisen, and J. Bowling. 2015. *What caused the crime decline?* New York: Brennan Center for Justice.

Romo, D. D. n.d. *Jan. 28, 1917: The Bath Riots*. https://www.zinnedproject.org/news/tdih/bath-riots (accessed May 25, 2023).

Roodman, D. 2017. *The impacts of incarceration on crime*. San Francisco, CA: Open Philanthropy Project.

Ross, D., D. Goble, J. H. Franklin, S. Ellsworth, R. Warner, C. Snow, R. Brooks, A. H. Witten, L. Rankin-Hill, P. Stubblefield, L. O'Dell, A. Brophy, and M. Horner. 2001. *Tulsa Race Riot: A report by the Oklahoma Commission to Study the Tulsa Race Riot of 1921*. Oklahoma City, OK: Oklahoma Commission to Study the Tulsa Race Riot of 1921.

Rothstein, R. 2017. *The color of law: A forgotten history of how our government segregated America*. New York, NY: Liveright Publishing Corporation.

Rovner, J. 2021a. *Black Disparities in Youth Incarceration*. https://www.sentencingproject.org/fact-sheet/black-disparities-in-youth-incarceration/ (accessed March 18, 2023).

Rovner, J. 2021b. *Disparities in Tribal Youth Incarceration*. https://www.sentencingproject.org/app/uploads/2022/10/Disparities-in-Tribal-Youth-Incarceration.pdf (accessed March 18, 2023).

Rovner, J. 2021c. *Latinx Disparities in Youth Incarceration*. https://www.sentencingproject.org/fact-sheet/latinx-disparities-in-youth-incarceration/ (accessed March 18, 2023).

Running Bear, U., C. D. Croy, C. E. Kaufman, Z. M. Thayer, and S. M. Manson. 2018. The relationship of five boarding school experiences and physical health status among Northern Plains Tribes. *Quality of Life Research* 27(1):153–157.

Running Bear, U., Z. M. Thayer, C. D. Croy, C. E. Kaufman, and S. M. Manson. 2019. The impact of individual and parental American Indian boarding school attendance on chronic physical health of Northern Plains Tribes. *Family & Community Health* 42(1):1–7.

Sai, K. 2018. *The Illegal Overthrow of the Hawaiian Kingdom Government.* https://www.nea.org/advocating-for-change/new-from-nea/illegal-overthrow-hawaiian-kingdom-government (accessed March 18, 2023).

Schilling, E. A., R. H. Aseltine, Jr., and S. Gore. 2007. Adverse childhood experiences and mental health in young adults: A longitudinal survey. *BMC Public Health* 7(30).

Schleimer, J. P., S. A. Buggs, C. D. McCort, V. A. Pear, A. D. Biasi, E. Tomsich, A. B. Shev, H. S. Laqueur, and G. J. Wintemute. 2022. Neighborhood racial and economic segregation and disparities in violence during the COVID-19 pandemic. *American Journal of Public Health* 112(1):144–153.

Sebastian, T., H. Love, S. Washington, A. Barr, I. Rahman, B. Paradis, A. M. Perry, and S. Cook. 2022. *A new community safety blueprint: How the federal government can address violence and harm through a public health approach.* Washington, DC: The Brookings Institution.

Siegel, M., R. Sherman, C. Li, and A. Knopov. 2019. The relationship between racial residential segregation and Black–White disparities in fatal police shootings at the city level, 2013–2017. *Journal of the National Medical Association* 111(6):580–587.

Siegler, A. 2021. *End Mandatory Minimums.* https://www.brennancenter.org/our-work/analysis-opinion/end-mandatory-minimums (accessed March 18, 2023).

Sims, J., R. Baird, M. J. Aboelata, and S. Mittermaier. 2023. Cultivating a healthier policy landscape: The Building Healthy Communities initiative. *Health Promotion Practice* 24(2):300–309.

Stemen, D. 2017. *Vera evidence brief: The prison paradox: More incarceration will not make us safer.* New York: Vera Institute of Justice.

Stern, A. M. 1999. Buildings, boundaries, and blood: Medicalization and nation-building on the U.S.–Mexico border, 1910–1930. *Hispanic American Historical Review* 79(1):41–81.

Stern, A. M. 2020. *Forced Sterilization Policies in the U.S. Targeted Minorities and Those with Disabilities—and Lasted into the 21st Century.* https://ihpi.umich.edu/news/forced-sterilization-policies-us-targeted-minorities-and-those-disabilities-and-lasted-21st (accessed March 18, 2023).

Taylor, L., and M. Jorgensen. 2022. *Landback policy briefs: Considerations for federal and state landback.* Cambridge, MA: Harvard Univeristy, Ash Center for Democratic Governance and Innovation.

Thompson, C. E. 2020. *Returning the Land.* https://grist.org/fix/justice/indigenous-landback-movement-can-it-help-climate/ (accessed June 6, 2023).

Thriving Together. n.d. *Belonging and Civic Muscle.* https://thriving.us/vital-conditions/belonging-civic-muscle/ (accessed June 7, 2023).

Townsley, J., U. M. Andres, and M. Nowlin. 2021. *The Lasting Impacts of Segregation and Redlining.* https://www.savi.org/2021/06/24/lasting-impacts-of-segregation/ (accessed March 18, 2023).

Tribal Budget Formulation Workgroup. 2022. *Advancing health equity through the federal trust responsibility: Full mandatory funding for the Indian health service and strengthening nation-to-nation relationships.* Washington, DC: National Indian Health Board.

U.S. Commission on Civil Rights. 2018. *Broken promises: Continuing federal funding shortfall for Native Americans.* Washington, DC: U.S. Commission on Civil Rights.

UCLA Center for Health Policy Research. n.d. *Building Healthy Communities.* https://health-policy.ucla.edu/chis/bhc/Pages/default.aspx (accessed June 8, 2023).

University of Chicago Crime Lab. 2018. *Preventing youth violence: An evaluation of Youth Guidance's Becoming a Man program*. Chicago, IL: University of Chicago Crime Lab.

University of Chicago Crime Lab. n.d. *"Becoming a Man"—Improving Decisions, Reducing Crime*. https://www.bhub.org/project/becoming-a-man-improving-decisions-reducing-crime/ (accessed March 18, 2023).

University of Hawai'i at Mānoa. n.d. *Imua, me ka hopo ole: Forward, Without Fear*. https://coe.hawaii.edu/territorial-history-of-schools/ (accessed March 18, 2023).

University of Wisconsin Population Health Institute. 2023. *County Health Rankings National Findings Report 2023: Cultivating civic infrastructure and participation for healthier communities*. Madison, WI: University of Wisconsin Population Health Institute.

Urban Indian Health Institute. 2018a. *Missing and murdered Indigenous women & girls: A snapshot of data from 71 urban cities in the United States*. Seattle, WA: Urban Indian Health Institute.

Urban Indian Health Institute. 2018b. *Our bodies, our stories*. Seattle, WA: Urban Indian Health Institute.

Urban Institute. 2023. *Criminal Justice Expenditures: Police, Corrections, and Courts*. https://www.urban.org/policy-centers/cross-center-initiatives/state-and-local-finance-initiative/state-and-local-backgrounders/criminal-justice-police-corrections-courts-expenditures (accessed March 18, 2023).

USDA (United States Department of Agriculture). 2021. *USDA Opens Signup for Clear30, Expands Pilot to Be Nationwide*. https://www.fsa.usda.gov/news-room/news-releases/2021/usda-opens-signup-for-clear30-expands-pilot-to-be-nationwide (accessed March 18, 2023).

VA (Department of Veterans Affairs). 2022. *Agent Orange Exposure and VA Disability Compensation*. https://www.va.gov/disability/eligibility/hazardous-materials-exposure/agent-orange/ (accessed March 14, 2023).

Villanova University. n.d. *The Equal Rights League and Voting Suffrage*. https://exhibits.library.villanova.edu/institute-colored-youth/community-moments/equal-rights-league-and-suffrage (accessed March 18, 2023).

Wailoo, K. 2018. Historical aspects of race and medicine: The case of J. Marion Sims. *Journal of the American Medical Association* 320(15):1529–1530.

Wall, L. L. 2006. The medical ethics of Dr. J. Marion Sims: A fresh look at the historical record. *Journal of Medical Ethics* 32(6):346–350.

Washington, H. A. 2006. The black stork: The eugenic control of African American reproduction. In *Medical apartheid: The dark history of medical experimentation on Black Americans from colonial times to the present*. New York, NY: Harlem Moon. Pp. 189–215.

Welburn, J. W., P. N. d. Lima, K. B. Kumar, O. A. Osoba, and J. Lamb. 2022. *Overcoming compound racial inequity: Policies and costs for closing the Black–White wealth gap*. Santa Monica, CA: RAND Corporation.

Wertheimer, J., and E. Hill. 2022. *The intersection of domestic violence, race/ethnicity, and sex*. New York, NY: NYC Mayor's Office to End Domestic and Gender-Based Violence.

Whitbeck, L. B., G. W. Adams, D. R. Hoyt, and X. Chen. 2004. Conceptualizing and measuring historical trauma among American Indian people. *American Journal of Community Psychology* 33(3–4):119–130.

The White House. 2022a. *Justice40*. https://www.whitehouse.gov/environmentaljustice/justice40/ (accessed March 7, 2023).

The White House. 2022b. *White House Releases First-of-a-Kind Indigenous Knowledge Guidance for Federal Agencies*. https://www.whitehouse.gov/ceq/news-updates/2022/12/01/white-house-releases-first-of-a-kind-indigenous-knowledge-guidance-for-federal-agencies/ (accessed March 18, 2023).

The White House OSTP and Council on Environmental Quality. 2022a. *Guidance for federal departments and agencies on Indigenous knowledge*. Washington, DC: Executive Office the President.

The White House OSTP and Council on Environmental Quality. 2022b. *Implementation of guidance for federal departments and agencies on Indigenous knowledge*. Washington, DC: Executive Office of the President.

WHO (World Health Organization). 2002. *World report on violence and health*. Geneva, Switzerland: World Health Organization.

Wildeman, C., and H. Lee. 2021. Women's health in the era of mass incarceration. *Annual Review of Sociology* 47(1):543–565.

Williams, M. T., A. M. Haeny, and S. C. Holmes. 2021. *Posttraumatic stress disorder and racial trauma*. White River Junction, VT: National Center for PTSD, Department of Veterans Affairs.

Wilmington Race Riot Commission. 2006. *1898 Wilmington Race Riot report*. Wilmington, NC: Office of Archives and History, North Carolina Department of Cultural Resources.

8

Roadmap to Racial, Ethnic, and Tribal Health Equity

INTRODUCTION

The charge for this committee was to identify how past and current *federal* policies (or features/components of federal policies) considered neutral or even created to promote health and well-being instead operate in ways that create, maintain, and amplify racial, ethnic, and tribal health inequities. Moreover, the committee worked to identify key features of past and current policies that have served to reduce inequities and consider other factors to inform the creation of future policies to not only further reduce and eliminate inequities but also create equity.

As illustrated in this report, policies in numerous domains can positively or negatively impact racial, ethnic, and tribal health equity. The committee provided examples in each chapter that highlight aspects of policies, or lack of a policy in a given area, that contribute to health inequities. Many recurring themes stood out in the committee's review of the available evidence; these themes are highlighted and discussed in Chapters 2–7 and include the following:

- A lack of prioritization of racial, ethnic, and tribal health equity in policy agenda setting;
- A lack of, inconsistent, and incorrect data, which undermines policy makers' and researchers' ability to fully understand the state of health inequities;
- Access and eligibility restrictions in federal policy that stifle the ability to further health equity or achieve equitable outcomes;

- Inequitable budgeting among federal programs;
- Implementation and governance issues, including federalism and how laws that could advance health equity are systematically undermined;
- A lack of enforcement of existing laws and policies;
- Inadequate community voice and expertise in federal policy making, including in policy creation and implementation;
- Inadequacy of a one-size-fits-all approach—different populations (whether that is based on race, ethnicity, ancestry, geography, sex/gender, or other intersections of identity) need different tools and resources;
- A lack of coordination among federal agencies to address the structural and social determinants of health (SDOH); and
- Insufficiency of federal regulatory change; funding, guidelines, incentives, enforcement, and data collection for evaluation and governmental capacity building are also needed.

Executive Order (EO) 13985 *Advancing Racial Equity and Support for Underserved Communities Through the Federal Government*[1] (see Chapter 1), underscores many of these crosscutting needs. As directed by the EO, in 2021 the Office of Management of Budget (OMB) conducted a study in partnership with the heads of federal agencies to identify methods to assess equity (OMB, 2021), with these overall findings:

- Finding 1: A broad range of assessment frameworks and data and measurement tools have been developed to assess equity, but equity assessment remains a nascent and evolving science and practice.
- Finding 2: Administrative burden exacerbates inequity.
- Finding 3: The federal government needs to expand opportunities for meaningful stakeholder engagement and adopt more accessible mechanisms for co-designing programs and services with underserved communities and customers.
- Finding 4: Advancing equity requires long-term change management and a dedicated strategy for sustainability.
- Finding 5: The scale of initiatives by the federal government creates an opportunity to advance equity by ensuring that resources are made available equitably though its core federal management functions including financial management and procurement.

OMB issued a request for information to seek input, and recommendations from a broad array of stakeholders in the public, private, advocacy, not-for-profit, and philanthropic sectors, including state, local, tribal, and

---

[1] Exec. Order No. 13985, 86 FR 7009 (Jan. 2021).

territorial entities, on available methods, approaches, and tools (Performance.gov, 2021). The input aligns with the opportunities and barriers identified by the committee in Chapters 2–7 (see Box 8-1 for summary of the comments).

The EO and public comments responding to OMB are major advancements in federal policy making focused on equity. However, EOs are political and so risk lack of sustainability through changing administrations.

In Chapters 1–7, the committee focused on both the upstream and downstream impacts of federal policies (including policies that have legacies of trauma, such as theft of land and displacement from ancestral lands; see Chapters 2 and 7). To be most effective, federal policies, programs, and services need to focus on the upstream, population-level preventive issues that might impact root causes, using a "whole-of-government," "whole person," and "whole community" approach that increases intentional planning and coordination among departments and agencies and across programs and services to better meet both the short- and long-term whole person/family/community needs in more comprehensive, integrated, and aligned ways. For example, the Supplemental Nutrition Assistance Program (SNAP) (see Chapter 3) seeks to mitigate food insecurity and is an essential program for doing so, but it does not address the root causes, such as lack of employment opportunities and access to fresh food. Another example is health insurance. Access is predominantly linked to employment and incentivized by the federal government through tax benefits, leaving hundreds of thousands of people who lack employer-provided insurance with limited public insurance options. Many of these individuals are unable to afford private coverage and ineligible for public options.

These employees are more likely to be racially and ethnically minoritized people in service and other industries, which are unlikely to offer health insurance benefits (small companies are not required to offer health insurance benefits). These populations have also been excluded from employment opportunities due to employment discrimination, immigration policies, and other factors (see Chapters 2 and 3). Furthermore, employment opportunities are dependent on educational opportunities, which are disproportionately less available to racial and ethnic populations that are minoritized (see Chapter 4). One reason for racial and ethnic disparities in educational opportunities is public elementary and secondary schools largely being financed by local property taxes (supplemented by federal and state funding), which depend on the value of the local housing stock. Due to the legacy of housing segregation (including redlining and the disproportionate impact of the 2007–2010 subprime mortgage crisis on minoritized and underserved people and communities) (Badger, 2013), these populations are more likely to live in areas with lower average property values, which results in lower property taxes to support public education (Rugh and Massey, 2010).

BOX 8-1
Summary of Comments Received by the Office of Management and Budget from Methods and Leading Practices for Advancing Equity and Support for Underserved Communities Through Government Request for Information

- Many agencies underestimate the **volume, variety, and significance of barriers** that individuals face when learning about and attempting to access public benefits and services. From assessing the usefulness of work requirements to strengthening outreach and improving coordination across agencies, stakeholders identified multiple opportunities to reduce burden and prioritize equitable access when looking at how programs are administered.
- There is a strong desire for a **"no-wrong door" or one-stop shop** approach to benefit program administration and streamlining/standardizing/modernizing application processes and offices to account for as many Federal programs as possible at once (increasing both experience and efficiency).
- Importance of **enhancing access to opportunities** by
  1. simplifying application processes and reporting requirements;
  2. reviewing and, as needed, revising grant scoring norms, rubrics, and processes to be more equitable;
  3. conducting targeted, culturally responsive outreach to underserved communities and smaller organizations; and
  4. coupling flexible grant funding programs with capacity-building activities and technical assistance from trusted and experienced intermediaries.
- **Make meaningful, long-term community engagement** a priority and recommend actions such as
  1. engaging community members, especially those with lived experience, from the very early stages of program discussion and design and in any decision-making processes;
  2. establishing advisory boards, task forces, and commissions that include (and compensate) representatives from underserved communities; and
  3. including participatory budgeting processes where feasible to ensure communities can indicate collectively how resources should be spent and directed.
- Stakeholders also encourage Federal agencies to **"meet people where they are at"** through steps such as
  1. taking on the responsibility to initiate and maintain contact;
  2. making whatever accommodations (technological, physical, and otherwise) are needed to facilitate community participation, especially from underserved communities;
  3. offering multiple, accessible avenues (including virtual) to provide public comment; and
  4. reaching out via organizations and partner agencies that are trusted in the community.

SOURCE: Excerpts from Performance.gov, 2021.

Conclusion 8-1: The widespread inequities in education, income, and other factors that impact health are the result of the disparate and harmful impact of trauma, laws, and policies at all levels of government, both past and present. Health inequities are prevalent, persistent, and preventable and federal policy is an important tool for correcting historical and contemporary harms.

On the path to eliminating health inequities, both short-term strategies (e.g., mitigation by getting people what they need now to thrive) and long-term structural and systems change strategies that address the root causes (e.g., employment and economic development) will be needed. Based on the committee's guiding principles laid out in Chapter 1, its review of federal policies across the SDOH in Chapters 2–7, the crosscutting issues identified, and its information gathering, the committee identified four action areas that include both short- and long-term strategies for improvement of federal policy making, using a panoramic view across the SDOH to improve these vital conditions for all:

1. Implement Sustained Coordination Among Federal Agencies
2. Prioritize, Value and Incorporate Community Voice in the Work of Government
3. Ensure Collection and Reporting of Data Are Representative and Accurate
4. Improve Federal Accountability, Enforcement, Tools, and Support Toward a Government That Advances Optimal Health for Everyone

The committee presents 13 recommendations organized by these four action areas. Some will not be budget neutral, but they will address many costly inefficiencies in current federal policies and programs.

RECOMMENDATIONS

Many of the policy shortcomings the committee identified at the institutional level could be addressed in the short term. Some of the structural-level needs will require broad societal-level change and long-term effort. Both levels of action are required to get on the path to eliminating—versus only mitigating—racial, ethnic, and tribal health inequities, which are tied to accumulated inequities over generations that need to be unwound to truly achieve health equity. National Academies reports have made relevant recommendations to improve federal policies to advance racial, ethnic, and tribal health equity that have not yet been implemented and should also be considered (see, for example, Boxes 3-1, 4-2, 5-9, 6-2, 7-5). The broad

Statement of Task for this report created the opportunity to consider recommendations to address systems affecting the breadth of federal policy contributing to racial, ethnic, and tribal health inequities.

Action 1: Implement Sustained Coordination Among Federal Agencies

The federal policy landscape is complex, with 15 executive-level departments, over 100 agencies, and the legislative and judiciary branches. The policies of many of these agencies affect health, even if health is not their main purview and they focus, for example, on housing, transportation, or homeland security. Coordination among federal agencies is critical to advance health equity. It is encouraging that some collaborations are underway, such as the Federal Plan for Equitable Long-Term Recovery and Resilience (ELTRR) (ELTRR Interagency Workgroup, 2022), a major interagency effort that has transcended administrations (see Chapter 1 for more information).

The importance of a whole-of-government approach to advance equity is central to EO 13985. Similar to a Health in All Policies Approach (see Chapter 1), the committee recommends a parallel "whole person" and "whole community" approach. Just as health equity is not only about health care access and quality—as laid out in this report—it is the responsibility of not only the Department of Health and Human Services (HHS) but multiple departments, such as the Departments of Housing and Urban Development, Education, Transportation, Commerce, and Agriculture, all of which impact individual health and well-being. Therefore, achieving racial, ethnic, and tribal health equity requires centering equity in federal policy creation, decision making, implementation, and regulation (including accountability standards) and a sustained effort to ensure equity in agency processes and outcomes.

The recent release of the Federal Plan for ELTRR, led by the Office of Disease Prevention and Health Promotion within HHS, which lays out a whole-of-government approach to strengthen resilience and improve well-being in communities nationwide, provides an important framework for interagency coordination. The committee reviewed the plan's recommendations to amplify and add to strategies intended to eliminate racial and ethnic health inequities and improve well-being. As discussed in Chapter 7, the ELTRR plan includes 10 crosscutting recommendations to improve agency coordination and infrastructure and support better alignment and collaboration (ELTRR Interagency Workgroup, 2022).

However, as discussed by OMB, "experts note that changing systems and organizations is notoriously challenging—so much so that the work of sponsoring large-scale change is often referred to as a 'wicked problem.' The 'wickedness' of the challenge lies in the fact that problems often persist because of complex interdependencies, where solving one aspect of the problem reveals or creates new challenges. . . Systems change becomes feasible when a sense of urgency prevails and the status quo becomes untenable" (OMB, 2021, p. 35). In addition, federal programs can have different legal responsibilities, many of which cannot be easily coordinated around. The OMB report adds that equity specialists explain that the work typically involves complex, long-term change management and that this sustained attention is needed because many forms of "systemic bias flourish in practices that appear to be neutral on the surface" and that applying equity and justice to specific practices can mean different things to different people based on their lived experiences (OMB, 2021, p. 36). OMB notes that the implications of these divergent perspectives are significant, as agency stakeholders "may differ in their view of equity challenges across different agencies, just as stakeholders within government may not always agree on how to advance equity optimally. Thus, even when agencies subscribe to a common value—for example, of allocating resources fairly—different agency teams (or even different people on the same team) may have different ideas about how to make policies and procedures more equitable" (OMB, 2021, p. 36).

> **Recommendation 1: To improve health equity, the president of the United States should create a permanent and sustainable entity within the federal government that is charged with improving racial, ethnic, and tribal equity across the federal government. This should be a standing entity, sustained across administrations, with advisory, coordinating, and regulatory powers. The entity would work closely with other federal agencies to ensure equity in agency processes and outcomes.**

Multiple options exist to configure this entity, with advantages and disadvantages.

- Option 1: The president could establish a Racial, Ethnic, and Tribal Equity Council (RETC) by EO. It would be added to the president's executive office and similar to the recently created Gender Policy Council.[2] The RETC would need to be vested with the authority to ensure needed actions are undertaken by federal agencies to address equity. It would work in coordination with the other White House policy councils and across all federal offices and agencies to drive a strategic, whole-of-government approach to advance racial and ethnic equity. The RETC would include racial, ethnic, and tribal equity policy experts. Given the central

---

[2] See https://www.whitehouse.gov/wp-content/uploads/2021/10/National-Strategy-on-Gender -Equity-and-Equality.pdf (accessed March 9, 2023) for more information.

role of community involvement and engagement for racial, ethnic, and tribal equity, a Senior Advisor on Community Engagement could be created as part of this office. It is important to note that all presidential advisory bodies are subject to the authority of the president to continue, amend, or terminate. Strong partnerships with OMB in its oversight of agency performance in relationship to racial, ethnic, and tribal equity and with the Domestic Policy Council (DPC) in the crafting and implementation of policies can further solidify this role. Moreover, creating a new council would require a significant investment of resources. If established, the RETC would not replace the White House Council on Native American Affairs; and/or

- Option 2: The president could establish a Racial, Ethnic, and Tribal Equity Policy Team within the DPC. The DPC comprises numerous policy teams and offices that work to implement the president's domestic policy priorities. This team would align with the role of the DPC, and start-up costs would be lower compared to creating a council (see Option 1), but this is also subject to the priorities of the president in office; and/or

- Option 3: The president could appoint a senior staff member to OMB with the responsibility of overseeing implementing the president's vision for racial, ethnic and tribal equity across the executive branch. OMB is already involved in this process, so this position would be a natural extension of its work on equity oversight and coordination.

This recommendation builds upon EO 13985, which created task forces and working groups related to these efforts that are synergistic with this recommendation (e.g., Interagency Working Group on Equitable Data) and would work in collaboration with this council (similar to what is being done for the Gender Policy Council). The entity developed would work with all federal agencies with attention to all SDOH.

Research of organizational effectiveness in improving equity outcomes suggests that structures that embed accountability, authority, and expertise are essential to reduce/eliminate inequities across race, ethnicity, gender, and other demographic characteristics (Kalev et al., 2006). Moreover, a growing body of research and research expertise exists on measuring equity, designing and implementing more equitable policies and evaluating their impact, and holding institutions accountable for achieving equity goals. As efforts to advance coordination and accountability are implemented, those leading this work can draw from this research and practice capacity. This recommendation reflects the accountability, authority, and expertise required to achieve equity based on the research evidence.

A cost analysis was beyond the scope of the committee's work, but the committee notes that the monetary cost to implement this recommendation would vary by option.

Leadership for the Equitable Long-Term Recovery and Resilience Plan

A major component of the ELTRR Plan is establishing an executive steering committee to guide and compel coordination across federal agencies at multiple levels. After final consensus on the plan from agencies involved in its drafting, the committee will be established and provide guidance for implementing recommendations, agency commitment, actionable steps, and milestones. Executive steering committee "decisive leadership is required to compel coordination, within and across federal departments and subordinate agencies, in service of policies and programs that strengthen what works well and re-engineer what no longer serves" (ELTRR Interagency Workgroup, 2022, p. 35). The ELTRR Plan notes that the committee will be composed of senior executive leaders from a significant number of departments and agencies and will set a vision of the role of the federal government in building community and individual resilience and guide implementation of the plan. The Assistant Secretary for Health and one non-HHS agency lead (to be determined) will serve as committee cochairs. The initial committee charge is the following:

- Deliberate on the plan's recommendations,
- Prioritize strategies for implementation,
- Delegate actions to respective agencies,
- Assess the progress and identify opportunities to go further or redirect, and
- Formally charge and empower the ELTRR Interagency Workgroup with implementation support and monitoring (ELTRR Interagency Workgroup, 2022).

The committee affirms the crucial role of the executive steering committee:

Recommendation 2: The president of the United States should appoint a senior leader within the Office of Management and Budget (OMB) who can mobilize assets within OMB to serve as the cochair of the Equitable Long-Term Recovery and Resilience Steering Committee.

This configuration is ideal because, unlike HHS, OMB has the capacity and authority to oversee implementing ELTRR across the executive branch (i.e., executive departments and agencies), including oversight of agency performance. Moreover, given that the plan has a 10-year horizon,

OMB is made up mainly of career-appointed staff who provide continuity across changes of party and administration to ensure plan implementation is sustainable. An OMB-led committee also better reflects the interagency nature of the ELTRR Plan.

Equity Audit and Scorecard

"As policies and budgets are designed and policy alternatives are debated" for racial, ethnic, and tribal equity, policy makers should consider the "potential to remediate or exacerbate inequitable outcomes and design policies and budgets accordingly" (Ashley et al., 2022, p. 5). However, as discussed in a recent Urban Institute and PolicyLink report, data are needed during policy making for Congress to better prioritize racial, ethnic, and tribal equity and improve the design and budgets of proposed policies (Ashley et al., 2022). Congressional Budget Office (CBO) analysts are not required to score legislation for its effect on racial, ethnic, or tribal equity, "though CBO is starting to present analyses disaggregated by race and ethnicity. CBO recently noted that showing income, taxes, and transfers by race is sometimes not possible because of limited data disaggregated by race or privacy concerns regarding whether race and ethnicity data can be matched to common administrative data sources" (Ashley et al., 2022 p. 5). Policies are often adopted that unintentionally contribute to unfair outcomes related to the SDOH—sufficient data and analysis are needed to understand the different effects of policies across racial, ethnic, and tribal groups (Ashley et al., 2022).

> Recommendation 3: The federal government should assess if federal policies address or exacerbate health inequities by implementing an equity audit and developing an equity scorecard. Specifically,
>
> a. Federal agencies should engage in a retrospective review of federal policies that had a historical impact on racial and ethnic health inequities that exist today to address contemporary impacts.
>
> b. The Office of Management and Budget should develop, and federal agencies should conduct, an equity audit of existing federal laws. The federal laws reviewed should be identified via public input obtained by a variety of means. The equity audit should include a review of how the laws are implemented and enforced by federal agencies and state and local governments. The audit should also include criteria related to equity in process, measurement, and outcomes.
>
> c. Congress should develop and implement an equity scorecard that is applied to all proposed federal legislation, similar to the requirement of a Congressional Budget Office score.

> d. The process and results from the equity audit and scorecard should be transparent and made publicly available.

Implementing this recommendation will help ensure the equitable and effective distribution of resources across the SDOH, including for the policies and programs discussed in Chapters 3–7. If a health equity coordination entity is created per Recommendation 1, it could oversee and coordinate this process; however, such an entity is not required to implement this recommendation.

The equity audit of existing federal policies in Recommendation 3b would build on the work currently underway by federal agencies under EO 13985, updated by EO 14091,[3] that directs each federal agency to develop health equity teams to implement its equity initiatives. Given the numerous federal policies and programs, a mechanism will need to be developed to identify which should be prioritized and reviewed for Recommendations 3a and 3b, but it could include factors such as programs with known barriers to enrollment or access or that have shown inequitable outcomes in the past. This should be done with broad public input. In addition, when an existing policy is reviewed for other reasons,[4] an equity audit can be conducted simultaneously. The coordination entity from Recommendation 1 could undertake this role. Another important factor is how accountability will be applied after these audits are conducted. For example, if a policy does not meet the equity criteria used, a plan should be developed and put in place to ensure needed changes are enacted (or, when appropriate, the policy may need to be stopped if causing harm or rethought through new legislation). Similarly, if lack of enforcement is identified as contributing to racial, ethnic, or tribal health inequity, a plan to address this would be needed. For example, federal agencies have a critical role to play in enforcing civil rights protections (especially under Title VI of the Civil Rights Act of 1964).[5]

Elements for consideration to develop measures for the equity audit reflect concerns identified in this report on structure, process, and outcomes: does the structure of the policy exclude groups that would benefit and are disproportionately minoritized (such as immigrants or people with disabilities); does the process streamline administration to avoid additional barriers for minoritized groups; has community voice and expertise been included to improve the program; and are final outcomes assessed with appropriate

---

[3] Exec. Order No. 14091, 88 FR 10825 (Feb. 2023).

[4] For example, the Presidential memorandum in 2021 directing Department of Housing and Urban Development to review discriminatory housing practices and policies (The White House, 2021b).

[5] Title VI Statute, 42 U.S.C §§ 2000d - 2000d-7.

data for accountability to achieve program goals equitably across racial, ethnic, and tribal groups?

The Urban Institute notes that "equity measurement is multifaceted and cannot be reduced to a single construct" and a multifaceted approach is needed (Martin and Lewis, 2019, p. 3). Martin and Lewis (2019) identified six main components that could be taken into consideration for the equity audit: (1) historical legacies (e.g., implications of how past inequities might impact effectiveness of a law); (2) awareness of populations (e.g., procedural fairness and equal protections); (3) inclusion of other voices; (4) access discrimination (e.g., access is available equally, including removal of any financial, perceptual, or behavioral barriers that different groups may face); (5) output differences (e.g., a process assures that services and benefits are either delivered consistently or enhanced for underserved populations); and (6) disparate impacts (e.g., quantifying the potential outcomes in different populations while controlling for other contributing factors, such as the SDOH).

Developing a scorecard to assess future proposed legislation (Recommendation 3c) will provide a guardrail yet still offer flexibility. It is beyond the expertise of the committee to prescribe how the equity audit is undertaken, but considerations for this process include who is best placed to conduct the audits—for example, the Government Accountability Office, researchers, a newly appointed government standing committee, or perhaps a combination of governmental and nongovernmental actors.

Legislation is the "bare bones" of a policy or program, and implementation through regulations and adjustments in the field to address unanticipated complications determine its implementation. Therefore, even if an equity score is implemented for proposed legislation, an equity audit would still be required once the program or policy has been fully implemented.

Although there is no existing or ready to use method for determining or rating equity in this manner, sources are available to inform the development of the equity audit and scorecard (for example, see Ashley et al., 2022; Martin and Lewis, 2019; MITRE, n.d.; OMB, 2021; Urban Institute, n.d.)—for example, OMB identified several tools in its 2021 review (OMB, 2021), and the Urban Institute and PolicyLink *Scoring Federal Legislation for Equity* report also provides strong elements that should be considered (Ashley et al., 2022) (see Box 8-2 for components of equity scores). The report also poses questions for consideration for an equity scorecard that would apply here that would assess whether the proposed law centers equity in its design and intent:

- Does the proposed policy specify eligibility, access, and experiences and aim to overcome current inequities? If the policy is not implemented as intended, could this lead to inequitable outcomes?
- Will the policy close gaps in access and reduce disparities in outcomes across groups, and does it increase access to opportunity for all?

BOX 8-2
Components of Equity Scores

Design versus outcomes: Equity scores focus on outcomes. Equity assessments can have a broader focus. They can consider outcomes but may also analyze justice, fairness, and other aspects of policy or program design. Assessments may consider historical evidence and other research on known constraints, systemic barriers, and outcomes from similar efforts, among other factors.

Measured outcomes: Some equity issues can be analyzed with precise, quantitative measures. Others may be best done as descriptive analysis. Equity scores sit at the quantitative end of this spectrum. Equity scores will likely include quantitative measures that contextualize how potential policies affect subgroups of interest and for the population as whole.

Policy processes: Equity assessments can be performed in many contexts, including research, advocacy, and policy development. One particularly important context is the use of analytic information in formal policy making. Examples include the use of budget estimates in the congressional budget process and benefit-cost analyses in developing and reviewing regulations. Lawmakers could decide to include equity outcome measures in official policy processes. If so, analyses that estimate effects or measure outcomes would be called equity scores.

SOURCE: Excerpt from Ashley et al., 2022.

Various mechanisms can be used for the scorecard and could vary based on available data, evidence, and process. For example, point estimates could be used when data are available, or quantitative measures could be used to provide more context for lawmakers (Ashley et al., 2022).

An equity score needs to be provided early enough in the legislative process for members of Congress to have time to consider its implications (Ashley et al., 2022). "In the case of budget scoring, for example, CBO is required by law to provide cost estimates on legislation that is reported by full committee, which allows more informed consideration of budget issues in advance of action by the full House or Senate" (Ashley et al., 2022).[6] In some cases, CBO provides informal advice on the proposed legislation throughout the process to members of Congress on the budgetary impact of alternatives that are suggested during the legislative process (Ashley et al., 2022). Improved data collection would allow an equity scorecard to better assess the impact of legislative proposals (see Recommendations 5–9).

---

[6]For more information, see https://www.cbo.gov/about/processes (accessed May 26, 2023).

Although the equity audit of existing policies could be implemented in the short term, the equity scorecard for proposed legislation will likely be a long-term effort, as it faces several barriers to implementation. One aspect that should be considered while developing the scorecard is the potential to slow down legislation—however, investing the time to assess equity impacts will make legislation stronger. As noted, a framework and metrics to assess legislation specifically on equity would need to be developed, which could take considerable time, as stakeholders would have to agree on the questions and measures. Having the correct metrics in place will be critical to the success of the scorecard and assuring adequate vetting of proposed legislation. In addition, federal resources and employee staff time would be required. However, given the large impact that federal policies can have as documented in this report—to both advance and hinder racial, ethnic, and tribal equity—it is imperative to assure that future legislation is vetted and then audited once implemented. Structural changes are needed to move from mitigating to eliminating health inequities.

Proposals for an equity scorecard or similar have been introduced by legislators, and CBO occasionally does assess the equity impact of legislative proposals (Ashley et al., 2022). As noted in the 2022 Urban Institute and PolicyLink report, certain legislative proposals would require CBO to take steps toward developing equity scores for new proposals. For example, H.R. 2078 (2021), among other actions, would require CBO to provide an analysis of the equity impact of a bill or resolution in each of the first 4 years that it would be effective; and the CBO FAIR Scoring Act (S. 2723 and H.R. 5018, 2021) would require CBO ". . .estimate the distributional impacts by race and income—in dollar terms and as a percent change in after-tax-and-transfer-income—for bills that have a gross budgetary effect of at least 0.1 percent of GDP in any fiscal year within the 10-year budget window" and ". . .provide such scores to relevant congressional committees before the bills are reported to the floor, to the extent possible)" (Ashley et al., 2022 p. 22).

Summary

The committee offers recommendations for sustained coordination and accountability:

- Create a permanent and sustainable entity within the federal government that is charged with improving racial, ethnic, and tribal equity across the federal government (Recommendation 1).
- Appoint a senior leader of OMB to serve as the cochair of the Equitable Long-Term Recovery Plan (Recommendation 2).

- Undertake a equity analysis of existing and past policies (Recommendation 3).
- Develop and implement an equity audit and an equity scorecard to assess federal policies and identify needed changes (Recommendation 3).

Implementing Recommendations 1–3 would signal that racial, ethnic, and tribal equity is a national priority and advance equity in domestic policy development, implementation (including accountability standards), and evaluation (of current federal policies) across domains including health, economic security, the criminal legal system, and education.

Action 2: Prioritize, Value, and Incorporate Community Voice in the Work of Government

It is essential to base federal policy for all SDOH on the best available evidence—this includes communities' experiences, knowledge/expertise, and needs (Farrell et al., 2021). The reasons to value, prioritize, and incorporate community voice in the work of government are ethical, practical, and related to accountability and achieving intended outcomes.

Affected communities need to be an integral part of the legislative process from beginning to end and in deciding how laws, regulations, programs, and policies are administered. Racial, ethnic, and tribal communities have been consistently left out of the federal policy-making process, and the effects have sometimes been egregiously inequitable. The voices of communities are needed to redress past harms and earn trust (ethical imperative), secure partnership, buy-in, and collaboration (practical imperative), and ensure policies are fully responsive to their needs and advance health equity (accountability and effectiveness).

Studying the relationship between engaging communities in policy making that will affect them and the resulting policy outcomes (e.g., the relationship between community-engaged interventions and health outcomes) involves navigating complex human and social systems and extensive mixed methods research, including of subjective and hard-to-measure factors. Over the past decade, study of these relationships has begun to yield evidence of positive effects. For example, a systematic review by Haldane and colleagues (2019) concluded there was "promising evidence that community engagement has a positive impact on health, especially when supported by a strong organizational and community foundation." An earlier meta-analysis found that "public health interventions using community engagement strategies for disadvantaged groups are effective in terms of health behaviours, health consequences, health behaviour self-efficacy, and perceived social support. . . . There are also indications from a small number of studies that community engagement interventions can improve outcomes for the community" (O'Mara-Eves et al., 2015).

Many examples, especially from recent history, illustrate the need for trusted community representatives to inform, codesign, and often assist with implementing federal programs and priorities. This is especially true for leaders or organizations representing minoritized racial, ethnic, and tribal communities. For example, in early 2020, greater investment in community advisory groups, including regional Census 2020 Complete Count Committees, could have helped avoid many of the racial disparities that arose with the speedy rollout of COVID-19 vaccines in early 2021 (Schoch-Spana et al., 2021). Similarly, the disbursement of hundreds of billions of dollars from the American Rescue Plan, designed to help communities recover from the health and economic consequences of the pandemic, relied on the decisions of elected representative institutions. In many instances, however, racial, ethnic, tribal, communities had little opportunity to inform or influence the disbursement of these funds (CPEHN, 2022).

The importance of working with communities and centering their voices and knowledge is discussed throughout this report. It includes extensive discussion of data issues (e.g., data sovereignty for Tribal Nations) and data collection, and examples of advocacy that achieved changes in federal policy. Although the examples of organized advocacy for policy change are compelling, integrating community voice in the federal policy-making process more expansively would imply more proactive engagement, rather than reactive and slow response to community needs and requests.

Chapter 4 outlines several channels for involving communities in federal education policy, by supporting states and local school districts and communities with resources and guidance to work together to improve educational achievement and health. The federal government has provided resources for community schools, and national-level efforts have identified "four core pillars of work that drive improved student outcomes" (Task Force on Next Generation Community Schools, 2021): after-school, summer, and other curriculum-enriching programming; active engagement of families and community members; collaborative and coordinated community school services and leadership; and support of students through integrated, holistic services (e.g., ranging from mental health care to housing) provided by strategic community partnerships (Task Force on Next Generation Community Schools, 2021).

Engaging community voice in federal policies that shape health care (see Chapter 5) is challenging, but existing models do work, and recent developments are promising. Federally qualified health centers are required to have at least 51 percent of their boards include center patients and be demographically representative of the communities they serve. Recent efforts to ensure representation on clinical trials are part of a broader attention to the issue of mistrust in the biomedical establishment and the recognition that community participation and engagement in health care are essential.

In Chapter 6, the committee provided the example of advocacy organizations whose efforts decades ago yielded the "socially disadvantaged farmer and rancher" designation in the 1990 Farm Bill, to inform targeting of specific Department of Agriculture programs (e.g., guaranteed loans, assistance under the American Rescue Plan) to racially and ethnically minoritized farmers.

The discussion of social and community context in Chapter 7 includes two major promising frameworks for community engagement. The OMB report on assessing equity outlined how key strategies across all domains of federal work would center community needs, expertise, and voice (on issues ranging from data collection to communication to codesign of programs and services) (OMB, 2021). The federal ELTRR Plan uses the Seven Vital Conditions Framework (which was first introduced in the 2021 Surgeon General's Report *Community Health and Economic Prosperity* [HHS, 2021]). It centers "belonging and civic muscle"—a term of art describing the range of community and civic engagement activities and opportunities (for example, see Box 7-1 [One Million Experiments, n.d.]).

A promising strategy to improve policies that do not promote health equity is to elevate and empower community voice and expertise to influence outcomes through the following design principles:

1. Prioritize meaningful community input by moving from the level of inform toward the more substantive levels of consult, involve, collaborate, and empower in the International Association for Public Participation Framework whenever possible (IAP2, 2018);
2. Ensure effectiveness, efficiency, and equity in the way that community input is collected;
3. Maximize coordination and sharing of information and insights on implementation across federal agencies while maintaining data privacy and client confidentiality; and
4. Within each federal agency, maximize coordinating and sharing information and insights on implementation among federal, state, local, and tribal government counterparts.

While there are many technical and scientific advisory bodies at federal departments and agencies, few recognize the unique perspectives of communities—including the recipients and beneficiaries of federal programs and services—as the "expertise" and (lived) experience as essential for designing, implementing, and evaluating those programs and services.

Recommendation 4: The federal government should prioritize community input and expertise when changing or developing federal policies to advance health equity. Specifically,

1. The president of the United States should require federal agencies relevant to the social determinants of health to generate and sustain community representation and advisory practices that are integrated with accountability measures and enforcement mechanisms.

2. Congress should request a Government Accountability Office report to document across federal agencies whose work impacts the social determinants of health, as well as federal statistical agencies, that

   a. Assesses how community advisory boards are positioned within their agencies, whom they are composed of, how often they meet, how they report back, and how that work influences the agencies' policies and programs; and

   b. Identifies promising and evidenced-based practices, gaps, and opportunities for community advisory boards that could be applied by other agencies.

Several mechanisms for community input at the federal level exist to learn from, improve, and/or implement more broadly—for example, community engagement associated with the decennial census, the White House Initiative on Asian Americans and Pacific Islanders Regional Interagency Working Group, and Tribal Consultation and Urban Confer (see Chapter 7).

Action 3: Ensure Collection and Reporting of Data Are Representative and Accurate

To advance health equity, data need to better capture the experiences and needs of tribal and smaller racial and ethnic groups. As discussed in Chapter 2, lacking representation in data collection and inaccurate or imprecise reporting have meant that government agencies have been unprepared to understand, let alone reduce or eliminate, health inequities. It is essential to collect and use high-quality data to understand the full extent of inequities and appropriately distribute resources. Federal government data collections have, at times, occurred without accountability or consideration of their effects and demands on communities (e.g., time and other resources), matters of tribal sovereignty, and community interest in the use of the data. Below, the committee provides four recommendations to improve federal data sources to advance health equity.

These are not the only recommendations on this topic. Numerous reports outline data gaps, needs, and priorities related to racial, ethnic, and tribal health inequities (for example, see AAPI Data and National Council of Asian Pacific Americans, 2022; Bhakta, 2022; Kauh et al., 2021; Moy et al., 2005; NRC, 2004; RWJF, 2022; Yom and Lor, 2022). The committee builds on existing recommendations and tailors them specifically to data needs and actions related to federal policy making and decision making and for use by communities and other advocates to advance racial, ethnic, and tribal health equity.

Data Equity for Small Minimum Reporting OMB Categories

Sample sizes in national surveys are often too small to obtain reliable nationally representative estimates required to monitor issues of health equity for all the minimum reporting OMB categories of race and ethnicity.[7] The issues are more pronounced the smaller the category and/or survey. For the current minimum reporting OMB race and ethnicity categories, the 2020 Census counts 1.6 million Native Hawaiian and Pacific Islander (NHPI), 9.7 million American Indians and Alaska Native (AIAN), 21 million Asian, 38 Black or African American, 62 million Hispanic/Latino/a, and 204 million White people. The omission of high-quality and accurate nationally representative data for these minimum reporting OMB categories perpetuates inequities and promotes inaction—particularly when these groups are invisible in federal datasets.

For example, studies from both the California Health Interview Survey, which has included oversamples of Asian detailed-origin groups that are lacking in the National Health Interview Survey (NHIS), and the representative NHPI NHIS found significant Asian and NHPI differences in rates of chronic diseases, disease comorbidity, disability, and self-reported physical health (Adia et al., 2020; Galinsky et al., 2017, 2019; Zelaya et al., 2017). The data currently collected on these smaller minimum OMB categories are often biased due to incomplete representation, poorly designed sampling frames, inadequate collection approaches, language barriers (including failure to administer instruments in the person's primary language), and culturally inappropriate question design. Despite recognition that health outcomes are generally worse for these populations, the lack of representative data makes it impossible to understand the full extent of inequities and where to focus interventions. A federal and federal tribal-consulted data system is needed that is intentionally committed to support data equity, particularly for the smallest minimum OMB categories. The statements in this paragraph are also true for detailed-origin categories within OMB

---

[7]OMB requires five minimum reporting categories: American Indian or Alaska Native, Asian, Native Hawaiian or Other Pacific Islander, Black or African American, and White, and an ethnicity category of Hispanic or Latino (OMB, 1997).

minimum categories—the committee addresses issues specific to detailed-origin categories in the subsequent recommendation.

> **Recommendation 5:** The Office of Management and Budget (OMB) should require the Census Bureau to facilitate and support the design of sampling frames, methods, measurement, collection, and dissemination of equitable data resources on minimum OMB categories—including for American Indian or Alaska Native, Asian, Black or African American, Hispanic or Latino/a, and Native Hawaiian or Pacific Islander populations—across federal statistical agencies. The highest priority should be given to the smallest OMB categories—American Indian or Alaska Native and Native Hawaiian or Pacific Islander.

Detailed-Origin Categories and Data Disaggregation

Each OMB minimum reporting category has important differences based on origin and/or tribe. The need to collect and disseminate data at this level of disaggregation has been discussed for decades. Unfortunately, all federal agencies have not undertaken a concerted effort to address it. Recently, the Census Bureau has made positive strides, and many expert panels and committees have provided recommendations regarding how to disaggregate data and accomplish this goal (see Chapter 2). This need is recognized across multiple racial, ethnic, and tribal populations, and especially American Indian or Alaska Native, Asian, Black or African American, and Native Hawaiian or Pacific Islander detailed-origin groups.

Countless examples exist of the value of deeper disaggregation. In one, the Census Bureau, in collaboration with the National Center for Health Statistics, employed the American Community Survey (ACS) sampling frame to identify a representative sample of NHPI households for the 2014 NHPI NHIS. It found significant racial differences between NHPI and other racial groups and detailed-origin differences within the NHPI population on outcomes ranging from serious psychological distress to asthma, cancer, and diabetes (Galinsky et al., 2017, 2019).

Meaningful Tribal Consultation and Urban Confer (IHS, n.d.) will be needed when developing methods, surveys, and equity assessments to produce accurate and meaningful estimates for disaggregated tribal populations. These methods could be expanded to other OMB minimum categories, such as Asian, Black or African American, Native Hawaiian or Pacific Islander, and Latino/a, for greater granularity, particularly at the subnational level, including states and counties that help administer federal programs.

Disaggregating racial and ethnic minimum category data takes many forms. It is not only by origin and/or tribe; these communities contain many important intersecting identities, including lesbian, gay, bisexual, transgender, queer (or questioning), and other sexual identities people, people of varying immigrant statuses, people with disabilities, women, and children.

To enhance data systems to produce accurate and meaningful estimates of disaggregated data for all minimum OMB categories, the committee recommends:

> **Recommendation 6: The Office of Management and Budget (OMB) should update and ensure equitable collection and reporting of detailed-origin and tribal affiliation data for all minimum OMB categories through data disaggregation by race, ethnicity, and tribal affiliation (to be done in coordination with meaningful tribal consultation), including populations who self-identify as American Indian or Alaska Native, Asian, Black or African American, Hispanic or Latino/a, and Native Hawaiian or Pacific Islander.**

Implementing this recommendation will increase racial, ethnic, and tribal health equity through the uniform use of detailed-origin and tribal affiliation data to be collected, analyzed, and disseminated for all groups. This data should also be accessible to the affected communities. Important considerations for this recommendation include the following:

- It may be difficult to share results for some groups because the small samples may create large margins of error or privacy concerns. Disseminating data by detailed origin should be done to the maximum extent possible, weighing the benefits of doing so against the risk of privacy violations for individuals and households. Disseminating point estimates by population group should include margins of error at the 95 percent confidence interval, with no predetermined cutoff on sample size as long as data privacy concerns are addressed.

- To the fullest extent possible, checkboxes should be provided on detailed origin and federal- and state-recognized tribes rather than write-in boxes for Black or African American and AIAN populations (OMB is considering this).[8] Evidence from the Census Bureau's 2010 Alternative Questionnaire Experiment indicated a reduction in detailed-origin identification among some Asian groups when the write-in format was provided in lieu of checkboxes (Compton et al., 2013). Agencies should provide as many checkboxes as possible for detailed-origin groups, and electronic

---

[8] See https://www.federalregister.gov/documents/2023/01/27/2023-01635/initial-proposals-for-updating-ombs-race-and-ethnicity-statistical-standards (accessed March 11, 2023).

data collection could include more checkbox categories than might be permissible in paper forms that comply with the Paperwork Reduction Act. From an equity perspective, having checkboxes for some but not all categories can lead to disparate results because of the greater likelihood of coding errors and higher burdens posed by write-in responses.

- Expanding sampling frames to generate accurate statistical information on detailed-origin groups (such as Chinese, Haitian, Hmong, Chamorro, Native Hawaiian, Nigerian, Samoan, Tongan, and Vietnamese people) where prior evidence—such as findings on health inequities by race and detailed origin from scientific publications, and on housing and socioeconomic inequities from federal data sources, such as the ACS—justify producing statistically reliable estimates of the population at varying levels of geography. Decisions to expand sampling frames to detailed-origin populations need to weigh the balance of factors, such as the size of the population, the magnitude of the disparity based on scientific research, and the cost and feasibility of producing such samples.

- Decisions on allocating agency staff and financial resources to collect, analyze, and disseminate detailed-origin data need consideration with a view toward equity and the program coverage and effectiveness implications of providing such data. For example, distinguishing between self-identified German-origin versus Welsh-origin respondents is less likely to be a significant concern for racial equity with respect to service delivery or population-based outcomes. By contrast, groups identifying as Middle East and North African, Cambodian, Laotian, African American, Haitian, Dominican, Nigerian, Tongan, Marshallese, Samoan Navajo, and Cherokee have varying language access needs and significant historical and contemporary patterns of inequitable service delivery and so require disaggregated data to inform policy decisions.

As described in Chapter 2, in January 2023, OMB released a Federal Register notice with proposed changes to data collection on race and ethnicity (OMB, 2023). Several of these proposed changes are in line with the committee's recommendation, such as requiring federal agencies to collect detailed race and origin data by default unless they determine that the benefit of doing so would not justify the additional burden or risks to privacy. However, the proposal has several shortcomings. For example, the categories set forth are sociopolitical constructs and not an attempt to define race and ethnicity biologically or genetically. The examples of Indo-Fijians counted toward NHPI and Indo-Caribbean counted toward Black reflect the problem faced in bridging identity and achieving comparable data by race or ethnicity. In addition, "minority" and "majority" have been removed to reflect changing demographics in the United States. However, due to the sustained differences in health and other outcomes for the populations currently referred to as minorities, it is important to differentiate these populations. Populations who have been "racially and ethnically minoritized" or similar could be used to account for populations who may be the largest racial or ethnic group in a jurisdiction but nevertheless continue to face barriers and cumulative burdens based on race or ethnicity (such as Latino/a people in California). Furthermore, the AIAN population does not appear to have six checkboxes assigned to represent detailed categories as other racial and ethnic groups do—all detailed information is collected through write-in. Finally, removing "who maintain tribal affiliation or community attachment"[9] for the AIAN definition is problematic because not all AIAN people are enrolled members of federally recognized tribes (see Chapter 2), so this would lead to further undercounting this population, perpetuating inequities.

Measures of Social and Structural Inequities

Interpretations of racial and ethnic health inequities without proper social and environmental context may inadvertently emphasize individual-level biological and behavioral explanations of the inequities and risk blaming individuals and groups for poor health outcomes. Including measures of racialized social and structural inequities at multiple levels of influence in national health surveys and other federal health data sources can contextualize the data and promote the investigation of the effects of social and structural factors on these inequities. For example, Chapter 2 points out that national health surveys and other federal administrative and surveillance data sources will have greater potential for informing the development of interventions that address the root causes of racial, ethnic, and tribal health inequities in their proper social, economic, and historical context if such measures are collected.

Recommendation 7: The Centers for Disease Control and Prevention should coordinate the creation and facilitate the use of common measures on multilevel social determinants of racial and ethnic health inequities, including scientific measures of racism and other forms of discrimination, for use in analyses of national health surveys and by

---

[9] Those with community attachment are AIAN people who are not enrolled members of a federally recognized tribe. There are racial AIAN people whose tribes were never recognized, unrecognized (during termination era), or are state recognized; they may still identify as AIAN but are in a different legal category.

other federal agencies, academic researchers, and community groups in analyses examining health, social, and economic inequities among racial and ethnic groups.

Such measures should pertain to racism and other forms of discrimination and include:

- Social, economic, educational, political, and legal indicators of racial and ethnic inequities in a range of societal domains (e.g., employment, housing, health insurance, homeownership, incarceration) for diverse racially and ethnically minoritized groups; and
- Measures of interpersonal racism, individual-level experiences of structural racism, and sociocontextual measures of structural racism at the federal, state, county, local, and neighborhood levels (for examples of such measures see, Agénor et al., 2021; Greenfield et al., 2021; Krieger, 2020; Mesic et al., 2018; Williams, 2016).

These measures should also be usable at the state, county, and neighborhood levels and developed in partnership with academic researchers, community groups and members, and other key stakeholders (see Chapter 2 for additional discussion). Some of this work is already underway,[10] and the health equity coordinating entity from Recommendation 1 could facilitate these efforts.

There has been an increasing level of understanding of and attention to the SDOH within public insurance and healthcare programs, including Medicare, Medicaid, the Children's Health Insurance Program, veteran's healthcare, and federally qualified health centers. Measuring and addressing the SDOH in healthcare is important (NASEM, 2019). However, SDOH has been conflated with individual "social needs," including among people working within the health care system (Green and Zook, 2019). Public insurance and health care programs are increasing their ability to address individual patient social needs, which is a positive development (NASEM, 2019). However, the upstream drivers of the SDOH operate above and beyond individuals and cannot be addressed by merely attending to the resulting social and health needs downstream. The use of 1115 waivers, Medicaid payment reforms, accountable care organizations, and others (see Chapter 5 for more information) is important but does not fundamentally address the primary upstream drivers of socioeconomic and health inequities. Federal health care programs may not be the most effective governmental area to

---

[10] See, for example, https://hdpulse.nimhd.nih.gov/data-portal/home (accessed May 29, 2023).

address the fundamental causes of social, economic, environmental, housing, and health inequities.

Budget Needs

Oversampling and targeted data collection are admittedly costly. However, identifying health, socioeconomic, and environmental inequities that negatively affect outcomes for minoritized groups across the life span is essential for identifying solutions to achieve health equity goals. A classic example of this cost–benefit argument is seen in the prevalence of chronic noncommunicable diseases (NCDs) among AIAN, NHPI, and Southeast Asian populations. Avoiding many NCDs or minimizing their impacts can be achieved through screening, early diagnosis, and health interventions. Without reliable information on NCD clusters, interventions cannot be targeted, with consequences that include increased medical costs, increased emergency room visits, medication compliance, surgical interventions, and the costs of lifelong disability. High-quality, accurate, representative, and reliable data will ensure equitable access to health care and effective planning to address populations with special needs. Furthermore, as discussed in Chapter 2 and Recommendation 7, context on social factors when interpreting racial and ethnic health inequities is crucial to understand the multiple levels of influence that impact health-related outcomes (such as social, demographic, economic, educational, housing, environmental, political, and legal indicators).

> **Recommendation 8: Congress should increase funding for federal agencies responsible for data collection on social determinants of health measures to provide information that leads to a better understanding of the correlation between the social environment and individual health outcomes.**

These data will more accurately identify the specific needs of underserved populations and improve overall equity in health and socioeconomic outcomes by identifying where policy change or interventions are needed to inform government investments to advance health equity. In the immediate term, increased funding is especially needed for the following:

- The Census Bureau, the Centers for Disease Control and Prevention, and the National Center for Health Statistics to collect relevant, high-quality, accurate, nationally representative data to monitor the health and nutritional status of the total AIAN and NHPI populations and provide comparable statistics to larger

racial and ethnic populations according to the revised OMB minimum categories for data on race and ethnicity.
- A permanent budget for ACS. A continuous and national survey, it
  was introduced in 2010 to replace the long form[11] for the decennial
  census (which had important data on important social and economic factors) so that these critically important data could be more
  timely and useful. ACS is the most comprehensive, robust, and
  current source of information on social, economic, housing, and
  demographic data on large and small communities. Census-guided
  federal spending uses ACS data to inform spending on government services, other stakeholders also use it (e.g., businesses, local
  planners, and state/local officials). However, ACS has documented
  operational challenges (The Census Project, 2022) that have led
  to delays in data release[12] and reliability (partly due to declining
  response rates and therefore data stability and reliability). This is
  in part due to delayed investments (the budget has not increased
  in several years) to allow for innovation to improve response rates
  and modernization.

However, other funding will also be needed to improve data systems to
advance health equity. For example, funds need to be dedicated to conduct
a second iteration of the NHPI NHIS in 2024. It was introduced in 2014
and added a wealth of baseline data. Like NHIS, which is conducted annually to monitor the health of the U.S. population since 1957, follow-ups of
the NHPI NHIS would provide useful nationally representative evidence to
inform policy and intervention programs to address disparities. In addition,
inclusion of a robust sample of the NHPI population in the National Health
and Nutrition Examination Survey is vital to assessing their health and
nutritional status and biomedical health information, which is nonexistent.

Equitable Data Working Group

In April 2022, the Equitable Data Working Group (established under
EO 13985) developed a report with recommendations for improvements
in data equity, including the areas covered in Recommendations 5 and 6.
The report was delivered in April 2022 to the assistant to the president for
domestic policy and cochaired by senior leadership in OMB and the Office

---

[11] The long-form questionnaire includes the same six population questions and one housing
question that are on the Census 2000 short form, plus 26 additional population questions and
20 additional housing questions (Census Bureau, 2021b).

[12] Data quality challenges prevented the Census Bureau from releasing standard 2020 ACS
1-year estimates in 2021, and the 2016–2020 ACS 5-year estimates were delayed until March
2022 (Census Bureau, 2021a)

of Science and Technology Policy (OSTP) (Equitable Data Working Group, 2022). That report identified inadequacies in existing federal data collection programs, policies, and infrastructure across agencies (see Chapter 2 for more information). Since then, OSTP has also worked with federal interagency working groups to ensure timely and effective implementation of policies, programs, practices, and investments, to ensure progress on data equity. To ensure that this important work is enduring, the committee recommends:

> **Recommendation 9: The president of the United States should convert the Equitable Data Working Group, currently coordinated between the Office of Management and Budget (OMB) and the Office of Science and Technology Policy, into an Office of Data Equity under OMB with representation from the Domestic Policy Council, with an emphasis on small and underrepresented populations and with a scientific and community advisory commission, to achieve data equity in a manner that is coordinated across agencies and informed by scientific and community expertise.**

Although the Equitable Data Working Group has made significant progress in identifying data barriers to racial equity and solutions to overcome them, it is temporary by design. In addition, federal agency working groups do not typically have a scientific or community advisory commission to provide guidance. To make this work more enduring, and benefit from the guidance of scientific and community experts, the federal government should make interagency coordination on data equity a permanent feature across statistical agencies. By situating the Office of Data Equity under OMB, the federal government will be able to ensure cross-agency coordination and collaboration on data improvements that advance health equity in all federal agencies and policies.

Action 4: Improve Federal Accountability, Tools, and Support Toward a Government That Advances Optimal Health for Everyone

Although states and other levels of government need to tailor their health equity efforts to the needs of their populations, they need the federal-level tools and support to do so. Often, politics can stand in the way of or stall good policy, so processes and guardrails need to support state, local, tribal, and territorial needs. For example, guidance that has been vetted for health equity effects at the federal level needs to be in place to implement policies, access requirements, and set expectations. Accountability mechanisms and processes can play a vital role in driving progress for health equity and require engaging with multiple diverse actors using dynamic accountability processes. The committee provides recommendations related to federal accountability, tools, and support to advance optimal health for everyone. However, aspects of Recommendations 1–3 will also advance accountability and could work hand-in-hand with the recommendations provided here.

Program Implementation and Access

Chapters 3–7 pointed to numerous examples of barriers around implementation and access to federal programs that exacerbate inequities. Administrative burden—the challenges of accessing a public benefit (Burden et al., 2012)—is one example of an access barrier. This can include time spent on applications and paperwork and navigating systems, verifying eligibility, and navigating web interfaces. The 2021 OMB report notes that these administrative burdens do not fall equally on all individuals and groups, which leads to inequitable underuse of supportive services and programs for the populations most in need (Ashley et al., 2022). OMB pointed out that a fundamental "leading practice" that needs to be scaled government-wide is the "completion of administrative burden audits that can identify points resulting in drop-off, and in particular, increased drop-off among sub-groups" (OMB, 2021, p. 21). Another barrier is how programs are implemented; state implementation can vary, which can sometimes lead to people having access to different programs based on where they live. For example, this variation has occurred in Medicaid expansion (see Chapter 5) and participation in social benefits programs, such as SNAP (see Chapter 3).

> **Recommendation 10: Congress and executive agencies should leverage the full extent of federal authority to ensure equitable implementation of federal policies and access to federal programs.**
> a. Relevant federal departments and agencies should design and implement policies to improve the administration of assistance programs to facilitate access to the benefits to which individuals and families are entitled. Such activities should include implementation and delivery processes, including administrative burden, eligibility, enrollment, enforcement, and client experience; and, where applicable, the creation of performance standards in federal programs administered by other (state, local, and tribal) governments.
> b. Congress should ensure that sufficient funding is made available to conduct these activities.

Equitable implementation supports government efficiency and effectiveness and can improve outcomes for all and decrease inequities across populations. Implementation of this recommendation should take into account the unique challenges in rural areas and for Tribal Nations. Although implementation is not dependent on Recommendation 3, it could be one of the processes for that effort. The goal of this recommendation is to deliver federal programs and services to those who need it for all SDOH—where a person lives in the United States or its territories should not impact access. Inequitable access contributes to racial, ethnic, and tribal inequities. It is beyond the scope of this committee's work to recommend the specific action steps; however, it provides some of the many examples discussed in the report related to implementation and access in Chapters 3–7. This recommendation builds on work underway by federal agencies to identify mechanisms to reduce administrative burden for underserved communities (The White House, 2021a, 2023). To enable agencies to leverage the full extent of their authorities, additional funding may be needed—for example, for enforcement of civil rights protections.

When implementing this recommendation, federal agencies should consider effective approaches across sectors (e.g., housing, transportation, environment), as well as existing authority to enforce civil rights provisions that are not currently prioritized and enforced. For example, the Fair Housing Act requires that grantees take steps to affirmatively further fair housing. Equality directives, a civil rights regulation, are used in regulatory frameworks for federal transit funding and function "by placing positive duties on state actors to promote equality and inclusion" (Amri, 2017). This places the affirmative requirements on state and local grantees when using federal funds and uses "ex ante" regulatory power rather than "ex post" court enforcement (that is, equality directives use regulatory rather than judiciary power). Even without express statutory language establishing affirmative obligations, existing law offers underpinnings for an obligation to affirmatively further health equity. For example, antidiscrimination legislation (Title VI of the Civil Rights Act, ACA Section 1557, and the Americans with Disabilities Act) offers legal authority for a health-focused equality directive; legal and regulatory frameworks relating to tax exemption and the federal government's funding of Medicare and Medicaid are models for how such an equality directive might be implemented.

Streamlining eligibility criteria variation may be difficult given the "block" of funding by state and variation in need for nonentitlement programs (e.g., child care subsidies eligibility vary greatly due to different demand volume by state); however, the federal government could standardize the approach for eligibility criteria, conditions of participation related to administrative burden, and enrollment by streaming eligibility and enrollment processes with coordination across federal programs. This aligns with the health equity assessments and equity plans undertaken by EO 13985 and Finding 2 of an OMB report ("administrative burden exacerbates inequity") (OMB, 2021; The White House, n.d.). To address this recommendation and the goal of EO 13985 to "expand opportunities for meaningful stakeholder engagement," the federal government could require community-involved processes. One area to review is the Administrative Procedure Act[13] regarding public comment. This is more accessible to academics and interest groups with resources and less accessible to communities. The federal movement could also include incentives to states that include accessible, meaningful community involvement processes in laws and implementation.

Implementing this recommendation could also reduce participation churn in federal programs administered by states; in social benefits programs, such as SNAP and Medicaid, this is when otherwise eligible participants fail to recertify and are removed from the program, but subsequently reapply as a new case within a short period, such as in a few months or a year. Churn drives up administrative costs, because new cases are more expensive to process than recertifications, and reduces program effectiveness when families lose benefits due to administrative burdens. The federal government could monitor rates of churn and set performance standards. For example:

- **SNAP.** Administrative burdens have been shown to reduce recertification among eligible individuals, and reforms that simplify recertification can increase retention (see Chapter 3). Federal policy could authorize, without the need for states to apply for waivers, administrative procedures that make it easier to enroll in and stay on SNAP. These included the extension of certification periods, reduced paperwork and interview burdens, telephonic signatures, and electronic filing of paperwork.
- **Medicaid.** Federal policy could allow (without a waiver) or mandate that states permanently maintain continuous enrollment, specifying that all individuals enrolled in Medicaid and/or the Children's Health Insurance Program are guaranteed 12 months of coverage regardless of what happens to income during those 12 months.[14] Under this policy, some people would get Medicaid for a part of the year where they are no longer eligible, but many people who are eligible but not enrolled would be covered. Such a

---

[13] Pub. L. 79–404, 60 Stat. 237 (1946).

[14] New York and Montana have such a continuous eligibility policy for adults, allowed via waiver under the Medicaid law. In an evaluation of New York's 12-month continuous eligibility policy for adults, Liu and coauthors (2021) found that it increased Medicaid coverage duration by 8.2 percent in the population enrolled through the ACA Marketplace and 4.2 percent among those enrolled through local social service departments. Medicaid costs increased just 2.6 percent and 3.1 percent, respectively, as some of the increased duration was offset by lower per-member monthly costs.

policy would also help address health inequities and lower administrative costs associated with constantly checking eligibility and processing claimants as they churn on and off the rolls. For children, multiyear continuous eligibility could be allowed or mandated.[15]

As described in Chapters 3, 4, and 5, participation rates vary widely overall and across groups in social benefits programs, such as SNAP, Special Supplemental Nutrition Program for Women, Infants and Children (WIC), the National School Lunch Program, and Medicaid. Administrative burdens contribute to incomplete participation among eligible populations. The federal government could monitor participation rates and set performance standards where it is not already doing so. To increase transparency, state-by-state performance could be published. For example:

- **WIC.** Federal policy makers could establish performance metrics for cross-enrollment in WIC of eligible SNAP and Medicaid participants.
- **SNAP.** Although overall participation is high, fewer than half of eligible older adults participate. The Elderly Simplified Application Project is a federal demonstration project that allows streamlined administrative policies for elderly SNAP participants and has been shown to increase participation. Mandating this program or allowing it without a waiver could advance health equity.
- **Medicaid.** Even small premiums discourage Medicaid participation. Barring states from requiring premiums or copayments for Medicaid, which discourage participation, would increase coverage, as would increasing customer service focused on helping people sign up for and maintain Medicaid.

An existing tool that aims to reduce administrative burden for children is Express Lane Eligibility, which intends to facilitate enrollment in health coverage (OIG, 2016) by permitting "states to rely on findings, for things like income, household size, or other factors of eligibility from another program designated as an express lane agency" (Medicaid.gov, 2021). Express Lane agencies may include SNAP, Temporary Assistance for Needy Families, Head Start, National School Lunch Program, and WIC. "A state may also use information from state income tax data to identify children in families that might qualify and so that families do not have to submit income information" (Medicaid.gov, 2021).

---

[15] Oregon received a waiver from CMS to provide multiyear continuous eligibility for children in October 2022, and Washington and California are seeking such a waiver. States are already able to provide 12 months of continuous coverage for children without a waiver.

Eligibility for Federal Program and Services

Access to federally funded programs for everyone who meets requirements is essential to move toward health equity. For example, formerly incarcerated people and immigrants have restricted access to SNAP, WIC, and the Earned Income Tax Credit (see Chapter 3), and those who are incarcerated are not eligible for Medicaid benefits; immigrants are not eligible for Medicaid until they have completed 5 years of legal residence in the United States (see Chapter 5). To increase access to federally funded programs to those who are categorically excluded, the committee recommends:

Recommendation 11: The president of the United States should direct the Office of Management and Budget to review federal programs that exclude specific populations, such as immigrants and those with a criminal record and, in some cases, currently incarcerated people (e.g., Medicaid coverage), to assess the rationale and implications for equity of excluding these populations, including potential impacts on their families and communities. A report on the findings and suggested changes (when applicable) should be made publicly available.

For each excluded category in federally funded programs, both the pros and cons, including cost and health equity implications, should be weighed. An example of an eligibility barrier being removed is the Pell Grants program. In 2020, the Higher Education Act of 1965 and the Free Application for Federal Student Aid program reinstated Pell Grant access for incarcerated people enrolled in qualifying prison education programs (see Chapter 4). This is a promising example of how removing erected barriers to access for specific populations can address unequal access to federal programs that are linked to SDOH and health inequities. This recommendation aligns with the *Second Chance Opportunities for Formerly Incarcerated Persons* effort, announced in April 2022, which includes a proposal to establish a special Medicare enrollment period of 6 months postrelease for people who missed an enrollment period while incarcerated, which would reduce potential gaps in coverage and late enrollment penalties and expand access (The White House, 2022b).

Advance American Indian and Alaska Native Health Equity

Although the committee was expansive in its attempt to incorporate all racial, ethnic, and tribal communities impacted by federal policies, it paid special attention to AIAN communities who are often overlooked in large national reports. Some recent positive steps forward have occurred, but the committee urges further and bigger strides be urgently taken to make up for the gaps and losses in health and health equity that AIAN people experienced for hundreds of years.

As detailed in Chapters 2, 5, 6, and 7, the United States has a complex relationship with the AIAN population. The traumas that have unfolded over generations have resulted in untold cumulative harm, the effects of which are still felt today. Unlike other racial and ethnic groups in the United States, AIAN Tribal Nations are sovereign governments and have legal rights via a trust responsibility that has not been fully upheld. For example, federal responsibility for AIAN health care was codified in the Snyder Act of 1921 and the Indian Health Care Improvement Act of 1976, which form the legislative authority for the Indian Health Service (IHS). Funding for IHS is the lowest of any federal per capita health program dollars as compared to Medicare, Medicaid, Veterans Affairs, and for federal prisoners (see Chapter 5 for a detailed discussion).

Community voice Through most administrations, whether Democrat or Republican, few AIAN voices have been in leadership or influence in the executive branch. In one notable step forward, on September 22, 2022, OMB named Elizabeth Carr as Tribal Advisor to the Director. As stated in its press release,

> This position is historic—the first of its kind at OMB, created out of conversations with tribal leaders — and will be instrumental in coordinating tribal priorities across OMB's budgetary, management, and regulatory functions, while working with other key leaders at the White House and across the entire administration. (The White House, 2022a)

The appointments of Deb Haaland (Laguna Pueblo) as the Secretary of the Department of the Interior, Chief Marilyn Malerba (Mohegan) as U.S. Treasurer, and Carr (Sault Ste. Marie Tribe of Chippewa Indians) bring welcomed and previously absent AIAN perspectives to these areas of policy and governmental concern. Secretary Haaland created the Federal Indian Boarding School Initiative, and she and Secretary Vilsack (Department of Agriculture) have signed off on a number of costewardship agreements (per Joint Secretarial Order 3403 on *Fulfilling the Trust Responsibility to Indian Tribes in the Stewardship of Federal Lands and Waters* they launched in 2021) (Bendery, 2023). These appointments are a source of confidence and furtherance of reconciliation, which happens when space is made in the usual dominant culture structures to purposively allow Indigenization, which is adding Indigenous people, thought, and actions to areas that have been completely devoid of these. However, in the realm of achieving AIAN *health equity*, further adjustments are necessary to close the inequity chasm.

Another appointment is necessary to advance health equity—the elevation of the Director of IHS to an Assistant Secretary of HHS. This appointment has been introduced in legislation by the Senate Committee on Indian Affairs (S. Rept. 106-148) to "to further the unique government-to-government relationship between Indian tribes and the United States, facilitate advocacy for the development of Indian health policy, and promote consultation on matters related to Indian health" (Congress.gov, 1999), which argued that this stature was needed for IHS because of the failure to incorporate tribal recommendations in final budget requests and that because IHS is the largest direct health care provider in HHS, it should answer directly to the HHS Secretary to ensure that tribes' needs are addressed. Establishing an Assistant Secretary of IHS will ensure there is a senior official in future administrations who is knowledgeable about the U.S. legal and moral obligations to AIAN people and the mission of IHS and has the status to advocate within HHS and OMB. Similar legislation was introduced in 2003 by Senator McCain (S.558) (Congress.gov, 2003).

Similarly, because of the special government-to-government relationship and the historical lack of voice for AIAN people, representation is needed in the House and Senate. In 1946, a legislative reorganization act abolished both the House and Senate Committees on Indian Affairs; in 1977, the Senate reestablished its committee.[16] It has jurisdiction to study the unique problems of AIAN and Native Hawaiian peoples and propose legislation to alleviate them. These issues include Indian education, economic development, land management, trust responsibilities, health care, and claims against the United States. In addition, legislation proposed by members of the Senate that pertains specifically to AIAN or Native Hawaiians is under the jurisdiction of the Committee (Committee on Indian Affairs, n.d.-b). The committee has given voice to the AIAN community and helped to pass legislation to advance AIAN priorities (Committee on Indian Affairs, n.d.-a). A recent striking example is in the *Consolidated Appropriations Act, 2023* (H.R. 2617). On September 30, 2022, six members of the Senate Committee on Indian Affairs sent a letter to House leadership, Senate leadership, and the Appropriations Committee urging that congressional leadership include advance appropriations for IHS for FY2024 in the final FY2023 omnibus bill to forestall temporary lapses in appropriations and continuing resolutions. The letter emphasized that during the 2019 government shutdown, "IHS was the only federal health care entity forced to operate without appropriations, causing some Urban Indian Organizations to close their doors completely. This funding disruption resulted in some health providers being unable to provide patients with critical care

---

[16]The committee was created in 1977 as a temporary Select Committee (February 4, 1977, S. Res. 4, Section 105, 95th Congress, 1st Sess. [1977], as amended). It was to disband at the close of the 95th Congress, but following several term extensions, the Senate voted to make it permanent on June 6, 1984.

and medication" (Raimondi, 2022). In a groundbreaking change, H.R. 2617 authorized $6.96 billion for IHS for FY2023, a $360 million increase above the FY2022 enacted level; advance appropriations for IHS totaling $5.13 billion for FY2024; and $90.42 million for urban Indian health for FY2023. However, the act only assures advanced appropriations for 2 years, and it is not clear whether this will continue past 2024. Tribes, tribal organizations, and others have advocated for advance appropriations for IHS for over a decade. The support by the Senate Indian Affairs Committee gave this work a platform and community voice (National Indian Health Board, n.d.). A congressional Committee on Indian Affairs is needed to further raise community voice.

> Recommendation 12: The federal government should undertake the following actions to advance health equity for American Indian and Alaska Native communities in both urban and rural settings by raising the prominence of the agencies that have jurisdiction. Specifically,
> a. The president of the United States and Congress should raise the level of the Director of Indian Health Service (IHS) to an Assistant Secretary.
> b. Congress should authorize funding of IHS at need/parity with other health care programs. This funding should be made mandatory and include advance appropriations.
> c. The House of Representatives should re-establish an Indian Affairs Committee.

Although these actions will not address all barriers to health equity for the AIAN population, together, they will give more voice and prominence to AIAN people, which will help advance health equity for a population that is inadequately resourced and ignored. Other government agencies support AIAN health and address elements of the SDOH. For example, the Bureau of Indian Affairs' mission is to enhance quality of life, promote economic opportunity, and carry out the responsibility to protect and improve the trust assets of AIAN people. It provides resources that can be used to address many SDOH, including education, disaster relief, Indian child welfare, tribal government, Indian self-determination, and reservation roads programs. Just as the committee assessed whether IHS was meeting the needs of AIAN people, a similar assessment is needed for the Bureau of Indian Affairs to assure it is fully resourced to meet its trust obligations.

Health Care Access

Chapter 5 provides an overview of the U.S. health care system and describes how it helps to advance health equity and areas for improvement.

One major aspect is access—this includes insurance coverage and the availability of and access to culturally appropriate, high-quality care, including preventive care, primary care, specialist care, chronic disease management, dental and vision care, mental health treatment, and emergency services. Health care access is an essential element of promoting health equity. Furthermore, affordable health care is necessary for quality care and has been shown to improve health outcomes. Lack of insurance access leads to adverse health outcomes and economic effects that exacerbate racial and ethnic inequities. However, health insurance is just one piece of the equation.

> **Recommendation 13: The Departments of Health and Human Services, Defense, Veterans Affairs, Homeland Security, and Justice, as federal government purchasers and direct providers of health care, should undertake strategies to achieve equitable access to health care across the life span for the individuals and families they serve in every community. These strategies should prioritize access to effective, comprehensive, affordable, accessible, timely, respectful, and culturally appropriate care that addresses equity in the navigation of health care. While these strategies have a greater chance of success when everyone has adequate health insurance, there are ways the executive branch can improve and reinforce access to care for the adequately insured, the underinsured, and the uninsured.**

There are a multitude of approaches that federal agencies can use to achieve this outcome, including ensuring access to health insurance coverage, primary care, enhancing inclusivity of language and communication/health literacy, engendering trust, and other innovative approaches. Although it is not a panacea for health care access, access to insurance remains critical for all U.S. residents regardless of immigration status, state of residency, or employment status. Example mechanisms to increase access are persuading Medicaid nonexpansion states to adopt federal financial support for their uninsured residents and federal directed strategies, such as expanding the Health Resources and Services Administration portal used during the COVID-19 pandemic. The committee notes AIAN people have a legal right to quality physician-led health care under their treaty and trust responsibility. Further integration across the federal health system will also help achieve this recommendation—implementing Recommendation 1 would facilitate the needed integration (Khullar and Chokshi, 2016).

CALL TO ACTION

This report points to both the positive and negative impacts federal policy has had on racial, ethnic, and tribal health equity. Although federal policy has played an important role in correcting past harms and advancing equity, substantial opportunities remain. The four action areas outlined are connected and impact each other. For example, without data that are accurate and representative of a population, it is more difficult to identify where resources and tools are needed and policy efforts should be focused. The lack of community voice and expertise in policy development, even with the best of intentions, can lead to omissions and unintended consequences. Vigilance for this in implemented policies is an essential equity component that needs to be built into feedback monitoring loops and measured in equity audits, as per committee recommendations. Furthermore, as the federal government continues its path to advance health equity, it should keep front and center this report's guiding principles:

1. Health is more than physical and mental well-being—it also includes well-being in social, economic, and other factors, all of which are necessary for human flourishing;
2. All federal policies have the potential to affect population health;
3. Evidence is informed by quantitative, qualitative, and community sources (all of which should be equally valued);
4. Federal policies should center health equity; and
5. To advance health equity, structural and systems change are needed.

Addressing the recommendations in this report will bring the federal government past acknowledging past harms (which is needed but not sufficient) and their impacts on racial, ethnic, and tribal health inequities, to concerted action to expedite the elimination of inequities. It will also improve the circumstances in which people, families, and communities live, play, work, pray, and age so that all people living in the United States have the opportunity to meet their full health potential.

Conclusion 8-2: Federal policy can play a key role in eliminating health inequities by collecting and employing high-quality and accurate data, doing a better job of including and empowering communities that are most affected, and coordinating and holding those who implement policy accountable.

REFERENCES

AAPI Data and National Council of Asian Pacific Americans. 2022. *2022 Asian American, Native Hawaiian, and Pacific Islander (AA and NHPI) roadmap for data equity in federal agencies.* Washington, DC: National Council of Asian Pacific Americans.

Adia, A. C., J. Nazareno, D. Operario, and N. A. Ponce. 2020. Health conditions, outcomes, and service access among Filipino, Vietnamese, Chinese, Japanese, and Korean adults in California, 2011–2017. *American Journal of Public Health* 110(4):520–526.

Agénor, M., C. Perkins, C. Stamoulis, R. D. Hall, M. Samnaliev, S. Berland, and S. Bryn Austin. 2021. Developing a database of structural racism–related state laws for health equity research and practice in the United States. *Public Health Reports* 136(4):428–440.

Amri, S. 2017. Fighting for fair fares in New York City through civil society enforcement of title VI. *Journal of Law and Policy* 26(1):165–224.

Ashley, S., G. Acs, S. Brown, M. Deich, G. MacDonald, D. Marron, R. Balu, M. Rogers, M. McAfee, J. Kirschenbaum, T. Ross, A. Gardere, and S. Treuhaft. 2022. *Scoring federal legislation for equity: Definition, framework, and potential application.* Washington, DC: Urban Institute and PolicyLink.

Badger, E. 2013. *The Dramatic Racial Bias of Subprime Lending During the Housing Boom.* https://www.bloomberg.com/news/articles/2013-08-16/the-dramatic-racial-bias-of-subprime-lending-during-the-housing-boom (accessed February 23, 2023).

Bendery, J. 2023. *After Centuries of Stealing Land, the U.S. Govt. Is Actually Inviting Tribes to Help Manage It.* https://www.huffpost.com/entry/biden-administration-deb-haaland-interior-department-land-costewardship-tribes_n_63b86e01e4b0d6f0b9face1a (accessed March 11, 2023).

Bhakta, S. 2022. Data disaggregation: The case of Asian and Pacific Islander data and the role of health sciences librarians. *Journal of the Medical Library Association* 110(1).

Burden, B. C., D. T. Canon, K. R. Mayer, and D. P. Moynihan. 2012. The effect of administrative burden on bureaucratic perception of policies: Evidence from election administration. *Public Administration Review* 72(5):741–751.

Census Bureau. 2021a. *Census Bureau Announces Changes for 2020 American Community Survey 1-Year Estimates.* https://www.census.gov/newsroom/press-releases/2021/changes-2020-acs-1-year.html (accessed May 29, 2023).

Census Bureau. 2021b. *Decennial Census of Population and Housing Questionnaires & Instructions.* https://www.census.gov/programs-surveys/decennial-census/technical-documentation/questionnaires.2000_Census.html (accessed May 29, 2023).

The Census Project. 2022. *New Report Raises Alarm That Essential Data for the Nation Is at Risk.* https://censusproject.files.wordpress.com/2022/03/censusprojectpressreleaseonacsreport3-8-22final.pdf (accessed March 11, 2023).

Committee on Indian Affairs. n.d.-a. *117th Congress Accomplishments.* https://www.indian.senate.gov/sites/default/files/117th%20Congress%20SCIA%20Accomplishments.pdf (accessed March 11, 2023).

Committee on Indian Affairs. n.d.-b. *About the Committee.* https://www.indian.senate.gov/about-us (accessed March 11, 2023).

Compton, E., Michael Bentley, Sharon Ennis, and S. Rastogi. 2013. *2010 Census Race and Hispanic Origin Alternative Questionnaire Experiment.* https://www2.census.gov/programs-surveys/decennial/2010/program-management/5-review/cpex/2010-cpex-211.pdf (accessed March 11, 2023).

Congress.gov. 1999. *S. Rept. 106-148—A Bill to Elevate the Position of Director of the Indian Health Service Within the Department of Health And Human Services to Assistant Secretary for Indian Health, and for Other Purposes.* https://www.congress.gov/congressional-report/106th-congress/senate-report/148 (accessed March 11, 2023).

Congress.gov. 2003. *S.558—a Bill to Elevate the Position of Director of the Indian Health Service Within the Department of Health and Human Services to Assistant Secretary for Indian Health, and for Other Purposes.* https://www.congress.gov/bill/108th-congress/senate-bill/558/text (accessed March 11, 2023).

CPEHN (California Pan-Ethnic Health Network). 2022. *American Rescue Plan Act Scorecards for California Counties.* https://www.cpehn.org/ARPAscorecards/ (accessed June 1, 2023).

ELTRR (Equitable Long-Term Recovery and Resilience) Interagency Workgroup. 2022. *Federal plan for equitable long-term recovery and resilience for social, behavioral, and community health.* Washington, DC: Department of Health and Human Services.

Equitable Data Working Group. 2022. *A vision for equitable data: Recommendations from the Equitable Data Working Group.* Washington, DC: The White House.

Farrell, L., Mel Langness, and E. Falkenburger. 2021. *Community Voice Is Expertise.* https:// www.urban.org/urban-wire/community-voice-expertise (accessed March 11, 2023).

Galinsky, A. M., C. E. Zelaya, C. Simile, and P. M. Barnes. 2017. Health conditions and behaviors of Native Hawaiian and Pacific Islander persons in the United States, 2014. *Vital and Health Statistics Series. Series 3, Analytical and Epidemiological Studies*(40):1–99.

Galinsky, A. M., C. Simile, C. E. Zelaya, T. Norris, and S. V. Panapasa. 2019. Surveying strategies for hard-to-survey populations: Lessons from the Native Hawaiian and Pacific Islander national health interview survey. *American Journal of Public Health* 109(10):1384–1391.

Green, K., and M. Zook. 2019. *When Talking About Social Determinants, Precision Matters.* https://www.healthaffairs.org/content/forefront/talking-social-determinants-precision-matters (accessed October 29, 2022).

Greenfield, B. L., J. H. L. Elm, and K. A. Hallgren. 2021. Understanding measures of racial discrimination and microaggressions among American Indian and Alaska Native college students in the southwest United States. *BMC Public Health* 21(1).

Haldane, V., F. L. H. Chuah, A. Srivastava, S. R. Singh, G. C. H. Koh, C. K. Seng, and H. Legido-Quigley. 2019. Community participation in health services development, implementation, and evaluation: A systematic review of empowerment, health, community, and process outcomes. *The Public Library of Science* 14(5):e0216112.

HHS (Health and Human Services). 2021. *Community health and economic prosperity: Engaging businesses as stewards and stakeholders—a report of the surgeon general.* Atlanta, GA: Department of Health and Human Services, Centers for Disease Control and Prevention, Office of the Associate Director for Policy and Strategy.

IAP2 (International Association for Public Participation). 2018. *IAP2 Spectrum of Public Participation.* https://cdn.ymaws.com/www.iap2.org/resource/resmgr/pillars/Spectrum_8.5x11_Print.pdf (accessed March 9, 2023).

IHS (Indian Health Service). n.d. *Tribal Consultation and Urban Confer.* https://www.ihs.gov/dbh/consultationandconfer/ (accessed March 11, 2023).

Kalev, A., E. Kelly, and F. Dobbin. 2006. Best practices or best guesses? Assessing the efficacy of corporate affirmative action and diversity policies. *American Sociological Review* 71(4):589–617.

Kauh, T. J., J. G. Read, and A. J. Scheitler. 2021. The critical role of racial/ethnic data disaggregation for health equity. *Population Research and Policy Review* 40(1):1–7.

Khullar, D., and D. A. Chokshi. 2016. Toward an integrated federal health system. *Journal of the American Medical Association* 315(23):2521–2522.

Krieger, N. 2020. Measures of racism, sexism, heterosexism, and gender binarism for health equity research: From structural injustice to embodied harm—an ecosocial analysis. *Annual Review of Public Health* 41:37–62.

Liu, H. H., A. W. Dick, N. S. Qureshi, S. M. Baxi, K. J. Roberts, J. S. Ashwood, L. A. Guerra, T. Ruder, and R. A. Shih. 2021. *New York State 1115 demonstration independent evaluation: Interim report.* Santa Monica, CA: RAND Corporation.

Martin, C., and J. Lewis. 2019. *The state of equity measurement: A review for energy-efficiency programs.* Washington, DC: Urban Institute.

Medicaid.gov. 2021. *Express Lane Eligibility for Medicaid and CHIP Coverage.* https://www.medicaid.gov/medicaid/enrollment-strategies/express-lane-eligibility-medicaid-and-chip-coverage/index.html (accessed May 30, 2023).

Mesic, A., L. Franklin, A. Cansever, F. Potter, A. Sharma, A. Knopov, and M. Siegel. 2018. The relationship between structural racism and black–white disparities in fatal police shootings at the state level. *Journal of the National Medical Association* 110(2):106–116.

MITRE. n.d. *A Framework for Assessing Equity in Federal Programs and Policy.* https:// www.mitre.org/news-insights/publication/framework-assessing-equity-federal-programs-and-policy (accessed March 7, 2023).

Moy, E., I. E. Arispe, J. S. Holmes, and R. M. Andrews. 2005. Preparing the national health-care disparities report: Gaps in data for assessing racial, ethnic, and socioeconomic disparities in health care. *Medical Care* 43(3 Suppl):I9–16.

NASEM (National Academies of Sciences, Engineering, and Medicine). 2019. *Integrating social care into the delivery of health care: Moving upstream to improve the nation's health*. Washington, DC: The National Academies Press.

National Indian Health Board. n.d. *Advance Appropriations*. https://www.nihb.org/legislative/advance_appropriations.php (accessed March 11, 2023).

NRC (National Research Council). 2004. *Eliminating health disparities: Measurement and data needs*. Washington, DC: The National Academies Press.

O'Mara-Eves, A., G. Brunton, S. Oliver, J. Kavanagh, F. Jamal, and J. Thomas. 2015. The effectiveness of community engagement in public health interventions for disadvantaged groups: A meta-analysis. *BMC Public Health* 15(1):129.

OIG (Office of Inspector General). 2016. *State use of express lane eligibility for Medicaid and CHIP enrollment*. Washington, DC: HHS.

OMB (Office of Management and Budget). 1997. Revisions to the standards for the classification of federal data on race and ethnicity. *Federal Register* 62(210):58782–58790.

OMB. 2021. *Study to identify methods to assess equity: Report to the president*. Washington, DC: Office of Management and Budget.

OMB. 2023. *Initial proposals for updating OMB's race and ethnicity statistical standards*. Washington, DC: Office of Management and Budget.

One Million Experiments. n.d. *About One Million Experiments*. https://millionexperiments.com/about (accessed March 23, 2023).

Performance.gov. 2021. *Methods and Leading Practices for Advancing Equity and Support for Underserved Communities Through Government*. https://www.performance.gov/equity/rfi-summary/#takeaways (accessed March 11, 2023).

Raimondi, M. 2022. *Senators Request Congressional Leadership Support Advance Appropriations to Stabilize the Indian Health Service*. https://ncuih.org/2022/10/14/senators-request-congressional-leadership-support-advance-appropriations-to-stabilize-the-indian-health-service/ (accessed March 11, 2023).

Rugh, J. S., and D. S. Massey. 2010. Racial segregation and the American foreclosure crisis. *American Sociological Review* 75(5):629–651.

RWJF (Robert Wood Johnson Foundation). 2022. *Transforming public health data systems*. Santa Monica, CA: Robert Wood Johnson Foundation.

Schoch-Spana, M., E. K. Brunson, R. Long, A. Ruth, S. J. Ravi, M. Trotochaud, L. Borio, J. Brewer, J. Buccina, N. Connell, L. L. Hall, N. Kass, A. Kirkland, L. Koonin, H. Larson, B. F. Lu, S. B. Omer, W. A. Orenstein, G. A. Poland, L. Privor-Dumm, S. C. Quinn, D. Salmon, and A. White. 2021. The public's role in COVID-19 vaccination: Human-centered recommendations to enhance pandemic vaccine awareness, access, and acceptance in the United States. *Vaccine* 39(40):6004–6012.

Task Force on Next Generation Community Schools. 2021. *Addressing education inequality with a next generation of community schools*. Washington, DC: The Brookings Institution.

Urban Institute. n.d. *Quantitative Data Analysis*. https://www.urban.org/research/data-methods/data-analysis/quantitative-data-analysis/microsimulation (accessed March 7, 2023).

The White House. 2021a. *Executive Order on advancing racial equity and support for underserved communities through the federal government*. Washington, DC: The White House.

The White House. 2021b. *Memorandum on Redressing Our Nation's and the Federal Government's History of Discriminatory Housing Practices and Policies*. https://www.whitehouse.gov/briefing-room/presidential-actions/2021/01/26/memorandum-on-redressing-our-nations-and-the-federal-governments-history-of-discriminatory-housing-practices-and-policies/ (accessed March 11, 2023).

The White House. 2022a. *Announcing OMB's First Ever Tribal Advisor*. https://www.whitehouse.gov/omb/briefing-room/2022/09/12/announcing-ombs-first-ever-tribal-advisor/ (accessed March 11, 2023).

The White House. 2022b. *Fact Sheet: Biden-Harris Administration Expands Second Chance Opportunities for Formerly Incarcerated Persons*. https://www.whitehouse.gov/briefing-room/statements-releases/2022/04/26/fact-sheet-biden-harris-administration-expands-second-chance-opportunities-for-formerly-incarcerated-persons/ (accessed March 11, 2023).

The White House. 2023. *Executive Order on Further Advancing Racial Equity and Support for Underserved Communities Through the Federal Government*. https://www.whitehouse.gov/briefing-room/presidential-actions/2023/02/16/executive-order-on-further-advancing-racial-equity-and-support-for-underserved-communities-through-the-federal-government/ (accessed March 15, 2023).

The White House. n.d. *Advancing Equity and Racial Justice Through the Federal Government*. https://www.whitehouse.gov/equity/ (accessed March 21, 2023).

Williams, D. R. 2016. *Measuring Discrimination Resource*. https://scholar.harvard.edu/files/davidrwilliams/files/measuring_discrimination_resource_june_2016.pdf (accessed March 8, 2023).

Yom, S., and M. Lor. 2022. Advancing health disparities research: The need to include Asian American subgroup populations. *Journal of Racial and Ethnic Health Disparities* 9(6):2248–2282.

Zelaya, C. E., A. M. Galinsky, C. Simile, and P. M. Barnes. 2017. Health care access and utilization among Native Hawaiian and Pacific Islander persons in the United States, 2014. *Vital and Health Statistics, Series* 3(41):1–79.

Appendix A

Public Meeting Agendas

FIRST PUBLIC MEETING

June 2, 2022

VIRTUAL MEETING VIA ZOOM

12:00 p.m.	Welcome SHEILA BURKE and DANIEL POLSKY, *Committee Cochairs*
12:05–1:00	Presentation of the Statement of Task, Background, and Discussion RDML FELICIA COLLINS Deputy Assistant Secretary for Minority Health; Director, Office of Minority Health, Department of Health and Human Services
1:00	Adjourn

SECOND PUBLIC MEETING

July 26, 2022

VIRTUAL MEETING VIA ZOOM

11:00–11:05 a.m.   Welcome
                   SHEILA BURKE and DANIEL POLSKY, *Committee Cochairs*

11:05–12:05   Public Comment

The National Academies of Sciences, Engineering, and Medicine invites the public to provide comments to be considered by the Committee on the Review of Federal Policies that Contribute to Racial and Ethnic Health Inequities.

The committee welcomes input on federal policies that contribute to racial and ethnic health inequities and potential solutions.
- What are examples of federal policies that create racial and ethnic health inequities?
- What are examples of federal policies that promote racial and ethnic health equity?
- What are the most important considerations when prioritizing action regarding federal policies to advance racial and ethnic health equity?

Participants:
- **Cevadne Lee,** Director, Office of Community Outreach and Engagement, Chao Family Comprehensive Cancer Center
- **Ruqaiijah Yearby,** Professor of Law, Moritz College of Law, The Ohio State University
- **Winston F. Wong,** Chair and acting CEO, National Council of Asian Pacific Islander Physicians Associate; National Research Council
- **Cynthia Adinig,** SolveMe
- **Amanda J. Calhoun,** Yale Psychiatry Resident/Child Psychiatry Fellow
- **Timothy Thomas,** Captain, U.S. Public Health Service
- **Kelsey Runge**
- **B. Suzi Ruhl,** Senior Research Scientist, Child Study Center, Yale School of Medicine

- **Harald Schmidt,** Assistant Professor, Department of Medical Ethics and Health, Policy Perelman School of Medicine, University of Pennsylvania
- **Tiffany Green,** Assistant professor, Departments of Population Health Sciences and Obstetrics and Gynecology, University of Wisconsin School of Medicine and Public Health
- **Diana Zuckerman,** President, National Center for Health Research

12:05–12:15	**Break**

12:15–12:45   **Racial and Ethnic Health Inequities and Socioeconomic Differences in Health**
JANET CURRIE
Henry Putnam Professor of Economics and Policy Affairs; Codirector, Center for Health and Wellbeing, Princeton University

12:45–1:15   **Housing Policy**
RICHARD CHO
Senior Advisor—Housing Services, Department of Housing and Urban Development

1:15   **Closing Remarks/Adjourn**

August 1, 2022

VIRTUAL MEETING VIA ZOOM

12:00–12:10 p.m.   Welcome
SHEILA BURKE and DANIEL POLSKY, *Committee Cochairs*

12:10–1:00   **Community Infrastructure Challenges and Solutions**
TOM MORRIS
Associate Administrator for Rural Health, Policy Health Resources and Services, Administration Department of Health and Human Services

BARBARA MASTERS
Director, California Accountable Communities for Health Initiative

1:00–1:50	**Housing Policy** Ananya Roy Professor, Urban Planning, Social Welfare, and Geography; Meyer and Renee Luskin Chair in Inequality and Democracy, University of California, Los Angeles
	Liz Osborn Vice President of Public Policy Advocacy, Enterprise Community Partners
1:50–2:00	**Break**
2:00–3:00	**Transportation Policy** Megan Ryerson UPS Chair of Transportation, Professor, and Associate Dean for Research, Weitzman School of Design, University of Pennsylvania
	Kamilah Martin-Proctor Member, Board of Directors, WMATA Board; Commission Chair, D.C. Commission on Persons with Disabilities
3:00	**Closing Remarks/Adjourn**

August 3, 2022

VIRTUAL MEETING VIA ZOOM

11:00–11:05 a.m.	Welcome Sheila Burke and Daniel Polsky, *Committee Cochairs*
11:05–11:35	**Federal Indian Law, Constitutional Law, and Available Policy Levers** Maggie Blackhawk Professor of Law, NYU School of Law
11:35–12:05	**Community Infrastructure and Development in Urban Environments** Sue Polis Director, Health and Wellness, Institute for Youth, Education, And Families, National League of Cities

STEPHANIE MARTINEZ-RUCKMAN
Legislative Director for Human Development,
National League of Cities

12:05–12:35   **Health Policy Processes and Levers and Interagency Collaboration**
ALLISON ORRIS
Senior Fellow, Center on Budget and Policy Priorities

12:35–12:45   **Break**

12:45–1:45   **Health Care and Public Health Policy**
LORETTA CHRISTENSEN
Chief Medical Officer, Indian Health Service

CINDY MANN
Partner, Manatt, Phelps & Phillips, LLP

J. NADINE GRACIA
President and CEO, Trust for America's Health

1:45–2:30   **Racial and Ethnic Health Inequities**
GAIL CHRISTOPHER
Executive Director, National Collaborative for Health Equity

JOHN A. RICH
Director, Rush BMO Institute for Health Equity, Rush University Medical Center

2:30   **Closing Remarks/Adjourn**

THIRD PUBLIC MEETING

September 9, 2022

VIRTUAL MEETING VIA ZOOM

2:00–2:05 p.m.   **Welcome**
SHEILA BURKE and DANIEL POLSKY, *Committee Cochairs*

2:05–3:30   **Public Comment**

The National Academies of Sciences, Engineering, and Medicine invites the public to provide comments to be considered by the Committee on the Review of Federal Policies that Contribute to Racial and Ethnic Health Inequities.

At this meeting (September 9, 2022), the committee welcomes input on federal policies that contribute to racial and ethnic health inequities and potential solutions.

The committee is interested in hearing about lived experiences navigating federal programs and systems including barriers and solutions from community members and organizations.

Additional questions the committee would like input on are
- What are examples of federal policies that create racial and ethnic health inequities?
- What are examples of federal policies that promote racial and ethnic health equity?
- What are the most important considerations when prioritizing action regarding federal policies to advance racial and ethnic health equity?

Participants:
- **Juliette Blount,** Nurse Practitioner and Health Equity, Speaker Health Equity NP, LLC
- **Grace Wickerson,** Policy Entrepreneurship Fellow, Federation of American Scientists
- **Willa Truelove,** Councilperson for People with Disabilities
- **Richard Schulterbrandt Gragg III,** Professor of Environmental Science and Policy, Florida A&M University, School of Environment
- **Mahin Khatami,** Retired Immunologist NCI/NIH
- **Tobi Oloyede,** Step Up Savannah, Georgia Southern University
- **P. Fadwah Halaby,** Chairperson, ACNM Home and Birth Center Committee
- **Monica R. McLemore,** Associate Professor, University of California, San Francisco
- **Michael Ellenbogen**
- **Earnest Davis,** President, Community Psychology Health Collaborative
- **Linda Shosie,** Founder, Environmental Justice Task Force, Tucson
- **Lisa Schlager,** Vice President of Public Policy, Facing Our Risk of Cancer Empowered
- **Keegan Warren-Clem,** Health Management Associates

- **JoAnn Yánez,** Executive Director, Association of Accredited Naturopathic Medical Colleges
- **Nicole T. Rochester,** Founder and CEO, Your GPS Doc LLC
- **Gina Currie,** Registered Nurse CureRx
- **Asma Jafri**
- **Gnora Gumanow,** Partnerships Manager, Healthy Democracy, Healthy People
- **Heather Sauyaq Jean Gordon,** Research Scientist II Child Trends
- **Jessica Nickrand,** Manager, Programs, Child Neurology Foundation
- **Malaak Elhage,** Changemaker, CLASP New Deal for Youth
- **Cody Rooney,** Changemaker, CLASP New Deal for Youth

3:30   Closing Remarks/Adjourn

Appendix B

Committee Member and
Staff Biographies

COMMITTEE

Sheila P. Burke, M.P.A., R.N., FAAN (Cochair), is an adjunct lecturer at the J. F. Kennedy School of Government at Harvard University, where she was executive dean. Ms. Burke is vice chair of the Commonwealth Fund Board of Directors. She also serves as a senior public policy advisor and chair of the Government Relations and Policy Group at Baker Donelson. Ms. Burke had been chief of staff to the Senate Majority Leader Bob Dole and deputy staff director of the Senate Committee on Finance and the Secretary of the Senate, the chief administrative officer of the body. She has served as a commissioner on the Medicare Payment Advisory Commission and chair of the Kaiser Foundation Board. Early in her career, she was a staff nurse in California. Ms. Burke was the deputy secretary and chief operating officer of the Smithsonian Institution, where she received the Secretary's Gold Medal for Exceptional Service. Ms. Burke is a member of the National Academy of Medicine (NAM), where she was a member of the NAM Council and received the David Rall Award. She is also a fellow of the American Academy of Nursing and member of the National Academy of Public Administration. She has honorary degrees from Marymount University and the Uniformed Services University of the Health Sciences. She is a graduate of the University of San Francisco and Harvard University.

Daniel E. Polsky, Ph.D. (Cochair), is the Bloomberg Distinguished Professor of Health Economics and Policy at Johns Hopkins University. He holds primary appointments in the Department of Health Policy and Management,

Bloomberg School of Public Health, and Carey Business School. As the director of the Hopkins Business of Health Initiative and former executive director of the Leonard Davis Institute for Health Economics, Dr. Polsky has extensive experience in leading interdisciplinary teams advancing research to inform U.S. health policy to address challenges of access, affordability, value, and equity. He was the Robert D. Eilers Professor at the Wharton School and the Perelman School of Medicine, University of Pennsylvania, where he was faculty (1996–2019). Dr. Polsky is a member of NAM and on the HMD Committee for the National Academies. He was the senior economist on health issues at the President's Council of Economic Advisers. He received his MPP from the University of Michigan in 1989 and a Ph.D. in economics from the University of Pennsylvania in 1996.

Madina Agénor, Sc.D., M.P.H., is an associate professor in the Department of Behavioral and Social Sciences and Center for Health Promotion and Health Equity at the Brown University School of Public Health. She is also adjunct faculty at the Fenway Institute and leads the Sexual Health and Reproductive Experiences Lab at Brown University. As a social epidemiologist, Dr. Agénor investigates health inequities in relation to multiple social positions and power relations—especially sexual orientation and heterosexism, gender and (cis)sexism, and race/ethnicity and racism—using an intersectional lens and a mixed-methods research approach. Specifically, she uses quantitative and qualitative research methods to investigate the structural and social determinants of sexual and reproductive health and cancer screening and prevention among marginalized populations, especially sexual minority women, transgender and gender diverse young adults, Black women, and Black and other LGBTQ+ racially and ethnically minoritized people. Her current research seeks to elucidate how multiple, intersecting forms of structural and interpersonal discrimination, including racism, heterosexism, and (cis)sexism, independently and jointly influence access to and use of these preventive services and related health outcomes among multiply marginalized groups. Her research has been published in leading public health and medical peer-reviewed journals, including *American Journal of Public Health*, *Social Science & Medicine*, *American Journal of Preventive Medicine*, and *Annals of Internal Medicine*. Dr. Agénor completed postdoctoral research training in cancer prevention equity as part of the Harvard Educational Program in Cancer Prevention and was visiting research faculty at the Center for Interdisciplinary Research on AIDS at Yale University. Before joining Brown University, she was the Gerald R. Gill Assistant Professor of Race, Culture, and Society at Tufts University and an assistant professor at Harvard T.H. Chan School of Public Health. She holds an Sc.D. in social and behavioral sciences with a concentration in women, gender, and health from Harvard T.H. Chan School of Public Health, an M.P.H. in sociomedical sciences from Columbia University Mailman School of Public Health, and an A.B. in community health and gender studies from Brown University.

Camille M. Busette, Ph.D., is a senior fellow in governance studies with affiliated appointments in economic studies and the metropolitan policy programs at the Brookings Institution. She is the director of the Race, Prosperity, and Inclusion Initiative, focusing on issues of equity, racial justice, and economic mobility for low-income and racially and ethnically minoritized communities. Earlier, Dr. Busette was an executive at the World Bank, where she led its financial inclusion innovation arm. She was the inaugural CEO of the Consumer Financial Protection Bureau's Office of Financial Education, where she was a member of the policy and executive Management teams. Dr. Busette has held executive positions at PayPal, Intuit, and NextCard and is a public governor of FINRA, the self-regulatory agency for the broker-dealer industry. She holds a Ph.D. and M.A. in political science from the University of Chicago and a B.A. in political science from the University of California, Berkeley and is former Ford Foundation postdoctoral fellow.

Mario Cardona, J.D., is professor of practice and director of policy at the Children's Equity Project based out of Arizona State University. He served as Child Care Aware of America's chief of policy and practice, where he provided leadership and outreach to the government, its members, and the general public on issues relating to the early childhood education (ECE) system. He also led its policy, advocacy, and practice strategy. In December 2021, Mr. Cardona was selected for a Pahara Fellowship, a 1-year program that identifies exceptional leaders in the educational excellence and equity movement, facilitates their dynamic growth, and strengthens their collective efforts to dramatically improve public education, especially those programs serving low-income children and communities. He was in the Obama Administration as a senior policy advisor on the White House Domestic Policy Council and held senior roles in the Senate, including as a principal advisor to the chair of the Health, Education, Labor and Pensions Committee. While in Congress, he wrote and led staff negotiations to pass the Child Care & Development Block Grant Act of 2014, which comprehensively updated the quality and safety standards in federally subsidized child care for the first time in nearly 20 years. He earned a B.A. from the University of Texas at Austin, an Ed.M. from Harvard University, and a J.D., with honors, from the George Washington University Law School. *Resigned from the committee on October 5, 2022.*

Juliet K. Choi, J.D., is the president and CEO of the Asian & Pacific Islander American Health Forum, a national health justice organization that influences policy, mobilizes communities, and strengthens programs and organizations to improve the health of Asian American and Native Hawaiian and Pacific Islander (NHPI) people. She is an accomplished cross-sector leader and coalition builder who specializes in change management, system reform, and stakeholder relations, particularly in the areas of immigration, civil rights, health care and disaster relief. She served in the Obama administration as the chief of staff and senior advisor of two federal agencies: U.S. Citizenship and Immigration Services at the U.S. Department of Homeland Security and the Office for Civil Rights at the Department of Health and Human Services. Before that, she led disaster relief operations and strategic partnerships at the American Red Cross as a member of the disaster leadership team. She has worked at the Partnership for Public Service, Asian American Justice Center, Mental Health America, and a Fortune 500 corporation. Ms. Juliet received her law school's Alumni Association Award for Leadership and Character and Rising Star Alumnus Award. The proud daughter of South Korean immigrants, she is on the Presidential Advisory Council on HIV and AIDS, Robert Wood Johnson Foundation Commission on Data Modernization, Office of Minority Health Subject Matter Experts Group on Asian American, Native Hawaiian and Pacific Islanders, and boards of the National Asian Pacific American Bar Association Law Foundation and national YWCA USA. She received her J.D. from University of Maryland School of Law and clerked for the Hon. Dennis M. Sweeney (ret.) of the Circuit Court for Howard County, Maryland. She received her B.A. in economics from University of Virginia.

Juan De Lara, Ph.D., M.A., is associate professor of American studies and ethnicity at University of Southern California Dornsife College of Letters, Arts, and Sciences. He is a human geographer who studies race, space, and power. Dr. De Lara is the inaugural director of the Center for Latinx and Latin American Studies. His research focuses on three broad themes: urban political economy, racialization, and the politics of space; the use of data science and technology to reorganize how various state agencies are restructuring the social relations of race, immigration, and labor; and research that supports community-based organizations in their efforts to resolve social disparities. Dr. De Lara authored the book *Inland Shift: Race, Space, and Capital in Inland Southern California*, which uses logistics and commodity chains to unpack the black box of globalization by showing how the scientific management of bodies, space, and time produced new racialized labor regimes inside modern warehouses. He received his B.A. in sociology and labor studies from Pitzer College, an M.A. in urban planning

from University of California, Los Angeles, and a Ph.D. in geography from University of California, Berkeley.

Thomas Dobbs III, M.D., M.P.H., is dean of the John D. Bower School of Population Health at the University of Mississippi Medical Center. He also teaches epidemiology for the School of Population Health and School of Health-Related Professions and has a clinical position within the Division of Infectious Disease, working specifically on HIV and sexually transmitted infections with a focus on the intersection of disease and the social determinants of health. He was the state health officer for Mississippi from 2018 through July 2022. Dr. Dobbs served in other public health roles at Mississippi State Department of Health, including district health officer and state epidemiologist. He is a board-certified internal medicine and infectious diseases physician, working at the intersection of public health and patient care, both domestically and internationally, with specific expertise in HIV, tuberculosis, public health, and health equity. He has won numerous awards for work in public health and education, including Mississippi Senate and House resolutions for his work through the COVID pandemic. He received his M.D. and M.P.H. from the University of Alabama at Birmingham.

Megan D. Douglas, J.D., is an associate professor in the Department of Community Health and Preventive Medicine and director of research and policy in the National Center for Primary Care at Morehouse School of Medicine. She is a licensed attorney, and her research focuses on studying how laws and other policies improve population health and advance health equity. She has expertise in legal epidemiology, which uses scientific methods to study the effects of laws on health outcomes, and has applied this approach for policies related to primary care, behavioral health, developmental disabilities, digital health tools, and structural racism. Ms. Douglas has been awarded funding from OMH, the Patient-Centered Outcomes Research Institute, Centers for Disease Control and Prevention, and the National Institutes of Health. She received her B.S. in biology from Virginia Tech and her J.D. from Georgia State University College of Law. She was the first attorney to complete the Health Policy Leadership Fellowship in the Satcher Health Leadership Institute at Morehouse.

Abigail Echo-Hawk, M.A., is the executive vice president of Seattle Indian Health Board and director of its data and research division, Urban Indian Health Institute. She serves on the Robert Wood Johnson Public Health Data National Commission, University of Washington Population Health Initiative External Advisory Board, Data for Indigenous Justice Board, and many other boards and committees related to data justice and health equity. She also served on the National Academies committee A Framework for Equitable Allocation of Vaccine for the Novel Coronavirus in 2020. Since the COVID-19 pandemic began, Ms. Echo-Hawk's voice has been front and center on a national level, ensuring that the urban Native community is represented in data collection. The Seattle Indian Health Board has been a leader in the COVID-19 response directly because of her leadership and vision. She has coauthored numerous peer-reviewed articles, including two for CDC's *Morbidity and Mortality Weekly Report* on COVID-19 among AIAN people, and was lead author on a report about their data genocide in COVID-19 data. Ms. Echo-Hawk has also led the way in bringing the issue of missing and murdered Indigenous women and girls to the forefront, leading directly to federal, state, and local legislation working to protect Native women. She is on the Washington State Missing and Murdered Indigenous Women and People Taskforce, which she was instrumental in creating. She is a researcher and policy professional specializing in tribal government and urban Indian relations. She successfully leads teams of public health professionals to develop culturally competent and culturally relevant NIH-, CDC-, and HHS-funded health and policy interventions with tribal and urban communities across the country. She earned a B.A. in American Studies with a minor in human rights and M.A. in policy studies from the University of Washington.

Hedwig (Hedy) Lee, Ph.D., is a professor of sociology at Washington University in St. Louis and holds a courtesy joint appointment at the George Warren Brown School of Social Work. She is also the associate director of the university's new Center on the Study of Race, Ethnicity, and Equity and Scholar in Residence of Sociology, Duke University. Earlier, she was a professor at the University of Washington Department of Sociology in Seattle. Her research focuses on the SDOH and consequences of population health and health disparities, with a particular focus on the role of structural racism (e.g., mass incarceration) in racial/ethnic health disparities. She serves on the board of the Population Association of America and the research advisory board for the Vera Institute for Justice. She is also a member of the General Social Survey Board of Overseers and the National Academies, Division of Behavioral and Social Sciences and Education, Committee on Population. She received her Ph.D. in sociology at the University of North Carolina at Chapel Hill and was a Carolina Population Center Predoctoral Trainee and a Robert Wood Johnson Foundation Health and Society Postdoctoral Scholar at the University of Michigan.

Margaret P. Moss, Ph.D., J.D., R.N., FAAN, is an enrolled member of the Mandan, Hidatsa, and Arikara Nation and also Dakhóta. She is a professor and director at the First Nations House of Learning at the University of British Columbia. Previously she was also the interim associate vice president of equity and inclusion. She has been a nurse for 32 years and a fellow in the American Academy of Nursing since 2008 and was recently elected to its board of directors. Dr. Moss is the first and only American Indian to hold both nursing and juris doctorates. She was appointed to the Board on Population Health and Public Health Practice at the National Academies. She was named on the inaugural Forbes 50 over 50 Impact List 2021, in part due to her editing and authoring the first nursing text on American Indian health, which won two book-of-the-year awards. Her second text, *Health Equity and Nursing*, was published in 2020. Dr. Moss has been a Robert Wood Johnson Foundation Health Policy Fellow, staff on the Senate Special Committee on Aging 2008; a Fulbright Research Chair at McGill University on Indigenous contexts since 2014; and on the British Columbia Minister of Health's investigation team and report *In Plain Sight: Addressing Indigenous-Specific Racism and Discrimination in B.C. Health Care.* She received her Ph.D. from the University of Texas Health Science Center at Houston and her J.D. from Mitchell Hamline School of Law.

Sela V. Panapasa, Ph.D., is an associate research scientist at the Research Center on Group Dynamics at the University of Michigan's Institute for Social Research. As a social demographer, Dr. Panapasa studies population dynamics, family demography, and racial and ethnic health disparities and conducts mixed-methods research on the health and well-being of hard-to-survey populations. Specific areas of expertise include the life-course perspective on health outcomes and quality of life among NHPI populations. Dr. Panapasa received her Ph.D. in sociology and was a Population Studies and Training Center trainee at Brown University and postdoctoral scholar at the University of Michigan.

S. Karthick Ramakrishnan, Ph.D., is professor of public policy at the University of California, Riverside and executive director of California 100, a transformative statewide initiative focused on building a shared vision and strategy for California's next century that is innovative, sustainable, and equitable. Dr. Ramakrishnan also founded the Center for Social Innovation at Riverside and AAPI Data, a national publisher of demographic data and policy research. He has published many articles and seven books, most recently *Citizenship Reimagined* and *Framing Immigrants*. Dr. Ramakrishnan was named to the Frederick Douglass 200 and is working on projects related to racial equity in philanthropy and regional development. He serves on the Board of The California Endowment and Association of Princeton Graduate Alumni, chairs the California Commission on APIA Affairs, and is on the U.S. Census Bureau's National Advisory Committee. Dr. Ramakrishnan also founded Census Legacies, which builds on the foundation of census outreach coalitions to build more inclusive and equitable communities, and the *Journal of Race, Ethnicity, and Politics*, an official section journal of the American Political Science Association. He holds a B.A. in international relations from Brown University and a Ph.D. in politics from Princeton University.

Diane Whitmore Schanzenbach, Ph.D., is director of the Institute for Policy Research at Northwestern University. She is also the Margaret Walker Alexander Professor in the School of Education and Social Policy at Northwestern. She is a research associate at the National Bureau of Economic Research, nonresident senior fellow at the Brookings Institution, and research associate at the Institute for Research on Poverty at the University of Wisconsin—Madison. Dr. Schanzenbach is an economist who studies policies aimed at improving the lives of children in poverty, including education, health, and income support policies. Her work traces the impact of major public policies, such as Supplemental Nutrition Assistance Program, school finance reform, and ECE, on long-term outcomes. Dr. Schanzenbach was the director of the Hamilton Project at the Brookings Institution. She is an elected member of the National Academy of Education and the National Academy of Social Insurance. She graduated magna cum laude from Wellesley College with a B.A. in economics and religion and received a Ph.D. in economics from Princeton University.

Lisa Servon, Ph.D., is the Kevin and Erica Penn Presidential Professor department chair in the Weitzman School of Design at the University of Pennsylvania. Dr. Servon was professor of management and urban policy at the New School, where she also served as dean at the Milano School of International Affairs, Management, and Urban Policy. She conducts research in the areas of urban poverty, community development, economic development, and issues of gender and race. Her specific areas of expertise include economic insecurity, consumer financial services, and financial justice. She holds a B.A. in political science from Bryn Mawr College, an M.A. in history of art from the University of Pennsylvania, and a Ph.D. in urban planning from the University of California, Berkeley.

Vivek Shandas, Ph.D., is a professor of climate adaptation and founder and director of the Sustaining Urban Places Research at Portland State University, where he brings a policy-relevant approach, including evaluating environmental stressors on human health, developing indicators and tools to improve decision making, and constructing frameworks to guide the growth of urban regions. He specializes in developing strategies for addressing the implications of climate change on cities. His teaching and research examine the intersection of exposure to climate-induced events, governance processes, planning mechanisms, and relevant implications on the public's health. As an interdisciplinary scholar, Dr. Shandas studies the emergent characteristics that generate vulnerability among communities and infrastructure. He teaches courses in environmental planning, urban ecology, health impact assessments, and climate adaptation. Funding for his research comes primarily from federal agencies, and he focuses on understanding the disparate health impacts emerging from the built environment, planning policies, and coping capacities of communities for the increasing effects of climate change. Dr. Shandas has written articles on water quality and use, climate justice, air quality, and interdisciplinary education for diverse publications, including *Urban Geography, Journal of the American Planning Association, Landscape and Urban Planning, BioScience, International Journal of Environmental Research and Public Health, Urban Climate,* and *Journal of Environmental Management.* Earlier, he was a school teacher in Oregon (Vernonia); curriculum developer in California (San Jose); and a health and environmental policy analyst for the governor of New York State (Albany). He serves on several national and local advisory boards and is an advisor to CAPA Strategies, a global consulting firm specializing in preparing communities for climate-induced extreme events. He earned his Ph.D. at the University of Washington.

Melissa A. Simon, M.D., M.P.H., is the George H. Gardner Professor of Clinical Gynecology and vice chair of Research in the Department of Obstetrics and Gynecology at Northwestern University Feinberg School of Medicine. She is also the founder and director of the Center for Health Equity Transformation and the Chicago Cancer Health Equity Collaborative. She serves as the Robert H. Lurie Comprehensive Cancer Center's associate director for community outreach and engagement. She is an expert in implementation science, women's health across the life-span, minority health, community engagement and health equity. Dr. Simon has been recognized with numerous awards for her substantial contribution to excellence in health equity scholarship, women's health, and mentorship, including her election to NAM and the Association of American Physicians. She has received the Presidential Award in Excellence in Science, Mathematics, and Engineering Mentorship and is a Presidential Leadership Scholar. Dr. Simon is a former member of United States Preventive Services Task Force and on the NIH Office of Research in Women's Health Advisory Committee. She is a member of the National Academies Board on Population Health and Public Health Practice and the Roundtable on the Promotion of Health Equity.

NATIONAL ACADEMY OF MEDICINE
GREENWALL FELLOW IN BIOETHICS

Kavita Shah Arora, M.D., M.B.E., M.S., is an associate professor with tenure and the division director for general obstetrics, gynecology, and midwifery at the University of North Carolina—Chapel Hill. Her clinical, research, and education interests center around reproductive justice and ensuring evidence-based and equitable reproductive health policy, with a focus on sterilization disparities. She has authored over 90 peer-reviewed publications and been funded by the NIH, Health Resources and Service Administration, and Society for Family Planning. At the National Academies, she is the Greenwall Fellow in Bioethics. She has served as Chair of the national ethics committee of the American College of Obstetricians and Gynecologists, on the national ethics committee of the American Medical Association, and on the board of directors of the American Society for Bioethics and the Humanities. She has served on the Governing Council for the Young Physicians Section of the American Medical Association. She was named as a 40 under 40 leader in minority health by the National Minority Quality Forum in 2022. She received her B.S. with a minor in philosophy from the Pennsylvania State University. In 2009, she graduated with both an M.D. from Jefferson Medical College and a master's degree in bioethics from the University of Pennsylvania. She completed her residency in obstetrics and gynecology at McGaw Medical Center of Northwestern University and an M.S. in clinical research at Case Western Reserve University.

STAFF

Amy Geller, M.P.H., is a senior program officer in HMD on the Board on Population Health and Public Health Practice. During her 20 years at the National Academies, she has staffed committees spanning many topics, including advancing health equity, reducing alcohol-impaired driving fatalities, workforce resilience, vaccine safety, reducing tobacco use, drug safety, treating post-traumatic stress disorder, and prevention and control of STIs. She is the study director for the Committee on the Review of Federal Policies that Contribute to Racial and Ethnic Health Inequities. She also directs the DC Public Health Case Challenge, a joint activity of HMD and NAM that aims to promote interdisciplinary, problem-based learning for college students at universities in the DC area.

Alina B. Baciu, M.P.H., Ph.D., is a senior program officer in HMD and on the Board on Population Health and Public Health Practice. She has directed the activities of the Roundtable on Population Health Improvement since 2013. After joining the National Academies in 2001, Dr. Baciu staffed or directed several consensus studies, including those that produced the reports *Leading Health Indicators 2030: Advancing Health, Equity, and Well-Being* (2020), the *For the Public's Health* series of reports on measurement, law, and funding (2010–2012), and *The Future of the Public's Health in the 21st Century* (2003). From 1997 to early 2001, she worked at the Orange County (California) Health Care Agency; later, she served at the Public Health Agency as a health educator in maternal, child, and adolescent health. In 2010, she received a Ph.D. in human sciences (an interdisciplinary program in culture, language, and society) from George Washington University. After earning her M.P.H. (international health) in 1996 from Loma Linda University School of Public Health, she spent 1 year as training coordinator on a United States Agency for International Development-funded maternal and child health project in Zambia. She was born in Romania and emigrated as a child.

Aimee Mead, M.P.H., is an associate program officer in HMD and on the Board on Population Health and Public Health Practice. She has staffed National Academies consensus reports on a variety of public health challenges, including eliminating hepatitis B and C in the United States, reducing alcohol-impaired driving, reviewing the public health consequences of e-cigarettes, preventing STIs, and reviewing the health effects and patterns of use of premium cigars. She has also supported the Roundtable on Environmental Health Sciences, Research, and Medicine. Earlier, she worked at the National Heart, Lung, and Blood Institute. She received her M.P.H. from the Yale School of Public Health and her B.S. from Cornell University.

L. Brielle Dojer, M.P.H., is a research associate in HMD and on the Board on Population Health and Public Health Practice. Earlier, she worked on health equity issues as an intern with the Access Challenge, a 501(c)(3) nonprofit, and as a volunteer with the student-founded organization ContraCOVID NYC. She also worked in research laboratories at NYU Langone and Mount Sinai Hospital before pursuing a career in public health. She holds an M.P.H. from the Icahn School of Medicine at Mount Sinai and a B.A. in biology from Boston University.

Maggie Anderson is an HMD research assistant and on the Board on Population Health and Public Health Practice. Earlier, Ms. Anderson worked at Program Savvy Consulting as an independent contractor and as an intern with the Food Policy Council of Buffalo and Erie County. She received a B.A. in biology with a minor in environmental studies from Mount Holyoke College.

G. Ekene Agu was born and raised in Houston, Texas. He is a recent graduate from Georgetown University. He majored in human science and graduated in May 2021. He served as an EMT for Georgetown EMS. He also worked at the Students of Georgetown Inc., which is the largest student-run nonprofit organization in the United States. He has a passion for biomedical sciences and music. He plays the violin and served as part of an orchestra for 4 years.

Grace Reading is a senior HMD program assistant on the Board of Population Health and Public Health Practice. Earlier, she was an activist in Missouri and Kansas. She founded the Strip Your Letters Campaign, a multicampus initiative to combat institutional violence in all forms on college campuses and in Greek letter organizations. Ms. Reading served on the KU Culture of Respect team to perform a comprehensive analysis on university policies to address institutional responses to sexual violence. For 3 years, she volunteered as an advocate for victim-survivors of sexual violence at the Sexual Trauma and Abuse CARE Center, where she logged over 3,000 hours of community service. She holds a B.S. in marketing from the University of Kansas School of Business and a minor in women, gender, and sexuality studies.

Rose Marie Martinez, Sc.D., has been the director of HMD (formerly the Institute of Medicine) Board on Population Health and Public Health Practice since 1999. Dr. Martinez was a Senior Health Researcher at Mathematica Policy Research (1995–1999), where she conducted research on the impact of health system change on the public health infrastructure, access to care for vulnerable populations, managed care, and the health care workforce. She is a former assistant director for Health Financing and Policy with the Government Accountability Office and served for 6 years directing research studies for the Regional Health Ministry of Madrid, Spain.

Y. Crysti Park is a program coordinator on the Board on Population Health and Public Health Practice. Earlier, she was in marketing and sales management for over 15 years, working on creating catalogs, merchandising, and production in the garment industry. She attended the Fashion Institute of Technology and Cornell University.